Anatomy of a Hospital

Hospital for Special Surgery 1863–2013

Anatomy of a Hospital

Hospital for Special Surgery 1863–2013

Editor-in-Chief

David B. Levine, MD

Director

Alumni Association & Archives

Hospital for Special Surgery

Emeritus Professor

Clinical Orthopaedic Surgery

Weill Cornell Medical College

Executive Administrator

Laura Robbins, DSW

Senior Vice President

Education & Academic Affairs

Designated Institutional Officer, GME

Associate Scientist, Research Division

Hospital for Special Surgery

Senior Administrator

Marcia Ennis

Director

Education Publications & Communications

Education & Academic Affairs

Hospital for Special Surgery

Hospital for Special Surgery

New York, New York

Published in 2013 by Hospital for Special Surgery
Education & Academic Affairs
535 East 70th Street
New York, NY 10021
www.hss.edu

Additional copies available at www.hss.edu/store.

Produced by Print Matters, Inc.
Cover design by Christina Fisher, MFA

Printed in the United States of America by Thomson-Shore, Inc.

ISBN: 978-0-9796685-2-4

For my wife, Janet

CONTENTS

PART II
ASSOCIATED SPECIALTIES

PART III
CHALLENGES

PREFACE

In Perspective

TO TELL THE STORY OF the 150-year history of the nation's oldest orthopaedic hospital in an abbreviated saga would likely exclude distinguished names of pioneers of medicine, renowned scientists, discoveries of new syndromes, advances in diagnostic skills and treatments (both surgical and nonsurgical), and educational initiatives. I have done my best to recount this story in as comprehensive a way as possible, putting the history of Hospital for Special Surgery (HSS) in the context of the history of our country and the world.

I have organized Part I of this book (chapters 1–14) on the periods of the surgeon-in-chief, his life, his influence on the developing hospital, changes in patient healthcare and prevention, and the evolution of medicine from the years of "Heroic Medicine" (1780–1850) to the post-Civil War period of emerging scientific-based approaches (1865–1890). Briefly, I have touched upon the workings of the hospital within a rapidly developing city, in a country at war and at peace, and as a nation in a changing world.

Although Hospital for Special Surgery wasn't the first orthopaedic hospital in this country, it remains the oldest. There were other earlier orthopaedic institutions, most of them very small. The first in this country was the "Orthopedique Infirmary" (later called the Boston Orthopaedic Institution), which was founded in Boston by John Ball Brown in 1838.

As early as 1842, James Knight, MD, who was a medical visitor of the Association for Improving the Condition of the Poor and who was not a surgeon, saw the need for a hospital tending to the crippled and the ruptured. (Incorporated in 1848, the New York Association for Improving the Condition of the Poor eventually became the Community Service Society of New York.) In the early 1860s, many neglected cripples—both children and adults—roamed the streets of New York, exposing their deformities to trigger sympathy as they begged for alms.

Knight was a pioneer in both vision and action who was able to organize the support of prominent New York citizens to fund his hospital—the Hospital for the Ruptured and Crippled (R&C) the forerunner of HSS—and enlist distinguished physicians and surgeons to join its staff. The ruptured and the crippled would finally get the help they needed.

This book begins with two forewords by gentlemen with important roles in the history of HSS:

- Richard L. Menschel, who was not only a member of the HSS Board of Trustees but is also a major donor to the hospital, a surviving postpolio patient treated at HSS, and more importantly, a good friend of the hospital and its professional staff. He shared the position of co-chair of the board for 11 years—first with Winfield P. Jones, and then later, with Aldo Papone.

- Philip D. Wilson Jr., MD, who, from the age of 14, grew up at R&C when his father, Philip D. Wilson, MD, moved from Boston with his family to New York in 1934 to become the fifth surgeon-in-chief. Wilson Jr. trained as an orthopaedic surgeon at HSS and other teaching institutions. He followed in his father's footsteps to become the 11th surgeon-in-chief and carried on the "Wilson" tradition for 17 years until 1989, when he stepped down to continue to treat patients, and later to consult on patients with challenging diagnoses.

Although we have referred to the Hospital for the Ruptured and Crippled when it opened in 1863 as an orthopaedic hospital, it was far from that, relative to what we know of orthopaedic institutions today. The first two hospitals treated only children as inpatients, with adults cared for in outpatient clinics. A comparison of the typical inpatient length of stay in the nineteenth century (which sometimes extended up to 2 years) with the same-day surgery of today makes one appreciate how dramatically a century and a half of medicine has changed. Although orthopaedics remains the major focus of HSS, patient care, education, and research have exploded into various facets of comprehensive musculoskeletal care, and are now supported by a variety of sophisticated subspecialties.

Appreciating the major influence of "nonorthopaedics" in the evolution of this hospital as it changed from the Hospital for the Ruptured and Crippled to Hospital for Special Surgery, the five chapters (chapters 15–19) of Part II have been written by five department heads (specialists in their fields) and an administrator. These chapters describe the analogous history of the growth of these departments, which was critical in helping to make this institution a top leader in the musculoskeletal world. Even I, a student of R&C/HSS history for over 30 years, encountered surprising, historical facts, unknown to me before.

The intermediate chapters (chapters 11–14), although still focusing on the surgeon-in-chief as the central theme, more accurately expose the true modern day anatomy of a hospital as government and private regulators have influenced the daily delivery of patient care. Escalating costs of healthcare have demanded changes in its delivery, prompting administrators to become more closely allied with medical, nursing, and scientific staff.

To help the reader of this book recall more than 200 names, I have included a list entitled "Names from the Past" of many persons referenced in the book, some directly involved with the hospital and others a part of the associated changing times and who are now deceased.

Part III includes two chapters by the hospital's chief executive officer and surgeon-in-chief focusing on the strengths of the hospital and what makes Hospital for Special Surgery so special.

This book is the second published on the history of our hospital, the first being written by Fenwick Beekman, MD, in 1939, when the hospital celebrated its 75th anniversary. It has been an honor for me to chronicle all 150 years as the hospital approaches its sesquicentennial celebration.

David B. Levine, MD
December 2012
For the Sesquicentennial Celebration
May 2013

FOREWORD

One Hundred Fifty Years

HOSPITAL FOR SPECIAL SURGERY OFFERS the City of New York—and indeed the world—specialized care and research in orthopaedics and rheumatology. As we look back at our evolution over 150 years, we can take pride in the contributions of HSS to advances in musculoskeletal surgery, noninvasive treatments, radiology, neurology, physical therapy, and research.

Having my own orthopaedic issues as a result of contracting polio years ago, I have been a frequent patient at HSS. I have received superb nursing care as well as surgical and physician care. The patient floors provide a level of comfort and efficiency that *all* of our clients experience. I have been impressed by the carefully orchestrated teamwork of our staff—beginning in the examination and consultation rooms, then in the surgery and recovery areas, and finally on patient floors.

During my 22 years of experience with HSS, we have enlarged and modernized our physical facilities while also expanding our investments in research. Today we spend over $30 million in research annually. Our patients benefit from the advances developed by our investigators working in concert with practicing physicians and surgeons—and, in return, research is informed "real time" by actual patient conditions. Collectively, the translational benefits of scientific inquiry have enhanced our physicians' worldwide leadership in their subspecialties.

Everyone associated with HSS can take pride in our celebration of 150 years of serving patients—not many institutions can claim this longevity. We are able to do so because of our culture of striving for excellence in surgical practice, patient care, hospital management, and innovation.

The Board of Trustees, of which I was the co-chair for 11 years, has worked successfully with management to steer through the uncertainties and challenges of changing insurance reimbursement practices and government regulations. We have an engaged board whose members make substantive contributions through working committees, often as a result of their own medical issues or professional experiences. The board committees successfully involve doctors, nurses, and other professional staff as well as trustees, all working collaboratively in planning and financial management.

Our specialization and size have enabled us to remain agile and to forge a spirit of community, binding together physicians, nurses, support staff, management, and trustees. For me, seeing people on the HSS staff taking pride in their work and the hospital, whether as an attendant or a doctor, is as gratifying as our earning the coveted number one spot in the *U.S. News and World Report* "Best Hospital" rankings in orthopaedics, as well as significantly high rankings in rheumatology, neurology, and geriatrics.

For 28 years, David B. Levine, MD, was one of our leading physicians and is internationally known for his skills as an orthopaedic spine surgeon. Recently, as a professor emeritus, he has written, in collaboration with fellow HSS physicians, this story of our 150-year history. It is a compelling recital of compassion and human endeavor, from the hospital's first response to crippled children roaming the streets of New York City, to the treatment of people of all ages today with conditions ranging from congenital to sports-related.

As we move forward, we can never become complacent and instead must continue to look for ways to improve our care, advance our research, conserve our resources, and enhance education. We also need to maintain our responsiveness to changes in the healthcare environment. The coming years will be challenging as the public demands reductions in healthcare costs, but will also be highlighted by improvements in the quality of care and advances made possible by research. I am confident that we can manage these sometimes conflicting goals through professional dedication, ingenuity, and continued solid financial management—and by educating the public on the value of investing in research as well as excellent care.

Richard L. Menschel
Emeritus Co-Chair
Board of Trustees
Hospital for Special Surgery
July 2012

FOREWORD

A View from an Emeritus Surgeon-in-Chief

I AM PROUD TO HAVE BEEN ASKED to write a foreword to this book commemorating the sesquicentennial of Hospital for Special Surgery. Yet at the same time, I am humbled by the actual task. I can attest to the quality of the research and accuracy that has gone into the writing of *Anatomy of a Hospital* as presented by David B. Levine, MD. Its depth is impressive, and the personal asides of selected leading staff members characterize the feeling of family that we experience when we refer to "HSS."

Over the years, the staff of HSS has included not only those from medical, educational, and scientific professions but also volunteers and employees who have contributed much in thought and time to the benefit of the hospital. For example, I will never forget Tommy Cannon, a lame hemiparaplegic from birth, who cheerfully greeted everyone who entered the halls of the old R&C on East 42nd Street.

Organized into 21 chapters, this book is both instructive and pleasing. Levine wrote the first 14 chapters himself, based on existing documentation as well as conversations (when possible) he had with the leaders involved. He was assisted by eight colleagues in writing the remaining chapters. All friends of HSS are grateful for their industrious work and careful documentation. I know that I am very grateful for their labor. We admire their courage and achievement.

Chapter 15 on anesthesiology, written by Gregory Liguori, MD, and Mary Hargett contains a brief preliminary historical review, which comes alive when Nigel Sharrock, MB, ChB, was recruited in 1986 to lead and revolutionize the department. Sharrock's adoption of the concepts of regional anesthesia with close patient monitoring set new standards at HSS. The staff gradually increased to smoothly manage rapidly increasing caseloads, and preoperative and postoperative close monitoring have provided additional safeguards. An effective pain control service was also established.

Helene Pavlov, MD, begins chapter 16 with a brief historical summary of the development of radiology at HSS. She then follows with the presentation of newer techniques such as MRI, under the direction of Hollis G. Potter, MD, as well as interventional radiography with reduced radiation exposure, ultrasonic localization, and interventional ultrasound-guided biopsy and injection procedures. The conversion from analog to digital imaging capture has permitted speedy imaging for use by staff without record room delay.

Adele Boskey, PhD, the Starr Chair in Mineralized Tissue Research and director of the Musculoskeletal Integrity Program at HSS, is also closely identified with Weill Cornell Medical College in New York City and Cornell University's School of Mechanical and Aerospace Engineering in Ithaca. She has always been mindful of the mission to maintain a close relationship between basic laboratory and clinical research divisions. She is highly respected on both sides of the bridge connecting the two.

In chapter 17, Boskey details the history of the development of the Research Division, going back to its formal beginning in 1955—5 years before a separate building was erected but connected to the hospital by a bridge. The bridge has been highly traveled and the connection well practiced.

Biomechanics has also grown significantly over the years and for some time has been under the direction of Timothy Wright, PhD. He has dovetailed his interests and those of the Sibley School of Engineering at Cornell University in Ithaca into a stronger unified effort.

With the new appointment of a chief scientific officer in 2006, Steven R. Goldring, MD has been assigned the Richard L. Menschel Research Chair. Among his many plans is an in-depth study of osteoarthritis. More information can be found in chapter 14.

In chapters 18 and 19, Charles L. Christian, MD, and Steven M. Paget, MD, impressed me greatly with their presentation and discussion of the creation of the Division of Rheumatology from what was initially just an outpatient service focused on arthritis. Christian's ambition was to build a division with impressive local, national and international recognition, and build it he did. Paget carried on this effort, and initiated a more formalized staff of rheumatologists to provide 24/7 care for patients undergoing surgery or those requiring hospitalization for other reasons. He was succeeded by Mary K. Crow, MD, who now serves as chair of the Division of Rheumatology as well as physician-in-chief of HSS. Further details and the latest development plans are also provided in greater detail in chapter 14.

I recommend careful reading of *Anatomy of a Hospital* to friends of HSS, whether they are already involved or are thinking of becoming involved in its future. This historic document demonstrates how medicine, education, and research can only improve with time, as long as we maintain adequate funding to support our endeavors.

Sustaining the accelerated pace of the growth of the clinical, scientific, and educational staff of HSS and the productivity of the institution requires continued support of our web of creativity. Such support is critical for HSS to maintain our leadership position in clinical care, teaching, and research in the fields of orthopaedics and rheumatology.

Philip D. Wilson Jr., MD
Surgeon-in-Chief, 1972–1989
Attending Orthopaedic Surgeon
Member, Board of Trustees
Hospital for Special Surgery
Professor of Orthopaedic Surgery
Weill Cornell Medical College

PART I

FROM THE HOSPITAL FOR THE RUPTURED AND CRIPPLED TO HOSPITAL FOR SPECIAL SURGERY 1863–2013

The only thing new in
the world is the history
you don't know.

Harry S. Truman (1884–1972)

CHAPTER 1
JAMES KNIGHT, MD
FOUNDER AND FIRST SURGEON-IN-CHIEF (1863–1870)

DAVID B. LEVINE, MD

IN THE MIDDLE OF THE Civil War, with disease, poverty, and unemployment rampant in New York City, a relatively unknown physician—a general practitioner hailing from Maryland, James Knight, MD—was able to persuade a group of prominent local citizens to form a society to establish and support an orthopaedic hospital. Neither a nation at war nor a city confronted with uncontrolled disease, overwhelming disabilities, poverty and suffering, medicine in its infancy, the growth of new large hospitals, civil unrest, and political corruption could discourage this physician, who held steadfast to his vision to establish a hospital for the treatment and rehabilitation of the crippled and disabled.

Little did he know that this hospital, eventually to be known as The Hospital for the Ruptured and Crippled (R&C), would one day become one of the world's leading institutions in musculoskeletal research, education and treatment. It would be renamed in 1940 as The Hospital for Special Surgery (HSS), and now stands as the oldest existing orthopaedic hospital in this country.[1]

James Knight (1810–1887)

Born on February 14, 1810, in Taneytown, Maryland, Knight graduated from the Medical-Chirurgical Faculty (of Maryland) in Baltimore in 1832. In 1835, at age 25 years, he moved to New York City to open his office as a general practitioner. It must have been a very big step—coming from a small hamlet in the rolling foothills of the Catoctin Mountains in Central Maryland, with a population just under 400, to an expanding city of more than 700,000.

Taneytown's only other claim to fame was Francis Scott Key, author of "The Star Spangled Banner," who was born there in 1779.[2]

Early in his career, Knight became obsessed with treating patients using what he called "surgicomechanics"—otherwise known as "bracing." Bandaging and supports were used to manage hernia, varicose veins, hemorrhoids, and prolapsed uteri.

This became Knight's introduction to orthopaedics, and, eventually, his incentive to design and construct appliances to restore impaired locomotion in children. Such deformities included congenital disorders, sequelae from infantile paralysis, constitutional impairments, and other pathological conditions, such as caries of the spine.[3]

Knight witnessed the poor, the helpless, the deformed, and the crippled on the streets of New York. Citizens of the city—afflicted with ruptures, varicose veins, and ulcerated legs—became professional beggars. They often exposed their bodies to further their needs. Mothers carried their deformed and sick children while begging. No known cures for these conditions existed, and hospitals would not admit them, as they were not considered "sick." They depended on charity to survive. They could not gain any employment. Sometimes a brace or truss would help them to become more functional.[4]

Soon after coming to New York, Knight was appointed a visitor to the Association for Improving the Condition of the Poor. In this era, there were limited ways to accurately diagnose diseases and few proven methods of treating them. Medicine was far from being a science. At best, there were a few evolving theories explaining the pathogenesis of infectious diseases with varied agreement. In 1860, Louis Pasteur proved that living organisms, not chemical reactions, caused fermentation, furthering the followers of the "germ theory." Influenced by Pasteur, Joseph Lister applied these principles to surgery, developing antiseptic procedures in the operating room and significantly reducing infection.

Meanwhile, in France, medicine was emerging from the dark periods. In Paris, Pierre Louis was applying arithmetic to analyze the treatment of patients in large numbers of charity hospitals and correlating various diseases and different therapies with their outcomes—the birth of systematic databases. In England, others used mathematics to promote the discipline of epidemiology. In Germany, Rudolph Virchow, MD, was establishing the field of cellular pathology.

However, in America, these medical advances ironically triggered skepticism and engendered resistance, resulting in a neglect of new treatments for disease. In Europe, doctors were embracing thermometers, stethoscopes, and other diagnostic instruments to enhance their practices. Yet by the time of the Civil War, few in America were using such novel tools.

Surgery only grew in popularity as a major method of treatment after the introduction of ether anesthesia by William Morton in 1846 and chloroform by James Simpson, MD, the following year. There would be no operating room at R&C until 1889, although the first anesthetist at R&C appointed on a part-time basis was Thomas L. Bennett, MD (see Chapter 15 for more information).

Early New York City Hospitals

The oldest and most famous hospital in New York City, Bellevue Hospital, was formed in 1736 as the Almshouse Infirmary. It was a "Publick Workhouse and House of Correction," with an upper floor housing an infirmary containing six beds. It was also a rehabilitation center with areas for sewing, spinning, weaving, and working on iron and leather, and even an adjacent farm (an early form of occupational therapy).

As New York grew rapidly, public health was essentially nonexistent. At the beginning of the nineteenth century, yellow fever epidemics occurred annually, with filth and plague abounding and uncontrolled sewage in the streets. In 1811, the city purchased six acres of the Kip's Bay Farm along the East River. Bounding it on one side was Belle Vue Place. Building construction, delayed due to the War of 1812, proceeded with the new institution, which finally opened in 1816 as Bellevue Hospital. Home of the first school of nursing in the country (1873), Bellevue Hospital was also the first in the city to deal with the medical needs of the poor and the destitute.[5]

New York Hospital came later in the century, opening in 1791 and generously supported by the Dutch gentry, with many of its trustees of Dutch ancestry. The Lying-In Hospital was founded in 1798 after a yellow fever epidemic of that year. In Brooklyn, Kings County Hospital originated, like Bellevue, from an almshouse in 1831. Brooklyn City Hospital was incorporated in 1845, supported by the Brooklyn Association for Improving the Conditions of the Poor.

By the beginning of the Civil War, there would be twelve more large hospitals. The upper and middle classes preferred to be treated at home or in small private hospitals. They did not wish to be associated with the stigma of large charity institutions.

Conservatism versus Surgery

Bellevue Medical College opened in 1859. One of its cofounders, Lewis Sayre, MD, was interested in paralysis and tuberculosis of the bones and joints. He was appointed as the first chair of orthopaedic surgery and became the first professor of orthopaedic surgery in the country.

Five years earlier, Sayre performed the first resection of a hip joint for tuberculosis. He was considered an excellent surgeon and visionary and formulated many new approaches to the causes of deformities. If he could not operate, he used plaster casts and other forms of immobilization. He was the first to use plaster of paris jackets for scoliosis and Pott's disease (tuberculosis of the spine).

Another large group of practitioners preached conservative treatment, however, and considered Sayre's surgery to be "adventurous" and of no possible use for this disabled population. These physicians preferred to use braces, trusses, bandages, and other mechanical methods to rehabilitate their patients.

Prominent among this latter group was Knight (Fig. 1), who not only favored the conservative approach but also vehemently opposed any surgical intervention. He defined his conservative program as "expectant treatment" in contrast to the "adventurous" surgical approach.

In addition to his use of surgicomechanics, his regimen included properly enforced hygiene, good food and tonics, exercise, fresh air, education, and religious principles. Some questioned other methods he employed, such as mercury for cachectic cases, direct local application of molasses or cod liver oil for corneal ulcers, and Spanish fly blisters for acute stages of hip diseases.[6]

Turbulent Times

At the beginning of the Civil War in April 1861, the 33 states and territories had a population of about 31 million, with 23 million living in the 22 northern states and 9 million in the southern states. The Battle of Chancellorsville, Virginia

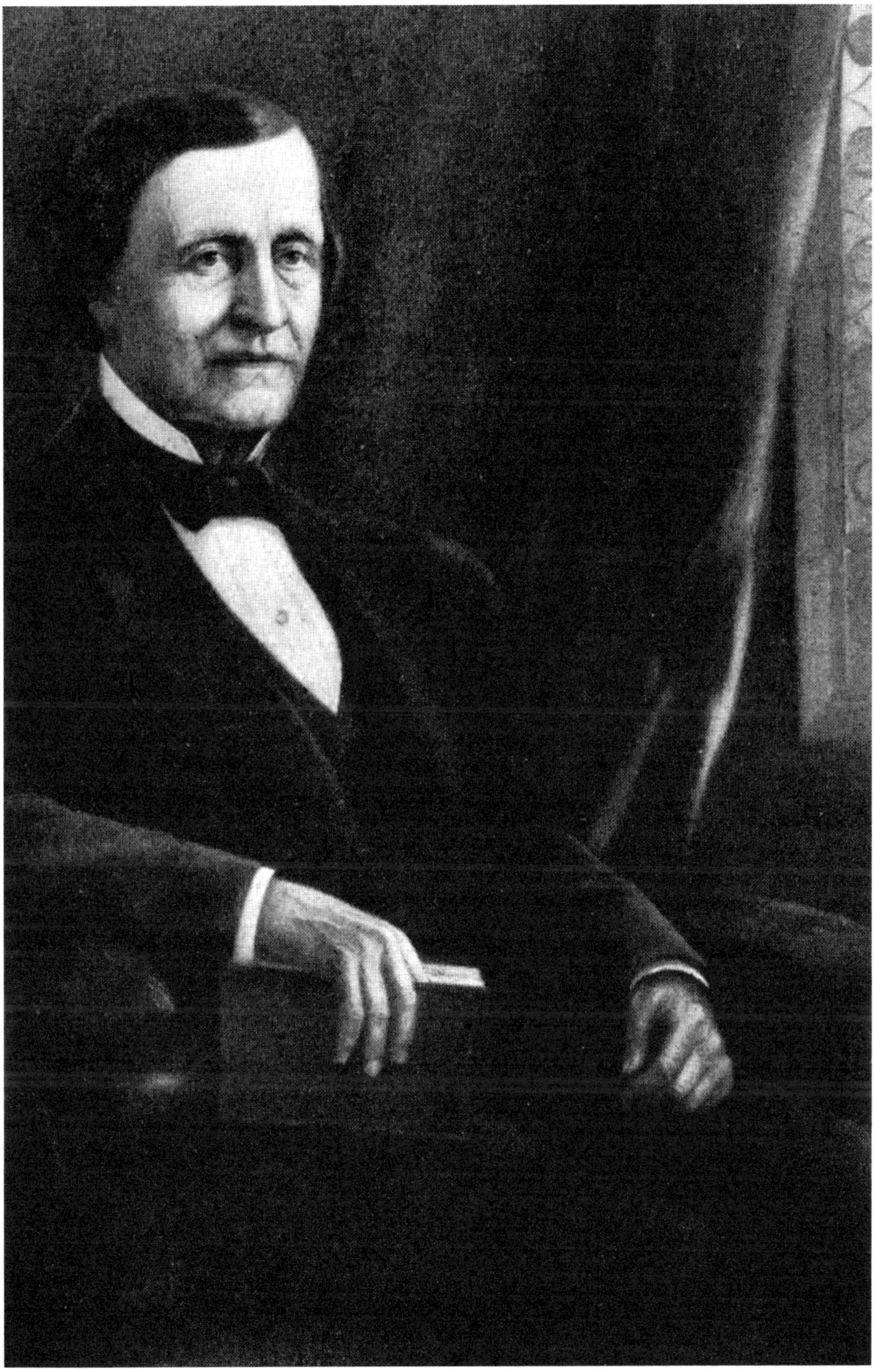

Fig. 1 This portrait of James Knight hangs in the Richard L. Menschel Education Center of Hospital for Special Surgery. In his hand is his text entitled *Orthopaedia*. (From Hospital for Special Surgery Archives)

was a great victory for Gen. Robert E. Lee, but it eventually led to the beginning of the end for the Confederate army. Lee and Gen. Thomas J. (Stonewall) Jackson met in the deep woods near Chancellorsville on the evening of May 1, 1863 (the day R&C opened). They planned their attack on the Federals for the next day, resulting in a large success, but it was a bloody battle, with Union casualties exceeding 17,000 and Confederates more than 12,000—including the loss of Jackson himself, who was accidentally shot by his own men and died three days later of pneumonia.[7]

Buoyed by this win, on July 2, 1863, Lee ordered a massive assault at Gettysburg, which ended in a major loss for the South. Casualties were devastating, with some from the Union army eventually being treated at R&C.

New York City was going through the Draft Riots, the largest civil insurrection in American history apart from the Civil War itself. In March 1863, Congress had passed the Enrollment (Draft) Act, which forced men between the ages of 20 and 45 years into military service. New York State Gov. Horatio Seymour and other Democratic leaders felt the conscription act was unconstitutional, supporting resistance and inciting the populace to action. The spark that ignited the grievances of the working class (mostly Irish living in poverty) was the provision in the law that conscription could be avoided by paying $300 to the government.

For four days (July 13–16, 1863), there were large-scale bloody riots, known as Draft Week, which local police could not control. It took New York troops, including the famous 7th Regiment (sent to the front at Gettysburg)—with the aid of the militia, Navy, West Point cadets, and police—to finally squelch the uprisings.[8]

By the latter half of the nineteenth century, political corruption in New York City was already flourishing, with Tammany Hall electing its first mayor, Fernando Wood, in 1855. The Tammany Society—founded in 1789 by William Mooney, a Revolutionary War veteran—was originally created as a patriotic and charitable organization. In the early 1800s, the Irish managed to force their way into the society, and the practice of exchanging votes for benefits led to extreme corruption in the city.

The New York Society for the Relief of the Ruptured and Crippled

Knight's great ambition was to establish a hospital for rehabilitation. In March 1862, he enlisted the help of Robert M. Hartley,[a] secretary of the Association for Improving the Condition of the Poor. Hartley conferred with Knight, stating that in his involvement with the poor, he realized the necessity for such a hospital and was only waiting for the appropriate circumstances. He promised his influence and personal cooperation.

Consequently, on April 15, 1862, Mr. Hartley arranged a meeting at No. 39 Bible House, the office of the association, "to consider the expediency of forming a society for the relief of the Ruptured and Crippled." Attending this meeting with Knight and Hartley were Stewart Brown, Robert M. Minturn, John C. Green, William Bibbins, Joseph B. Collins, and Apollos R. Wetmore.

In reference to that meeting, Knight would later describe the following in the First Annual Report of the Society for the Ruptured and Crippled:

> I became more familiar with the prevalence of the maladies among the laboring population. The necessity for an Institution for their relief was impressed upon my mind when attending the late professor Mott's clinics, held in 1842 in the University Medical College; and from that period I made efforts from time to time to effect an organization for that purpose by means of printed circulars.
>
> In January 1862, I obtained the approval, by signatures, which I have in my possession, of Professors Valentine Mott, Willard Parker, J. M. Carnochan and James R. Wood; George Opdyke, then Mayor of the City of New York; R. A. Witthaus, Wilson G. Hunt, Robert L. Stuart, T. B. Stillman and Peter Cooper.
>
> The plan was so well accepted by these gentlemen, that the present society was organized the next year establishing twenty members of the Board of Managers. A Certificate of Intention to Incorporate in the State of New York was filed March 27, 1863 and certified April 13, 1863. However, the charter of incorporation was not enacted until April 23, 1867.

Article I (Objects of the Society) of the Constitution[9] stated,

> The objects of the Society are to supply skillfully constructed surgico-mechanical appliances, and the treatment of in and out-door patients requiring trusses or spring supports; also bandages, lace stockings and other apparatus for the cure of cripples, both adults and children, on such conditions which will make their benefits available, so far as is possible to the poorest in the city.

The events leading to the establishment of a hospital devoted to orthopaedics based on conservative principles were entirely the results of Knight's vision, perseverance, and ability to gain the confidence of prominent members of local society. R. M. Hartley was the catalyst, which completed the equation.

The Hospital for the Ruptured and Crippled—1863

Organization of the new institution proceeded. It was to be located in Knight's private residence at 97 Second Avenue at Sixth Street, in lower New York City. It would be a 28-bed hospital with a conservatory to make braces. Knight arranged with the Board of Managers to lease his house for $1,200 per year[b] (Fig. 2). He was appointed the resident physician and surgeon.

On May 1, 1863, the new hospital admitted its first patient: a 4-year-old boy of destitute parents who had paralysis of his left leg since 18 months of age. He lived in the hospital with Mrs. Knight, who supervised domestic affairs, and their daughter, who volunteered teaching the children. Knight, who also acted as superintendent, saw some private patients and turned over all fees to the hospital. In return, he had an annual salary of $2,000[c] and was very instrumental in raising large sums of money to support the hospital.

In addition to Knight and his family, his staff included four consultants, all prominent surgeons at that time: Valentine Mott, MD, William H. Van Buren, MD, Willard Parker, MD, and John M. Carnochan, MD.

Knight was in absolute control as head of his household. There were no trained nurses or other paraprofessionals. He was said to have been immune to criticism. Because of his residence in the hospital, he had ideal conditions to observe and make conclusions regarding treatment and outcomes.

In retrospect, the solid foundation of the first hospital, its growth, its continued existence, and its eventual emergence as a leader in orthopaedics, rheumatology, and related fields of medicine in this country and worldwide could not have been accomplished without the close collaboration of prominent, philanthropic, and supportive members of the Board of Managers (Board of Trustees). The founding Board was comprised of persons with such qualifications. John C. Green[d] was elected their first president, serving from 1864 to 1874.

Membership on the Board of Managers through the years was often comprised of family descendants. One of the founding members of the Board was Jonathan Sturges (1802–1874), a grandson of a member of Congress from Connecticut. Sturges was a director of the Illinois Central Railway and

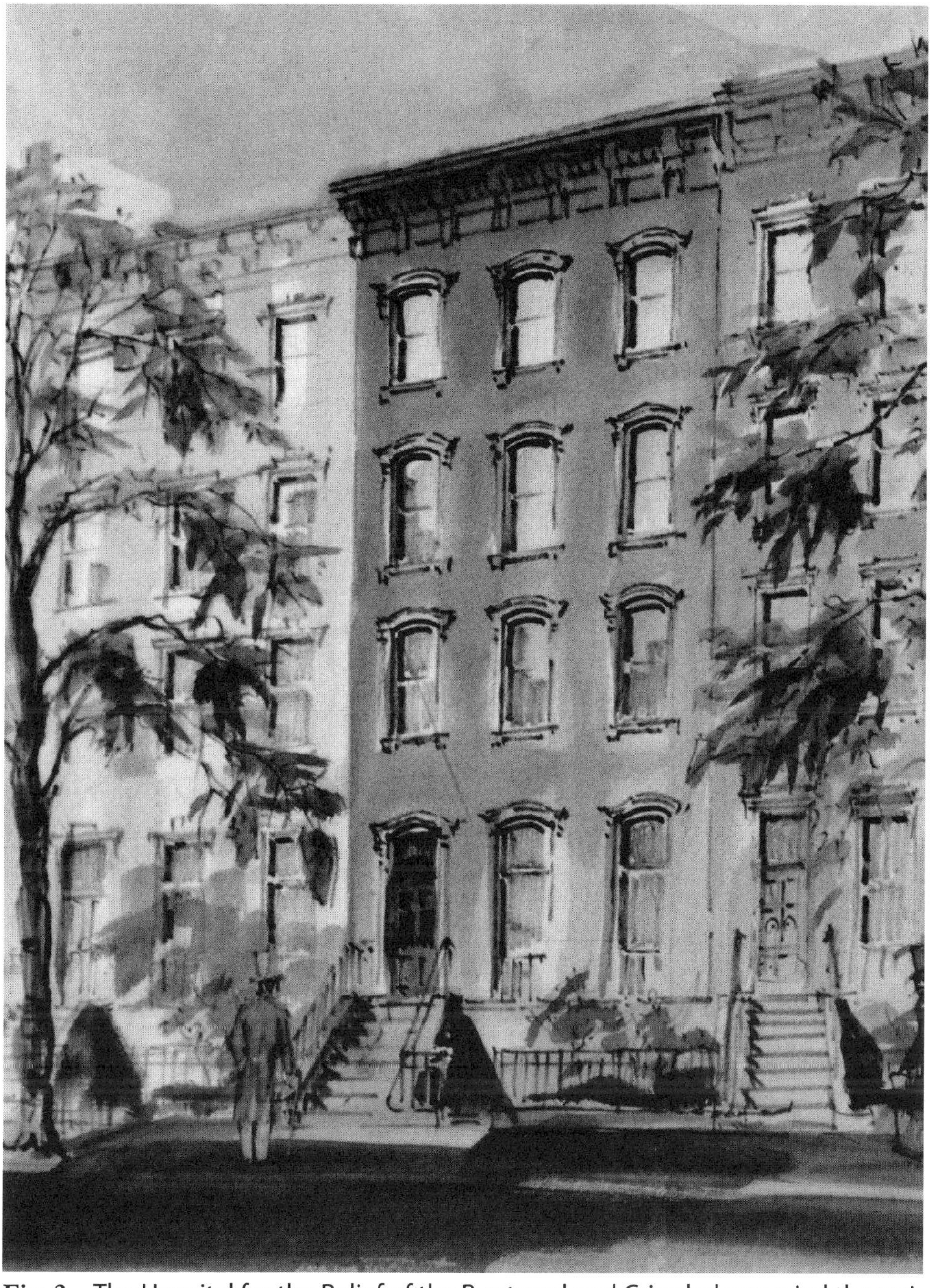

Fig. 2 The Hospital for the Relief of the Ruptured and Crippled occupied the residence of James Knight at 97 Second Avenue, just south of Sixth Street in lower New York City, from its founding in 1863 until 1870. Above is an artist's reproduction of Knight's home. (From Hospital for Special Surgery Archives)

during the Civil War was among the most liberal and outspoken supporters of the government. He eventually retired in 1868 from a mercantile house, with a large fortune.

There have been eight other members who followed in Sturges' lineage on the board, all descendants of the Osborn family. The latest member, Katherine O. Roberts, was made a life trustee in recent years.

In his First Annual Report, Knight listed the number of patients received in May 1863 as 66, of which 10 were "in-door" patients with the following conditions:

- one case of contracted leg from extensive ulceration
- two cases of caries of the spine (humpback)
- three of hip disease
- one of lateral curvature of the spine
- three of clubfeet

Three surgical procedures were performed:

- one removal of a portion of a crochet needle from the knee joint
- two divisions of tendons

Knight informed the board that expanding the hospital was critical for the optimal treatment of in-door patients. He concluded his first report[9] with the following:

> As I have already stated, the augmenting number of these cases will, ere long, so fully occupy our present limited accommodations for in-door patients, that they will exclude that class of patients who are in the incipient stage of disease, and whose cases, if taken in time, promise a speedy recovery, while if restricted to our ordinary out-door treatment, and subjected to the influences of insufficient care, clothing and nourishment, and unwholesome air, they rapidly become worse. I cannot therefore too earnestly express hope that the Board may see their way clear to the enlargement of their in-door accommodations.

The board was impressed by this need for larger accommodations and responded accordingly and quickly.

From Sixth Street to 42nd Street

Following the end of the Civil War in 1865, life in New York City—the youngest of the world's greatest cities—was wrought with civil unrest, greed, crime, corruption, and tenements with cramped living space, disease, and despair. But the worst was to follow, as estate owners and property agents converted houses and buildings into small unbearable living areas. Cholera epidemics, barely touching clean residential areas, resulted in increased mortality rates from 1 in 42 in 1815 to 1 in 27 after 1855.

The tenement population swelled on the East Side, the most densely populated area in the world, to a rate of 290,000 to the square mile. Tenement housing became popular after the New York State Legislature passed the Tenement Housing Act of 1867, which defined multiple households of two to three families sharing common cooking facilities, hallways, yards, and privies. Swine roamed the streets until 1867, when owners of swine were prohibited by ordinance from letting them run freely.

It was in this climate that the Board of Managers supported Knight's proposal to move to larger facilities. In the spring of 1867, five lots were purchased for $40,000[e] on the uppermost border of the city, then considered the "country." Edward T. Potter[f] was employed as the architect. With large sums of money totaling $224,167,[g] contributed by John Green, Jonathan Sturges, and numerous other board members and friends, a new building on the corner of Lexington Avenue and 42nd Street was constructed.

In April 1870, to pay remaining bills and furnish the hospital, the building committee felt that the board would not be safe unless an additional $50,000 was raised. Rather than take out a mortgage, John Green, then board president and chairman of the finance committee, offered to give the society $50,000 if the board could raise the same amount in 30 days. Jonathan Sturges, as treasurer, informed Green a month later that they were successful and Green immediately handed him a check for $50,000.

Sturges reported:

> We have a hospital capable of accommodating 200–250 children.
> We owe no man anything but love.
> We have assets amounting to $100,000.

The new hospital opened to patients in May 1870.

Orthopaedic Institutions Followed

Charles Fayette Taylor, MD (1827–1899), another early orthopaedic surgeon in New York, was as ultraconservative as Knight. Born in Vermont, Taylor was very disturbed about the challenges of treating Pott's disease. One evening in 1858, he devised a way to construct a brace to immobilize the spine. This approach was enthusiastically received by his colleagues, who suggested to Theodore Roosevelt, Sr.[h] that he bring his 4-year-old daughter with spine disease to Taylor.

Taylor designed a brace, which allowed the child to develop a normal life. Although she needed to wear a brace for ten years, she grew up to marry and deliver a child. Roosevelt was so grateful to Taylor that he enlisted other prominent New Yorkers to give financial support to Taylor's work.

Recognizing the need for a second orthopaedic facility, Taylor founded the New York Orthopedic Dispensary in October 1866, a four-story building on Broadway between 35th and 36th Streets. The dispensary was moved to East 59th Street in 1873, and the next year, the name was changed to the New York Orthopedic Dispensary and Hospital.[10]

In 1872, the first orthopaedic service in a general hospital in the United States was formed at St. Luke's Hospital in New York City. Its first chief, Newton Melman Shaffer, MD (1846–1928), a great conservative trained by Knight, had been on staff at R&C until 1870. In 1876, he succeeded Taylor as surgeon-in-chief of the New York Orthopedic Dispensary and Hospital. He became clinical professor of orthopaedic surgery at New York University Medical College in 1882 and finally, in 1900, the first professor of orthopaedic surgery at Cornell Medical College in New York City. In February 1950, the New York Orthopedic Hospital merged with Columbia-Presbyterian Medical Center, where it remains today.

In November 1906, the Hospital for Deformities and Joint Diseases opened its doors at 1917 Madison Avenue in Harlem. Henry Frauenthal, MD, and his brother, Herman C. Frauenthal, MD, were the founders of the third orthopaedic hospital in New York. Graduating from Bellevue Hospital Medical College in 1890, Herman Frauenthal became the first surgeon-in-chief at the new Madison Avenue hospital. At Bellevue, he had studied with Lewis A. Sayre, serving as his assistant for eleven years.

The hospital's name was officially shortened on November 14, 1921, to the Hospital for Joint Diseases. Currently affiliated with New York University School of Medicine, it now stands on East 17th Street at Second Avenue.[11]

REFERENCES

1. Wilson PD Jr., Levine DB. Hospital for Special Surgery. A brief review of its development and current position. *Clin Orthop*. 2000;374:90–105.
2. Boone TJ. *Images of America Taneytown*. Charleston, SC: Arcadia Publishing; 2004.
3. Wilson PD Jr. James Knight (1810–1887) of the Hospital for the Ruptured and Crippled. *Clin Orthop*. 1958;11:1–8.
4. Beekman F. *Hospital for the Ruptured and Crippled. A Historical Sketch Written on the Occasion of the Seventy-Fifth Anniversary of the Hospital*. New York, NY: privately printed; 1939.
5. Knights EM Jr. Bellevue Hospital. History Magazine: http://www.history-magazine.com/bellevue.html. Accessed Feb. 22, 2005.
6. Whitman R. A critical estimation of the personal influence of four pioneers on the development of orthopaedic surgery in New York. *J Bone Joint Surg*. 1934;16:331–342.
7. Murray AR. *Edit Civil War and Leaders*. New York, NY: DK Publishing; 2004:7–57.
8. Jackson KT. The Encyclopedia of New York City. New Haven, CT: Yale University Press; 2010.
9. Knight J. *First Annual Report of the New York Society for the Relief of the Ruptured and Crippled*. New York, NY: New York Society for the Relief of the Ruptured and Crippled. May 1864.
10. Shookster L. The role of Theodore Roosevelt's family in the founding of the New York Orthopedic Hospital. *Theodore Roosevelt Assoc J*. 2007(Summer).
11. McDowell B, Green WS, Zuckerman. *J Hosp Joint Dis*. 1905–2005.

NOTES

a. Robert M. Hartley (1796–1881), born in England, followed his father in the woolen business, although he had ministerial ambitions. In 1843, he was one of the founders of the Association for Improving the Condition of the Poor. He published many articles on religious, sanitary, and scientific subjects. He was happily married to Catherine Munson and had ten children.

b. In 2011 dollars = $21,000.

c. In 2011 dollars = $35,000.

d. John Clevis Green (1800–1875), born in New Jersey, attended the Lawrenceville School and became a very successful China Trader. Returning from Canton in 1839 with a sizable fortune, he settled in New York, became president of the Bleecker Street Savings Bank, and invested heavily in railroads. He was a trustee of New York Hospital and the Hospital for the Deaf and Dumb and a very charitable contributor to religious organizations. As a trustee of Princeton University, he endowed three chairs, the first School of Science named after him, the first library, and renovated the dining hall and chapel. His great-great-grandfather, Jonathan Dickinson, was the first president of the College of New Jersey, which would become Princeton University.

e. In 2011 dollars = $597,000.

f. Edward Tuckerman Potter, a specialist in ecclesiastical design, was born in Schenectady and was the son of Bishop Alonzo Potter, the former president of Union College. He studied under Richard Upjohn, then the foremost church architect in the country. He was the first architect for Lehigh University and designed buildings for Princeton as well as many churches. He died in 1901.

g. In 2011 dollars = $3.35 million.

h. Theodore Roosevelt, Sr. was the father of U.S. President Theodore Roosevelt and the paternal grandfather of America's First Lady, Eleanor Roosevelt.

CHAPTER 2

LEXINGTON AVENUE AND 42ND STREET (1870–1887)

DAVID B. LEVINE, MD

EMBARKING ON ITS SEVENTH YEAR since its opening in May 1870, the Hospital for the Ruptured and Crippled (R&C) moved from lower Second Avenue to its new home on 42nd Street and Lexington Avenue—the current site of the Grand Hyatt Hotel. It was considered the country, as the heart of the city at that time was due south, in lower Manhattan. A continuous exodus of people streamed from the Wall Street area, the lower Eastside, and Canal Street, moving north to the open country above the East 50s. Still, shanties remained near 42nd Street, and goats had the luxury of roaming free.

The new hospital must have been an imposing structure in that open space, with its "pointed style" of architecture, alternate *voussoirs*[a] of light olive-colored Ohio freestone and Connecticut brownstone in the arches of the windows and doors. Hollow brick walls aided heating and ventilation (Fig. 1). Although the exterior was designed by architect Edward Tuckerman Potter—a well-respected specialist in ecclesiastical design who was Lehigh University's first architect—the interior of the building was entirely planned by Knight.[1,2]

Knight's vision of an institution for the relief of maladies of the laboring population had finally come to fruition. From its first location in 1863 in his converted residence at 92 Second Avenue, to an impressive 200-bed hospital uptown, the location was not only ideal for access to rail in all directions, but was a very pleasant site that aided the rehabilitation of patients. It was situated high on a lot (125 × 100 ft), with a view west to New Jersey and in the opposite direction to the East River.[3]

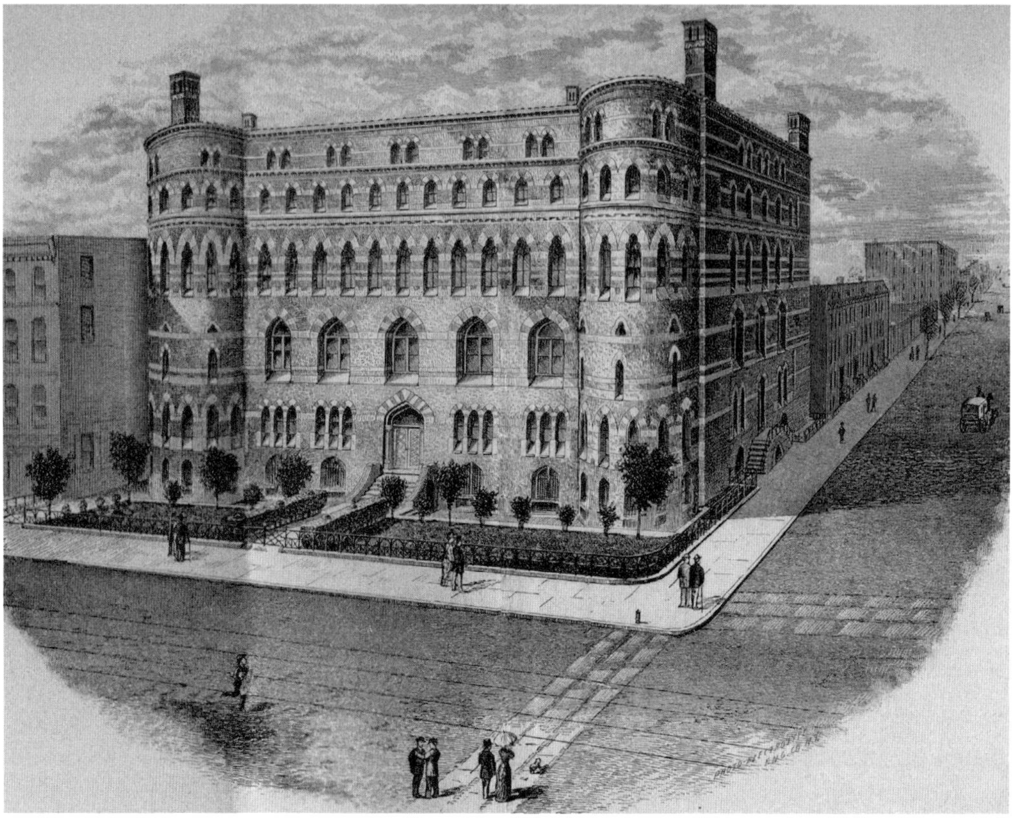

Fig. 1 The Hospital for the Ruptured and Crippled (1870) on the northwest corner of Lexington Avenue (right) and 42nd Street. (From Hospital for Special Surgery Archives)

In addition to a basement, the three-story building had a garden roof that could be opened in the summer and enclosed in the winter. Exposure to light and sun was paramount in the requirements of Knight. The structure was designed in the form of a parallelogram with three attached semicircular wings—two facing south on 42nd Street and one at the northeast corner on Lexington Avenue. At the northwest corner, there was a rectangular structure. These corner attachments housed nurses' rooms, bathing rooms, and so forth, while their rounded design allowed ample sun and light to penetrate.

The second and third floors were each limited to inpatient wards featuring 200 beds for children, with four ample fireplaces in each ward. The top floor was a combination gymnasium, garden, and playroom, airy and cheerful for the children—an advance for hospitals in those times.[1] Adults were treated in the outpatients' dispensary, which attended to 3,000 patients each year. Adult patients who required admission to the hospital were referred to other hospitals.

The first floor had furnished apartments for twenty private pay patients, as well as apartments for a resident physician and his family. The basement had a reception room for patients, kitchen, bakery, laundry, heating units, and a steam engine to run an elevator housed next to a fireproof staircase in a tower attached to the north side of the building.

Conspicuously missing was an operating room. Dogmatic in his conservative approach, Knight was strongly opposed to surgery. However, he allowed surgical tendon and fascia releases for fixed deformities.

Coping with Expansion

With the enlargement of the building came an expansion of the medical staff, as well as all departments and manufacturing services. The number of patients treated declined somewhat during the year of the move due to the change from a well-known location to a lesser-known site. The new hospital took months to have its interior completed for functional use, and there were not sufficient finances to treat a large number of patients. Building of the hospital and furnishing it, as was planned, had to proceed without debt.

Although the progress of the undertaking had not been delayed because of lack of funds, particularly because so many persons contributed generously, it was not possible to maintain an operating budget solely by relying on contributions. According to the annual report of John C. Green, the first president of the Board of Managers, this was very disturbing. The inpatient beds were only half filled. The hospital's annual outlay far exceeded its income; however, the board realized that the cost per capita of inpatients would decrease as the patient load rose over time.

Green, a China Trader, railroad entrepreneur, banker, and philanthropist, contributed heavily to Princeton University as well as R&C, other hospitals, and educational institutions, including libraries.[2] He made a serious commitment to the New York Society for the Relief of the Ruptured and Crippled and was deeply devoted to the goals of the institution. His conviction to help needy children may have been influenced by the fact that his own three children died young. He served as board president from 1864 until his death in 1874.

Green wrote,

> Have the friends of humanity duly appreciated the claims of these unfortunates? Should they not be cared for because they are *unfortunates?* The blind, the deaf, the dumb and even the morally corrupt, are provided for by legislative enactments. While all this is right, how few, comparatively, think of the poor cripples? Yet, who can witness their sufferings and helplessness without having his sympathy drawn out in their behalf? The children in question are often the offspring of parents too poor to pay for professional treatment, so that, however curable their ailments, their case is hopeless unless charity interposes for their rescue.
>
> In many instances, the apparatus applied costs fifty dollars, and this has to be worn and kept in repair perhaps for several years. For these obvious reasons, many mechanics and laboring people, having children with deformities, which may be relieved if not wholly cured because of the expense, cannot have them treated at their homes. This, however, is but a very partial view of the facts. The same is substantially true of thousands of adults of both sexes afflicted with hernia, varicose veins and analogous complaints, requiring costly appliances and dispensary treatment. Four-fifths of them being in indigent circumstances, they are unable to pay for the trusses, bandages, spring-supports and other surgico-mechanical apparatus their cases require. Hence, without such gratuitous relief as this Institution provides, they are doomed to life-long wretchedness, and often to premature death.

To produce a stream of revenue, the board devised a plan of annual subscriptions. The subscriber had a right to place a child under hospital treatment for one year for every hundred dollars paid, with the right to terminate the subscription at the end of each year.[3]

Building the Team

Before moving into the new hospital, the professional staff consisted of James Knight and four consultants.[2] Knight's official appointment was listed as resident physician and surgeon. This title remained until 1878, when Knight first appeared in the annual reports as surgeon-in-chief. In 1871, as part of the staff expansion, a resident junior assistant, Richard W. Allen, MD, an apothecary, Andrew J. Dowe, and an instructor in gymnastics, Herman Fleugal, were appointed. Later that year, a new assistant physician and surgeon, Virgil P.

Gibney, MD, age 24 years, was recruited. This would be an unusual appointment, as Gibney was a disciple of Lewis H. Sayre, MD, who represented everything that Knight was not.

Complexities of James Knight, MD

In 1871, Knight was 61 years old and had the personality of a surgeon but ironically remained vehemently antisurgery. His attributes as a caring physician, devoted to rehabilitating the poor and disabled, and as an organizer, leader, and philanthropist were in direct contrast to his dogmatic approach to his profession. An open discussion of methods of treatment was not allowed, and he insisted on complete loyalty from all his staff.[5] Although he read widely, he rejected new approaches in medicine, such as plaster of paris, bed rest, traction, and surgery. He published very little: two textbooks on nutrition and one on orthopaedics and one article on scoliosis, which was only a brief statistical analysis.

With his wife and daughter caring for the patients (there were no trained nurses employed), Knight resided in the hospital, thus devoting his entire professional and personal life to the poor crippled children whom he loved and treated. This allowed him to follow his patients very closely and evaluate his methods of treatment. He rarely kept detailed records, leaving such facts to memory. Statistical analyses were sketchy.

The hospital environment lent itself to religious and educational facilities. There was a public school system run by the city of New York (likely the first in a New York City hospital). Singing was encouraged, and patients learned trades. Exercises were important to Knight, who had designed the fourth-floor gymnasium as part of his total treatment program. Rehabilitation was bolstered through educational, religious, moral, physical, and occupational avenues.

He had complete faith in the use of bracing and felt that all physicians should be able to fit a brace. His interest in using static electricity as a tool in treatment was exemplified in a paper read before the New York Academy of Medicine in 1882. Knight was faced with many patients having rickets and other nutritional diseases and was an advocate of healthy food and sound nutrition.[6]

Outpatients most often suffered from hernias, varicose veins, hemorrhoids, and prolapsed uteri and were treated with braces, supports, and bandages. A majority of the inpatients were afflicted with tuberculosis, and thus their

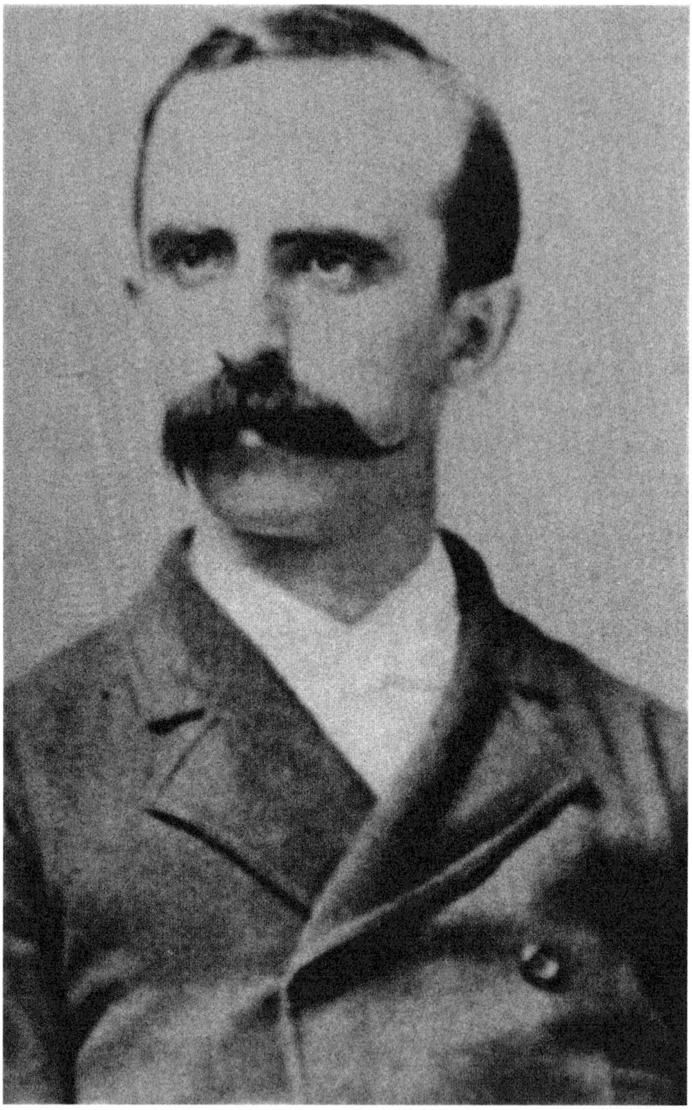

Fig. 2 Virgil P. Gibney, MD, was appointed assistant physician and surgeon to the R&C in 1871, at age 24 years. (From Hospital for Special Surgery Archives)

length of stay was protracted. Every child who could function out of bed participated during the day in Knight's rehabilitation program. Wheelchairs were used when necessary.

Eventually, Knight's model hospital became self-supporting through contributions, financial reimbursement from the city, and proceeds from private patients, which Knight turned back to the hospital since he received a substantial salary. Of course, this was very comforting for the trustees, who were relieved of much of the financial burden.

Knight was in full control of the hospital, his patients, and his family. Consequently, the board had complete confidence in him and his management style. They were well aware that James Knight was able to carry out the intentions of the incorporation and supported him fully.[7] The R&C soon became known as Dr. Knight's Hospital.

Virgil P. Gibney, MD

In late 1871, Virgil Pendleton Gibney, MD (Fig. 2), was appointed by Knight to the professional staff as assistant physician and surgeon—an appointment never fully explained in the annals of this hospital's history.

Gibney had just received his MD degree that year from Bellevue Medical College after one year of medical education there and a previous year spent at the University of Louisville. While at Bellevue, he became very impressed with Sayre, the first professor of orthopaedic surgery in the United States and a founder of Bellevue Medical College in 1859. Sayre—who performed the first resection of a hip joint for tuberculosis and used plaster of paris jackets for scoliosis and tuberculosis—was considered an "adventurous" surgeon. The conservative Knight, however, considered Sayre's treatment of no use to the crippled population. Knight was not only adamant about his methods of treatment but became militant toward anyone whose opinion differed with his own.[8]

Conversely, Sayre, called the father of American orthopaedic surgery, was open-minded and progressive and welcomed new ideas and methods of treatment. He was not the first American surgeon to devote his entire practice to orthopaedics, however; that distinction belongs to Buckminster Brown, MD, of Boston.[9] Sayre almost always attended meetings at the New York Academy of Medicine, where he often argued with Charles Fayette Taylor, MD, another pioneer in orthopaedics and a master of mechanical bracing. Taylor subsequently became the first director of the New York Orthopaedic Hospital and Dispensary, which was founded in 1866. The honor of beginning the third orthopaedic hospital in the country goes to Henry Frauenthal, MD, who founded the Hospital for Deformities and Joint Disease.[10] Knight, meanwhile, rarely appeared at these meetings. The one exception was the only time he read his paper on static electricity in 1882. Knight had met William J. Morton, MD, who had just returned from Paris, very enthused about static electricity. Morton stimulated him to prepare and present the paper. That was a memorable night, as the paper was received with applause.[11]

Sayre had little respect for Knight. Gibney admired both of his mentors and had great loyalty for Knight, never confronting him over the next 13 years as his assistant. "I grew to manhood under Doctor James Knight, living under the same roof for thirteen years, and while my early instructor, Doctor Sayre, disapproved, our friendship continued to the time of his death," wrote Gibney in 1912.

Gibney was a conservative surgeon who was ambitious, honest, and well respected by his peers and his patients, and he was always concerned about his assistants. He was a stimulating teacher and keen observer, studying large numbers of cases of hip disease. He kept copious notes and often discussed his beliefs of the best methods of treatment with his surgical friends and at meetings of the academy.

For tuberculosis of the hip, he advocated bed rest and traction, and surgery for more advanced cases. Finally, he decided to publish a book, *The Hip and Its Diseases*. Although Knight was aware that Gibney was interested in this subject, he was startled to learn of this book. He immediately asked Gibney for his resignation, and their relationship ended in 1884.

The Gilded Age

Mark Twain called the decades after the Civil War *The Gilded Age*.[b,12] It was a time of accumulation of tremendous wealth by a few, including John D. Rockefeller, Andrew Carnegie, and J. Pierpont Morgan. In 1867, Cornelius Vanderbilt consolidated the New York Central Railroad, and the first elevated line was constructed. In 1870, Morgan and Company developed syndicated banking, and John D. Rockefeller opened the New York office of Standard Oil Company.

New York was going through profound changes in its financial world and experienced social upheaval, extreme poverty, and critical public health challenges. The city grew at a staggering rate as immigrants continued to flock in

Table 1 Post–Civil War Growth in New York

1867—First elevated rail line is constructed.
1869—The American Museum of Natural History is incorporated.
1870—The Metropolitan Museum of Art is established.
The New York City Health Department is created.
1874—The 92nd Street Y is founded as the Young Men's Hebrew Association by German Jewish professionals in the home of Simeon Newton Leo.
1877—Alexander Graham Bell introduces the telephone to New York.
1882—The New York Philharmonic, founded in 1842, takes its first domestic tour.
1883—The Brooklyn Bridge is completed by George Washington Roebling.
Gounod's *Faust* is performed at the opening of the Metropolitan Opera House.
1884—The Statue of Liberty, a gift by France to the United States, is installed on Bedloe's Island.
1887—*Evening World* newspaper is established by Joseph Pulitzer.
1888—A commission is created by Mayor Abraham Hewitt to select a site and ask for bids for the eventual Manhattan Municipal Building, which would become the largest office building in the world.
1891—Carnegie Hall opens, with Tchaikovsky conducting *Marche Solennelle.*
1892—The New York City Bureau of Laboratories opens.
The New York City Buildings Department is founded.
Ellis Island Immigration station admits its first immigrant to be processed, Annie Moore, a 15-year-old Irish girl.
1895—William Randolph Hearst establishes the *New York Journal.*
1896—The first movies in the United States are shown at Koster & Beal's Music Hall.
Williamsburg Bridge construction commences and is finished in 1903.
1898—New York City becomes five boroughs in a new charter.
The New York City Art Commission is established.
1900—Construction of the first New York City subway begins.

from other countries and settle in distinct enclaves. There was a significant rise in real estate values, driving the wealthy from the center of the city up Broadway to sites far and apart from communities of immigrants and blue color workers. In 1880, the "model tenement" became the accepted standard for the crowded apartments.

Even with such political corruption, poverty, public health problems, and financial upheaval, the city grew at a staggering rate, and with it came many physical, cultural, and technical changes that benefited society (Table 1).

The Period of the Inter-regnum

In the 21st Annual Report of the Board of Managers of the New York Society for the Relief of the Ruptured and Crippled (1884–1885), there was no mention by Knight that Virgil Gibney was no longer on staff.[13] Yet the board had great faith in Gibney and often relied on him for medical and administrative advice during these years. Gibney called these years the *Period of the Inter-regnum.*

In December 1883, Gibney married and rented a home at 23 Park Avenue, directly across the street from William H. Osborn, a member and subsequent president of the Board of Managers.[8] Because there were no telephones, Osborn arranged with Gibney that when the board wished his advice, Osborn would hang a white handkerchief in his window signaling the need for a hospital conference at the Osborn home.

On July 10, 1884, the board, realizing the importance of Gibney and disappointed to see him leave, passed a resolution expressing a statement of esteem of Gibney. At about that time, Henry S. Terbell, the oldest member of the board, wrote to Frank H. Hamilton, MD, questioning the effectiveness of Knight's "expectant treatment" regimen. Hamilton replied that he had great confidence in Knight and his program.

Over the next couple of years, Knight's health declined, and he died on October 24th, 1887 at age 77 years. In a resolution, the board stated in part: "Dr. Knight was in the highest sense the friend of the needy and the afflicted....His aim in the work of this institution has been to treat the poor and afflicted in such a manner as to accomplish the greatest good with the least possible pain....We recall with gratitude his presence among, and his affection for, the little children confined to his care and skill and his exertions for their moral as well as their physical welfare."[4]

Gibney Assumes the Helm

A new era emerged. The board recalled Virgil P. Gibney and appointed him as surgeon-in-chief. The R&C would grow under Gibney (1887–1924), for the first time extending its reach into the world of surgery. Gibney chose to reside out of the hospital and would establish, in 1887, the first orthopaedic residency program (open to medical school graduates) in the United States.[14]

Osborn wrote in his 1887 report that although the usual systematic patient records of those treated, relieved and discharged could be retrieved, the thoughtful views, hopes, and explanations that Knight had been accustomed to express were missing. Despite his many shortcomings, however, James Knight's accomplishments became etched in the history of orthopaedics in this country.

REFERENCES

1. Sturges J. *Seventh Annual Report of the New York Society for the Relief of the Ruptured and Crippled.* New York, NY: New York Society for the Relief of the Ruptured and Crippled; 1870:21–22.
2. Levine DB. Hospital for Special Surgery: origin and early history. *HSS J.* 2005;(1):1–6.
3. Green JC. *Eighth Annual Report of the New York Society for the Ruptured and Crippled.* New York, NY: New York Society for the Relief of the Ruptured and Crippled; 1871:11–23.
4. Beekman F. *Hospital for the Ruptured and Crippled. A Historical Sketch Written on the Occasion of the Seventy-Fifth Anniversary of the Hospital.* New York, NY: privately printed; 1939.
5. Wilson PD Jr. James Knight (1810–1887) of the Hospital for the Ruptured and Crippled. *Clin Orthop.* 1958;11:1–8.
6. Knight J. *The Improvement of the Health of Enfeebled Children and Adults by Natural Means, Including a History of Food and a Consideration of its Substantial Qualities.* New York, NY: Sackett & Mackey; 1868.
7. Whitman R. A critical estimation of the personal influence of four pioneers on the development of orthopaedic surgery in New York. *J Bone Joint Surg.* 1934;16:331–342.
8. Gibney RA. *Gibney of the Ruptured and Crippled.* New York, NY: Meredith Corporation; 1969.
9. Sherk HH. *Getting It Straight: History of American Orthopaedics*, 1st ed. Rosemont, IL: American Academy of Orthopaedic Surgeons; 2008.
10. Bick EA. *Source Book of Orthopaedics.* New York: Hafner Publishing; 1968.
11. Gibney VP. Reminiscences of the orthopedic surgeons of the latter half of the nineteenth century. *New York Med J.* 1912;18:913–915.
12. Twain M, Warner CD. *The Gilded Age. A Tale of Today.* Hartford/Cincinnati: American Publishing Company; 1873.
13. Wilson PD Jr., Levine DB. Hospital for Special Surgery. A brief review of its development and current position. *Clin Orthop.* 2000;374:90–105.

NOTES

a. An architectural term, borrowed from the Old French and used in late Middle English, to describe a wedge-shaped or tapered stone used in the construction of an arch.

b. A satirical term; a gold covering but with a harsh reality, referring to corruption, dishonest politicians, robber barons, and land speculators.

CHAPTER 3

VIRGIL P. GIBNEY, MD SECOND SURGEON-IN-CHIEF (1887–1900)

DAVID B. LEVINE, MD

WITH THE DEATH OF DR. KNIGHT, in October 1887, the hospital took on a new and expanding course when the Board of Managers appointed Virgil Pendleton Gibney as their second surgeon-in-chief. Although Gibney was named the second surgeon-in-chief, for all practical purposes, he was truly the first surgeon to hold this title because Knight was not a surgeon.

Trained at Bellevue Medical College, under Dr. Lewis A. Sayre, the first professor of orthopaedic surgery in this country, Gibney introduced surgical treatment for the first time at the Hospital for the Ruptured and Crippled (R&C).

Born in Kentucky

Virgil Gibney was born September 29, 1847, on a farm in Jassamine County, Kentucky, the elder son of a general practitioner, Robert A. Gibney, MD (Fig. 1), and his second wife, Amanda Weagley. Robert Gibney's first wife, Pamela Pendleton, after 3 years of marriage, had died along with Virgil Gibney's baby brother. The two women had been very good friends, and Virgil Gibney's middle name was taken from Pamela Pendleton. Although there was no record why he was named Virgil, a youngest brother was named Homer.

His son, Robert A. Gibney, in a book published in 1969 and edited by Alfred R. Shands Jr., MD, medical director of the Alfred I. Dupont Institute for Crippled Children in Wilmington, Delaware, recalled much of Virgil Gibney's personal life. Dr. Shands' father, Alfred R. Shands, MD, had trained

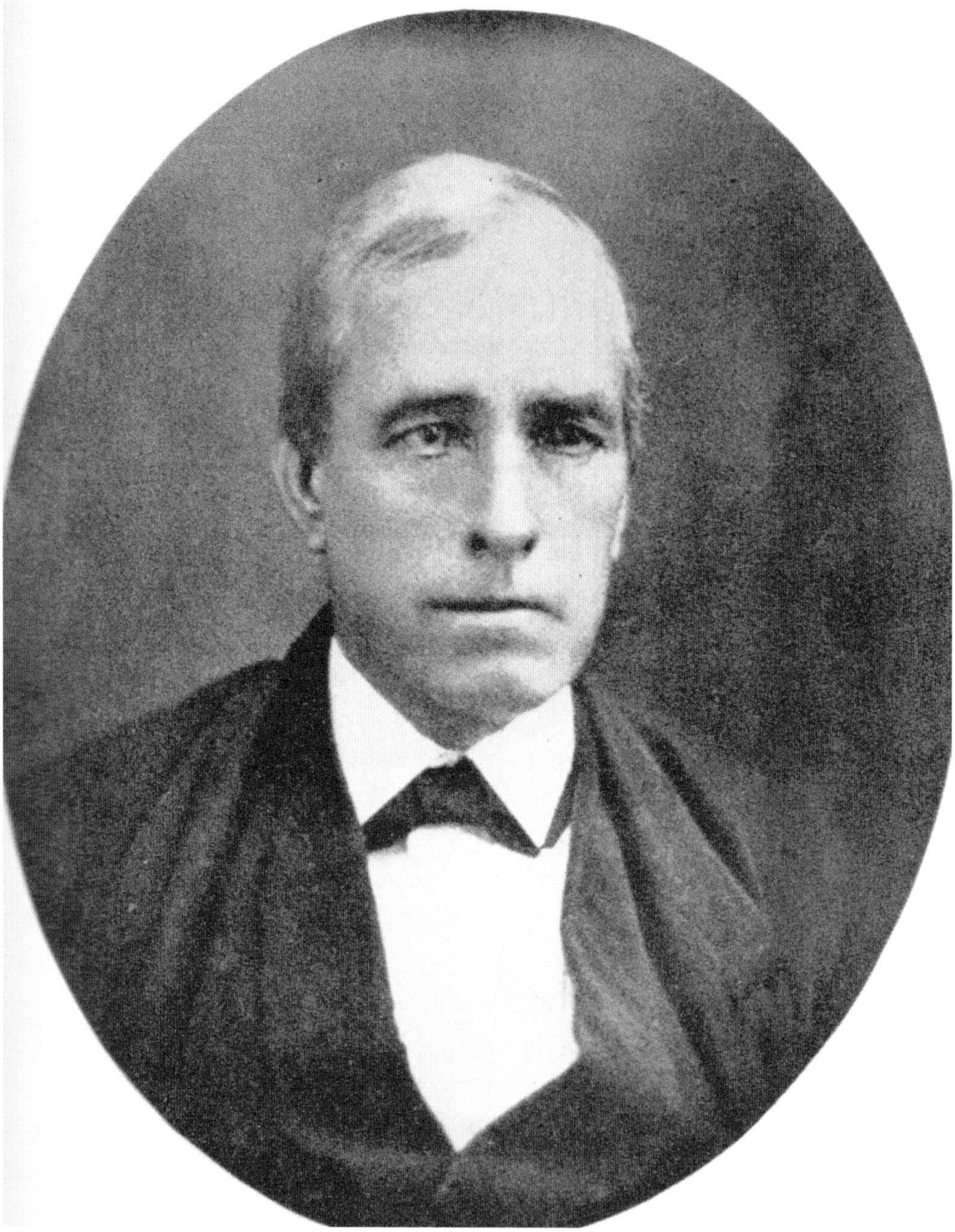

Fig. 1 Robert A. Gibney, MD (1816–1874), father of Virgil P. Gibney, MD. (From Hospital for Special Surgery Archives)

in orthopaedics under Gibney at R&C from 1892 to 1894 and was a good friend of his.

As described in the Foreword by Philip D. Wilson Sr., MD, the book was to be distributed to all graduates of the hospital's training program. Dr. Wilson called upon T. Campbell Thompson, MD, a former surgeon-in-chief and Dr. Robert Lee Patterson Jr., then the current surgeon-in-chief, to help find funding for this publication.[1]

In 1858, Virgil Gibney had lost his ring and little fingers of his right hand, when he was 11 years old, supposedly in an accident in his hometown, Nicholasville, Kentucky; however, this did not stop him from proceeding to study surgery. He was a student of Latin, Greek, and German but was less talented in mathematics. Consequently, in later years, he relied on others to manage his business affairs and investments.

Gibney's father emigrated from north of Ireland in the eighteenth century. As a physician, Dr. Robert A. Gibney needed to supplement his income, which he did by owning part of a retail store. Renting a small farmhouse on 5 acres from James McCampbell, he repaid the owner by providing medical care for the McCampbells. In 1860, the Gibneys bought a 200-acre farm for $110 per acre[1] near Lexington. It was reported to be a nice piece of land, well located with a pond. It was the beginning of the Civil War, and while Robert A. Gibney was a staunch Unionist, his son, Virgil, was a young rebel, too young to enlist.

The story told was when Morgan's Raiders came riding through, they heard of father Gibney's Union favoritism and they would raid the farm. Likewise, when a troop of Illinois or Ohio cavalry came storming through, they heard of Virgil's rebel sympathies and also raided the farm. A cloud of horsemen along the path would always mean trouble, whether the uniforms were blue or gray.

The farmhouse was eventually burned, and the family moved into the slave quarters. When that too was burned, they moved into empty chicken houses, finally moving to Lexington. As a result, young Gibney was eager to move from a farm and never ever return.

In 1869, Gibney obtained his AB degree from Kentucky University[2] in Lexington. The first year of his medical education was at Louisville University, after which he studied at Bellevue Medical College, receiving his MD degree in 1871.

Appointed to R&C Staff

Virgil Gibney's first appointment after medical school was assistant physician and surgeon at R&C. It was 1871, just a year after the hospital had moved from its first site, James Knight's residence on 2nd Avenue, into its new 200-bed building located on the corner of Lexington Avenue and 42nd Street. Gibney was to live in the hospital for the next 13 years as assistant to Knight.[1]

Knight held Gibney in great trust. In 1874, Knight wrote to the Board of Managers: "It is with pleasure I inform you of the very able assistance that has been rendered by my senior assistant, V. P. Gibney by his indefatigable attention to Hospital duties and scientific researches into the pathological conditions of patients, and especially to microscopic investigations."

In 1878, Knight's title was changed from resident physician surgeon to surgeon-in-chief, whereas Gibney's title, *assistant physician and surgeon*, became *house surgeon.*

Knight was becoming fatigued, and that year, at the age of 68 years, he took a few months off to regain his health. He turned over the leadership of the hospital to Gibney. Knight spent time in Europe, visiting hospitals similar to his, but seemed unimpressed of what he saw and returned with no new ideas or treatment methods.

Earlier in the history of the R&C, school classes in the hospital had been established by the Board of Education after Knight insisted that his inpatients needed daily learning in books, religion, and morals. Among the regular teachers employed was a Charlotte L. Chapin from Springfield, Massachusetts. Her mother and father had died when she was 6 years old, and she went to live with her aunt, eventually attending Mount Holyoke Female Seminary, where another aunt had been principal and from where her mother had graduated.

After two years at Mt. Holyoke, Charlotte Chapin left college and moved to New York, where she accepted a position as a schoolteacher at R&C. There she met the young, handsome surgeon, Virgil Gibney, and the two were married in 1883. Unfortunately, in 1889, a tragedy in Gibney's life occurred when both his wife and older son died of diphtheria.

A second son from this marriage, Robert A. Gibney, the collector of his father's history for this book, had been born only a month before this unfortunate event. It was strange that Gibney's father's first wife, Pamela Pendleton Gibney, had also died 3 years after their marriage.[1]

Four years later, Virgil Gibney at age 46 years, married for the second time, 24-year-old Julia A. Trubee of Bridgeport, Connecticut. From this marriage, they had two daughters.

At the R&C, Gibney studied over 2,000 cases of tuberculosis of the hip, all treated by expectant treatment as prescribed by Knight. Gibney was an excellent observer and took voluminous notes. He formulated his own approach to treating this condition. He advocated traction for mild cases and surgery for advanced cases. He never discussed these principles with his chief.[2]

In 1900, tuberculosis was the second leading cause of death over heart disease, cancer, and trauma.[3] Although very respectful of Knight and his conservative approach to treating patients, Gibney published a book on tuberculosis of the hip, advocating surgery in his last chapter. Knight discovered this publication and was astonished by its recommendations. Abruptly in 1884, he asked for Gibney's resignation.[2]

Establishing a Private Practice

When Gibney left the R&C in 1884, he established a private practice and opened an office in his home at 23 Park Avenue, seeing his first private patient February 3, 1884. For the next 3 years, he had no formal association with R&C, referring to this period from 1884 to 1887, as previously noted, as the *Inter-regnum*.[1]

Gibney's daily routine was to have morning office hours with his secretary, taking notes and making outside visits in the afternoon. He had a phenomenal memory for names of his patients and kept careful notes on them.

In his biography, his son, Robert A. Gibney, wrote:

> For years he carried a bright red leather cover into which was fitted his current memorandum book, changed every month and then filed. When he was unoccupied, he had a habit of taking out this memo book for reference as he thought things over, irrespective where he happened to be at the time.

> My stepmother, with long experience, was particularly careful when she and my father were in church. When she sensed Dr. Gibney was losing interest in the sermon, she would build up 4 or 5 hymnals and prayer books on the pew between them. When the memo book appeared, and he would start to raise it to the level of his eyes, she would topple over the prayer books against his leg. He understood the message, and with an apologetic shake of his head, the memo book would go back into his pocket, and his attention would return to the sermon.[1]

When Knight died on October 24, 1887, the board contacted Gibney to offer him the position of surgeon-in-chief. Gibney was visiting surgical clinics in England and Scotland with his wife and son. He received the wire from board member Cornelius Vanderbilt II, informing him of Knight's death and asking him to take charge of the hospital.

Gibney's European visit was very rewarding, as he met a number of notable surgeons. He made rounds with Hugh Owen Thomas (1834–1891) of Liverpool and became intimately acquainted with him at his home. Gibney also got to know his nephew, Sir Robert Jones (1857–1933) who was to become the most famous orthopaedic surgeon in Britain.

Resident Doctor

With the appointment of Gibney as the new surgeon-in-chief, major changes followed (Fig. 2).

Gibney established that the surgeon-in-chief's residence would move out of the hospital. His assistants would continue to live inside the hospital.

In 1888, he created the house staff as we know it today. Young doctors in training would apply for a 1-year position as house surgeon, senior assistant, and junior assistant. They became known as residents, a term now universally recognized in this country as a doctor in training.

So in 1888, the title resident doctor was used for the first time in this country at the R&C. There were both orthopaedic and surgical house staffs.

Candidates for these positions were required to be graduates in medicine. Depending on their hospital experience, they were assigned different positions. The junior assistants were appointed in January, May, and September. They served 4 months as junior, 4 months as senior, and 4 months as house

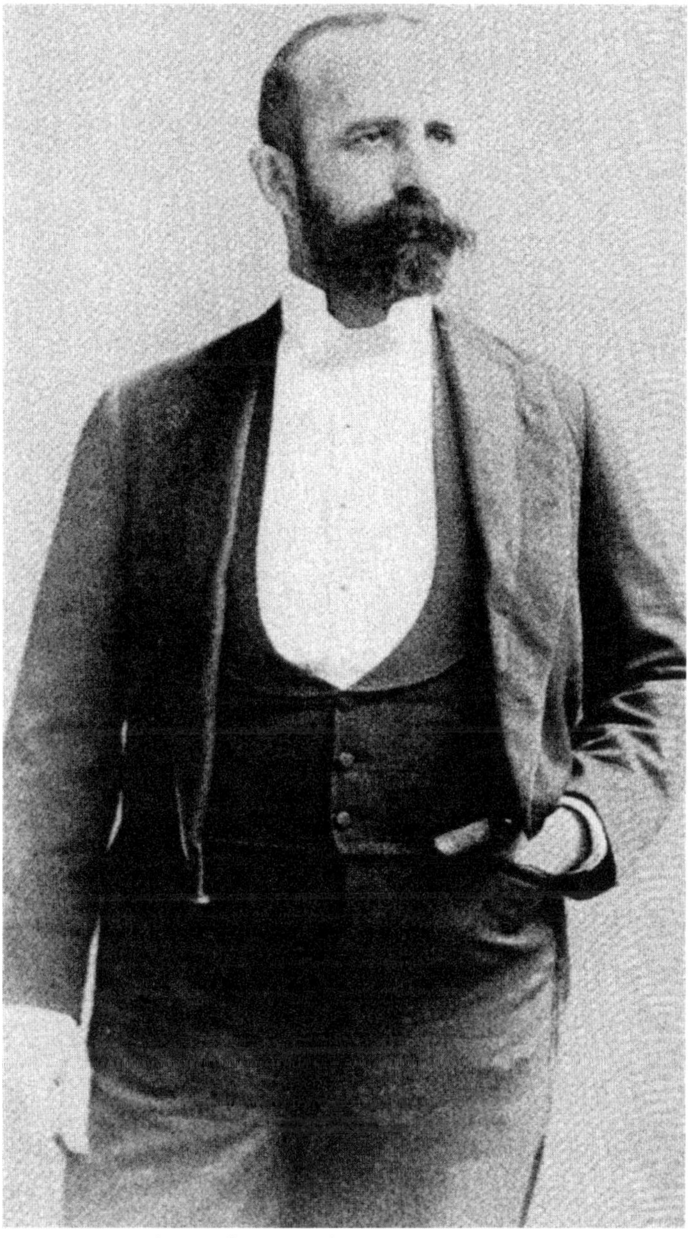

Fig. 2 Virgil Pendleton Gibney, MD, at age 40 years, in 1887 when he became surgeon-in-chief. (From Hospital for Special Surgery Archives)

surgeon. This procedural tract persisted into the 1960s when I was a junior orthopaedic resident in January 1961. At that time, a new resident was appointed in January, April, June, and September for a period of 3.5 years after serving 1 year of internship and 1 year of surgical residency in another hospital. It was unique to the Hospital for Special Surgery and a few other training programs.

Hospital Fire

In January 1888, a young, mentally challenged girl, who had been an inpatient for 2 years and obsessed with fire, succeeded in setting fire to the northwest wing of the hospital. All 120 children were safely relocated to the Vanderbilt Hotel, where the hotel received them free of charge. Seven others were taken into private homes. Unfortunately, there was one fatality; the cook, Mary Donnelly, suffocated in her room.[4]

Although insurance covered the extensive damages, the Board of Managers decided to improve hospital facilities, add the first operating room, expand the ward capacity, and add new outpatient facilities. It annexed the original building, expanding to 43rd Street. The new operating room was state of the art and met all the requirements of antiseptic surgery of those days.

Department of Hernia

Gibney realized the importance of separating patients with hernia conditions from orthopaedic problems. He gave his reasons as follows: "With a house staff which, of necessity, must change, it is difficult to command the kind of skill necessary for the treatment of hernia, even from a mechanical standpoint. However simple, it may seem to apply a truss, it must be remembered that there are many cases present where a truss should not be applied. I must congratulate the Board, therefore, on having secured the services of Dr. William T. Bull as Attending Surgeon to the Department of Hernia."

William Tillinghast Bull, MD (1849–1909), an 1869 graduate of Harvard College, received his medical degree from New York College of Physicians and Surgeons in 1872. He was one of the first in this country to devote himself entirely to surgery. He joined the surgical staff of the New York Hospital in 1883 and became renowned in surgical techniques. He was said to be the first to perform an emergency exploratory operation for an abdominal gunshot wound in 1884. He was a close colleague of Gibney who shared a private office with him.

Gibney's visit to Edinburgh and Glasgow was particularly eye opening, as he was exposed to the antiseptic techniques introduced by Lister in 1866. Such principles were slow to be accepted in America. Now that he was in charge of his own hospital with surgical patients, he needed advice and expertise in the field of surgery.

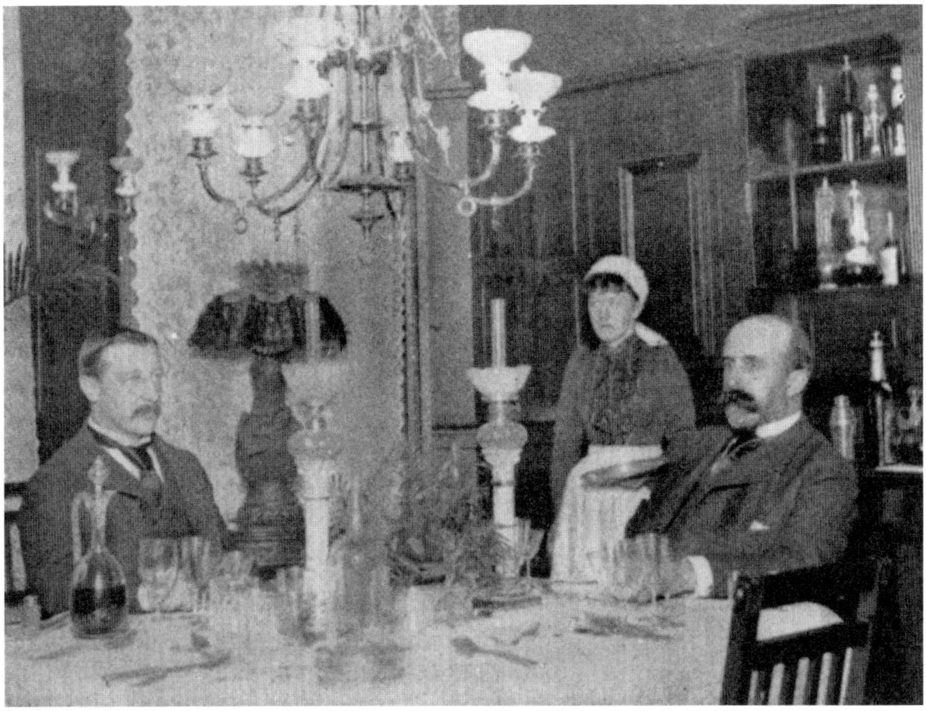

Fig. 3 Dr. Virgil P. Gibney (right) and Dr. Wisner Townsend (1895), in the dining room of Gibney's newer residence at 16 Park Avenue. (From Hospital for Special Surgery Archives)

Thus, Bull was an excellent choice to advise and direct the hospital's surgical service. Although Gibney represented the progressive group promoting surgery in contrast to others of the conservative group, his own qualifications hardly would have qualified him as an expert surgeon.

Gibney created a separate orthopaedic staff, appointing Wisner R. Townsend, MD, as assistant surgeon, with six clinical assistants in the Outpatient Department (Fig. 3). The board recognized in Gibney an accomplished physician with excellent administrative skills and the wisdom to be able to choose outstanding staff to work with him.

Royal Whitman

In 1889, Royal Whitman, MD (1857–1946), was appointed assistant surgeon of the Outpatient Department. Whitman, a graduate of Harvard Medical School in 1882, served a surgical internship at Boston City Hospital and trained further in England.

He was author of one of the most comprehensive orthopaedic text books in English history, *A Treatise on Orthopaedic Surgery*, first to be published in 1901 and revised six times, with the 7th edition published in 1923.[5] An accomplished surgeon, he was an expert anatomist who had meticulous surgical technique. As a result, his carefully planned operations led to excellent results with rare infections.

As a teacher, Whitman expected his house staff to be well-read on the subject; otherwise, he could be harsh and critical. Likewise, he was harsh on visitors, but his motives were not malicious, only to stimulate knowledge in the field of orthopaedics. He did the most to foster surgical treatment in contrast to the conservative approach of Knight and others. The American Orthopaedic Association (AOA), founded in 1887, supported increasing use of surgical treatment for orthopaedic conditions.

Samuel Kleinberg, MD (1885–1957), considered Whitman to be "the most accomplished orthopaedic surgeon of his day in our country."[6] Kleinberg had studied scoliosis under Whitman at R&C and was on its staff until Whitman's retirement in 1929. Kleinberg then became affiliated with the Hospital for Joint Diseases.

William Bradley Coley

William Bradley Coley, MD (1862–1936), was appointed clinical assistant to the Hernia Clinic in 1889, just 1 year after graduating Harvard Medical School. He then trained in surgery at the New York Hospital under Bull who considered him a unique physician. The New York Hospital at that time was located between 15th and 16th Streets in lower New York City. Coley's career would span 40 years at R&C and eventually become (in 1925) the third surgeon-in-chief. Bull also arranged his appointment to the attending staff of New York Hospital and the New York Cancer Hospital, then on the corner of 106th Street and Central Park West (now Memorial Sloan-Kettering Cancer Center).

Coley's lifelong professional career was to be shaped by one of his first patients. Little did he know that this event would not only determine his future in the world of medicine but it would establish his relationship with one of the most wealthy and influential men in our country.

The Legend of Elizabeth Dashiell

Seventeen-year-old, Elizabeth (Bessie) Dashiell, from New Jersey, incurred a minor injury to her hand in July 1890. While on vacation in Alaska, she caught it between two seats of a railroad car. She experienced increasing pain and was seen by a number of physicians. She was referred to William Coley, MD, a newly graduate surgeon, considered as an emerging star by his mentors. After examining Bessie on October 1, 1890, he diagnosed that her problem was an infection. The following week, using local cocaine injection (a common anesthetic at that time), he made a small incision, expressing a few drops of pus. Ten days later, when she returned for follow-up, she was experiencing increasing pain. Coley sought the advice of his mentors, Bull and Robert F. Weir, chief of surgery, at New York Hospital. Coley decided to take a biopsy and under ether anesthesia, he extended the incision down to the bone and scraped away some grayish tissue. On November 6th, the dreaded pathological report returned as round cell sarcoma, a very malignant cancer.

Bessie's older brother, Lefferts Dashiell, was a student at a private school, the Browning School, on the Upper East Side in New York. Among his very close friends was 16-year-old John D. Rockefeller Jr., with whom Bessie had developed a close relationship. Rockefeller, a shy boy, often rode horses with Bessie, walked with her in the park, enjoyed quiet conversations with her, and considered her as his sister (Fig. 4). After Bessie came under the care of Dr. Coley, Rockefeller was unaware that Bessie's condition was serious or that she was in the hospital.[7] When they were not together, he would write her long letters, which he then proceeded to do.

With a diagnosis of sarcoma, and consent of Bull and Weir, Coley performed a below-elbow amputation on November 8, 1890. Within a few weeks, Bessie experienced abdominal pain, enlarged lumps in her breasts and axillae, followed by further evidence of rampant metastasis. When Rockefeller heard how serious Bessie's illness was, he visited her in January at her home in New Jersey.

On January 23, 1891, with Coley at her bedside, Bessie, just 10 years younger than him, died at home. Coley signed her death certificate.

Returned to his home in Cleveland, Rockefeller, now 17, was devastated by the news and attended Bessie's funeral in New Jersey. Rockefeller, being so distraught, was unable to enter Yale College that fall. He postponed going to

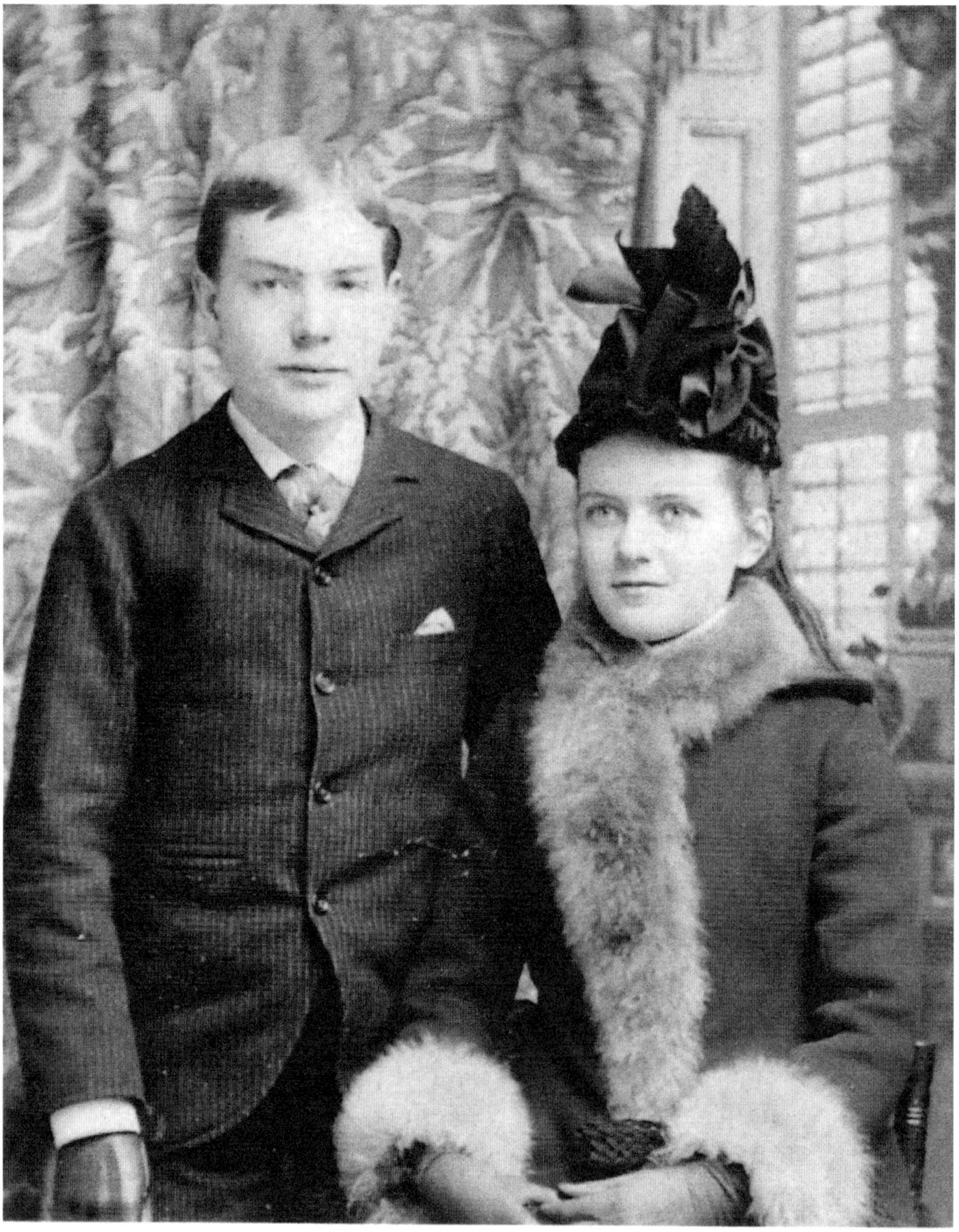

Fig. 4 John D. Rockefeller Jr. and Bessie Dashiell (circa 1888). (Courtesy of Rockefeller Archives Center)

college until the following year when he entered Brown University along with Lefferts Dashiell and their friends.

Rockefeller Jr. had developed a relationship with Coley, which would last for the rest of their lives, both having common interests in research and treatment of cancer. During this period, Coley also met the father, John D. Rockefeller. By 1896, John D. Rockefeller Jr. was seriously supporting cancer research including that of Dr. Coley. Subsequently, he opened the pathways for his father, John D. Rockefeller, to become a major supporter of medical research and particularly, cancer research, Rockefeller Institute for Medical Research was created, as well as millions of dollars given to New York Cancer Hospital (Memorial Hospital and now Memorial Sloan-Kettering Cancer Center).

So early in Coley's career, death confronted him as a physician, challenging the best of his medical knowledge. He faced one of his first patients, suffering with a minor injury that should have healed without incidence, follow a rapid fatal course. Coley realized how little was known in the medical field of the nineteenth century.

In April 1891, Coley read a paper before the New York Academy of Medicine, "Contribution to the Knowledge of Sarcoma," at which time he made it clear that he was going to devote his lifelong career to the study of cancer.[8]

American Orthopaedic Association

The AOA, the prestigious organization of the leaders of orthopaedic surgery in this country, was founded in New York in 1887. Depending on various sources, the preliminary meetings of organization differ. As written by John Ridlon, MD (1852–1936), and published in 1918 as "The Beginnings of the Transactions and Journal of the American Orthopaedic Association," Ridlon quoted Gibney, the first president of the AOA as follows: "My memory is that the late Dr. Steele, of St. Louis, (Aaron J. Steele 1835–1917) and Dr. Newton M. Shaffer, of this city, met at my house, 23 Park Avenue, and we organized the association. Dr. Steele was the prime mover, and the one who suggested the necessity for such an organization. I was chosen the first president."[9]

Thirty-six charter members were present at the first annual meeting in June 15, 1887, at the New York Academy of Medicine. The constitution and bylaws were adopted, and Gibney was elected president and Sayre was elected secretary.[10]

Newton Melman Shaffer, MD (1846–1928), trained by Knight and on staff at R&C until 1870, was appointed chief of the Orthopaedic Service at St. Luke's Hospital in 1872, the first orthopaedic service in a general hospital in this country. In 1876, he became the second surgeon-in-chief of the New York Orthopaedic Dispensary and Hospital (founded in 1866), succeeding Charles Fayette Taylor, MD (1827–1899). In 1900, Shaffer was to become the first professor of orthopaedic surgery at Cornell Medical College. He was a proponent of the conservative group and often would become adversely involved with Gibney at medical meetings.

In 1880, Shaffer appointed John Ridlon, MD, as his assistant in orthopaedics at St. Luke's Hospital. Ridlon, born in Vermont, had earned his MD degree from the College of Physicians and Surgeons in 1878. He was one of the first in this country to be attracted to the work of Hugh Owen Thomas, whom he visited in Liverpool in 1887 when he was 35 years old. When he returned to St. Luke's Hospital, he introduced the first Thomas splint to be applied for tuberculosis of the hip. Shaffer ordered the splint removed, but Ridlon refused.

At the end of the year, Shaffer prevented Ridlon's reappointment to the staff of St. Luke's. Ridlon left New York for Chicago in 1889, where he became professor of orthopaedic surgery at Northwestern University in 1890. He served as president of the AOA in 1895.

Gibney served a second time as AOA president in 1912, the only person ever to serve twice in that position. Royal Whitman was elected AOA president in 1896 and relished his membership in the AOA. He also was inducted as an honorary fellow of the Royal College of Surgeons and Royal Medical Society. In 1899, Wisner Townsend, MD, served as president of the AOA.

Tragedy and Expansion

Gibney continued to maintain a private practice and bought a brownstone in 1888 at 16 Park Avenue across the street from his previous residence. On the first floor was his office that he shared with Townsend and, at various times, with other colleagues and even his two brothers, both physicians.

It was in May 1889 when Gibney tragically lost his first son and then 5 days later, his wife from diphtheria. His second son, Robert A. Gibney, was only 6 weeks old. It was about the time that the hospital was annexed with the new

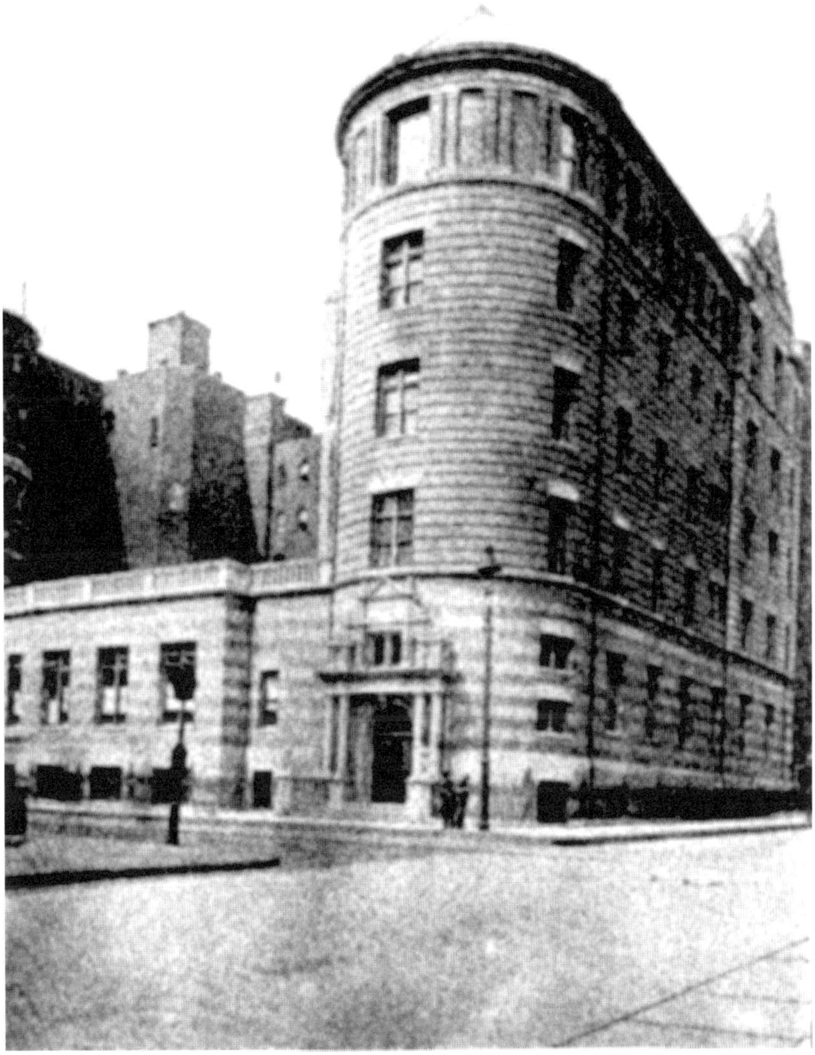

Fig. 5 Lexington Avenue and 43rd Street—in 1898, a new five-storied Outpatient Department was connected to the original building of the Hospital for the Ruptured and Crippled by a low structure (left) along Lexington Avenue. (From Hospital for Special Surgery Archives)

five-storied building (Fig. 5). The addition almost doubled the floor space with an operating suite on the fifth floor, additional wards for the children, an isolation room, gymnasium, and mortuary (Fig. 6).

The Office of Superintendent was created in 1898 with Sherman H. Le Roy filling this new position and relieving Gibney of many administrative duties. This office did not become a full-time position until 1902, when it was separated from the duties of the surgeon-in-chief.

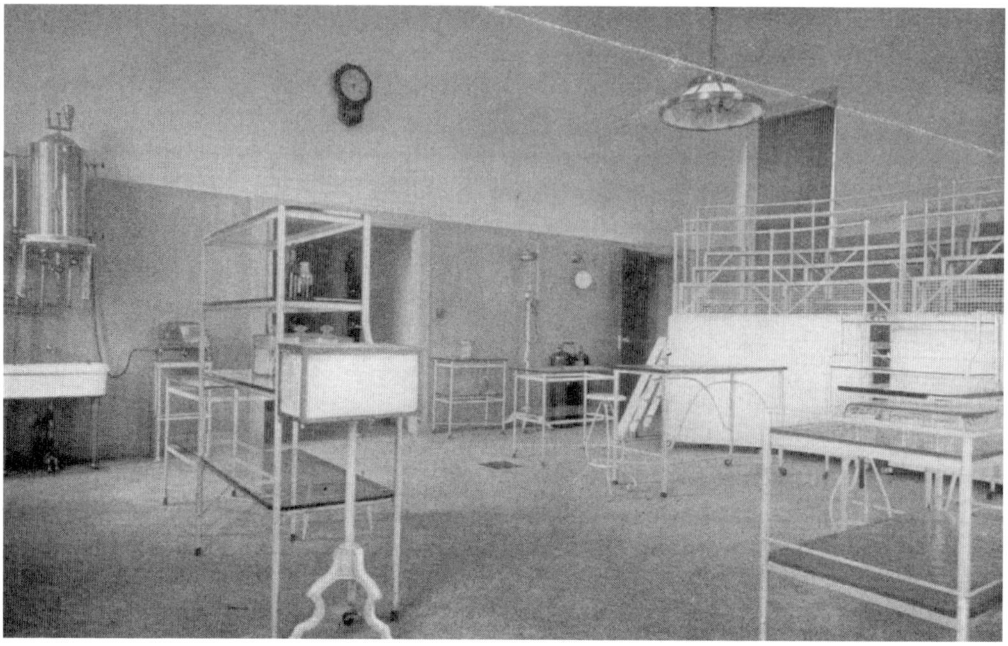

Fig. 6 The first operating room at R&C was built in 1889 as part of a building restoration after a fire. (From Hospital for Special Surgery Archives)

Two neurologists were appointed, and Walter Truslow, MD, took on the task of treating scoliosis. In 1899, a pathology laboratory was opened, and the first x-ray machine installed, just 4 years after Roentgen invented x-ray. With all these improved facilities, the annual number admissions to the wards were nearly doubled, and expenses rose proportionally. There were only enough inpatient beds for children, as there was no available funding for inpatient adults. The number of surgical procedures rose significantly. In 1894, Gibney was appointed the first professor of orthopaedic surgery at the College of Physicians and Surgeons.

Medicine in Contrast

With the changes introduced by the second surgeon-in-chief, the number of patients being treated in the outpatient department increased significantly, and long waiting lists resulted. Bed capacity was always full, but inpatients were all children with no limitation on length of stay. They were only discharged when they got better.

In 1893, Gibney reported to the Board of Managers:

> We still have a large waiting list for Orthopaedic and Hernia cases, and at times our inability to make room for an urgent case is very embarrassing. I need only refer you to the report of last year, while I make another appeal for increased facilities.
>
> Our institution has never exacted any limit for the stay of a patient in the hospital. The rule has been to give the child hospital care so long as it needs treatment. The aim is to shorten the stay ... but we have at present in the wards a large number of children whose parents have abandoned them or who have come from half orphan asylums and similar institutions. We must retain these children so long as their joints need protection.[11]

Even when the new addition on 43rd Street was completed, no adult patient beds were provided because of lack of funds; besides, there were no accommodations for private patients. Gibney and the physicians on staff continued treating private wealthy patients outside of the hospital. If they were outpatients, they would be examined in the physicians' private offices. If they needed to be admitted, Gibney and other physicians had established small private hospitals to fill this void. Together with Bull and John T. Walker, MD, Gibney took over six houses on East 33rd Street between Madison and Park where they established a Private Hospital Association equipped for medical and surgical care.

The wealthy in New York were treated differently from the indigent. Gibney had no reservations in charging the wealthy a healthy fee for his services; however, he was known to have high morals and excellent medical ethics.

The Country in Contrast

North of the tenements of Mulberry and Hester Streets were the mansions of Fifth Avenue—above 59th Street facing Central Park. William K. Vanderbilt, brother of Cornelius Vanderbilt II, lived in a large home on the corner of 57th Street. Mrs. William B. Astor, who lived in a mansion on Fifth Avenue and 65th Street, had given a ball, where invitations were limited to 400 guests. It was she who decided that there were only 400 eligible in the social register who should be invited—the origin of the *Four Hundred* of New York Society.[12]

Immigrants flooded this country, with over 2 million arriving between 1885 and 1895 (25 million between 1866 and 1915). Large groups of Italians and Jews settled in the Lower East Side. There were many from other countries including England, Russia, Poland, Germany, and Scandinavia. At one time, there were more Irish in New York City than in Ireland. Poverty, unemployment, and disease were rampant. Tenement slums took on the names of *Hell's Kitchen* or *Poverty Gap*. However, from these destitute areas came many who eventually were successful and even famous. One of these was Alfred E. Smith, four-time governor of New York and presidential candidate in 1928.

Parts of New York were festering sources of disease and deplorable public health conditions. Milk was sold from cows in the city, never to leave their stalls. Chalk was used to whiten the milk products.

Jacob Riis, a police reporter for the *New York Tribune*, wrote about slum life in New York in his famous book, *How the Other Half Lives*: "All the fresh air that enters these stairs comes from the hall door that is forever slamming.... The sinks are in the hallway, that all tenants may have access—and all be poisoned alike by the summer stenches...."[13,c]

In stark contrast, manufacturing in this country rose over 600% in the latter part of the nineteenth century. The growth of the railroad system was unbelievable, with over 100,000 miles of track being laid from 1870 to 1890. In the latter year, freight revenues totaled $1 billion, more than twice the annual revenue of our government. Steel, originally expensive and rare, was produced at the rate of 4 million tons per year in 1890 due to a new cost-effective process in refining it from iron ore. Andrew Carnegie made 70% of the country's steel in his Pittsburgh plants. In 1870, John D. Rockefeller from Cleveland merged five oil companies he owned into the Standard Oil Company. He controlled 90% of refining in 1892. Known to be a ruthless but brilliant businessman, he drove up the price of oil by buying out his competitors. He was said to have been worth $800 million by 1892.[4]

Such accumulation of money by a few promoted fraud, political graft, and crime, but also this was the land of opportunity. In 1879, Frank W. Woolworth opened the first five-cent store in Utica, New York. By 1913, he had accumulated enough wealth to build the Woolworth Building in New York, the tallest building in the world.

Then there was Robert Cheesbrough, a young chemist from Brooklyn, who in the 1870s invented petroleum jelly as a by-product of petroleum oil. He made much of it in his home, storing it in his wife's flower vases. From *vase* and *line*, he coined the name *Vaseline*. In 1893, at the Chicago World's Fair, Whitcomb Judson, a Chicago inventor exhibited the *clasp locker*, later to be called *zipper* by B. F. Goodrich who used it in overshoes. In 1908, Henry Ford produced the first Model T car.

As the R&C entered the twentieth century, medicine was changing rapidly. The hospital kept pace in growth, development, and expansion with its new addition on East 43rd Street (Fig. 5), its first operating room (Fig. 6) and its new wards.

It was a hospital that was financially secure under the able leadership of Virgil Pendleton Gibney and a fully supporting Board of Managers. It was ready to face the challenges of the twentieth century.

REFERENCES

1. Gibney RA. *Gibney of the Ruptured and Crippled. Meredith Corporation.* New York, NY; 1969.
2. Beekman F. *Hospital for the Ruptured and Crippled. A Historical Sketch Written on the Occasion of the Seventy-Fifth Anniversary of the Hospital.* New York, NY: privately printed; 1939.
3. Grob GN. *The Deadly Truth. A History of Disease in America.* Cambridge, MA; Harvard University Press; 2002.
4. Osborn WH. *Twenty-Fifth Annual Report of the New York Society for the Relief of the Ruptured and Crippled.* New York, NY: New York Society for the Relief of the Ruptured and Crippled; 1888:5–6.
5. Wilson PD Jr., Levine DB. Hospital for Special Surgery. A brief review of its development and current position. *Clin Orthop.* 2000;374:90–105.
6. Kleinberg S. Royal Whitman (1857–1946). *Orthopedics* 1960:16:1–4.
7. Hall SS. *A Commotion in the Blood, Life, Death and the Immune System.* New York, NY: Henry Holt & Co.; 1982.
8. Coley WB. Contribution to the knowledge of sarcoma. *Ann Surg.* 1891;14:199–220.
9. Brown T. The American Orthopaedic Association, a centennial history (no date).
10. Urbaniak JR. *A History of the AOA American Orthopaedic Association.* Rosemont, IL; American Orthopaedic Association; 2006.
11. Gibney VP. *Thirtieth Annual Report of the New York Society for the Relief of the Ruptured and Crippled.* New York, NY: New York Society for the Relief of the Ruptured and Crippled; 1893;13.
12. Lyman SL. *The Story of New York.* New York, NY: Crown Publishers; 1975.
13. Riis JA. *How the Other Half Lives.* New York, NY: Penguin Group; reprinted 1997.

NOTES

a. In 2011 dollars = $3,000.

b. The name was changed to Transylvania University (1799–1861) and then closed at the beginning of the Civil War.

c. Jacob Riis emigrated from Denmark in 1870 and was confronted with extreme poverty and unemployment until 1877, when he finally found a position on the *New York Tribune*. Along with other reformers, he brought about change for thousands of immigrants experien cing poverty and disease in New York. He continued his work through photography and became famous for his unique photojournalistic documentary approach for social reform. He died in 1914.

d. In 2011 dollars = $19.5 billion.

CHAPTER 4
THE TURN OF THE CENTURY (1900–1912)
DAVID B. LEVINE, MD

DISCOVERY. INNOVATION. EXPANSION. EXCITEMENT. As the new century approached, all could describe life in New York, in the country, and in medicine. In 1898, New York became five boroughs in a new charter. With the introduction of electricity, steel construction, and elevators in the 1800s, steel structures replaced concrete buildings—the first in New York City being the Tower building at 50 Broadway, completed in 1889, where Joseph Pulitzer's *New York World* was published.[1] Art, beauty, and classic architecture graced the New York scene.

Among the most prominent architects were Stanford White and his associates at McKim, Mead & White, who designed notable buildings—many still standing. Among them were the University Club, Harvard Club, Century Association Club, Metropolitan Club, and Madison Square Garden II, completed in 1890. However, as sometimes happens, where art traveled, drama followed: At a social gathering in 1906, while watching a show of dancing young ladies, White was shot in the face and killed by Harry K. Thaw. A well-known millionaire from Pittsburgh, Thaw was livid over a relationship his actress wife, Evelyn Nesbit, had been having with White.

By 1899, electric trolley cars began replacing horse-drawn carriages. Electric cars began to appear. The first subway line opened in 1904, running from City Hall to 42nd Street and Lexington Avenue—the site of the Hospital for the Ruptured and Crippled (R&C). Although it maintained its brace shop (Fig. 1), the hospital now had its new operating room and joined the trend of advancing the field of surgery. Better control of infections, coupled with the introduction of new medical techniques and tools such as the discovery of

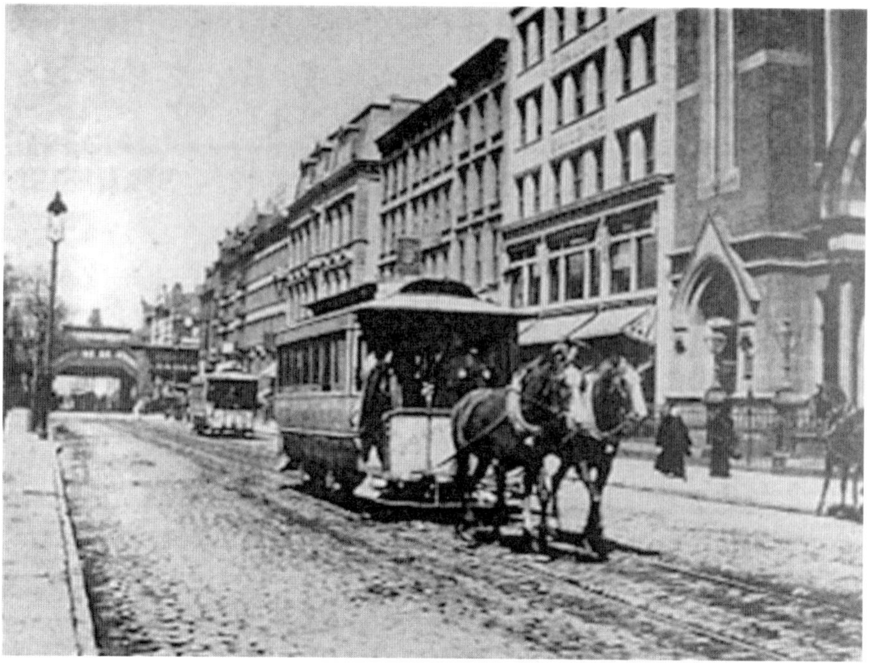

Fig. 1 After Gibney became surgeon-in-chief, he arranged with the City of New York to have the 42nd Street horse-drawn trolley stop in front of the hospital instead of at the corner to make it easier for his patients.

Table 1 Hospital Firsts

1887

1. The first orthopaedic residency program in this country was established.
2. The use of the name *resident*, to indicate a physician-in-training in this country, was first introduced by Virgil P. Gibney, MD.

1897

Thomas Linwood Bennett, MD, was appointed the first anesthetist and instructor in anesthesiology.

1898

1. An Office of Superintendent was created with the appointment of Sherman H. LeRoy. (The medical and administrative functions were not completely separated until 1902.)
2. Two neurologists were appointed to the orthopaedic clinic.
3. The first operating room was installed.

1903

Because of a generous woman's philanthropy, the first adult ward was opened exclusively for female inpatients.

Ellis Island Immigration station admits its first immigrant to be processed, Annie Moore, a 15-year-old Irish girl.

1905

Fred H. Albee, MD, was the first appointed radiologist, but he was not a radiologist. He was chief of surgery at New York Post-Graduate Medical School.

---

x-rays in 1895 by Roentgen,[a] helped enhance the rapid growth of surgery. Just 4 years later, the first x-ray machine was installed in R&C. It would be one of many "firsts" at R&C (Table 1).

After 12 years, as the second surgeon-in-chief, Gibney had nurtured R&C in its evolution from a home for the incurable to a modern hospital equipped with surgical facilities and the latest equipment.

The New York Central Railroad was also expanding and began to pressure its neighbor, R&C, to move. However, R&C was not ready to relocate . . . at least not yet.

Medical Staff

The R&C professional staff featured exceptionally trained physicians and surgeons who were active in teaching the house staff, delivering presentations at medical meetings, writing medical papers, and developing new surgical methods (Table 2). Prominent among the consultants were Charles McBurney, MD (1845–1913), who became surgeon-in-chief at Roosevelt Hospital in 1888 and who delivered a classic paper on the surgical approach to appendicitis at the New York Surgical Society in 1889; Edward G. Janeway, MD (1841–1911), New York City Health Commissioner from 1875 to 1881; and L. Emmett Holt, MD (1855–1924), the most prominent pediatrician of his time in this country, attending physician in 1888 at the newly opened Babies Hospital, and professor of diseases of children at the Columbia University College of Physicians and Surgeons from 1901 to 1922. His text, *The Diseases of Infancy and Childhood* (1896), became the definitive pediatric textbook in the English language, with 20 editions published by 1996. Holt began his career as a clerk at R&C and had been encouraged by Gibney to study medicine.[2]

Table 2 Medical Staff (1900)

SURGICAL AND MEDICAL STAFF.

VIRGIL P. GIBNEY, M. D., -	- *Surgeon-In-Chief.*
WILLIAM T. BULL, M. D., -	*Attending Surgeon to Hernia Department.*
AUSTIN FLINT, JR., M. D., -	- *Attending Physician.*

Assistant Surgeons.

Orthopedic Dept.	*Hernia Dept.*
WISNER R. TOWNSEND, M. D.	WILLIAM B. COLEY, M. D.
ROYAL WHITMAN, M. D.	JOHN B. WALKER, M. D.

Consulting Surgeons.

JOHN W. S. GOULEY, M. D.	CHARLES McBURNEY, M. D.
ROBERT ABBE, M. D.	CHARLES T. POORE, M. D.
JOSEPH D. BRYANT, M. D.	HENRY S. STEARNS, M. D.

Consulting Physicians.

EDWARD G. JANEWAY, M. D.	L. EMMETT HOLT, M. D.
F. P. KINNICUTT, M. D.	A. ALEXANDER SMITH, M. D.
ANDREW H. SMITH, M. D.	WALTER B. JAMES, M. D.

L. DUNCAN BULKLEY, M. D.,	*Consulting Dermatologist.*
DAVID WEBSTER, M. D.	*Consulting Ophthalmic and Aural Surgeon.*

Consulting Neurologists.

A. McLANE HAMILTON, M. D.	JOSEPH COLLINS, M. D.

D. BRYSON DELAVAN, M. D., - *Consulting Laryngologist.*

OUT-PATIENT STAFF.

ORTHOPEDIC SURGERY.

Chiefs of Clinic.

W. R. TOWNSEND, M. D. ROYAL WHITMAN, M. D.

Clinical Assistants.

HOMER GIBNEY, M. D. HENRY LING TAYLOR, M. D.
J. HILTON WATERMAN, M. D. CHARLES D. NAPIER, M. D.
WALTER TRUSLOW, M. D. ARTHUR H. CILLEY, M. D.
C. P. FLINT, M. D. P. W. NATHAN, M. D.
D. D. ASHLEY, M. D. THE SENIOR ASSISTANT.

Neurologists to Out-Patients,

JOSEPH F. TERRIBERRY, M. D. ERNEST W. AUZAL, M. D.

MISS KATHARINE B. PARK, - *Instructor in Gymnastics.*

DEPARTMENT FOR HERNIA.

WILLIAM T. BULL, M. D., *Attending Surgeon.*

Chiefs of Clinic.

WILLIAM B. COLEY, M. D. JOHN B. WALKER, M. D.

Clinical Assistants.

W. DUFF BULLARD, M. D. PRESTON SATTERWHITE, M. D.
E. E. WALKER, M. D. SHIRLEY E. SPRAGUE, M. D.
THE FIRST JUNIOR ASSISTANT.

HOUSE STAFF.

E. LEROY BARNETT, M. D., - - *House Surgeon.*
J. WILBERT STONE, M. D., - - - *Senior Assistant.*
EDWARD J. PARISH, M. D., - - *First Junior Assistant.*
THOMAS DELORCHE BURCKHALTER, M. D., *Second Junior Assistant.*

F. M. JEFFRIES, M. D., - *Pathologist and Bacteriologist.*
A. L. del CASTILLO, D. D. S., *Dental Surgeon.*
BERTHOLD E. KRYSTALL, M. D., *Masseur.*

On Gibney's orthopaedic staff was Royal Whitman, MD (1857–1946) (Fig. 2), acclaimed by Samuel Kleinberg, MD (1885–1957), to be "the most accomplished orthopaedic surgeon of his day in our country."[3] Whitman devised an operation to stabilize "flail foot" in patients who survived polio. He called this procedure "astragalectomy and backward displacement of the foot" in an article entitled "The Operative Treatment of Paralytic Talipes of the Calcaneous Type" in 1901, published in the *American Journal of Medical Sciences.* This article afforded him worldwide recognition in his field and also brought recognition to the hospital.

In the same year, Whitman first published his textbook, *Orthopaedic Surgery.* This volume would remain the most comprehensive and complete orthopaedic text in the English language for the next 40 years. Whitman went on to publish literature on a number of other subjects, including "The Diagnosis and Treatment of Incomplete Epiphyseal Fracture of the Hip," "The Treatment of Central Luxation of the Femur," and "The Reconstruction Operation for Ununited Fracture of the Femur."[5]

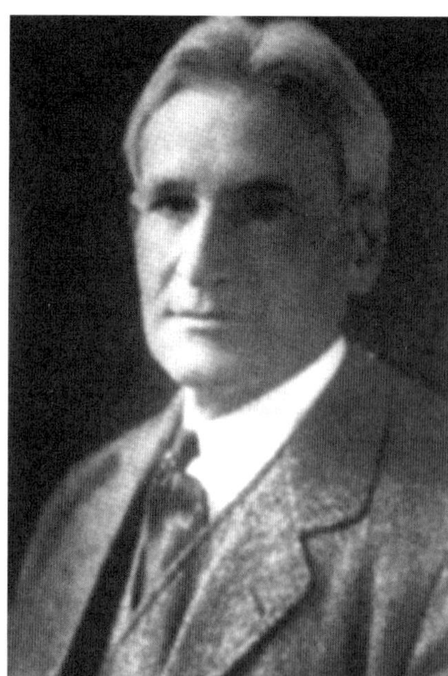

Fig. 2 Royal Whitman, MD, was an assistant surgeon in the Orthopaedic Department and a chief of the Outpatient Clinic in 1900. (From Hospital for Special Surgery Archives)

Whitman remained on staff for 40 years, until 1929, when he retired and moved to England. In 1943, after the death of his wife, he returned to the United States, where he lived for the remainder of his life.[3]

Surgeon-in-Chief, Physician, and Educator

In addition to being a very able chief surgeon, Gibney was also a prolific contributor to the orthopaedic literature, an avid teacher, and a caring physician.

Soon after being appointed surgeon-in-chief, he published several articles on the scope of orthopaedics and, later, case reports from the operating room. He also wrote about clubfoot, congenital dislocation of the hip, and tuberculosis of bone and the hip.[2]

Gibney realized the importance of making the institution a teaching hospital. He expressed such views in his Presidential Address before the American Orthopaedic Association in 1912, when he said: "Orthopaedic surgery is gaining a foothold in all medical colleges throughout the country. Not only are new orthopaedic hospitals being founded but orthopaedic adjuncts to the general hospitals are demanded, and there is no reason why a medical student should not be trained in early diagnosis. . . . I suggest, therefore, that those of us who hold hospital appointments should insist on teaching privileges and the educational use of the material at our command. . . . "[3]

Having elected to reside outside the hospital and establishing the training program for young physicians ("residents"), Gibney appointed the first house staff, consisting of three appointments of 4 months each. Soon, it was enlarged to four, for a total of 16 months of training. The next year, the 16-month program was abandoned and reverted back to a total of 12 months. The additional training period was thought to discourage the better class of medical student and hospital graduate applicants. However, medical students would soon be attracted to the hospital to observe orthopaedics and pathology, creating a larger pool of applicants for the training program.[5]

Medical Education in Reform

The turn of the century witnessed turbulent times in the medical world. Medical regulation was lacking. Medical education was proprietary (owned by the physician teachers), even in the best medical schools such as Harvard.

Standards and medical licensing blossomed in the latter quarter of the nineteenth century. To establish such recognition, the medical profession had to join with other sectarians to win licensing laws. There were two principal medical sects in America at that time: the Eclectics and the Homeopaths.[6]

The Eclectics were botanic doctors who took their name from their ability to take the best from various medical schools. They were founded by Wooster Beach in 1827, first as the United States Infirmary and then 3 years later as the Reformed Medical College of the City of New York. Born in Connecticut, Beach did receive a degree from an acceptable medical college, but he made it his mission to reform and improve existing methods in the practice of medicine. The Eclectics accepted scientific teaching, but in treatment methods they taught herbal medicine and opposed drugging and bleeding.

The Homeopaths took an entirely different approach to medicine. Founded by Samuel Hahnemann (1755–1843), a German physician, homeopathy taught that disease was a matter of spirit inside the human body, not governed by physical laws. They had three doctrines:

1. Disease could be cured by drugs that produced the same symptoms in a healthy person.
2. The more diluted the dose, the greater the effect.
3. All diseases were the result of a suppressed itch (psora).

Some of the appeal of homeopathy stemmed from the dependent and personal relationship that developed between the patient and the doctor—a trend away from today's practice of medicine.

The battle of the sects and traditional medicine was intense during this period. On the same night when Abraham Lincoln was shot—April 14, 1865—Secretary of State William Seward had an attempted assassination on his life by Lewis Powell, an associate of John Wilkes Booth. The Surgeon General was denounced for taking part in the treatment of Seward because Seward's personal physician was a homeopath.

The American Medical Association (AMA) was not in favor of these sects. A New York physician was expelled because he bought milk sugar at a homeopathic pharmacy. Collaboration with the sects was deemed a violation of the AMA's code of ethics. When the AMA revised the ethics code in 1903, this changed, and within a few years, orthodox medical societies were seeking out members of other sects.

Reformation in medicine was not easy to accept but was critical for the future of medicine. New licensing laws resulted in higher standards. Proprietary medical schools frowned on these changes. Requiring medical school applicants to have a high school or college degree or its equivalent encouraged medical schools to manufacture such fraudulent certificates.

Harvard, Hopkins, and Rockefeller Take the Lead

When the Baltimore merchant Johns Hopkins died in 1873 and left $7 million[b] to build a hospital and university, his philanthropy became a significant peg in the advancement of medical education. Before that time, even Harvard Medical School was not closely affiliated with a university. Harvard's faculty collected fees from the students, paid the school's expenses, and divided what was left. The Harvard system changed in 1871 when Charles Eliot, president of Harvard University, was able to prevail on the medical school faculty to become salaried under the control of the Harvard Corporation, which would then govern the medical school.

Johns Hopkins University opened its medical school in 1893 (lagging behind the opening of its hospital in 1889 due to a lack of funding). The 4-year program required applicants to have a college degree, be fluent in French and German, and have a background of science courses.

Not until 1901 did Harvard require its medical school applicants to have a college degree. In fact, before that time, Harvard's only requirement was that the applicant should be able to read and write. Medical schools at the University of Pennsylvania and Columbia University followed suit, requiring college degrees from their applicants. Like Harvard, Hopkins paid the faculty salaries; they were not paid by the students. These dramatic changes in medicine are prefaced in John Barry's epic story of the deadliest plague in history, *The Great Influenza*.[7]

The Big Four

The founding physicians at Johns Hopkins University Medical School were known as the "Big Four." They included:

- William Henry Welch, MD (1850–1934), pathologist, the son of a physician. He graduated from the Columbia University College of Physicians and Surgeons, one of the most prestigious medical schools of the time. He then trained in Germany in pathology and bacteriology, returning to Bellevue Medical College in a teaching and research position. He was the first of the Hopkins faculty, arriving in 1884. He established a laboratory in 1886 and trained 16 graduate students. It was the first graduate training program for doctors in this country.
- William Stewart Halstead, MD (1852–1922), was recruited by Welch. Battling a lifelong addiction to drugs, including cocaine, Halstead was a meticulous and careful surgeon with unusual technical skills. Welch strongly supported Halstead and appointed him to a research laboratory while he recovered from his addiction. Halstead was the first to require surgeons to wear rubber gloves when operating, to reduce the risk of infection.
- William Osler, MD (1849–1919), a British Canadian, arrived in 1888 as physician-in-chief. He was a premier physician who published a famous text in 1892, *Principles and Practice of Medicine.*
- Howard Kelly, MD (1859–1943), a gynecologist, was brought from Philadelphia in 1889 by Osler. He completed the Big Four.

Welch, the founding editor of the *Journal of Experimental Medicine*, became the most eminent physician in medicine in this country. He was described as "the glue that cemented the entire American medical community."[7] A national and international figure, he served as president or chairman of the AMA, the American Association for the Advancement of Science, and the National Academy of Sciences, as well as numerous other medical societies. His power to transform the lives of professionals was unchallenged. Welch's second skill was to cultivate major funding for research.

Hopkins's influence on other medical schools was soon felt. Those that did not change eventually failed.

The year 1910 was notable for the advancement of American medicine. That year, the Rockefeller Institute Hospital opened its doors to the scientific research of named diseases. In 1901, John D. Rockefeller (1839–1937) founded the Rockefeller Institute for Medical Research (the name being changed to the Rockefeller University in 1965). Its own laboratories were first opened in 1903.

Chairing both the institute's board and the Board of Scientific Directors, William Welch declined the offer to head the new institute. He asked Simon Flexner, MD (1863–1946), a pathologist who was previously at Hopkins, to assume that position. While Flexner took on that role in 1903, the Rockefeller Institute was clearly under the control of Welch for a number of years. Eventually, Flexner molded the institute to mirror his own shadow—sharp, edgy, and brutal. The institute came first, and its individuals were second. It admitted at no charge patients with known diseases that were being investigated at the institute to further study their conditions. As the only such institute in the world at the time, it propelled the field of clinical research.

Flexner Report

In 1904, the AMA formed a Council on Medical Education, whose charges were to inspect 162 medical schools in the United States and Canada—more than half of all medical schools in the world. In 1907, the council concluded that the better schools were improving, but the proprietary schools continued to be significantly substandard. There was a great dichotomy in medical education. With less than optimal cooperation and support from many of the physicians in the country, the AMA needed help and sought the assistance of the Carnegie Foundation.

Carnegie commissioned Abraham Flexner (1866–1959), an educator on staff, to survey medical education in this country. Flexner, brother of Simon Flexner, had graduated from Johns Hopkins University and studied at Harvard, but was not a physician.

Flexner's report was published in 1910. Fifteen thousand copies were printed. The muckraking report created havoc: It concluded that 120 medical schools should be closed.

The AMA's Council on Medical Education immediately rated all medical schools as:

- Class A: Fully satisfactory
- Class B: Redeemable
- Class C: Needed complete reorganization. All schools owned and operated by the faculty were automatically placed in this category.

Within 4 years, 31 states denied licensing to class C schools, which then closed. Almost 100 medical schools had closed by the late 1920s. Medical education would be forever changed.

First Female Ward at R&C

While the number of American medical schools shrank, R&C continued to expand. In the Surgeon-in-Chief's Fortieth Annual Report, Gibney announced a generous contribution from a good friend of the hospital to support an adult female ward for 2 years.[8] In 1903, an 18-bed ward admitted 85 women ranging in age from 14 to 48 years. Yet R&C still did not have the funding to provide beds for adult males.

Expansion in teaching also continued. In 1904, the hospital opened its doors to selected fourth-year medical students to learn on the wards and in the operating rooms. This, of course, improved the selection of house staff. The hospital became well known it its field and received applications from all over the United States and Canada.

The Vanderbilts and the New York Central Railroad

Grand Central, the hospital's friendly neighbor, opened in 1871—a year after R&C had moved to the corner of Lexington Avenue and 42nd Street. It was built by the shipping magnate Cornelius Vanderbilt (1794–1877). A descendant of the Dutch family van Der Bilts who arrived in 1650, Vanderbilt was born on Staten Island. His unscrupulous tactic of leasing nonseaworthy vessels to the federal government made him one of the many profiteers during the Civil War. He bought up railroad stocks, initially the New York and Harlem Railroad, which started operating horse-drawn trains in 1832, and then the Hudson River Railroad, followed by the New York Central Railroad in 1869. Soon after, Vanderbilt obtained permission from the New York City Council to build Grand Central (Fig. 3).

Vanderbilt commissioned the famous architect John B. Snook, who designed a house on Fifth Avenue and 40th Street for his son William H. Vanderbilt, to draft plans for the new depot.

The station was constructed at a cost of $6.4 million.[c] However, by the time it opened, it was virtually obsolete. Renovated in 1898 and again in 1900, the terminal was eventually reborn as Grand Central Terminal.

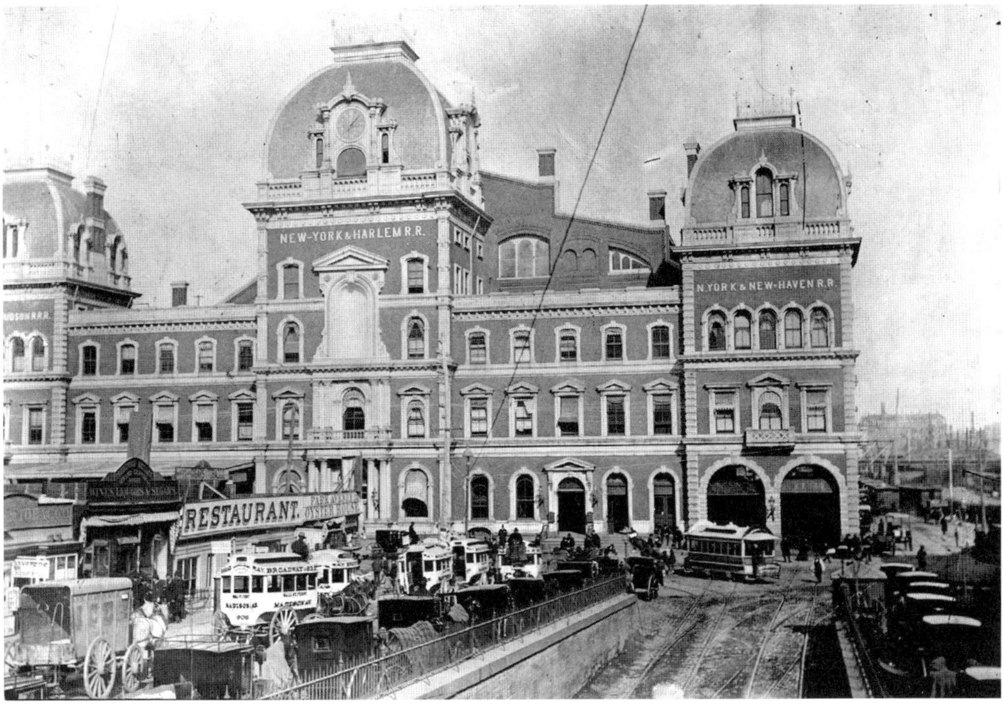

Fig. 3 The southern façade of Grand Central Depot (circa 1880), with a collection of hansoms and horse-drawn jitneys lined up. (Reprinted from the Collection of the New York Historical Society, negative #47557)

Due to a major train collision in 1902 in the Park Avenue tunnel, there was a public outcry for electric trains. The New York Central and Hudson River Railroad announced plans for a major expansion of Grand Central, increasing pressure on R&C to sell its property to the railroads. As in 1892, when other pressures by the railroad on the hospital to move had been attempted, prominent members of the hospital's Board of Managers were able to thwart those threats. Among those on the hospital board who defended the interests of R&C was Cornelius Vanderbilt II (1843–1899), favorite grandson of Cornelius Vanderbilt. Vanderbilt, the grandson, was the member of the board who personally invited Gibney back from Europe to accept the hospital's offer to become the second surgeon-in-chief when Knight died.

Besides befriending Vanderbilt, Gibney had extraordinary personal relations with many of the New York Central staff, including porters, baggage men, gatemen, and attendants. With the hospital situated right next to Grand Central, it was always open to those who worked at the railroad. Injured staff were seen at R&C at no charge. The chief of the Red Caps often sang Gibney's praises. Taking a train to his country home in Bridgeport, Connecticut, Gibney always had time to chat with railroad workers.

Mrs. Gibney also had a collegial relationship with the railroad and ancillary services. As she had her laundress in Bridgeport while the Gibneys spent the winter in New York, she was able to make the following arrangements: Jackson's Express Co. in New York would pick up her laundry at 16 Park Avenue and deliver it to the Baggage Master at Grand Central, where it was put in the baggage car for Bridgeport. There, Hicky's Express delivered it to the laundress in Bridgeport. Clean clothes were returned in the same manner, and all at no charge to the Gibneys.

A Time to Move

As work on the new terminal proceeded, Gibney realized the railroad's need for expansion and felt it was now time to look for a new site for R&C. The board responded quickly, and the hospital and New York Central Railroad reached an agreement in 1910. The hospital sold its property on 42nd and 43rd Streets to the railroad for $1.35 million[d] and purchased a new site further east on 42nd Street, between First and Second Avenues, extending through to 43rd Street, for $307,125.[e]

The plot was half as large as the old property. The new building, with its basement and six stories, officially opened on December 16, 1912—although the patients had been moved there on November 29, and in just one day.

The credit for this complex property change was primarily given to William Church Osborn, elected president of the board in 1911, who exhibited perseverance and good judgment (Fig. 4). Osborn came from a long line of family members involved with the hospital's board dating back to his grandfather, Jonathan Sturges, a founding member of the hospital in 1863 (Table 3).

The Birth of the Alumni Association

With the move to the new site in 1912 came, the establishment of an alumni association for R&C. That year, a constitution and bylaws of the society of the alumni of the R&C was drafted. The object was advancement of the branches of surgery represented at the hospital and promotion of social exchange. Membership was designated as (continued on page 64):

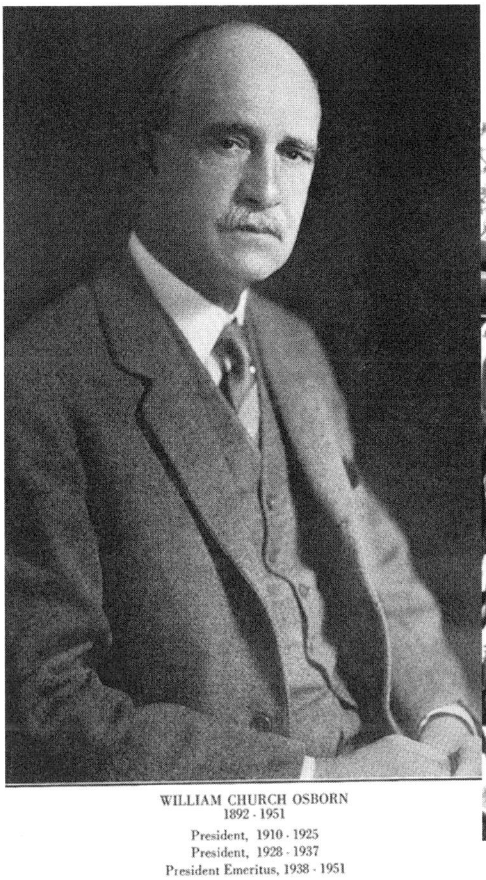

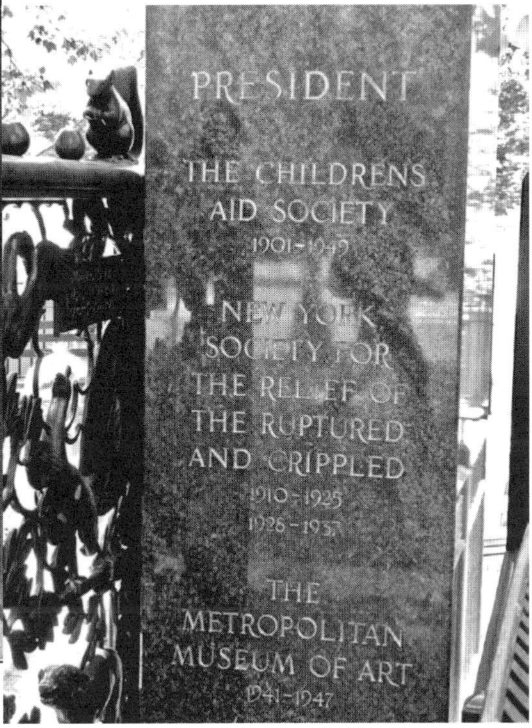

Fig. 4 William Church Osborn, former president of the R&C board, received much of the credit for the hospital's move in 1912. He served as president of the Metropolitan Museum of Art from 1941 to 1947. A children's park on the museum grounds was named after him. Osborn died in 1951 at age 59 years. (From Hospital for Special Surgery Archives)

Table 3 The Osborn Dynasty

BOARD OF TRUSTEES
1871–1891: William H. Osborn
1892–1951: William Church Osborn
1913–1928: Frederick H. Osborn
1941–1951: A. Perry Osborn
1951–1963: Earl D. Osborn
1957–1988: William H. Osborn Jr.
1982–2004: Katherine Osborn Roberts (life trustee)

1. Active members: Persons who have served on the house staff
2. Associate members: Persons who have served on the attending staff

The annual dues (as amended December 19, 1914) were $1 per member plus the cost of the annual dinner. The first meeting of this organization was held on December 29 and 30, 1913 (Table 4). Annual meetings since then have been held without interruption, except in the years of World War I (1917–1918), 1936–1937, and World War II (1943–1946). Alumni officers of the R&C (whose name was changed in 1940 to the Hospital for Special

Table 4a First Annual Alumni Meeting (1913)

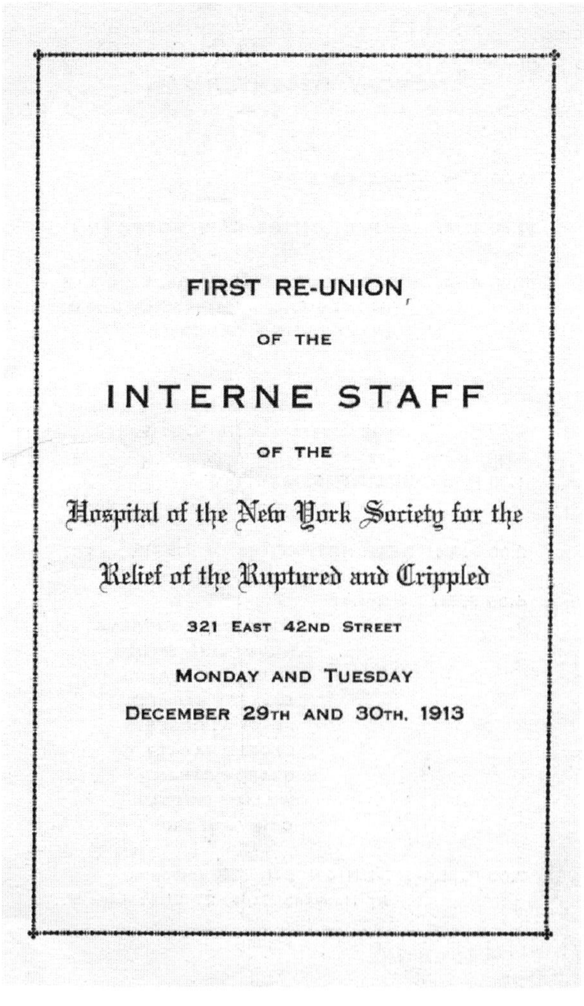

FIRST RE-UNION

OF THE

INTERNE STAFF

OF THE

Hospital of the New York Society for the

Relief of the Ruptured and Crippled

321 East 42nd Street

Monday and Tuesday

December 29th and 30th, 1913

Table 4b

MONDAY, DECEMBER 29TH

10.00 A. M.	ROLL CALL
10.30 A. M.	INSPECTION OF NEW HOSPITAL
11.00 A. M.	WARD ROUNDS WITH DR. VIRGIL P. GIBNEY AND DEMONSTRATION OF INTERESTING CASES
12.30 P. M.	LUNCHEON As Guests of the Hospital through the Courtesy of Dr. V. P. Gibney
1.30 P. M.	BUSINESS MEETING For Purpose of Organization, Etc.
2.00 P. M. to 4.00 P. M.	DEMONSTRATION OF CASES, ETC. By the following Members of the Staff: Doctors WISNER R. TOWNSEND HENRY LING TAYLOR WALTER W. STRANG E. LEROY BARNETT PERCY W. ROBERTS GEORGE HAWLEY GEORGE BARRIE WILLIAM FRIEDER C. H. SANFORD
7.00 P. M.	RE-UNION DINNER (informal) At Harvard Club, 27 West 44th St.

TUESDAY, DECEMBER 30TH

8.30 A. M. to 11.00 A. M.	ORTHOPEDIC OPERATIONS By Dr. V. P. Gibney and Members of the Attending Staff
11.00 A. M. to 12.30 P. M.	HERNIA OPERATIONS by Dr. William B. Coley and Dr. John B. Walker and Members of the Attending Staff
12.30 P. M.	LUNCHEON Guests of the Hospital through the Courtesy of Dr. V. P. Gibney
2.00 P. M. to 4.00 P. M.	DEMONSTRATION OF CASES, Etc. by the following Members of the Staff: Doctors ROYAL WHITMAN HOMER GIBNEY ARTHUR H. CILLEY CHARLTON WALLACE B. H. WHITBECK W. L. SNEED S. KLEINBERG JAS. P. MORRILL

Surgery, or HSS) have included many prominent orthopaedic surgeons over the past century (Table 5).

Alumni worldwide have returned at various times to attend the scientific programs provided annually at the alumni meetings, usually in November.

Table 5 Hospital for Special Surgery Alumni Association Officers

PAST PRESIDENTS

1913–1915: Virgil P. Gibney, MD
1916–1917: Clarence L. Starr, MD
1919–1920: A. R. Shands, MD
1920–1922: William T. Shields, MD
1922–1923: F. W. Gilday, MD
1923–1925: E. W. Hannock, MD
1925–1926: John A. Brooke, MD

1926–1928: A. Mackenzie Forbes, MD
1928–1930: Charlton Wallace, MD
1930–1931: Lewis Clark Wagner, MD
1931–1932: Earl Van Derweker, MD
1932–1933: Percy W. Roberts, MD
1933–1934: Lewis Clark Wagner, MD
1934–1935: Armitage Whitman, MD
1935–1936: Richmond Stephens, MD
1936–1937: No meeting
1937–1938: Andrew R. MacAusland, MD
1938–1939: Walter Craig, MD
1939–1940: Paul Colonna, MD
1940–1941: Earl Van Derwerker, MD
1941–1942: Frank A. Purcell, MD
1942–1943: Barney Owens, MD
1943–1946: No meeting (war years)
1947–1948: Francis J. Carr, MD
1948–1949: Theodore A. Willis, MD
1949–1950: Toufick Nicola, MD
1950–1951: Burr H. Curtis, MD
1951–1952: Rufus A. Aldredge, MD
1952–1953: Walter C. Graham, MD
1953–1954: Arthur A. Thibodeau, MD
1954–1955: J. Gordon Petrie, MD
1955–1956: Albert C. Schmidt, MD
1956–1957: John J. Flanagan, MD
1957–1958: Reginald C. Farrow, MD
1958–1959: Joseph H. Boland, MD
1959–1960: Donald W. Blanche, MD
1960–1961: Frank F. Parrish, MD
1961–1962: Paul C. Colonna, MD
1962–1963: John R. Cobb, MD
1963–1964: T. Campbell Thompson, MD
1964–1965: Frank W. Teague, MD
1965–1966: Theodore A. Lynn, MD
1966–1967: Lee Ramsay Straub, MD
1967–1968: William F. Donaldson, MD
1968–1969: Homer C. Pheasant, MD
1969–1970: Ernest M. Burgess, MD
1970–1971: Paul H. Curtiss Jr., MD
1971–1972: Vincent J. Turco, MD
1972–1973: Michael M. Donovan, MD

1973–1974: Richard P. Embick, MD
1974–1975: J. Paul Harvey Jr., MD
1975–1976: Robert L. Patterson Jr., MD
1976–1977: James A. Nicholas, MD
1977–1978: Charles H. Herndon, MD
1978–1979: Harlan C. Amstutz, MD
1979–1980: Philip D. Wilson Jr., MD
1980–1981: Peter V. C. Dingman, MD
1981–1982: Bernard Jacobs, MD
1982–1983: Americo A. Savastano, MD
1983–1984: Alexander Hersh, MD
1984–1985: John D. Haugh, MD
1985–1986: Allan E. Inglis, MD
1986–1987: Alan Pavel, MD
1987–1988: David B. Levine, MD
1988–1989: Victor M. Goldberg, MD
1989–1990: Leon Root, MD
1990–1991: Clifford W. Colwell Jr., MD
1991–1992: Russell F. Warren, MD
1992–1993: Chitranjan S. Ranawat, MD
1993–1994: Paul A. Lotke, MD
1994–1995: John P. Lyden, MD
1995–1996: Michael F. Rodi, MD
1996–1997: Thomas P. Sculco, MD
1997–1998: Merrill A. Ritter, MD
1998–1999: Eduardo A. Salvati, MD
1999–1900: Norman Johanson, MD
2000–2001: Patrick F. O'Leary, MD
2001–2002: Paolo Aglietti, MD
2002–2003: Joseph M. Lane, MD
2003–2004: Serena Hu, MD
2004–2005: Charles N. Cornell, MD
2005–2006: Gary M. Garstman, MD
2006–2007: Paul M. Pellicci, MD
2007–2008: Harry J. Robinson Jr., MD
2008–2009: Thomas L. Wickiewicz, MD
2009–2010: Patrick V. McMahon, MD
2010–2011: Jon B. Wong, MD
2011–2012: Domenick J. Sisto, MD
2012–2013: Daniel S. Rich, MD
Past Secretary/Treasurers
1913–1916: Charles Ogilvy, MD

Table 5 *(continued)*

1919–1920: Richmond Stephens, MD
1920–1921: Isadore Zadek, MD
1922–1923: Earle E. Van Derwerker, MD
1924–1925: Toufick Nicola, MD
1925–1927: Irwin Balensweig, MD
1928–1932: Lewis Clark Wagner, MD
1933–1938: Francis Carr, MD
1939–1940: Peter Cyrus Rizzo, MD
1940–1941: John J. Flanagan, MD
1941–1942: Frederick Vom Saal, MD
1942–1946: No meeting (war years)
1946–1948: Lewis Clark Wagner, MD
1948–1949: Henry P. Lange, MD
1949–1961: Lewis Clark Wagner, MD
1961–1968: Peter Cyrus Rizzo, MD
1968–1975: Bernard Jacobs, MD
1975–1982: David B. Levine, MD
1982–1989: Thomas D. Rizzo, MD
1989–1994: John P. Lyden, MD
1994–1901: Charles N. Cornell, MD
2001–2004: Paul M. Pellicci, MD
2004–2008: Riley J. Williams III, MD
2008–2011: Douglas N. Mintz, MD
2011–present: Shevaun Mackie Doyle, MD

This devoted alumni association has been a major force in strengthening the hospital and promoting it as a leader in the orthopaedic world.[9]

From this group—now numbering more than 1,500—alumni continued to encourage young physicians in training to apply for postgraduate residency and fellowship positions at HSS. As the size and composition of the house staff changed, the alumni association would become even stronger and more important to the future of HSS.

REFERENCES

1. Lyman SE. *The Story of New York*, 2nd ed. New York, NY: Crown Publishers; 1975.
2. Beekman F. *Hospital for the Ruptured and Crippled. A historical sketch written on the occasion of the seventy-fifth anniversary of the hospital.* New York, NY: privately printed; 1939.

3. Whitman R, Kleinberg S, Whitman A. *Publications of the First Orthopedic Division of the Hospital for the Ruptured and Crippled.* New York, NY: privately printed; 1922.
4. Osborn WH. *Thirty-Seventh Annual Report of the New York Society for the Relief of the Ruptured and Crippled.* New York, NY: New York Society for the Relief of the Ruptured and Crippled; 1900.
5. Gibney RA. *Gibney of the Ruptured and Crippled,* edited by AR Shands Jr. New York, NY: Meredith Corporation; 1969.
6. Starr P. *The Social Transformation of American Medicine.* New York, NY: Basic Books; 1982.
7. Barry JM. *The Great Influenza.* New York, NY: Penguin Group; 2004.
8. Osborn WC. *Fortieth Annual Report of the New York Society for the Relief of the Ruptured and Crippled.* New York, NY: New York Society for the Relief of the Ruptured and Crippled; 1903.
9. Wilson PD Jr., Levine DB. Hospital for Special Surgery. A brief review of its development and current position. *Clin Orthop.* 2000;374:90–105.

NOTES

a. Wilhelm Conrad Roentgen (1845–1923) was a German physicist who, on November 8, 1895, produced electromagnetic radiation in a wavelength range that he called x-rays. For this he won the first Nobel Prize in Physics, in 1901.

b. About $130 million in 2011 dollars.

c. About $116 million in 2011 dollars.

d. About $31 million in 2011 dollars.

e. About $7.14 million in 2011 dollars.

CHAPTER 5

THE THIRD HOSPITAL (1912–1925) 321 EAST FORTY-SECOND STREET

DAVID B. LEVINE, MD

VIRGIL PENDLETON GIBNEY ENTERED HIS 25th year as surgeon-in-chief of the Hospital for the Ruptured and Crippled in 1912, the year the hospital moved eastward to its new and third location at 321 East 42nd Street (Fig. 1). It was to remain at this location until 1955, when it would relocate to its current site on East 70th Street. Today, the site is occupied by the Ford Foundation (Fig. 2).

Situated in the middle of the block on the north side of 42nd Street between First and Second Avenues, the new hospital was very accessible to its patients. This was critical because the patients were mostly poor children and their parents who could reach the hospital from any part of the city on a five-cent fare.

Designed by the architectural firm of York and Sawyer, the newly constructed building consisted of a basement plus six stories. It officially opened on December 16th. The architectural partners of Edward York (1863–1928) and Philip Sawyer (1868–1949), both trained in the prestigious office of McKim, Mead & White, had established their own offices in 1898 in New York City.

York and Sawyer specialized in designing banks and hospitals, many of which were among the finest in the United States in the early decades of the twentieth century. Among some of their most famous buildings were the classical revival-style Greenwich Savings Bank (1922–1924) on Broadway at 36th Street, the Byzantine-inspired Bowery Savings Bank (1921–1923) on East 42nd Street, and the Federal Reserve (1919–1924) on Maiden Lane.

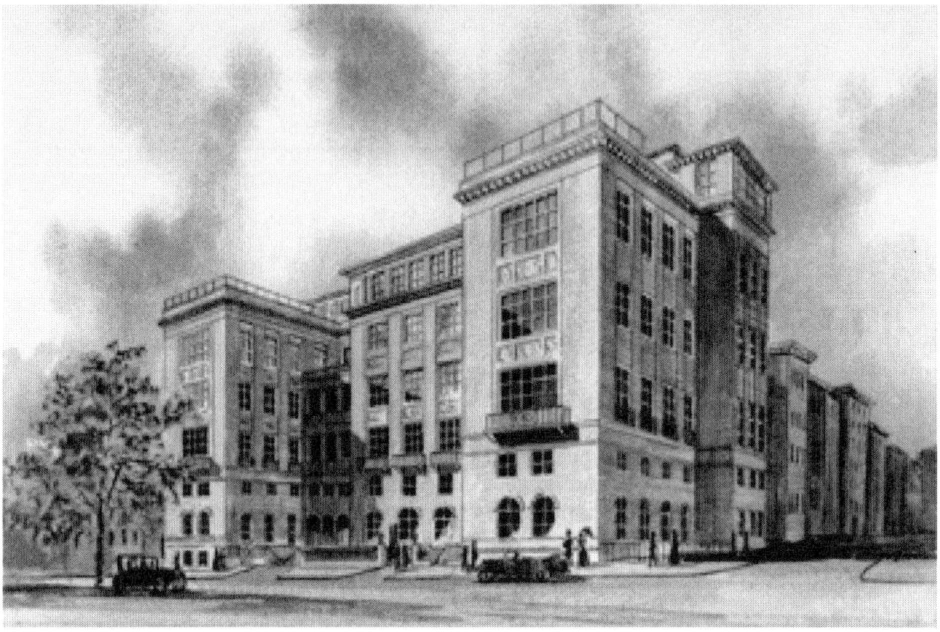

Fig. 1 The Hospital for the Ruptured and Crippled opened in 1912 on the north side of 42nd Street between First and Second Avenues. (From Hospital for Special Surgery Archives)

The firm also created designs for the New York Academy of Medicine on East 103rd Street, the New York Athletic Club on Central Park South, and the Beaux-Arts edifice of the New York Historical Society on Central Park West. From the end of the nineteenth century until World War I, many of New York's prominent landmarks exemplified Beaux-Arts Classicism,[a] including the central pavilion of the Metropolitan Museum of Art, the Statue of Liberty, and the main branch of the New York Public Library, to name a few.[2]

The basement of the new hospital housed utilities and service spaces such as the brace shop, leather room, sewing room, laundry, kitchen, and housing for male employees. The first floor provided the outpatient facilities and the matron's and surgeon-in-chief's offices. The second floor housed sections for residents, female employees, and graduate nurses. The third floor had three girls' wards and a female adult ward (Fig. 3). The fourth floor had three boys' wards, an operating amphitheater and support areas (Fig. 4). The fifth floor had space for a male adult ward, a large playroom, and classrooms, whereas the sixth floor featured two outdoor roof gardens and space for expansion.

Patients moved into the new hospital in one afternoon on November 29, just over 2 weeks before the official opening. The patients had lunch in the old

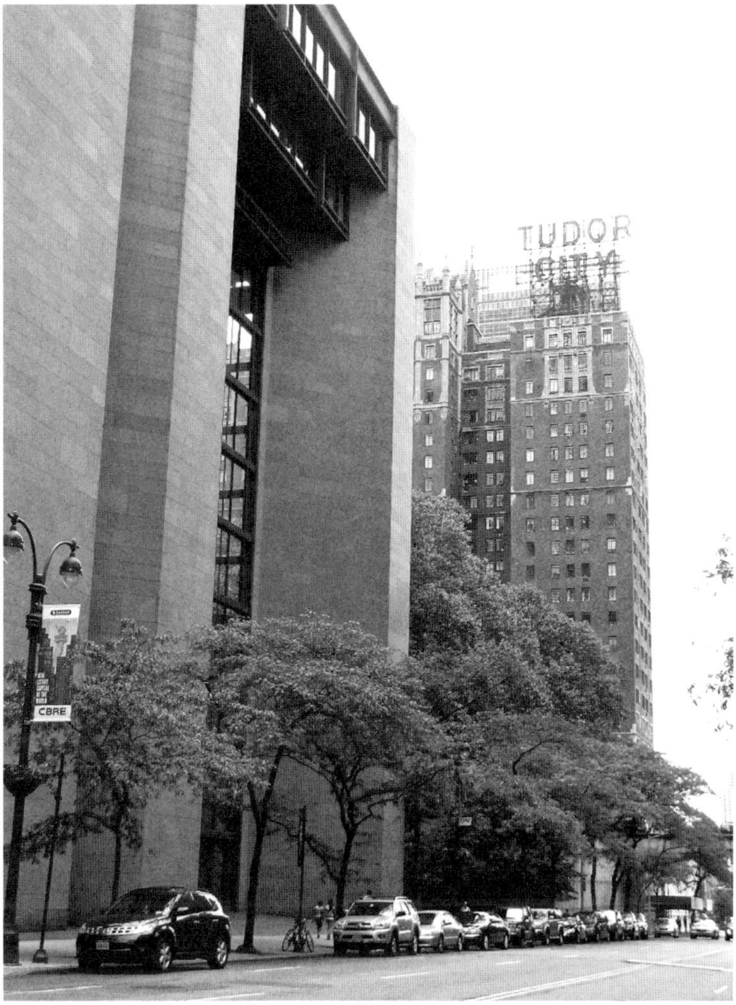

Fig. 2 In 2012, looking east on 42nd Street toward First Avenue, the Ford Foundation, seen on the left, occupied the site of the 1912 building of the Hospital for the Ruptured and Crippled. The area was known as Tudor City (defined in chapter 10, note 1a); see the top of the tall building in the background. (From Hospital for Special Surgery Archives)

hospital and dinner in the new one.[3] Although the plan was for all patients to be hospitalized in the new building, the adult male ward could not yet be opened due to lack of funds, and there were still no provisions for private patients.

Beginning in 1913, the Social Service Department was organized with one director, expanding the next year when an assistant was hired. The X-Ray Department was a small unit headed by Byron C. Darling, MD (1875–1926). His title (1911–1916) was changed from radiologist to roentgenologist in 1913.

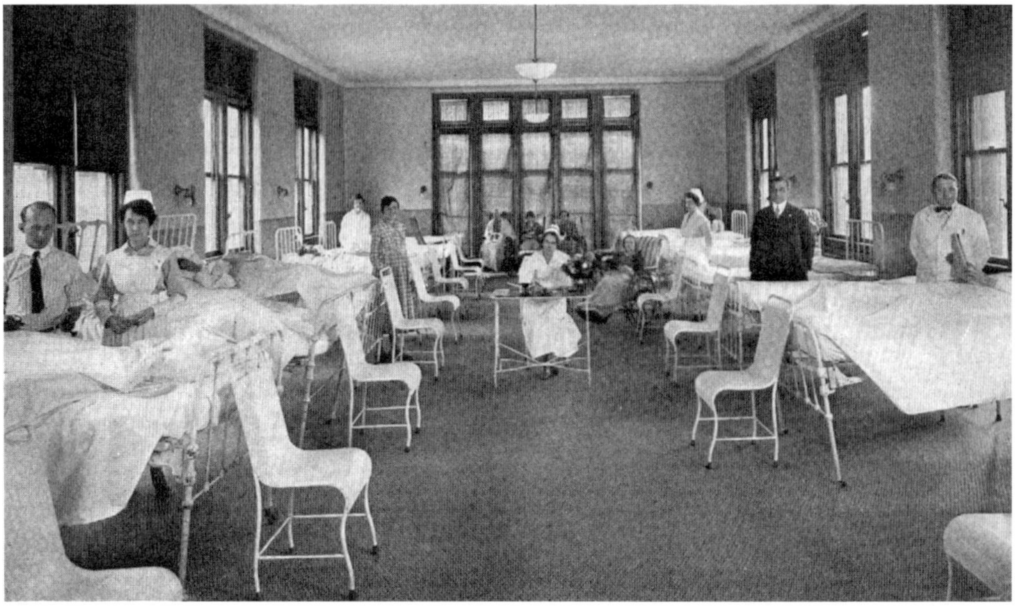

Fig. 3 When R&C opened on East 42nd Street in 1912, there was one female adult ward but no male adult wards. (From Hospital for Special Surgery Archives)

A laboratory was not yet equipped because of insufficient funds. F. M. Jeffries, MD (1865–1943), was the attending pathologist but was not employed full time. He conducted very minimal pathological examinations, but no routine inpatient work or autopsies.

The Birth of Nursing

When Hospital for the Ruptured and Crippled (R&C) was first located in the home of Knight (1863–1870), it was not staffed with any nurses. Nursing care was provided by Knight's wife, their daughter, and hired domestics.[3]

Just 3 years earlier, the first school of nursing in the world was established in 1860 by Florence Nightingale (1820–1910) at St. Thomas Hospital in London. As a pioneer of nursing and a reformer of hospital sanitation methods, Nightingale pushed for reform of the British military healthcare system. With that effort, the profession of nursing was born and gained respect.

In 1873, the first Nightingale-influenced school of nursing in the United States opened at Bellevue Hospital. The profession was quite different then. Nurses were expected to work 7 days a week to keep patient areas clean and to bring in coal to the furnaces, as well as to keep nurses' notes. A graduate nurse

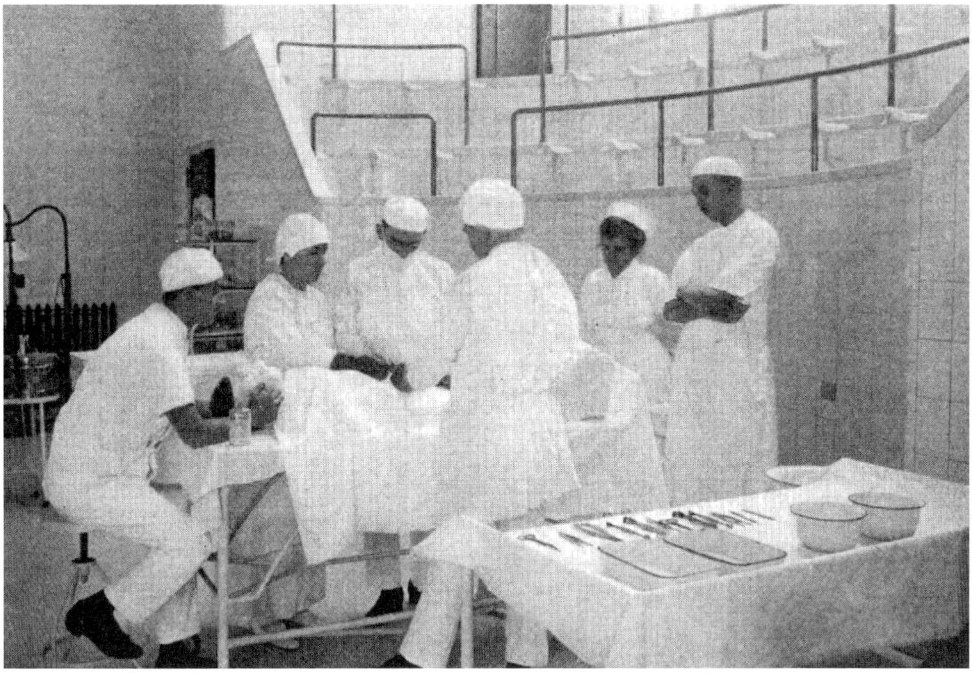

Fig. 4 The operating amphitheater with an observation gallery provided several operating tables for multiple procedures to be performed consecutively. (From Hospital for Special Surgery Archives)

received one evening off a week—two if she went to church. Nurses were expected to avoid smoking, drinking, dance halls, and beauty shops.[4]

The first Chief Nursing Officer at R&C was Ella Murdock in 1896, who was listed on staff as "matron". In 1909, there were only seven graduate nurses working 12-hour shifts. In 1912, the title of matron was expanded to include "directress of nursing," and Ella Patterson, RN, assumed that position. At that time, more than 18,000 patients had been cared for as inpatients and outpatients. Many children with crippling diseases remained as inpatients for years. School classrooms were provided, and Manhattan Public School 401 was established in the hospital. A public school continued to exist at Hospital for Special Surgery until the late 1960s.

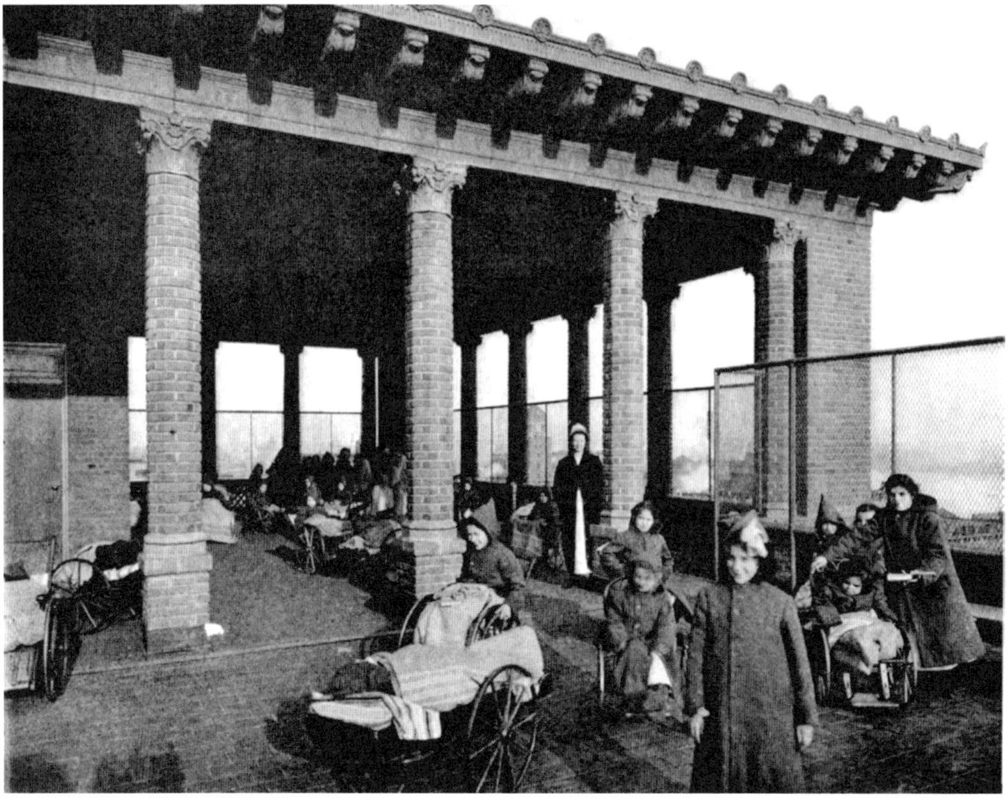

Fig. 5 Inpatient children, attended public school PS 401, the first public school in a New York City hospital.

Peddlers, Pushcarts, and Pickles

Immigration into New York City continued to be rampant well into the twentieth century, focusing mainly on the Lower East Side. It was bordered on the north by 14th Street, on the west by Broadway and Pearl, on the east by the East River, and on the south by Fulton Street. Immigrants clustered in sections such as Little Italy, Chinatown, the Jewish section north and east of Mulberry Street, and the German section around Tompkins Square at Second Avenue. Later, as the Germans moved on, the Jewish population expanded their culture and theatre, known as the "Jewish Rialto." The Italian population increased from over 44,000 in 1880 to more than 1.3 million in 1910. More Italians were located here than in any other location in North America.[5]

Families crowded into one-room living areas, sometimes with no toilets or bathing facilities. Public health was unregulated, and disease spread quickly among the tenements of New York. Tuberculosis, especially affecting the spine, flourished and became a major condition treated at R&C, probably the first hospital in the United States to concentrate on such a challenge. The hospital's mission further included rehabilitating children from poor families and the unemployed back to meaningful employment. When horses—used to transport ice and coal—would die, they often lay in the streets for days until the Society for the Prevention of Cruelty to Animals collected them. Children would play around the dead carcasses. Muck from these animals contaminated the streets; because of the stench, brownstone entrances were located above the end of a long flight of front stairs.

As immigrants poured into these areas, however, they brought with them hope and promises of golden dreams. They were escaping the poverty and endless toil their parents had experienced and sought freedom in a new land of opportunity. They shortened their first and last names, learned English, took advantage of free schools, bought new clothes to look American, deciphered the mysteries of the iron stove and washboard, learned not to fear policemen, and sought employment—particularly as street peddlers. Even schoolchildren would work after school to help support their families.

> We bought our pickles from a lady on the pushcart.... When she was finished, she brought them down to a rat-infested basement. The next day she went down to the rat-infested basement and brought up the same barrels. Those that had rat bites, she threw away.
>
> —A Lower East Side resident[5]

Working conditions cycled through changes, with improvement forced by ongoing events. In 1911, when fire raged through the Triangle Shirt Waist Company, 147 girls and women lost their lives. Blocked exits and no fire regulations accounted for the major part of this disaster. Following this tragedy, better safety regulations and safer working environments were legislated. In 1914, workers in the men's garment industry unionized into the Amalgamated Clothing Workers of America, founded by Sidney Hillman.[6]

The Progressive Era

Journalists, politicians, and crusaders led changes in social reforms during the first two decades of the twentieth century. They were known as "Progressives," and these muckrakers[b] were joined by many leaders at local, state, and national levels. Theodore Roosevelt (1858–1919), president of the United States from 1901 to 1909, ran again for president in 1912 on a Progressive ticket (Bull Moose Party) but was shot in the chest by a fanatic in Wisconsin. Although he recovered, he lost the election to a Democrat: Woodrow Wilson (1856–1924).

The Meat Inspection Act and the Pure Foods and Drug Act were passed in 1906, and the 16th Amendment (Federal Income Tax) and the Federal Reserve Act were passed in 1913. The progressive movement embraced the women who promoted temperance reform, led by the Woman's Christian Temperance Union (WCTU), the oldest continuing nonsectarian women's organization worldwide. As a result, the 18th Amendment (Prohibition) was passed on January 16, 1920.

Still not addressed in this country, however, was legislation to protect against disease. Such laws had been instituted in Western countries—first in Germany, where the first national system of compulsory health insurance was established, followed by similar systems in Austria (1888), Norway (1909), and Britain (1911). France and Italy provided assistance to pay for treatment in designated industries. Extensive aid was delivered in Sweden (1891), Denmark (1892), and Switzerland (1912).

Yet in the United States, this issue was not discussed in political arenas. In 1904, the Socialists were the first to support health insurance, led by the American Association for Labor Legislation (AALL). In the election of 1912, Roosevelt supported health insurance, but the election of Wilson was a blow to the Progressive Party. It would be another two decades before the national government debated many of these social issues.[7]

World War I (1914–1918)

In 1915, a German submarine sunk a British ship, the Lusitania, resulting in 128 American deaths. With the United States having close ties to Britain and France, Wilson eventually asked Congress for a resolution to declare war on Germany. It passed on April 6, 1917.

The U.S. military was ill equipped for war, with just 370,000 men in the Army and National Guard combined. By the end of the war in 1918, the military had swelled to 1.4 million, with a toll of 48,000 killed and 56,000 lost to disease (please refer to chapter 7). It cost our country $33 billion.[c]

Back in New York City, the youngest and one of the most honorable mayors the city had ever had was Mayor John P. Mitchel (1879–1924) who at age 34 years served one term (1914–1918). Unfortunately, when he ran for reelection, it was on a fusion ticket, and he lost to Tammany Hall candidate John F. Hylan (1868–1936). Mitchel enlisted in the Air Force, only to be killed in training. Hylan, a dark-horse candidate promoted by newspaper magnate William Randolph Hearst, went on to win a second term but was eventually defeated by State Senator James J. "Jimmy" Walker in 1925.

New Challenges to Face

The poliomyelitis epidemics of 1907 and 1916 brought an increased number of patients to R&C, not only from the city and suburbs but from upstate New York. Gibney wrote: "The treatment of those disabled by the 1916 epidemic continues with such success that the State Charities Aid Association appealed to us for aid for the paralytic crippled throughout the state and has sent during the year up-state cases requiring operation for correction of deformity to the number of 113, the larger number being of the 1907 epidemic."[3]

The war also had a major impact on R&C. The medical staff was depleted, with many physicians having enlisted in the military or joined other voluntary organizations to help the cause. Some saw active service in France.

A new ward was equipped and opened for treatment and surgery for U.S. Army recruits. In addition, 34 Army surgeons were taken on full-time to learn orthopaedics. The wards and the outpatient department were open to these military officers, and men in khaki were seen strolling throughout the hospital all day.

In 1917, 76 military personnel were treated in a new ward that opened in the solarium on the sixth floor. For the first time in the history of the hospital's 54 years of existence, adult male inpatients received treatment at R&C.

In March 1918, the Surgeon General of the Navy requested that sailors deferred for orthopaedic conditions be seen at R&C. Whitman was so successful in rehabilitating these patients that the hospital was soon called upon to treat sailors with hernias. Coley directed this program.

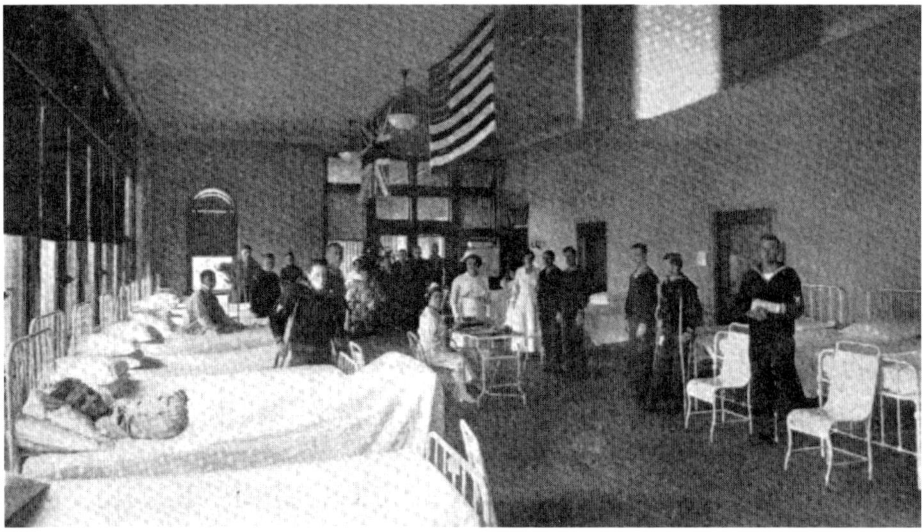

Fig. 6 The sailors' ward was one of the first adult male wards to open at R&C. (From Hospital for Special Surgery Archives)

Gibney reported that to accommodate all these military personnel, the hospital had to encroach upon the children's wards, women's wards, schoolrooms, gymnasium, and, in the summer, the roof. There were 120 beds provided for soldiers, sailors, and marines that were continuously filled[3] (Fig. 6).

The Arrival of a New Administrator

During these troubled times, the surgeon-in-chief was fortunate to have the able assistance of a new administrator, Joseph Flick (1872–1937). He was a comfort to Gibney and the Board of Managers. In its larger quarters in this time of conflict, the hospital required new regulations, had new financial needs, and needed to institute new policies.

Eminently fitted to handle these problems, Flick was born in Belgium and came to America in 1897 to better his condition. He was 44 years at the time of his appointment. With prior experience in a number of hospital administrative positions, he came to R&C after serving as superintendent of the New York Farm Colony on Staten Island. Gibney had more words of praise for Flick than his previous two superintendents (Fig. 7). He sensed that Flick had always been ready to cooperate in making the institution stand for the best interests of its patients.

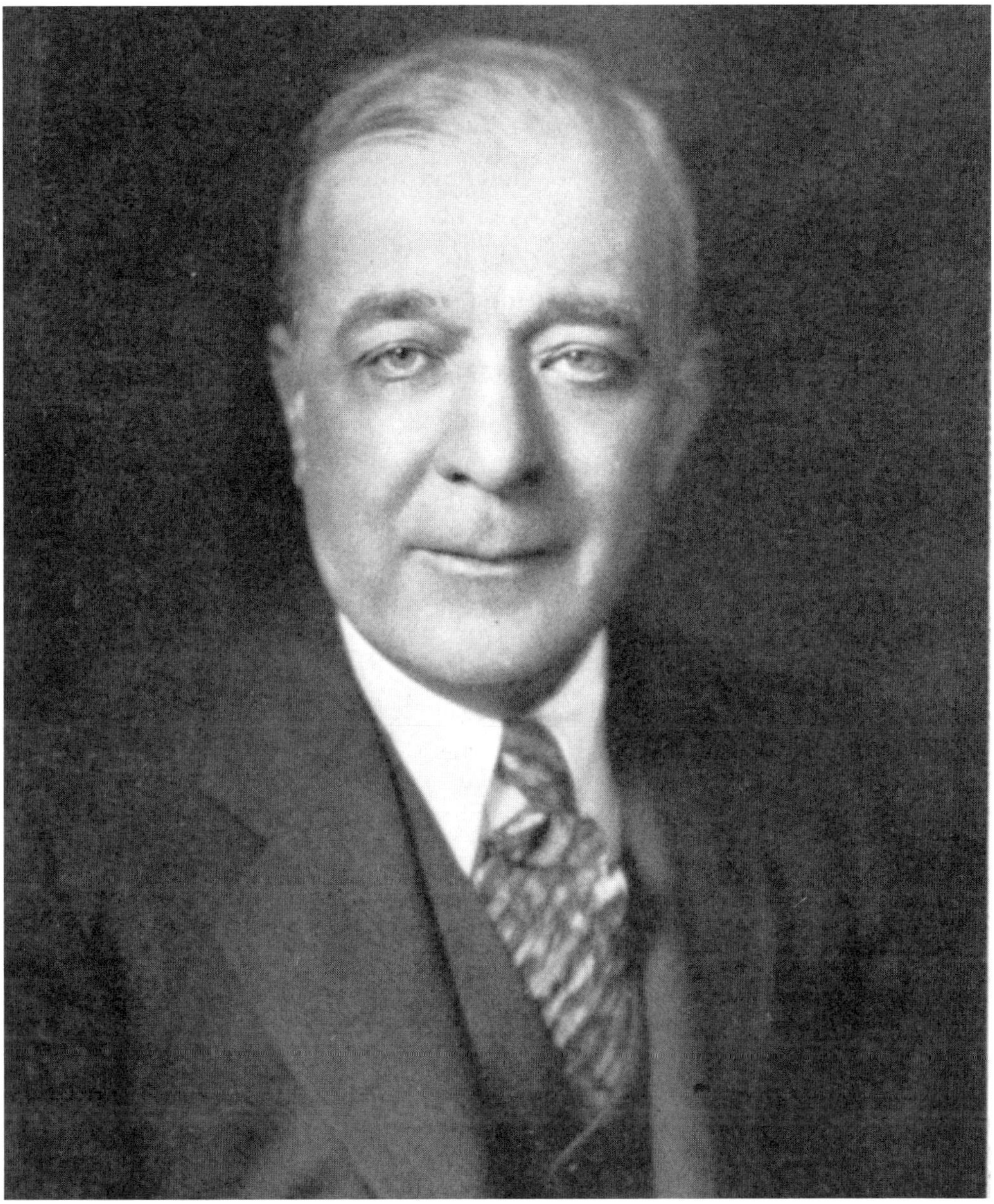

Fig. 7 Joseph Flick served as hospital administrator of R&C from 1917 to 1937. (From Hospital for Special Surgery Archives)

Following the war years, the hospital was pressed to balance its budget. The deficit for 1920 was $59,000,[d] and the board was at a loss to find ways of increasing revenue. To stem costs as much as he could, Flick practiced economy—but not at the expense of patients. He expanded the means of enrolling donors to the hospital. In his annual report of 1923, Gibney wrote about Flick: "I desire to

Table 1 Resident Staff (1921)

Surgeon-in-chief
Virgil P. Gibney, MD
Orthopaedic Department
First Division
James Wyant, MD
Robert E. Burns, MD
Louis Wagner, MD
William Horan, MD
Sherman Burns, MD
Second Division
Bernard Gaston, MD
Paul C. Colonna, MD
Robert Patterson, MD
Leon Slater, MD
Hernia Department
Irving Schwartz, MD
David Warsaw, MD
Russell Smith, MD

call to your attention the able way in which your superintendent, Mr. Joseph D. Flick, has added to the finances of the hospital by his untiring efforts."[9]

Following the war years, all the available spaces of the hospital were in use. There were five wards for children—one devoted to hernia cases—and three adult wards, including one for compensation cases. There was a desperate need for a section for private adult patients. In 1923, a new wing containing three floors for private patients, an operating room plant, and facilities for nurses was finally opened and quickly filled to capacity. Initially called the "Private Pavilion," its name was changed in 1931 to "The Gibney Pavilion for Private Patients." An additional resident was added to the house staff assigned to this pavilion.

In 1921, the orthopaedic department was reorganized into the First Division, whose chief was Royal Whitman, and the Second Division, led by Henry Ling Taylor (1857–1923). The Hernia Department had a separate staff, with its own residents. Because of expansion in the number of hospital beds, the number of residents was increased and now totaled 12 (Table 1).

Table 2 Orthopaedic Residents Serving Under Virgil Gibney (1887–1925)

Francis G. Aud (1910)	William E. Gallie (1905)
Georges Audet (1924)	Bernard Gaston (1921)
John Allen Balsley (1902)	Edwin O. Geckeler (1923–1924)
Edward LeRoy Barnett (1899–1900)	Moses Gellman (1923–1924)
David Beal (1920)	W. Travis Gibb (1887)
George E. Bennett (1909)	A. Lorne C. Gilday (1901)
William T. Berry (1901)	Frederick W. Gilday (1897)
James Bishop (1895)	Charles A. Goodrich (1896)
Harry Blair (1924)	Guy B. Grigsby (1907)
James Bost (1920)	Elwin W. Hannock (1910)
William A. Boyd (1908)	S. T. Harris (1894)
Frederick C. Bradner (1899)	Joseph D. Hartnett (1919)
Nathaniel Perkins Breed (1904)	Eugene Carson Hay (1890)
John A. Brooke (1914–1915)	Philip Heit (1923–1924)
Joseph Buchman (1923–1924)	Horace C. Holbrook (1918)
Charles P. Bull (1905)	William F. Holcomb (1923–1924)
James B. Bullitt (1889)	William Horan (1921–1922)
Thomas DeLorche Burckhalter (1900)	Robert L. Hull (1909)
Robert E. Burns (1921–1922)	Charles H. Jaeger (1896)
Sherman Burns (1921)	A. L. Johnson (1924)
F. F. Carr-Harris (1906)	G. Hewitt Johnson (1913)
Arthur H. Cilley (1897)	J. M. Johnston (1888)
C. C. Collins (1916)	S. Fosdick Jones (1904)
Paul C. Colonna (1921–1922)	Eli E. Josselyn (1887)
Ogden F. Conkey (1909–1910)	Ralph C. Kahle (1922–1923)
Thomas E. Cook (1924)	Edward Y. Kau (1919–1920)
John R. Coryell (1910)	Joseph R. Losee (1908–1909)
Frank T. Dare (1901)	Daniel F. Luby (1911)
Antonio E. DeMoya (1918–1919)	Andrew R. McAusland (1912)
Matthew DePass (1889–1890)	John J. McDermott (1922–1924)
Howard DuPuy (1917–1918)	Francis A. McGreen (1913)
E. R. Easton (1914–1915)	Henry J. McKenna (1911)
Charles F. Eikenbary (1903)	W. Ross Martin (1893)
Edward S. Farley (1918–1919)	Percival K. Menzies (1912)
Robert Felter (1924)	William J. Mersereau (1898)
P. H. Fitzhugh (1891)	Orville R. Miller (1914–1915)
C. A. Forgey (1892)	Samuel E. Milliken (1888)
C. F. Fowler (1917)	Barclay W. Moffat (1919–1920)
Clarence B. Francisco (1907)	Edmund J. Morrissey (1923–1924)
Thomas Moylan (1924)	Leon Slater (1921–1922)

Table 2 (*continued*)

Howard G. Myers (1888)	Russell Smith (1921–1922)
William A. Newman (1922–1923)	Samuel Smith (1890)
Toufick Nicola (1920)	W. Lent Sneed (1911)
Bernard S. O'Brien (1917–1918)	Shirley Erving Sprague (1899)
John B. O'Brien (1918)	C. L. Starr (1891)
John F. O'Brien (1917)	Frank H. Starr (1903)
Joseph F. O'Brien (1914–1915)	Richmond Stephens (1911–1912)
J. C. O'Neill (1915–1916)	J. Wilbert Stone (1900)
Charles Ogilvy (1898)	E. J. Strickler (1908)
W. Barnett Owen (1905)	F. P. Strickler (1915–1916)
Edward J. Parrish (1900–1901)	J. A. Taylor (1921–1922)
Robert Patterson (1921–1922)	Atha Thomas (1923–1924)
Seck Wah Phoon (1924)	W. B. Thompson (1894)
Robert T. Pirtle (1902)	C. A. Thomson (1892)
Charles E. Preston (1907)	Harlin Tucker (1913)
Frank A. Purcell (1922–1923)	Arthur H. VanDyke (1895)
Victor W. Purdy (1919–1920)	B. V. Van Meter (1897)
Joseph E. Raia (1916–1917)	Lewis Clark Wagner (1921–1922)
Abraham H. Rechtman (1923–1924)	R. B. Walker (1922–1923)
Charles A. Reed (1904)	Rawley V. V. Ward (1917)
W. G. Reynolds (1895)	George William Warren (1902)
John B. Richardson, Jr. (1903)	J. Hilton Waterman (1896)
W. B. Ryan (1916)	John W. Wheat (1894)
Judson J. Sales (1923–1924)	Henry G. Williamson (1898–1899)
Preston Satterwhite (1898)	Theodore A. Willis (1919–1920)
D. D. Saunders, Jr. (1893)	C. H. Wilson (1891)
Ben L. Schoolfield (1920)	Dale Wilson (1906)
Herman B. Schwatt (1906)	William E. Wirt (1889)
Irving Schwartz (1921)	W. E. Wolcott (1915)
Charles E. Sevier (1924)	James Wyant (1920–1921)
A. R. Shands (1892–1893)	I. Zadek (1916–1917)
William T. Shields, Jr. (1912–1913)	

The End of an Era

From 1887 until 1925, while Gibney was surgeon-in-chief, over 144 orthopaedic residents trained under him (Table 2). Of those, many became giants in their fields, including George Bennett, MD, Joseph Buchman, MD, Paul

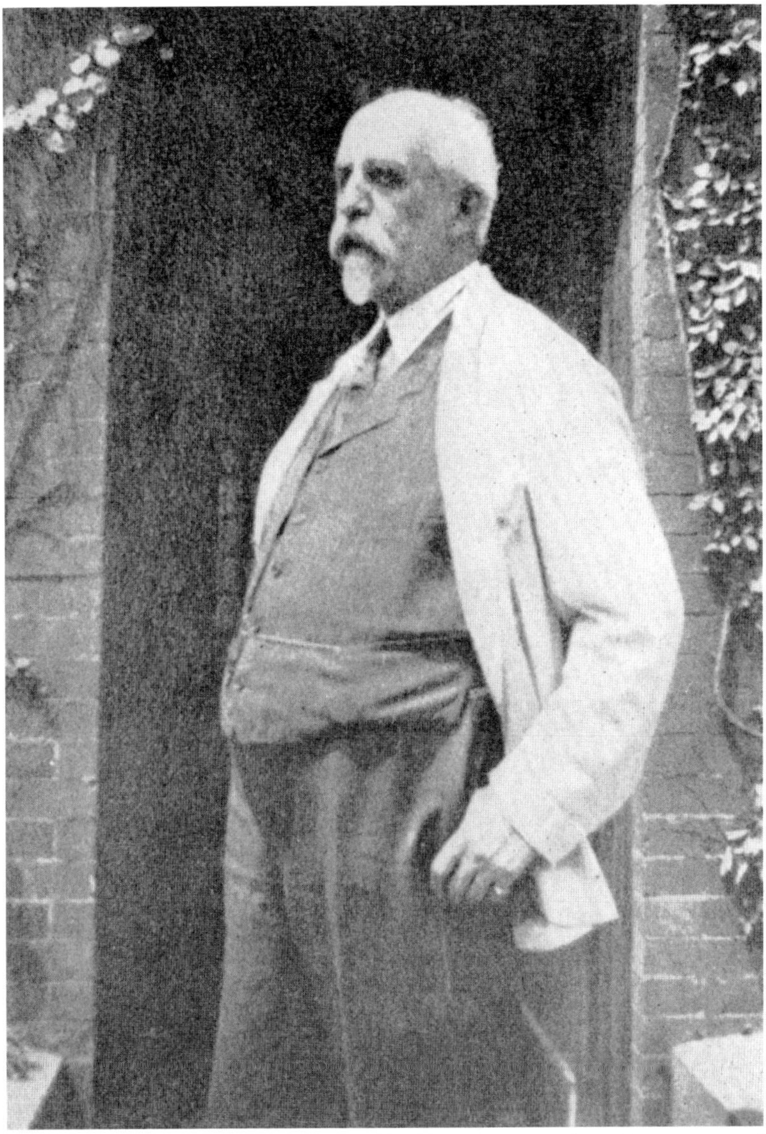

Fig. 8 Virgil Pendelton Gibney, MD, was 77 when he resigned as surgeon-in-chief in 1924. (From Hospital for Special Surgery Archives)

Colonna, MD, William Gallie, MD, Toufick Nicola, MD, A. R. Shands, MD, and L. C. Wagner, MD.

In the summer of 1922, which was particularly hot, there were many cases of polio. Gibney usually spent most of his summers at his Bridgeport, Connecticut home. However, this year he felt increasing responsibility to care for the many

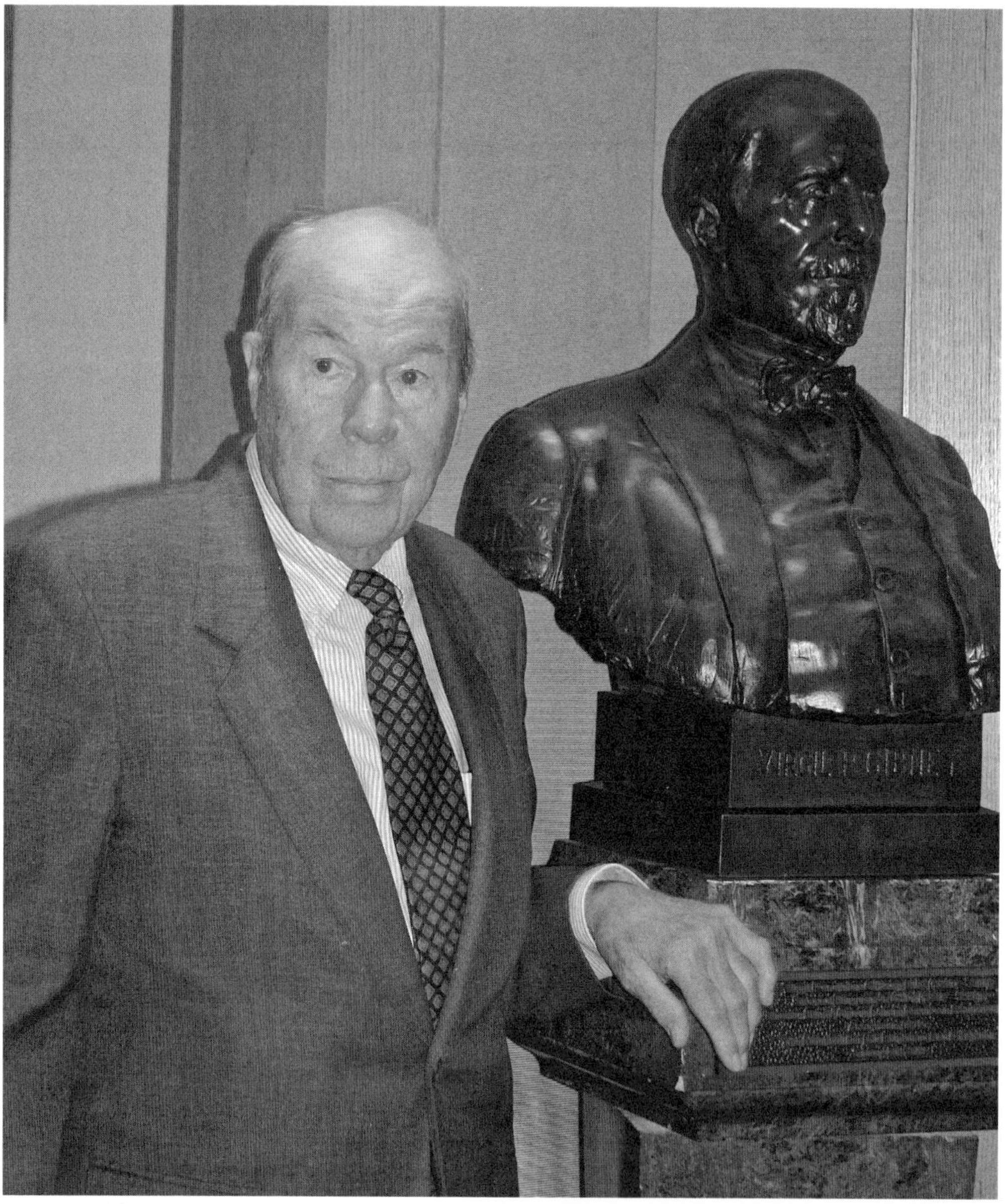

Fig. 9 Gibney Patterson, standing next to the bust of his grandfather, Virgil P. Gibney, in the Richard L. Menschel Education Center at Hospital for Special Surgery (2008). (See chapter 6 for information on Virgil Gibney's bust.) (From Hospital for Special Surgery Archives)

potentially crippled patients. He made a number of trips to his New York office, where he would often spend the night at his townhouse at 16 Park Avenue.

After one particular exhausting trip to New York that August, Gibney returned to his Bridgeport home, where he saw a post-polio patient in his reception area. As she was leaving, Gibney felt the early symptoms of a stroke. He bid her farewell and retired to his bedroom, where he lost consciousness.

His recovery was slow and never returned to normal. His wife realized that he would be unable to cope with their New York home (which lacked an elevator), so she winterized their Bridgeport home, which was originally built as a summer residence. The New York townhouse was sold the next year.

With continued improvement in his health, Gibney decided to return to his private practice. He sought the help of a recent R&C graduate orthopaedic resident, Lewis Clark Wagner, MD (1897–1974), who was then on staff at St. Luke's Hospital. Wagner, a Kentuckian and a graduate of Johns Hopkins Medical School, joined Gibney in private practice on July 1, 1923.

The establishment of a medical board that same year relieved other challenges for Gibney as surgeon-in-chief. Now with his private office under control, he approached the Board of Managers to discuss his resignation (Fig. 8). At first, the board felt he was able to carry on his hospital role, but in January 1925, they finally accepted his resignation.

The Board of Managers of R&C appointed William B. Coley, MD, as the third surgeon-in-chief of the hospital. At the same time, the board designated Gibney, then age 78 years and in deteriorating health, as surgeon-in-chief emeritus (Fig. 9).[e]

The original intention of the 20 organizers of the New York Society for the Relief of the Ruptured and Crippled in 1863—to care for the crippled, both children and adults, and to make these benefits available to the poorest in the community—continued to be practiced into the first quarter of the twentieth century.

REFERENCES

1. Gibney RA. *Gibney of the Ruptured and Crippled*, edited by AR Shands, Jr. New York, NY: Meredith Corporation; 1969.
2. Lowe DG. *Beaux Arts New York: the city in the gilded years.* New York, NY: Watson-Guptill; 1998.
3. Beekman F. *Hospital for the Ruptured and Crippled. A historical sketch written on the occasion of the seventy-fifth anniversary of the hospital.* New York, NY: privately printed; 1939.
4. Kahn BA. The evolution of orthopaedic nursing at the Hospital for Special Surgery. Orthop Nurs. 2005;24:343–348.
5. Hopkinson D. *Shutting Out the Sky.* New York, NY: Orchard Books; 2003.

6. Lyman SE. *The Story of New York*, 2nd ed. New York, NY: Crown Publishers; 1975.
7. Starr P. *The Social Transformation of American Medicine.* New York, NY: Basic Books; 1982.
8. Osborn WC. *Fortieth Annual Report of the New York Society for the Relief of the Ruptured and Crippled.* New York, NY: New York Society for the Relief of the Ruptured and Crippled; 1903.
9. Osborn WC. *Sixtieth Annual Report of the New York Society for the Relief of the Ruptured and Crippled.* New York, NY: New York Society for the Relief of the Ruptured and Crippled; 1923.

NOTES

a. Beaux-Arts Classicism originated at the famous Parisian school, École des Beaux-Arts, where many young architects from the United States studied. Favored materials included light-colored stones and bricks—particularly marble, limestone, and granite, lightening the color of the city from drab brownstones.

b. President Theodore Roosevelt often attached the name "muckraker" to journalists who seemed to expose the moral filth of life in this country. The term was originally used in the 17th century novel *Pilgrim's Progress.*

c. About $440 billion in 2011 dollars.

d. About $655,000 in 2011 dollars.

e. I have been fortunate to befriend Gibney's grandson, Gibney Patterson. He has recalled some of his memories of his grandfather with me.

CHAPTER 6

WILLIAM BRADLEY COLEY, MD THIRD SURGEON-IN-CHIEF (1925–1933)

DAVID B. LEVINE, MD

NOW IN ITS 62ND YEAR, The Hospital for the Ruptured and Crippled (R&C) was the oldest existing orthopaedic hospital in the country and had become the leading orthopaedic center under the skillful direction of Virgil Gibney. It was to remain at its third location on 42nd Street, just east of Second Avenue in New York, until 1955, when it would relocate to 535 East 70th Street as the Hospital for Special Surgery (HSS). Although founded by a general practitioner, James Knight, a general surgeon now occupied the office of surgeon-in-chief for the first time.

Upon the death of Gibney, "News Notes" in the *Journal of Bone and Joint Surgery* noted the following in 1927: "Gibney is dead. One of the fathers of Orthopaedic Surgery has been called away. The world is poorer by his loss … Dr. Gibney is dead, but his memory liveth and will live because he was more than a surgeon. He was a man with greatness in him."[1]

There were many other tributes recognizing Gibney. One was the naming of a private pavilion at R&C, *The Gibney Pavilion*, which was completed in 1923 and which remained until the hospital moved in 1955. Made possible by Lewis Clark Wagner, an anonymous patient donated a life-size bronze bust of Gibney that was unveiled on January 30, 1929. It was crafted by an American sculptress, Agnes Kemp, and set on a pedestal to replicate the exact height of Gibney. It presently stands in the reception area of the Richard L. Menschel Education Center in HSS. For many years, HSS resident physicians used to rub the nose of the bust before examinations for good luck, resulting in a shiny appearance.

As an assistant to Knight for 13 years, Gibney carefully examined his patients, systematically recorded his findings, and personally prescribed appropriate treatment. Although he was overshadowed by Knight's conservative principles, he respected Knight as a physician, educator, and administrator.

Gibney's patients revered him, were enamored by his winning smile, and sometimes felt overwhelmed just by his presence. Although he was an orthopaedic surgeon, he realized and accepted his own surgical limitations and appointed general surgeons to the staff who were great leaders in their fields.

Third Surgeon-in-Chief

The newly appointed surgeon-in-chief was William Bradley Coley, MD, age 63 years. At the time of Gibney's death, Coley remarked: "Dr. Gibney was highly fitted by nature for an orthopaedic surgeon.... Generations of house surgeons came and went and every one left with a feeling of great respect for Dr. Gibney's professional skills, and with a stronger feeling of friendship and affection that endured through all the years.... He will be remembered long as a distinguished surgeon and a great teacher, but even longer as a loyal and devoted friend."

Coley had been first appointed clinical assistant to the Hernia Clinic in 1889, just one year after receiving his medical degree from Harvard Medical School and while a house surgeon at New York Hospital (Fig. 1). It was William Bull, MD, Coley's mentor—who was on the surgical staff at New York Hospital, R&C, and the New York Cancer Hospital—who took a liking to Coley and arranged his appointments at these hospitals. Bull was a close colleague of Gibney's and shared an office with him.

Why a general surgeon received this appointment is not clear from hospital records or other sources of hospital history. There were certainly renowned orthopaedic surgeons on staff, the most famous probably being Dr. Royal Whitman, age 68 year, who had been on staff since 1889—the same year as Coley. It was also unusual that at the time of his appointment to R&C, Coley was recognized internationally as a pioneer in cancer research. Not many cancer patients were treated at R&C.

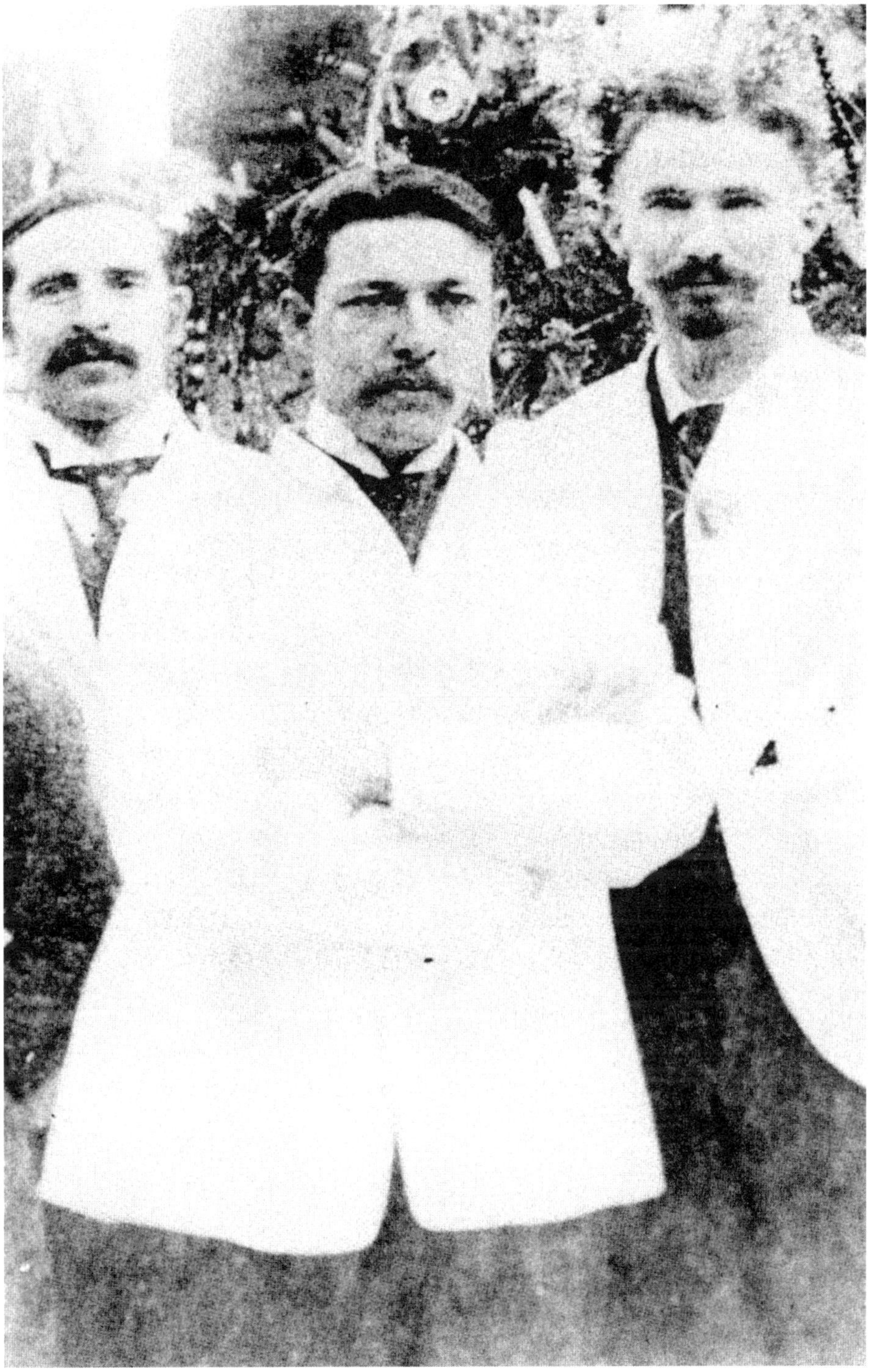

Fig. 1 William B. Coley, age 30 years, at a Christmas party in 1892 at the Hospital for the Ruptured and Crippled, seen with a house surgeon, C. A. Forgey, MD, on his left and an unidentified house surgeon on his right. (From Hospital for Special Surgery Archives)

From Saugatuck to New York

Born in the small village of Saugatuck, outside Westport on the Connecticut shoreline on the Long Island Sound on January 12, 1862, William B. Coley was the first surviving son of Horace Bradley Coley and Clarina Wakeman Coley. The family came from a long line of farmers, schoolmasters, and religious leaders from the west of England, dating back to the early part of the seventeenth century. The Civil War was entering its second year.

As a boy, Coley always wanted to go to Yale. When he was accepted in 1880, he was overjoyed, and he enrolled with a cousin. In those years, New Haven was a city of 78,000, with over 600 manufacturing companies.

Coley studied all the classics in a curriculum modeled after Oxford and Cambridge Universities. In his time away from the university, he either worked as a farm hand for neighboring farmers for $3.50 per day or for his father and grandfather for no pay.

Graduating from Yale College in 1884, he taught Latin and Greek in Oregon for 2 years (to be able to afford paying his college tuition) and then entered Harvard Medical School in 1886, graduating in 1888. During a previous summer, young Coley had visited some old Yale friends who were interning at New York Hospital. One of the resident physicians became sick, and Coley substituted for him for 5 weeks.

Coley then applied for an internship at New York Hospital, was accepted, and was appointed to the surgical services of Bull and Robert F. Weir, MD (1838–1927), another prominent surgeon at New York Hospital. The hospital had opened its doors in 1791 and became a major metropolitan hospital. In 1877, it had moved into a new building between West 15th and 16th Streets (Table 1).

In the early years of his professional practice, Coley divided his time between the New York Cancer Hospital on West 106th Street and R&C on 42nd Street and Lexington Avenue, probably a most formidable trip in those days. Coley was to relate in his later years, "I was favored by fortune in taking up the study of Medicine and Surgery at the most opportune time in a thousand years—that time when the old surgery, with high mortality from infection, was just beginning to be replaced by the new surgery, based on Lister's great discovery: antisepsis."[a]

Bull was a towering surgeon at the New York Hospital and an eminent surgeon in New York City, and his appointment at R&C in 1888 was very

Table 1 Timeline of Select Events at New York Hospital and Weill Cornell Medical Center

1771	King George III of England grants royal charter to the Society of the New York Hospital (current name)
1791	New York Hospital opens
1877	New York Hospital relocates between West 15th and 16th Streets
1898	Cornell University Medical College established
1913	New York Hospital and Cornell University Medical College affiliate
1927	New York Hospital–Cornell Medical Center agreement formed
1932	New York Hospital–Cornell Medical Center opens on East 68th Street
1951	The Hospital for Special Surgery (HSS) affiliates with New York Hospital–Cornell Medical Center
1955	HSS moves into a new building at 535 East 70th Street adjacent to New York Hospital
1979	Cornell University–New York Hospital School of Nursing closes
1997	New York Hospital merges with Presbyterian Hospital to form New York–Presbyterian Hospital
1998	Cornell University Medical College changes its name to Joan and Sanford I. Weill Medical College of Cornell University

important to Gibney, who needed guidance at the hospital during this new era of "aseptic" surgical principles. Bull was a perfect choice. He was appointed attending surgeon to a separate Hernia Department and reported only to Gibney as surgeon-in-chief.

In the nineteenth century, many adults and children became incapacitated by abdominal hernias, which had only been treated by braces and trusses, but Bull introduced modern surgery for the ruptured, and he and Coley eventually made the hospital the foremost hernia center in the country.

In 1889, Gibney reported to the Board of Managers: "The Hernia Department is no longer simply a dispensary. Dr. Bull has availed himself of the wards and our operating room to treat cases that need hospital care, so that your Hospital is now one for the ruptured and as well as the crippled."[2]

The earliest mention of surgery for hernias in children was reported by Bull and Coley in the *Annals of Surgery* in 1898, where they wrote that, in 1889 and 1890, 19 cases of hernia in children were operated on by the older method of Socin, Czerny, and Risel, and 50% relapsed during the first year.[3] So disappointing were the results that further hernia surgery was abandoned until the following year when Coley operated on a 15-year-old boy using the Bassini procedure (from Padua, Italy).

They then reported that the Bassini technique using kangaroo tendon produced excellent results in 400 procedures from 1895 to 1898. Of course, all operations were in children, as the hospital had no inpatient facilities for adults at that time. The report cited 34,271 cases of hernia treated at the R&C from 1890 to 1897. (The Hernia Department of R&C continued to be a major treatment center in the country until 1934, when it was renamed the Surgical Department by the fifth surgeon-in-chief, Philip D. Wilson, MD.)

A New Approach to Sarcoma

After treating one of his first patients, Elizabeth Dashiell (the story detailed in chapter 3), and with his professional future redefined, Coley immediately started investigating case histories of sarcoma at New York Hospital and in the private files of Bull and Weir.

Coley stumbled upon the case of a 29-year-old German immigrant, Fred Stein, who developed a growth on his face in front of his ear in 1880. This developed into an egg-sized mass, which eventually was excised at New York Hospital by Bull in 1883. In 1884, Bull operated twice more, but because of its large size, he could not obtain a primary closure. Pathological analysis revealed a round cell sarcoma. As a result of the ulcerated, open draining wound, a life-threatening infection—erysipelas (also known as "holy fire" and "St. Anthony's fire")—developed. (Erysipelas was first discovered in 1881 to be caused by *Streptococcus pyogenes*, or as it is better known today, "beta-hemolytic *Streptococcus* group A.") Bull deemed Stein to be "absolutely hopeless."

Over the next 5 months, however, the sarcomatous mass became smaller, until it finally disappeared. Stein was discharged in February 1885.[4]

It was exactly the type of case that Coley had been seeking. With much enthusiasm, energy, and perseverance, he began his hunt for Stein in the winter of 1891, searching for him in the tenements of the German section of the Lower East Side. For a number of weeks, Coley relentlessly canvassed the area, knocking on doors, and climbing stairs. Studying German at Yale probably made his search easier. No one knew if Stein was still in New York or if he had returned to Germany.

One day, Coley found his man. Face to face with a dark-haired man displaying the telltale scar below his ear, under a black beard, Stein was in good health, with no recurrence of his tumor. Coley brought Stein back to New York Hospital for Bull to examine. It had been 7 years since the patient had surgery for an "inoperable" and terminal malignancy, and he was now free of disease.

This was the beginning of William Coley's pursuit to find a cure for cancer, which one day would earn him the distinction to be remembered as the "father of cancer immunotherapy."

Coley searched the literature for cases of cancer regression and infection. As far back as 1725, Dedier, in Paris, noted that very few patients with syphilis developed malignant tumors.[4] He found other anecdotal reports, including the German physician Busch, who described a patient with erysipelas whose malignant tumor disappeared.[5]

Knowledge of immunology in 1890 was very scant. In about 1798, Edward Jenner, an English physician, noticed that milkmaids infected with the mild disease of cowpox never died from smallpox. He took the bold step of injecting several neighborhoods of children with the pus of a cowpox scab and then injecting them with live, lethal smallpox. The children survived any outbreaks of smallpox. This marked the beginning of the era of vaccination, although no one yet understood the mechanism.[6]

Mr. Zola

Coley speculated that if a *Streptococcus pyogenes*–producing infection could reverse cancer, then injections of this bacterium might be useful for treating other malignancies. In 1891, Coley asked Bull's permission to inject bacteria into patients with terminal cancer. Bull consented and referred to Coley a 35-year-old Italian immigrant drug addict named Mr. Zola, on whom he had operated twice for recurrent oral sarcoma. The man had only a few weeks to live.

Coley found Zola's throat blocked with tumor, rendering him unable to talk, eat, or drink. Emaciated and weak, Zola knew death was near.

Coley proposed a plan of injections of live *Streptococcus pyogenes* into the tumor, and with Bull's consent (as well as that of the patient, who was told of its experimental nature), Coley began his experimental series of injections. After 1 month, Zola's tumor shrank. After multiple injections over several months, the patient regained his health, with the tumor reduced in size. Zola lived in remission for another 8 years.[b]

By the end of 1892, Coley had treated a dozen patients with terminal cancer like Zola with injections. Yet two major problems remained: he was unable to predict whether a patient would develop erysipelas, and if so, he was unable to control the infection, and although some patients experienced tumor regression, two had died.

At age 22 years in 1884, Coley met 18-year-old Alice Lancaster at Miss Nott's Boarding School in New Haven. After an interrupted 7-year relationship, the two married, and they rented a walk-up apartment on East 33rd Street. In December 1892, Alice Coley gave birth to a boy, Bradley Lancaster Coley, and the couple moved to their first brownstone on East 35th Street.

Coley was rapidly becoming a well-known surgeon in New York, with a flourishing private practice and using new advances in cancer therapy. He had studied in only the best schools and hospitals in the country. Few physicians were even college graduates in those days, and it was not until 1901 that Harvard required a college degree to apply to its medical school.[7]

Coley was exposed to various life experiences in his worldly travels as a teacher in Oregon, a ship's surgeon in the Azores, and a lecturer in Europe. Besides a home in the city, he had a farm in Sharon, Connecticut, for many years, where he attempted to make a profitable business from farming. His medical writing included 19 papers published in international journals by 1896. He became a fellow of the American Surgical Association at age 36 years (the youngest ever elected) in 1897.

In 1908, Coley would be appointed the first surgeon of the New York Central Railroad. Financially, he would become very successful, reporting annual earnings of $33,000 in 1902.[c]

Coley's Toxins

Having become familiar with the work of Roux and Yersin at the Pasteur Institute in Paris, Coley concluded that it was not the living organism of *Streptococcus pyogenes*, but rather the secreted toxins that were destroying the tumors. If he could extract the toxins, he could apply them like a vaccine and attack the tumors. He learned of further work at the institute showing that certain bacteria could be enhanced with another harmless bacterium, *Bacillus prodigiosus* (*Serratia marcescens*).

With the help of a former classmate, Alexander Lambert, he created a mixture of one part *Serratia marcescens* and five parts *Streptococcus pyogenes.* The unique combination would become known as Coley's mixed toxins.

The first patient in whom he assessed this combination was a 16-year-old boy with an inoperable abdominal and pelvic sarcoma. In January 1893, he started giving injections of his mixed toxins to his teenage patient, gradually increasing the dosages. The boy responded with shaking chills, fever, local inflammation, and malaise—the classic symptoms of erysipelas. The tumor regressed; by May 1893, it had disappeared and the patient was discharged. The patient had no further evidence of disease and died 26 years later in 1919 of a heart attack.

In the next year, between this patient and 34 other patients treated with Coley's Toxins, there were 25 inoperable sarcomas. Nine showed marked improvement, eight had slight improvement, and six were declared cured. Of nine cases of carcinoma, there were less gratifying results—improvements, but no cures.

The New York Cancer Hospital

A place to carry out his investigations came in 1892, when Bull appointed Coley to the staff of the New York Cancer Hospital, which had opened 5 years earlier. Located at 106th Street and Central Park West, the hospital was the second in the world dedicated to cancer treatment. At that time, with little to offer in terms of effective therapy, cancer was a dreaded disease and was shunned by hospitals and particularly by the upper class. The Board of the New York Cancer Hospital had many wealthy New Yorkers, among whom was William Astor. He promoted changing the name in 1898 to the General Memorial Hospital, erasing the word "cancer" from the institution's name.[d]

Coley continued his friendship with John D. Rockefeller Jr., which dated back to the Bessie Dashiell event and also to his father, John D. Rockefeller, but his major source of funding would come through his introduction to the Huntington fortune. Arranged by Dr. John Walker at R&C, Coley met Archer Huntington. He soon became medical advisor, benefactor, and friend to

Archer's mother, Arabella. In 1901, Coley arranged for Arabella Huntington to make a gift of $100,000[e] to Memorial Hospital to establish the Collis P. Huntington Fund for Cancer Research. He reached out to new social contacts and eventually belonged to some 25 clubs in New York.

Coley now had a hospital to support his research work in developing what was to become a vaccine for the treatment of sarcoma. He befriended many of the wealthy families associated with the hospital, engineered significant financial support and received patient referrals from all over the world.

A Bumpy Road

In 1894, the Loomis Laboratory modified the method to produce killed bacteria, and this combination was used for the next 12 years. Beginning in 1899, Parke Davis & Company began producing Coley's Toxins for the next 30 years.

Coley's use of toxins for cancer treatment was heralded by many, particularly in Europe. There were opponents to his work, however, on the basis of inconsistencies in vaccine composition, the methods of administration, and varied results obtained by physicians throughout the world. Among them was his one-time close friend, James Ewing, MD (1866–1943), who would become the first professor of clinical pathology at Cornell Medical School in 1899. There was no doubt that Ewing was one of the most respected cancer investigators in the twentieth century, a man referred to in the newspapers as the "dean of American cancer authorities." Early in their careers, the Coley-Ewing relationship was one of respect and admiration. It later turned sour, however, with Ewing undermining Coley's work.

In the years to follow, the evolution of cancer therapy would progress through different pathways. Ewing became friendly with mining tycoon James Douglas, PhD (1837–1918), whose daughter, Naomi, was diagnosed with breast cancer in 1907. Douglas sought the help of Ewing, and Ewing accompanied Douglas and his daughter to London for treatment with the very rare radioactive element radium. As head of the Arizona mining company Phelps-Dodge, Douglas donated $100,000 to Memorial Hospital in 1912 with an additional pledge, bringing the total to $500,000.[6]

In 1913, Douglas and Ewing formed the National Radium Institute to extract radium from ore in Colorado. That same year, Ewing was named president of the Medical Board of Memorial Hospital, and in 1915, he instituted a policy that all ward cancer patients must be treated with radiation—a devastating blow to Coley. Toxins could still be used for private patients with cancer, however.[7]

Joining Ewing in his campaign opposing toxin treatment were Ernest A. Codman, MD (1869–1940), a Boston cancer specialist who founded the Bone Sarcoma Registry in 1920, and Joseph Colt Bloodgood, MD (1867–1935), a renowned cancer surgeon and adjunct clinical professor of surgery at Johns Hopkins Medical School. Despite the campaign against Coley, Coley's Toxins continued to be used extensively at Massachusetts General Hospital and the Mayo Clinic. The Mayo Clinic refused to contribute to Codman's registry, and Charles Mayo, MD (1865–1939), and his brother remained staunch Coley supporters.

Helen Coley Nauts

On September 2, 1907, Alice Coley gave birth to Helen Lancaster Coley in Sharon. Although she would have no medical training, Helen Coley in her later life became a major figure in her father's legacy of Coley's Toxins (Fig. 2). She married a banker, William Nauts, and they raised two children. At age 29 years in 1936, after her father's death, she began organizing and researching over 800 of Coley's medical records and case histories that were stacked away in their Connecticut barn.

In 1941, she contacted Cornelius P. "Dusty" Rhoads, MD (1898–1959), medical director of Memorial Hospital, for his advice in reviving interest in Coley's Toxins. Rhoads suggested she review 100 of his cases. Subsequently, she reviewed over 800 microscopically proven cases, but this was not enough to convince Rhoads. Little did she know that he, too, was a strong opponent of her father's toxins. He wrote a letter to John D. Rockefeller Jr. recommending that Rockefeller not support Coley.[8,h]

Her energy, perseverance, and knowledge, plus a grant of $2,000 from Nelson Rockefeller in 1953, led her to found—with her friend Oliver R. Grace (1909–1992)—the Cancer Research Institute in New York. Still going strong in 2011, over $14 million had been raised to support research in cancer immunotherapy the prior year. The annual William B. Coley Award for Distinguished

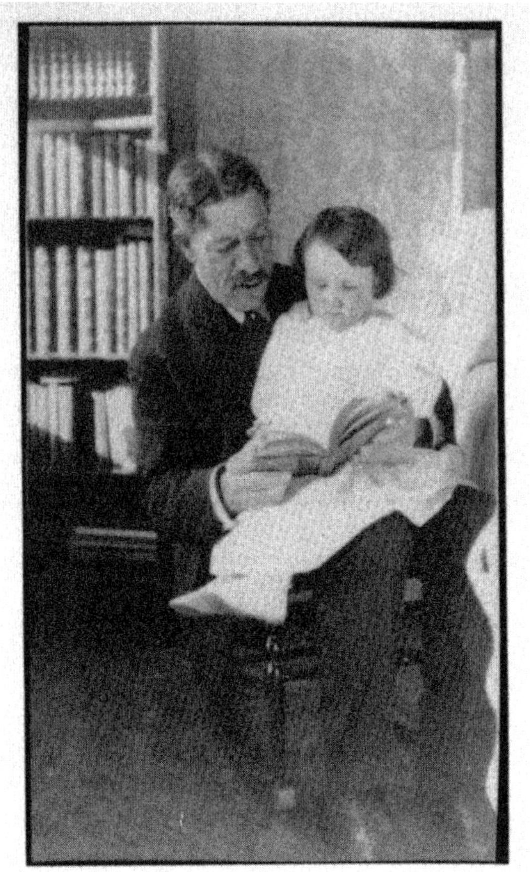

Fig. 2 Coley always made time for his family and is seen here reading a book to his daughter, Helen, circa 1910. (From Cancer Research Institute)

Research in Basic and Tumor Immunology (established in 1975) is presented yearly at the annual benefit. The institute, with its national headquarters in New York City, is a global leader in the advancement of immunology in general and cancer immunology in particular.

In 2010, two immunotherapies—a therapeutic vaccine for advanced prostate cancer and a monoclonal antibody for metastatic melanoma—were approved by the U.S. Food and Drug Administration for the first time.

Helen Coley Nauts died in 2000 at age 93 years, but her crusade to convince the medical establishment of the significance of her father's lifelong research in promoting cancer immunotherapy is going stronger than ever today.[i]

1925—The Roaring Twenties

When William Coley became surgeon-in-chief in 1925, the country was in its fifth year of Prohibition (1920–1933); organized crime was rampant, and social changes following World War I had exploded in the worlds of fashion, music, and literature. Jimmy Walker (1881–1946), known as "Beau James," was elected to his first term as mayor of New York. The flamboyant politician, friend of the stars and of the sports world, boasted a style that was synonymous with the Jazz Age.

This popular music, with roots in early Afro-American spirituals and New Orleans Dixieland, was coined in Chicago and moved to New York, concentrating in Harlem. Variations of this improvisational skill included introduction of the stride piano, popularized by the famous "Fats" Waller. During Mayor Walker's second term, an investigation in 1933 into possible bribes and corruption led him to resign from office. However, he was credited with establishing the first Department of Hospitals in the city and saving the 5-cent subway fare.

Prosperity was at every door—or if it was not, at least it was next door. After Woodrow Wilson's administration (1913–1921) dealing with World War I, the country was ready to return to normalcy. The next three presidents—Warren G. Harding (1921–1923), Calvin Coolidge (1923–1929), and Herbert Hoover (1929–1933), all Republicans—joined in a pursuit of financial wealth. They cut taxes for the wealthy, increased tariffs, and reduced interest rates. Harding died in office of a heart attack in 1923 and was succeeded by his vice president, Coolidge.

In March 1925, the country for the first time listened to their new president, Calvin Coolidge, take the oath of office on the radio. Broadcasting was at the pinnacle of its "golden age." It was first installed in the White House in 1922 by President Harding. The movie industry was among the top five industries in the country. Americans idolized their stars Rudolph Valentino and Charlie Chaplin and were overjoyed when talking movies began in 1927 with *The Jazz Singer*.

The New Surgeon-in-Chief

Luckily for Coley, in his first years as surgeon-in-chief, the era of the Roaring Twenties did not spill over into the hospital routine. The hospital administrator,

Joseph Flick, now in his eighth year, relieved a great deal of burden from the surgeon-in-chief's administrative duties—a welcome change from the time Gibney had assumed that office. Flick was a very able organizer, very congenial with the professional staff, and well liked by everyone.

In January 1926, in his first annual report as surgeon-in-chief to the Board of Managers, Coley cited a total of 3,143 operations performed during the year: 1,328 in the Orthopaedic Department, 817 in the Hernia Department, and 998 in the Private Pavilion. A new monthly staff conference was instituted, where the work done in the previous months was critically reviewed.[9]

Coley was very much aware of the need for physical and occupational therapy, an unusual appreciation for a surgeon. He worked closely with the Nursing Department under Ethel B. Ridley, RN, Directress of Nursing (1924–1942), and appointed the first graduate nurses to administer anesthesia in his first year.

Although there had been x-ray machines at the hospital for 27 years, the X-Ray Department was at first considered a technical specialty. In 1926, Raymond Lewis, MD, was appointed roentgenologist at R&C, and the specialty received departmental status.[10]

In 1928, Coley instituted the first hospital therapeutic pool in the city and persuaded the board to install a glass-covered solarium on the roof (Table 2).

He appreciated the need for a good records department, and the hospital records over the years were unusual, as all notes were typed. (It is well known that physicians' handwriting is invariably difficult to decipher. In the late 1970s, there was an attempt to abolish typing of HSS hospital records to reduce costs; luckily, this was overruled.)

In 1929, Coley established the first true Pathology Department and appointed John McWhorter, MD (1867–1936), as director and pathologist. McWhorter was an experienced pathologist who trained in the Surgical-Pathological Laboratory of the College of Physicians and Surgeons and who held important staff appointments at the French Hospital and Bellevue Hospital. In addition, Coley appointed his professional adversary, Ewing, as consulting pathologist in 1927.

Although Coley was the first nonorthopaedic surgeon to lead the hospital, he was very interested in advancing education, research, and treatment related to orthopaedic conditions. The records showed an increased number

Table 2 Significant Events at R&C Circa 1925

1923—First Medical Board established
1923—A private patients' pavilion opened, later in 1931, named in honor of Virgil Gibney
1924—The first Arthritis Clinic opened, with R. Garfield Snyder, MD, appointed its chief
1924—First Department of Physiotherapy opened, headed by Kristian G. Hansson, MD, a 1923 graduate of Cornell Medical College
1925—First graduate nurses at R&C appointed to administer anesthesia
1925—Occupational Therapy Department founded
1925—William Church Osborn resigns from as president of the Board of Managers, only to return to that position in 1928
1926—Alker Memorial Library founded by Mrs. Henry A. Alker, in memory of his mother and combined with the Arents Library for Children (founded 1905), both dedicated to servicing patients. The Library Committee was chaired by Helen Coley, William B. Coley's daughter.
1927—Fenwick Beekman, MD, appointed as associate surgeon to the Hernia Department and becomes first chair of HSS Library Committee in 1935
1928—Glass-covered solarium built on the roof
1928—First therapeutic pool opened in a New York hospital
1929—Hospital laboratory established with John McWhorter, MD, appointed director and pathologist
1929—An ambulance service was inaugurated in conjunction with the Department of Hospitals
1929—Royal Whitman, MD, resigns, later retiring to England

of patients with bone malignancies treated at R&C—not only by him, but by many others on staff during the late 1920s.

There were now three Orthopaedic Divisions working independently of each other, with each attending surgeon in charge of his own division. Royal Whitman headed the First Orthopaedic Division. Percy W. Roberts, MD (1867–1937), was the attending surgeon of Division Two. Charlton Wallace, MD (1872–1947), who had been professor of orthopaedic surgery at Cornell Medical College, was the attending surgeon of Division Three. The First Hernia Division was directed by Coley, and the Second Division by Joseph P. Hoguet, MD (1882–1946), who later lost one of his arms in a severe automobile accident.

Over the years, many other prominent orthopaedic surgeons on staff published new techniques for treatments in their subspecialties, including

Samuel Kleinberg, MD—scoliosis
Arthur Krida, MD—congenital dislocation of the hip
Paul Colonna, MD—hip reconstruction
Toufick Nicola, MD—recurrent dislocation of the shoulder
Lewis Clark Wagner, MD—paralytic drop foot

Coley's Health

In 1923, Coley had suffered two attacks of duodenal bleeding from ulcers. Ten years prior, he had learned that he was probably suffering from acromegaly (Fig. 3). Realizing the consequences of such a progressive condition originating from a pituitary tumor, he became very concerned that his life as a surgeon might become compromised in later years. He reappraised his financial status and began to reduce expenses in his real estate holdings and lifestyle.

In 1927, at age 65 years, his energy level was high—compromised only by repeated attacks of duodenal bleeding. Yet his acromegaly did not affect him, other than resulting in enlarging anatomy—such as his glove size increasing two sizes and an increasing head circumference, as well as diminished hearing.

By 1931, pyloric stenosis, resulting from his duodenal disease, caused him to undergo bypass surgery at New York Hospital. He recovered without complications at his home in Sharon. His political problems at Memorial Hospital added more stress to his life, as did financial pressures. His son Bradley L. Coley, MD, was appointed to the First Hernia Division in 1927 and was able to assist his father in surgery in later years.

On January 1, 1933, William Coley tendered his resignation at Memorial Hospital as chief of the Bone Tumor Service, and on February 1, he resigned as surgeon-in-chief of R&C. He continued to have admitting privileges at both hospitals where he operated. Bradley Coley was appointed successor to his father as chief of the Bone Tumor Service at Memorial Hospital (Fig. 4).

Memorial's Medical Board paid tribute to Coley by having a testimonial dinner at the Waldorf-Astoria Hotel for 350 people on January 12, 1933, Coley's 75th birthday. Speakers included Coley's friend Charles Mayo, MD, and Coley's adversary, Ewing.

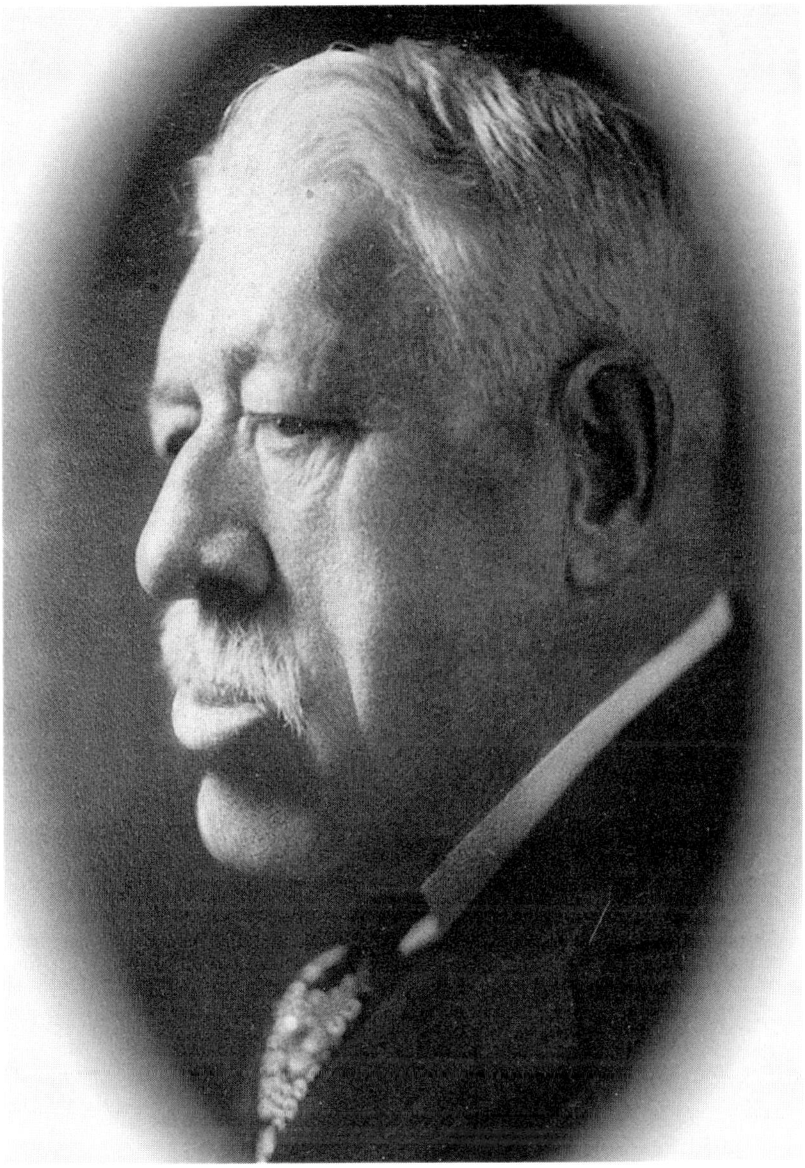

Fig. 3 William B. Coley in his later years showed typical enlarged facial features characteristic of acromegaly. (From Hospital for Special Surgery Archives)

What would probably be his most prestigious honor came in October 1935. At the Royal College of Surgeons of England, Coley reported a large number of patients with inoperable malignant tumors who had been treated with his toxins and survived 5 years or more. He was inducted as an honorary fellow, the fifth American so honored in that distinguished society.

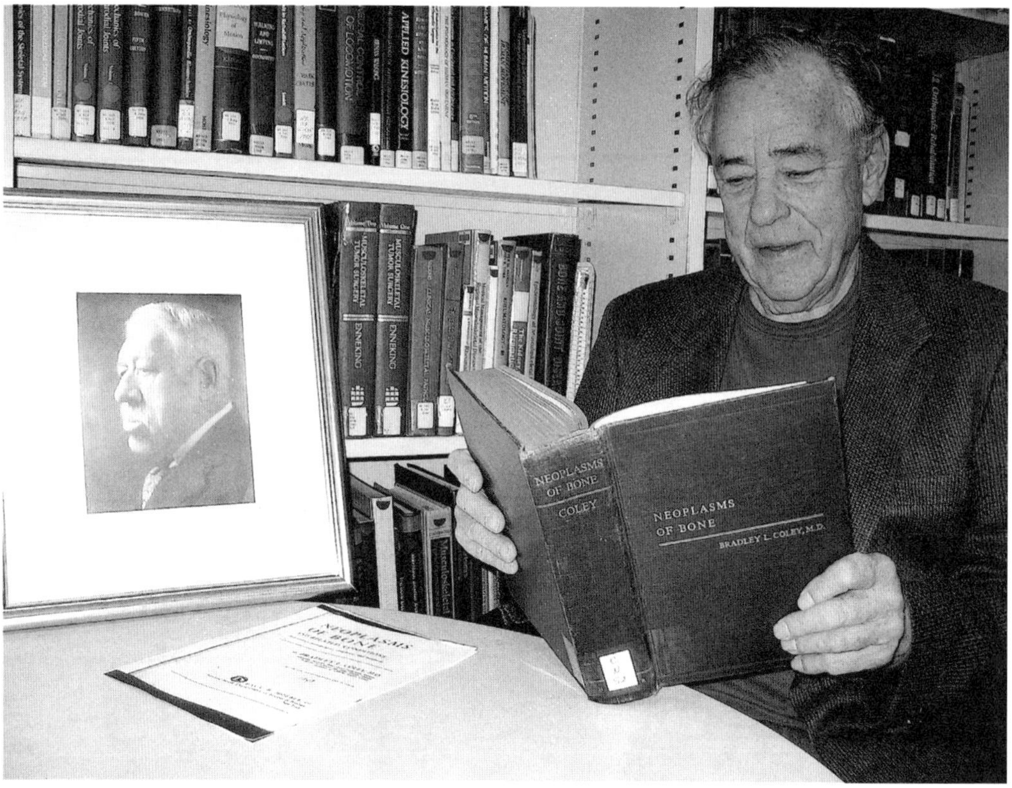

Fig. 4 Bradley L. "Pete" Coley Jr. sitting in the Hospital for Special Surgery Kim Barrett Memorial Library in 2009, reviewing his father Bradley L. Coley's book *Neoplasms of Bone*. Next to him is a framed photograph of his grandfather, William Bradley Coley.[j] (From Hospital for Special Surgery Archives)

In 1933, the Board of Managers appointed Eugene Hillhouse Pool, MD (1874–1949), as the fourth surgeon-in-chief at R&C. Pool—director of one of two surgical services at the New York Hospital, president of the New York Academy of Medicine, and president-elect of the American College of Surgeons—had been an associate of William Bull.

On April 15, 1936, William Coley suffered a recurrent attack of diverticulitis. He was operated on by Pool at R&C, but he died the next day. Seven months later, his widow, Alice Coley, who had been fighting cancer for many years, died in Sharon, where she was buried next to her beloved husband.

Working on a textbook at the time of his death, Coley published 143 papers or monographs between 1893 and 1936.

REFERENCES

1. Anonymous. News Notes, Virgil Pendleton Gibney. *J Bone Joint Surg Am.* 1927;9:781.
2. Gibney VP. *Twenty-Sixth Annual Report of the New York Society for the Relief of the Ruptured and Crippled.* New York, NY: New York Society for the Relief of the Ruptured and Crippled; 1889.
3. Bull WT, Coley WB. Observations upon the operative treatment of hernia at the Hospital for the Ruptured and Crippled. *Ann Surg.* 1898;28:577–604.
4. Dedier A. Dissertation Medicinal et Chirurgical sur les Tumeurs. Paris. 1725.
5. Busch W. Aus der Sitzung der medicinischen. *Berl Klin Wochenschr.* 1868;5:137.
6. Hall SS. *A Commotion in the Blood: Life, Death, and the Immune System.* New York, NY: Henry Holt & Co.; 1982.
7. Starr P Jr. *The Social Transformation of American Medicine.* New York, NY: Basic Books; 1982.
8. Nauts Coley H. An Honored Place in History. Unpublished manuscript. New York, NY; 1966.
9. Coley WB. *Sixty-Second Annual Report of the New York Society for the Relief of the Ruptured and Crippled.* New York, NY: New York Society for the Relief of the Ruptured and Crippled; 1925.
10. Beekman F. *Hospital for the Ruptured and Crippled. A historical sketch written on the occasion of the seventy-fifth anniversary of the hospital.* New York, NY: Statistical Press; 1939.

NOTES

a. Joseph Lister's first published work on antiseptic surgery in 1867 did not gain favor in the surgical world until about 1880. His antiseptic principles employed the use of carbolic acid to kill microorganisms; later, aseptic techniques included sterile methods to prevent infections.

b. Because of how seriously contagious the injections could be, all of the treatments were done outside of New York Hospital in Zola's home on the Lower East Side.

c. About $845,000 in 2011 dollars.

d. In 1916, the hospital's name was changed to Memorial Hospital. John D. Rockefeller Jr. donated land on York Avenue and $1 million for the relocation of the hospital beginning in 1936. The adjacent Sloan-Kettering Institute, established by Alfred P. Sloan and Charles F. Kettering, both of General Motors, was dedicated in 1948. In 1980, the two hospitals merged to become Memorial Sloan-Kettering Cancer Center (MSKCC).

e. About $2.6 million in 2011 dollars.

f About $11 million in 2011 dollars.

g. It was not known at that time of the potential deadly effects of the misuse and exposure to radium and radiation. Douglas used radium recreationally and drank so-called radium water as an elixir. He died in 1918 of probable radium poisoning. Other popular radium products of the 1920s were "Beanie Babies"—clocks and wristwatches with glow-in-the-dark dials. The timepiece industry employed over 4,000 women to paint these dials—licking their radium-contaminated brushes up to a 1,000 times a day.

h. Cornelius P. "Dusty" Rhoads, MD, who during World War II headed the medical division of the Army's Chemical Warfare Service, became medical director of Memorial Hospital in 1939. The next advance in the development of cancer treatment was the arrival of chemotherapy derived from the chemical poison mustard gas of World War I, which progressed to the nitrogen mustard of World War II. Rhoads, an avid opponent of Coley's Toxins, was labeled by historians as a leading "evangelist" promoting chemotherapy. In 1950, Rhoads wrote to Park Davis Pharmaceuticals suggesting that they discontinue the manufacture of Coley's Toxins because Memorial would make them. When Memorial ceased to make them, they were no longer made in the United States.

i. The final blow came in 1963. The U.S. Food and Drug Administration (FDA), given enhanced power and faced with the thalidomide scandal—a sedative causing birth defects in babies born to European women who took the drug during pregnancy—refused to "grandfather" Coley's Toxins without extensive clinical trials. The toxins were banned from manufacturing or use in the United States. Today, they are still manufactured in Canada, and clinical trials continue in other countries.

j. Bradley L. Coley Jr., grandson of William Bradley Coley, was kind enough to provide a copy of his aunt Helen Coley Nauts' 365-page unpublished manuscript, An Honored Place in History. It is a detailed story of her father's life and his pursuit of a vaccine for sarcoma. Nauts began a mission to carry on her father's crusade to treat cancer with vaccines. Reviewing 15,000 of her father's patient records, she eventually investigated over 800 case histories. In 1952, she founded the New York Cancer Research Institute (currently Cancer Research Institute) and worked relentlessly on her project until she died on December 2, 2000. Among her awards were the Commandeur de l'Ordre National du Mérite by French President Valery Giscard d'Estaing in 1981 for her "outstanding contributions to scientific research" and the 1997 National Institute of Social Sciences Gold Medal for Distinguished Service to Humanity, which has not been given to any other woman in science and medicine since Marie Curie.

CHAPTER 7
EUGENE H. POOL, MD
FOURTH SURGEON-IN-CHIEF
(1933–1939)
PHILIP D. WILSON, MD
FIFTH SURGEON-IN-CHIEF

DAVID B. LEVINE, MD

IN 1933, FOR THE SECOND time in the 70-year history of the Hospital for the Ruptured and Crippled (R&C), a general surgeon became surgeon-in-chief. Eugene Hillhouse Pool, MD, was appointed the fourth surgeon-in-chief by the Board of Managers of the New York Society for the Relief of the Ruptured and Crippled. A nationally known surgeon, Pool was director of the Second Surgical Service of New York Hospital and professor of surgery at Cornell University Medical College.

As the oldest orthopaedic hospital in the country, R&C's reputation as a leading institution in the field was further enhanced by the introduction of surgery in 1888 by Gibney and by the staff appointment of Royal Whitman. Despite this leadership, the reputation of the hospital started to show signs of decline in the first quarter of the twentieth century. As surgical techniques for treating hernias advanced significantly, the historical relationship between the treatment of rupture and crippling conditions deteriorated—even though the brace-maker continued to provide a common bridge for both conditions.

Support by the hospital's professional staff ebbed as the country faced the looming financial crisis. In 1929, a further blow to the hospital's status occurred when Whitman resigned at age 72 years. William Coley, not being an orthopaedic surgeon, added to the hospital's declining reputation in the orthopaedic world.[1]

With Coley's resignation in 1933, the Board of Managers realized the urgency of temporarily appointing a prominent surgeon from the academic community to the office of surgeon-in-chief to reestablish R&C as a leader in orthopaedics. The board persuaded Pool to accept this position on an interim basis.

For his first year in office, Pool critically observed the state of the hospital, its staff, its treatment of patients, teaching, education, and research, and he formulated a plan for improvement.

At the end of his first year in office, Pool reported the following to the Board of Managers:

> Since receiving the honor of being appointed Surgeon-in-Chief…I have been an observer rather than a worker, and have studied basic problems rather than details. In this connection, one is impressed by the extremely doubtful nature which a private, unattached hospital faces. Medicine and surgery have progressed so much during the three decades of the present century that the purely clinical institution finds itself handicapped in comparison with teaching and scientific centers as a result of lack of stimulus of scientific thought and the lack of laboratory facilities. The solution is an allegiance or affiliation with a university whereby the clinical workers may have access to the use of the laboratory facilities of a more highly developed institution and contacts with and the advice of the highly trained minds. Such an affiliation for the Hospital for Ruptured and Crippled is much to be desired.
>
> The Hospital for Ruptured and Crippled was in its early days the leading orthopaedic center of the country. It has not retained this position. We should therefore plan to regain it. If the institution is to develop on the lines suggested, a conspicuous leader should be chosen and placed in charge of the activities of the institution and all efforts should be centered upon the development of orthopaedic surgery and regaining the position of the institution, which it held under those great leaders Gibney, Bull, Whitman, and Coley.
>
> The interests of the institution are superior to those of the individual, and every one should feel that any sacrifice should be made to further its interests.
>
> He concluded, "The main weakness seemed to be a considerable number of attending surgeons, none of whom devoted a large part of their time to the Institution, with the result that there was no head, and little research work and teaching".[2]

The board received this report on February 8, 1934, and immediately took action to seek the best possible orthopaedic surgeon to fill this office.

The Education of Eugene Pool, MD

Eugene H. Pool was born June 3, 1874, in New York City. He graduated from St. Paul's School in Concord, New Hampshire, and received an AB from Harvard College in 1895. Awarded his MD degree in 1899 from the College of Physicians and Surgeons of Columbia University, Pool pursued a surgical internship at New York Hospital from 1900 to 1901.

He was greatly influenced by his mentor, Dr. William Bull, who later invited him to join his practice. Pool maintained a close association in practice with Bull for 7 years while rising through the ranks of the faculty of the College of Physicians and Surgeons, finally becoming professor of clinical surgery in 1915. Likewise, he maintained staff appointments at New York Hospital, becoming attending surgeon in 1932 when New York Hospital moved to the Upper East Side to become New York Hospital-Cornell Medical Center. Finally appointed clinical professor of Surgery at Cornell University Medical College, he ranked as a senior attending surgeon on the New York Hospital staff.

Pool assumed the position of chief of the Second Surgical Division of New York Hospital, and under his command, that department became one of the greatest surgical services in the country. His skills were taught, copied, and admired throughout the surgical world, and he encouraged his students to pursue research projects and further their education.

World War I

Many R&C surgeons were drawn into service during World War I. Pool served with distinction in France with Base Hospital No. 9 (New York Hospital Unit) located in Bitray, about 2 miles from Châteauroux (Fig. 1). The organization making up this hospital was mobilized in July 1917 on Governor's Island and Ellis Island in New York. It included, in part, 27 officers, 64 nurses, and 150 enlisted men.[3] In 1918, the hospital was converted to an orthopaedic hospital, and a staff of orthopaedic surgeons was selected under the direction of Lt. Col. Joel Goldthwait. Richmond Stephens, MD, of R&C headed one section.

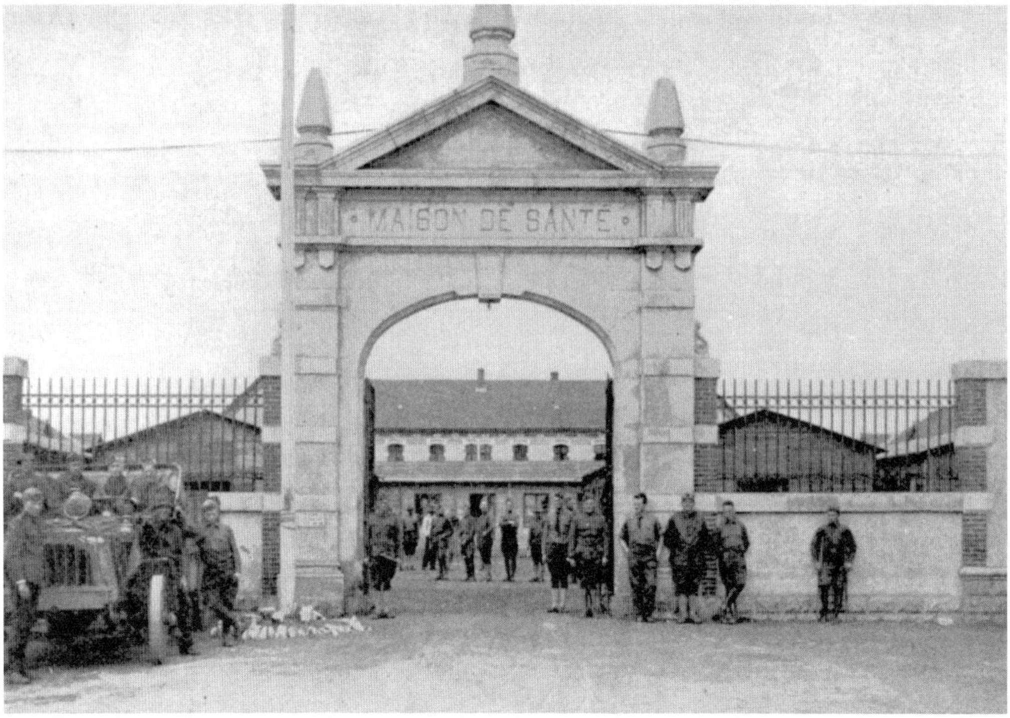

Fig. 1 Base Hospital No. 9 in Bitray, France, was located in a building originally built as an insane asylum. In 1917, it was used first as a general hospital, but in the spring of 1918, it became the Orthopaedic Centre of the American Expeditionary Forces.[3]

Pool was eventually appointed consulting surgeon to the First Army. Although a general surgeon, his wartime exposure to trauma, the treatment of joint injuries, and the principles of wound treatment allowed him to publish a number of articles in these fields. These experiences were particularly helpful in later years, when he assumed the leadership of R&C.

Discharged on January 30, 1919, with the rank of lieutenant colonel, Pool was awarded not only the Legion d'Honneur and the Distinguished Service Medal but also received a citation for meritorious services by the commander-in-chief, General John J. Pershing[a] (Fig. 2).

First Report to Board

In February 1934, Pool as surgeon-in-chief gave his first report for the year 1933 to the Board of Managers of the New York Society for the Ruptured and Crippled. The message had set clear goals to find the best orthopaedic

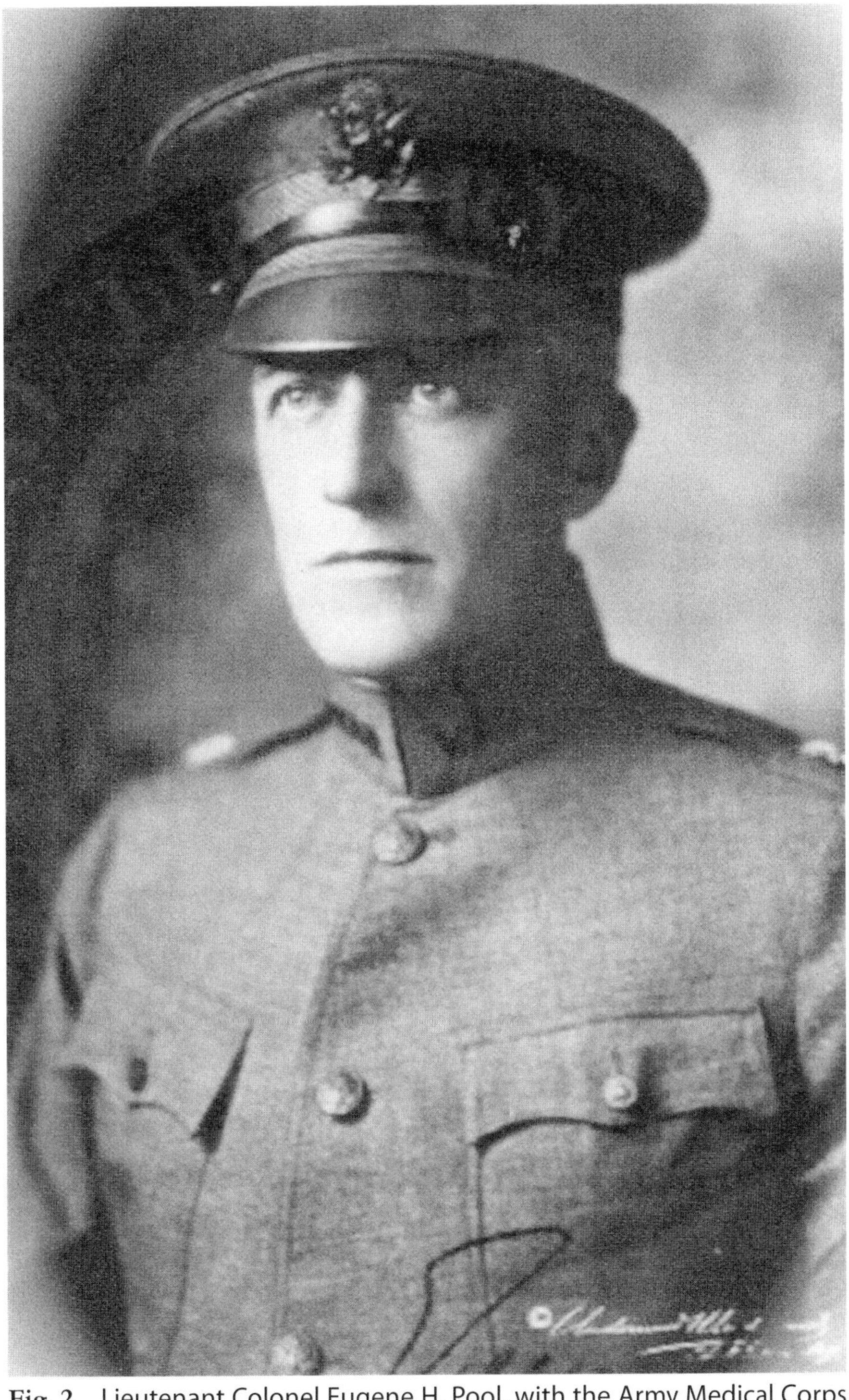

Fig. 2 Lieutenant Colonel Eugene H. Pool, with the Army Medical Corps in World War I, served during the St. Mihiel and Meuse-Argonne offenses in France. (Courtesy of the National Library of Medicine)

surgeon for the office of surgeon-in-chief, affiliate with a university, and expand the laboratories, research, and educational facilities. Additionally, it was vital to promote the interests of the hospital rather than emphasize an individual practitioner—a concept that has continued to challenge the academic medical world in present times.[2]

How could a reasonable financial arrangement be reached between an individual physician/surgeon and a hospital where such a close symbiotic relationship was advantageous? In the 1930s, most physicians and surgeons practiced independently, trying to make a living at the time of the Great Depression without concern for the health of their hospitals. It was key that both the individual physician and the institution needed to be successful, as well as remain players on the same team. Hospital for Special Surgery has attained that goal, being named number one in orthopaedics in the United States in 2012.[4] The formula may be very complex and difficult to achieve, but the end results

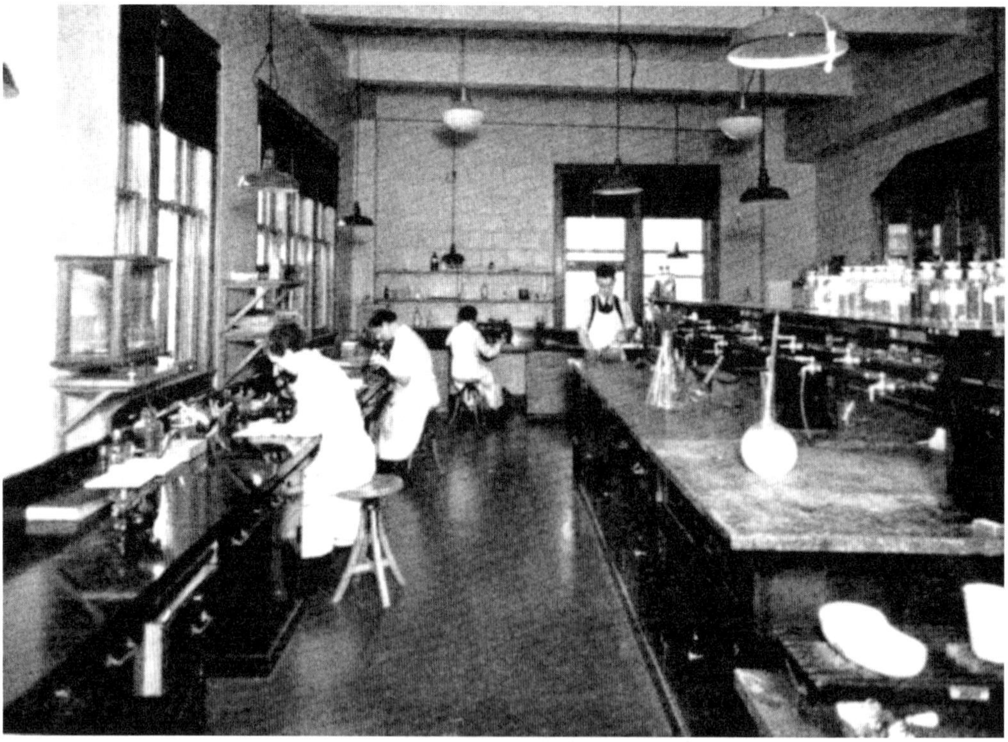

Fig. 3 A floor was added in 1934 to the East Wing of Hospital for the Ruptured and Crippled, featuring routine clinical and pathological laboratories and three laboratories for research. (From Hospital for Special Surgery Archives)

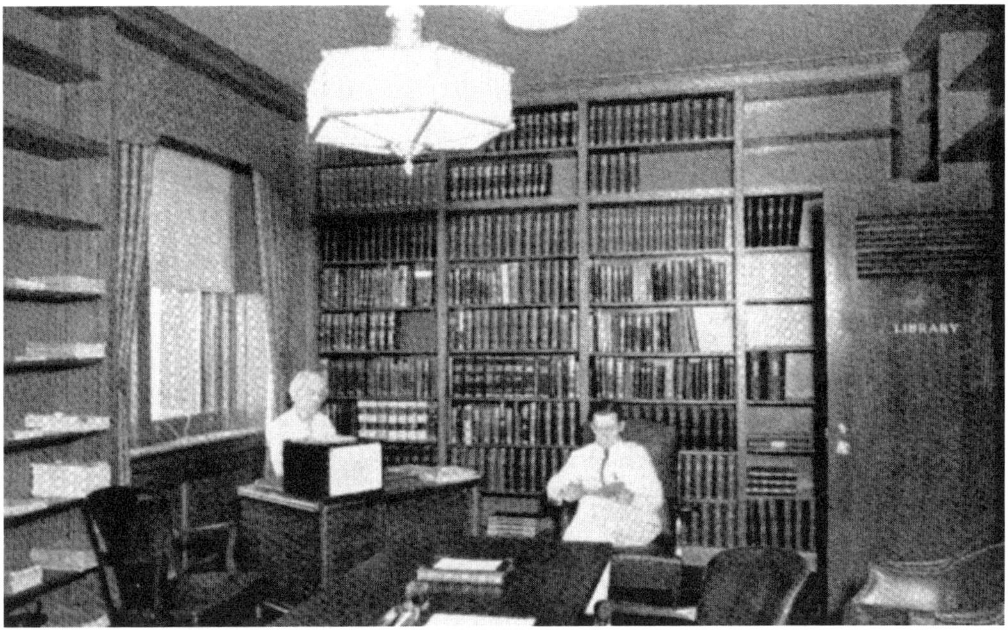

Fig. 4 Philip Wilson stressed the importance of a medical library and supervised and planned the building of a dedicated library in 1935 to house books and journals. The staff was financially supportive, which provided the library with a good foundation. (From Hospital for Special Surgery Archives)

need to be a mutual respect and mutual compensation benefiting both parties. Academic institutions and staff today continue to try to formulate this winning combination.

Pool's search ended with the appointment of Philip D. Wilson, MD, of Boston, a nationally known leader in orthopaedics, to fill the office of surgeon-in-chief. At age 48 years, Wilson resigned as chief of the Fracture Service at Massachusetts General Hospital (MGH) and from the faculty of Harvard Medical College. He became a staff member of R&C in May 1934 as director of orthopaedic surgery, while Pool retained the title of surgeon-in-chief. An affiliation was made with the College of Physicians and Surgeons of Columbia University, and Wilson received a university appointment as clinical professor of orthopaedic surgery.

On February 14, 1935, in the 72nd Annual Report of R&C, Pool gave his second and final report as surgeon-in-chief.[5] Wilson was to join the staff in 3 months. Two floors were added to expand the laboratories (Fig. 3), and a new X-Ray Department had been installed. A medical library was established with a secretary (Fig. 4).

Pool Resigns

With the appointment of Wilson as the fifth surgeon-in-chief at the R&C in 1935, Pool resigned from that office and was given the title of senior consulting surgeon and surgeon-in-chief emeritus (Fig. 5). Maintaining his private practice and staff privileges at New York Hospital and a number of other hospitals, he continued to attain many high honors in professional societies (Table 1).

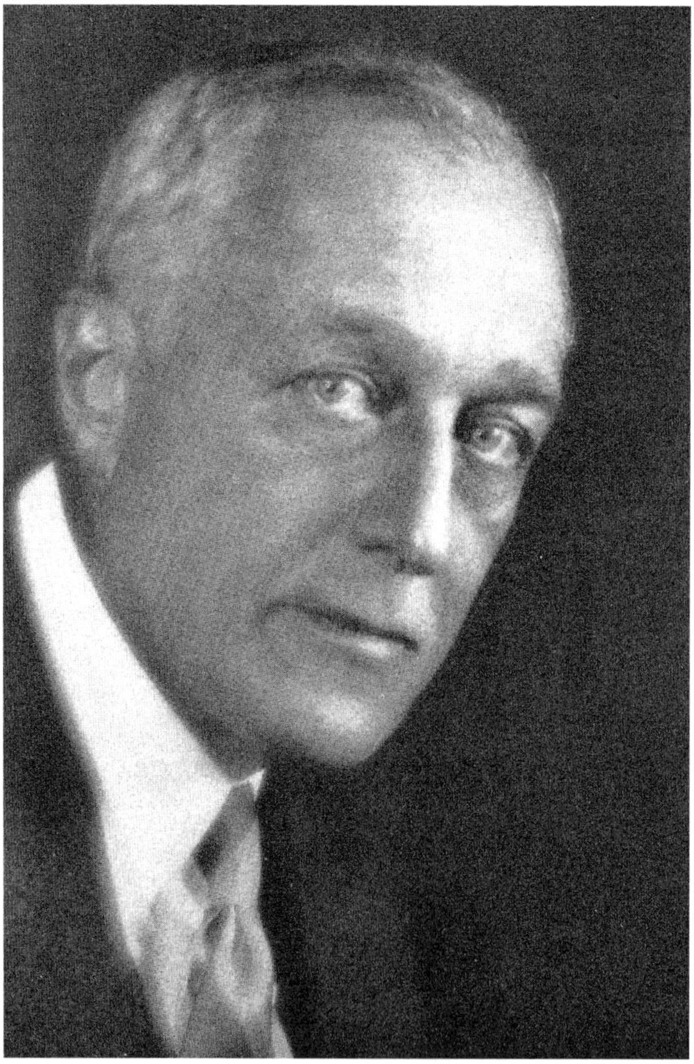

Fig. 5 Eugene Hillhouse Pool, when he served as surgeon-in-chief at the Hospital for the Ruptured and Crippled. (Courtesy of Medical Center Archives of New York–Presbyterian Hospital/Weill Cornell Medical Center)

Table 1 The Honors of Eugene Pool, MD

New York Surgical Society—president, 1923–1925
Society of Clinical Surgery—president, 1927–1929
New York Academy of Medicine—president, 1935–1936
American Surgical Association—president, 1936

S. S. Goldwater, MD, New York City Commissioner of Hospitals, appointed Pool as administrative consultant in surgery for the city hospitals in 1934. In 1935, New York Governor Herbert Lehman appointed Pool as chairman of the committee to rewrite the medical provisions of the Workmen's Compensation Act. This committee was created due to widespread abuses in this field, which were uncovered during the administration of the previous governor, Franklin D. Roosevelt. The committee completely rewrote all the provisions of the Workmen's Compensation Act, which were incorporated entirely in a bill presented by Governor Lehman to the State Legislature and passed with only minor revisions. In 1934, Pool received the Columbia University Alumni Federation's Gold Medal for distinguished contributions to the university.

Pool resigned from New York Hospital on April 7, 1947; he died on April 9, 1949, at age 75 years. He had been divorced from his first wife, Esther Hoppin Pool, in 1930, with whom he had two sons: J. Lawrence Pool, MD, and Beckman Pool.[b] His second wife, Kitty Lanier Harriman Pool, died in 1936, whereas his third wife, Frances Saltonstall Pool, survived him.

Upon his death, *The Evening Sun*, a leading newspaper in New York City, in a rare editorial on April 13, 1949, paid a superb tribute to Eugene H. Pool, concluding, "A man who habitually shunned the spotlight ... he left a shining example for doctors, present and future."

His career and his contributions were also memorialized by his surgical colleague Frank J. McGowan, MD, in an obituary published in the *Bulletin of the New York Academy of Medicine*:

> Dr. Pool was an extraordinarily able man. Endowed with a fine mind, he developed it to the highest degree. He was wise in counsel, discerning in judgment, unfailing in leadership, with a limitless capacity for work.... He had vision, was a straight thinker and was able to crystallize his thoughts.... He had a keen sense of kindly humor. He had a love of people and boundless kindness toward

people. That is why his patients believed in him, trusted him implicitly and never forgot him.[6]

Just like the many changes occurring during the early third decade at R&C, our nation was being challenged as it never had been before by the Great Depression. The economic slump took its toll on hospital operations and staff, particularly the physicians.

Beginning with the devastating crash of the stock market on October 29, 1929, the country did not begin to show any sign of recovery until the mid-1930s, after Franklin D. Roosevelt was inaugurated as the 31st president of the United States. Much of the country had blamed the previous Republican, President Herbert Hoover, for the Depression, although its roots reached further back to the administration of Calvin Coolidge. Hoover's big mistake was that he kept reassuring our country that "things were going to get better if they all had a little patience."

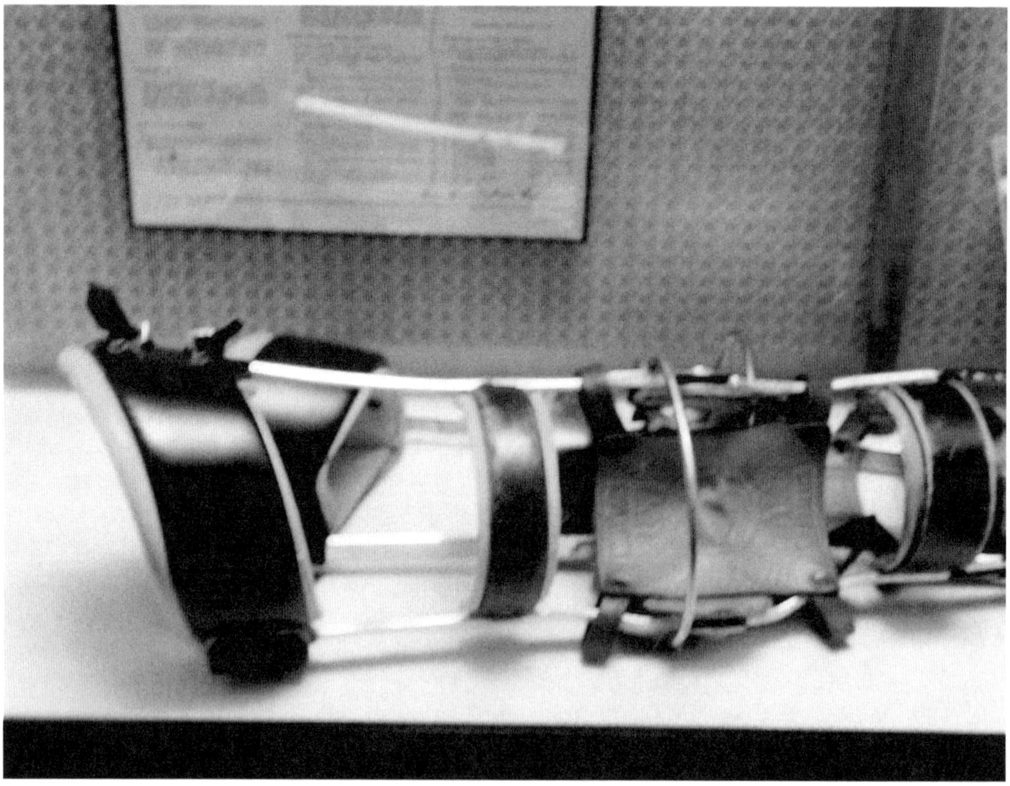

Fig. 6 One of Franklin D. Roosevelt's braces. He could only stand with some support or with his long leg braces locked using both of his crutches—a fact not realized by the nation. (From Hospital for Special Surgery Archives)

Roosevelt, who had been elected governor of New York in 1928, was afflicted with polio in 1922, leaving him essentially powerless in his lower extremities. Despite his physical frailties, he displayed invincible spirit while facing major challenges (Fig. 6). The unemployment rate, hovering as high as 25%, had caused palpable hardship to families, who were never before confronted with such overwhelming economic challenges. Job shortages led to the illegal deportation of 400,000 Mexican Americans, so that white males could get more jobs or receive relief from the government.[7]

Roosevelt's New Deal

In his first 100 days in office, Roosevelt—aided with help from a large southern-dominated Democratic majority in Congress—was able to introduce a considerable array of programs that began to turn the country around. Roosevelt's "New Deal" was what the country needed to pull itself up by its bootstraps (Table 2).

In 1935, Roosevelt introduced and encouraged Congress to pass the Social Security Act, the sweeping federal unemployment insurance and pension provision systems paid for by employers and their employees. New York City, with Wall Street at the eye of the storm, was experiencing troubled times, the like of which had never been seen before. The crash brought not only financial collapse, with wages and rents tumbling and long breadlines, but a significant increase in crime. There was a wave of gang warfare, murder, gambling, bribery, and corruption in politics, with links between the underworld and the police.[8]

Table 2 FDR's New Deal Programs in the First 100 Days

- Tennessee Valley Authority Act (TVA)
- Works Projects Administration (WPA)
- Homeowners Loan Act
- Agricultural Adjustment Act (AAA)
- Civilian Conservation Corps (CCC)
- Emergency Banking Act
- Federal Emergency Relief Act
- Civil Works Administration (CWA)

After spending seven terms in the House of Representatives as a Republican Congressman from the then-Italian East Harlem, Fiorello H. LaGuardia ran for mayor on an anticorruption fusion ticket as well as a nominee of the American Labor Party. He won a difficult election and served from 1934 to 1945.

Born in 1882 in the Bronx, Fiorello Enrico LaGuardia changed his middle name to Henry and affectionately was known by his constituents as "the little flower," the Italian translation of his first name. Raised as an Episcopalian, LaGuardia's nonpracticing Catholic father was from Cerignola in Apulia, a southeast region of Italy and his Jewish mother from Trieste, Italy.

LaGuardia was a fighter who aggressively pursued organized crime figures. The first thing he did when elected mayor was to order the Chief of Police to arrest the mobster Lucky Luciano. LaGuardia supported Roosevelt and his New Deal program and instituted a number of changes that helped address many issues created by the Depression in the city. Loved and trusted by his constituents, he was such a liberal Republican that he originally had difficulty enlisting party support.

One of his first appointments was that of Robert Moses (1888–1981) as commissioner of the New York City Department of Parks, a position Moses held until 1961. A 1909 graduate of Yale, Moses had entered college just before his 17th birthday. After Yale, he applied to Oxford University, where he was accepted and matriculated in Wadham College. There, conservatism prevailed, a political philosophy that would stay with Moses most of his life. Unsuccessful in seeking the nomination for mayor, Moses became the 1934 Republican nominee for Governor of New York but lost the election to Herbert Lehman. He went on to build New York City like no one else in history.[9, c]

He was responsible for establishing the concepts of "authorities," which would be independent from political pressures. His lifetime accomplishments of designing, building, and completing miles of highways, inspiring bridges, extensive parks, cultural centers, and a convention center were astonishing (Table 3). Moses brought jobs to the city in the Depression years and after, until the midcentury. He was a brilliant thinker with great vision. He had hoped to create New York City as a model for the rest of the nation. By the end of his career, he had built 658 playgrounds in New York City, 416 miles of parkways (more than all in Los Angeles), and 13 bridges.

Table 3 Creations and Influences of Robert Moses in New York City and Long Island

- Triborough Bridge
- Bronx-Whitestone Bridge
- Throgs Neck Bridge
- Cross Bronx Expressway
- Bruckner Expressway
- Henry Hudson Parkway
- Grand Central Parkway
- Northern State Parkway
- Southern State Parkway
- Belt Parkway
- Jones Beach State Park
- Orchard Beach
- Jacob Riis Park
- Lincoln Center
- Shea Stadium
- Co-op City
- New York Coliseum
- 1939 World's Fair

Reorganizing the Hospital

So it was a tumultuous period in New York City and in the nation when Wilson joined the R&C staff in May 1934. He took the rest of that year to assess and make necessary tactical changes (Fig. 7). Coley, as surgeon-in-chief emeritus, helped him reorganize the Surgical Department. The three independent orthopaedic divisions were abolished and replaced by a children's service and an adult service under the surgeon-in-chief. Members of the orthopaedic staff were to rotate on these services for equal periods. The Department of General Surgery, under the direction of Carl G. Burdick, MD (1880–1946), replaced the two hernia departments. The internists and pediatricians were combined into one service under Carlisle S. Boyd, MD (1881–1971).

Two Teaching Fellowships along with the Gibney Research Fellowship were designated to augment the incomes of newly practicing orthopaedic surgeons, who worked part time in teaching and research. At that time, training

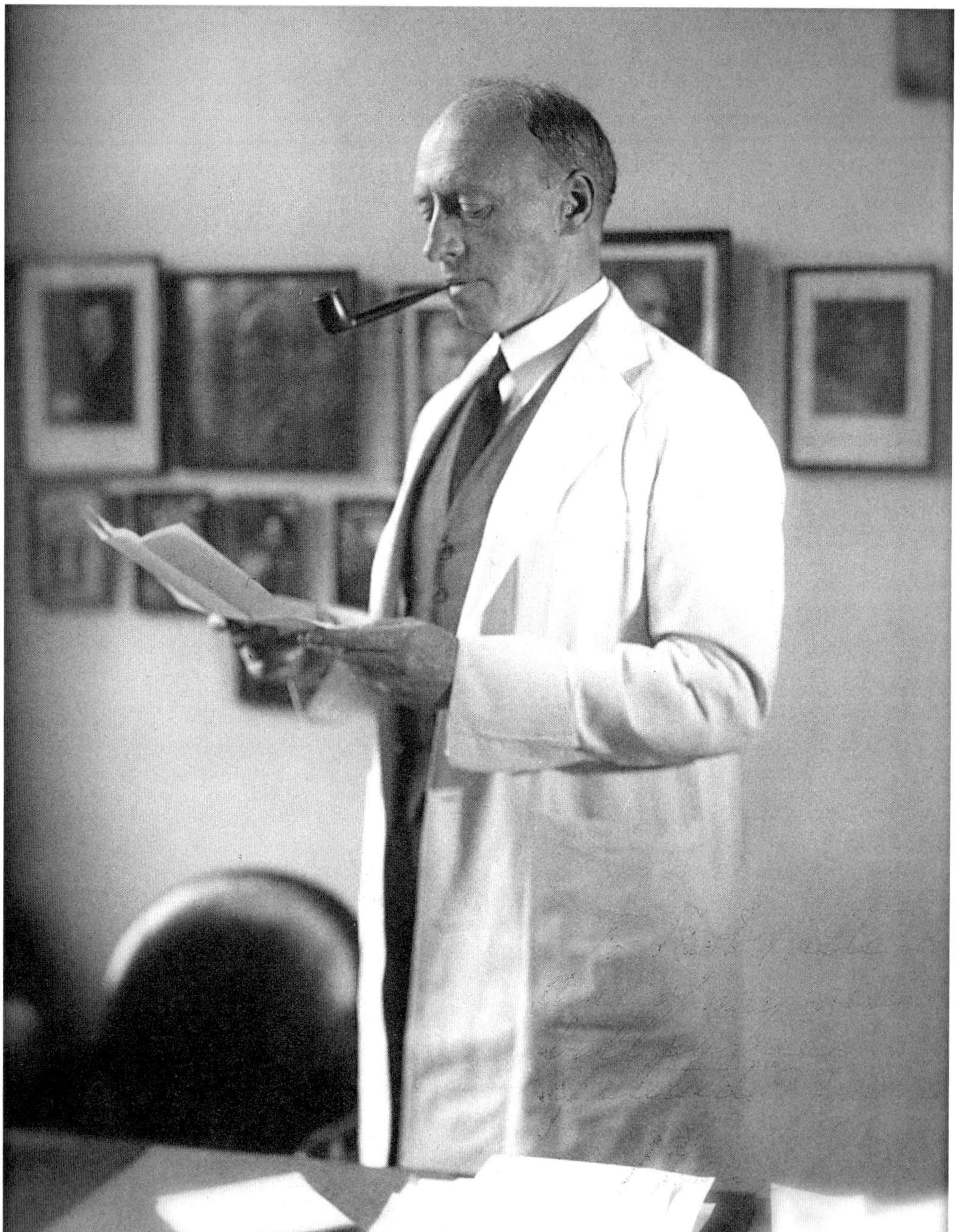

Fig. 7 Philip Wilson in his office circa 1934, when he moved from Boston to New York. (From Hospital for Special Surgery Archives)

requirements to become an orthopaedic surgeon were similar to what they are today. They included 4 years of college and 4 years of medical school, followed by 2 years of general surgery and 2–3 years of orthopaedic residency.

Realizing that graduating orthopaedists would have 2 to 3 lean years to cover expenses, the surgeon-in-chief proposed to the board a plan to appoint six additional fellows for 2 to 4 years at annual incomes of $2,000 to $3,000. This salary would not only support these new orthopaedic surgeons but would allow for replenishing the staff with new graduates. By the end of 1937, the major departments were reworked (Table 4a and b).[10]

Table 4a The Department of Orthopaedic Surgery staff in 1937 (as recorded in the Seventy-Fourth Annual Report of the Board)

HOSPITAL STAFF
Senior Consulting Surgeon and Surgeon-in-Chief Emeritus
EUGENE H. POOL, M.D.
Surgeon-in-Chief
PHILIP D. WILSON, M.D.
DEPARTMENT OF ORTHOPAEDIC SURGERY
Attending Orthopaedic Surgeons
RICHMOND STEPHENS, M.D
EARL E. VAN DERWERKER, M.D.
Associate Orthopaedic Surgeons
PAUL C. COLONNA, M.D.
LEWIS CLARK WAGNER, M.D.
Assistant Orthopaedic Surgeons
FRANCIS CARR, M.D.
PETER C. RIZZO, M.D.
T. CAMPBELL THOMPSON, M.D.
Executive Assistant to Surgeon-in-Chief
Teaching Fellows
ERNEST EDGAR MYERS, M.D.
Senior Research Fellow
JOHN R. COBB, M.D.
Gibney Research Fellow
Junior Research Fellows
J. NEILL GARBER, M.D.
(Completed January 1, 1938)

(continued)

Table 4a *(continued)*

ARTHUR A. THIBODEAU, M.D. (Completed January 1, 1938)
Visiting Fellow ARTHUR EYRE-BROOK, F.R.C.S. Bristol, England
In Charge of Plaster Room EDWARD LEROY BARNETT, M.D.
Orthopaedic Surgeons to Out-patient Department DAVID I. HORWICH, M.D. ROBERT L. PATTERSON, Jr., M.D.
Assistant Orthopaedic Surgeons to Out-patient Department WILLIAM FRIEDER, M.D. FRANCIS J. FADDEN, Jr., M.D. J. THEODORE GEIGER, M.D.

Table 4b The Hernia Department, Reorganized into the Department of General Surgery under Carl Burdick, MD

DEPARTMENT OF GENERAL SURGERY
Chief of Service CARL G. BURDICK, M.D.
Attending Surgeon FENWICK BEEKMAN, M.D.
Associate Surgeons DAVID GILLESPIE, M.D. RODERICK V. GRACE, M.D. BRADLEY L. COLEY, M.D. WALTER F. JONES, M.D. VINCENT HURLEY, M.D.
Assistant Surgeons ROLAND L. MAIER, M.D. JOSEPH SHAEFFER, M.D. VANSEL S. JOHNSON, M.D. NORMAN L. HIGGINBOTHAM, M.D. JOHN E. SULLIVAN, M.D. YOLANDE H. HUBER, M.D. W. ROSS McCARTY, M.D.

(continued)

Table 4b *(continued)*

DEPARTMENT OF MEDICINE AND PEDIATRICS
Chief-of-Service
CARLISLE S. BOYD, M.D.
Associate Attending Physicians
R. GARFIELD SNYDER, M.D.
FRANK G. PETTENGILL, M.D.
Assistant Attending Physician
CORNELIUS H. TRAEGER, M.D.
Physician to Out-patient Department
JOSEPH ALEXANDER, M.D.
LE MOYNE C. KELLY, M.D.
Assistant Physicians to Out-patient Department
FRANK ROSSOMONDO, M.D.
J. W. FORSTER, M.D.
LILLIAN HELLSTROM, M.D.
Clinical Assistant to Out-patient Department
WILLARD H. SQUIRES, M.D.
Pediatricians to Out-patient Department
RICHARD SCHORR, M.D.
FRANK H. ORR, M.D.
Assistant Pediatricians to Out-patient Department
WILLIAM WHEELER. Jr., M.D.

After William Coley's death in 1936, his son Bradley replaced his father as the second chief of the Bone Tumor Service at Memorial Hospital, serving on staff there from 1921 to 1959 (Fig. 8). His operation for replacing the hip joint for bone cancer became an accepted procedure throughout the country, as did many of his other procedures detailed in his classic text *Neoplasm of Bone and Related Conditions*, first published in 1949.

As an instructor at Cornell University Medical College and two other medical schools, Bradley Coley won the Legion of Merit during World War II, when he served in the Philippines as a surgical consultant to the Eighth Service Command. After the war, he was a founder of the Amputees Alliance, a self-help society.[d] In 1955, he turned the Amputee Alliance over to his friend Howard Rusk, whom he had known in the Army during the war and who

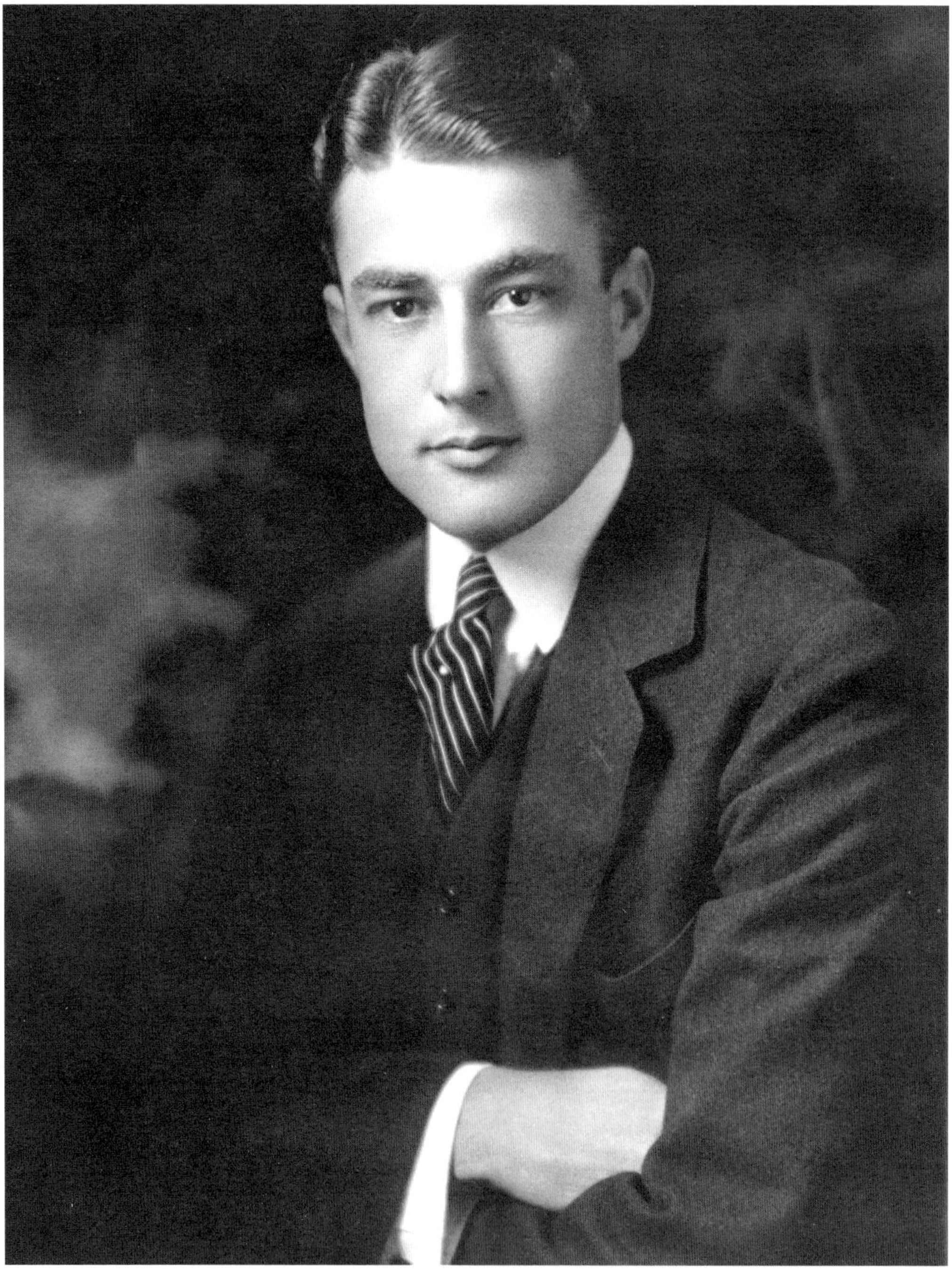

Fig. 8 Bradley L. Coley, MD, early in his professional life. (Courtesy of Bradley L. Coley Jr.)

founded the Rusk Institute of Rehabilitation Medicine at New York University School of Medicine.

Bradley Coley was married to Phyllis MacDonnell and had three sons: William B. Coley II, MD, Geoffrey M. Coley, MD, and Bradley L. Coley Jr. (nicknamed "Pete").[e] Bradley Coley died in 1960, at age 68 years.

Philip D. Wilson, MD

Born April 5, 1886 in Columbus, Ohio, Philip Duncan Wilson received his bachelor's degree from Harvard College and his medical degree from Harvard Medical School in 1912. Following training as a surgical house officer (1912–1914) at MGH, he returned to Columbus to join his father, Edward J. Wilson, MD, a well-known physician in practice.

With Europe at war, the young Wilson, along with Marius Smith-Peterson, MD (1886–1953), from Boston, was invited to join the Harvard Unit of American Volunteers under the leadership of Harvey Cushing, MD (1869–1939), to care for wounded French soldiers. He spent 3 months at the American Ambulance in Neuilly, where he treated many fractures. Wilson served under two senior medical officers—Robert E. Greenough, MD, and Robert B. Osgood, MD (1873–1956), both of whom took a liking to him (Fig. 9). In 1916, he spent another 3 months as a volunteer in a French Military Hospital on the coast of Normandy.

When the United States entered the war in April 1917, Wilson was commissioned as a captain in the Medical Corps and was sent overseas as a battalion medical officer assigned to the British Expeditionary Force. Later transferred to the No. 3 Australian Casualty Clearing Station, he was reunited with Osgood, who was organizing the orthopaedic service for the American Expeditionary Force (AEF). He had Wilson detached from the British and sent him for advanced war surgery to study amputation centers and the management of amputations in London, Paris, and Italy.

After reassignment at Base Hospital No. 9 near Châteauroux (Fig. 1), where Pool had been assigned, Wilson received his promotion to major and was assigned to the AEF as an orthopaedic consultant in amputations. He returned to America in February 1919 to assume the position of Chief of the Amputation Service at the Walter Reed General Hospital and served there until his honorable discharge in July 1919.

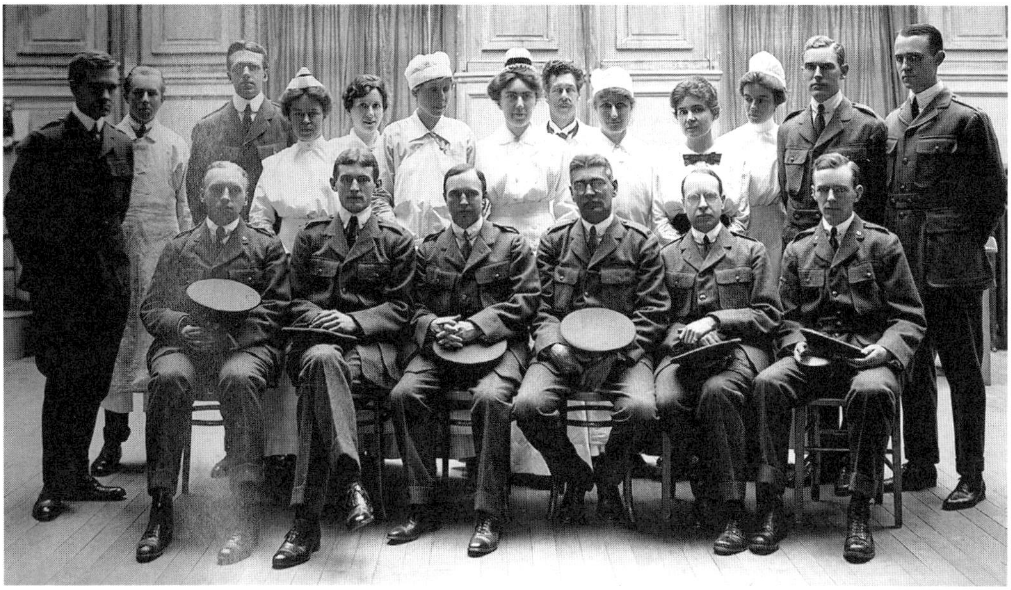

Fig. 9 During World War I in a military hospital, Philip Wilson is the first seated on the left, and Robert Osgood, MD, is the second seated on the right. (From Hospital for Special Surgery Archives)

A few months later, Wilson was invited to join the practice of Joel E. Goldthwait, MD (1961), and Osgood in Boston. He was appointed to the staff of MGH and to Harvard Medical School as instructor in orthopaedic surgery. In 1929, Wilson was deeply disappointed when he was passed over for chief of orthopaedics at MGH in favor of Smith-Peterson.[12] However, Wilson served as chief of the Fracture Service at the MGH and wrote the section on amputations in Nelson's *Loose-Leaf Living Surgery*. In collaboration with William A. Cochrane, FRCS, Edin. (1893–1944), Wilson authored the textbook *Fractures and Dislocations*.[2] In 1933, while still practicing in Boston, he became one of the founders of the American Academy of Orthopaedic Surgeons, serving as its president in 1934.

While on his first tour in France in 1915, Wilson met a 28-year-old French nurse's aide at the American Ambulance in Neuilly. They soon became engaged and were married in July 1916. Germaine Parfouru-Porel was the daughter of a famous actress. Her mother was also a successful producer and served as the head of the Odéon, the second state theater in Paris. Although Germaine Porel (the name was shortened by her father) was bilingual, she grew up in a home where her parents spoke only French. After returning to the United

Table 5 Chiefs of Specialty Clinics at Hospital for the Ruptured and Crippled (1936)

- Scoliosis Clinic—John Cobb, MD
- Clubfoot Clinic/Plaster Room—Leroy Barnett, MD
- Cerebral Spastic Clinic—Robert Lee Patterson Jr., MD
- Back Pain Clinic—Ernest E. Myers, MD
- Arthritis Clinic—R. Garfield Snyder, MD
- Obesity Clinic—Frank G. Pettingill, MD
- Bone Tumor Clinic—William B. Coley, MD, Bradley L. Coley, MD

States, the Wilsons eventually raised three children: Paul Wilson, Philip D. Wilson Jr., and Marianne Wilson Finkel.[f]

With R&C now under the leadership of a renowned orthopaedic surgeon, the organization of the hospital expanded. Wilson recruited new staff and introduced new programs in education and research. He successfully established an academic affiliation with the College of Physicians and Surgeons of Columbia University. He appointed three full-time fellows (including a Gibney Fellow) who were registered in Graduate Medical Education at the College of Physicians and Surgeons. After 2 years of study, T. Campbell Thompson, MD, John R. Cobb, MD (1903–1967), and Marvin Stevens, MD were awarded a degree in medical science in orthopaedics in June 1936. Wilson then created specialty clinics and assigned a staff member as chief (Table 5).

Medical Education

Resident education was very important and was originally established at the hospital by Gibney in 1887. The length of training for the eight orthopaedic residents was lengthened from 18 months to 2 years. General surgical residents trained for 1 year, and there was a medical residency for 1 year.

The annual surgeon-in-chief pro tempore program was inaugurated, with George Bennett, MD (1885–1962), professor of orthopaedic surgery at Johns Hopkins Medical School, becoming the first to occupy that role.

Wilson established the first medical library at the hospital in 1935. It had comfortable chairs, cases to house books and journals, and a secretary to assist with preparing bibliographies. It replaced a small area in the physicians' staff room where books and periodicals were collected but which often disappeared before residents had a chance to read them.

The X-Ray Department showed steady growth and for the first time had a full-time radiologist on staff. Raymond W. Lewis, MD (1889–1976), was appointed the department's director in June 1938.

The hospital suffered a major loss with the death of its administrator, Joseph D. Flick, on December 14, 1937. Appointed in 1917, Flick, at age 66 years,

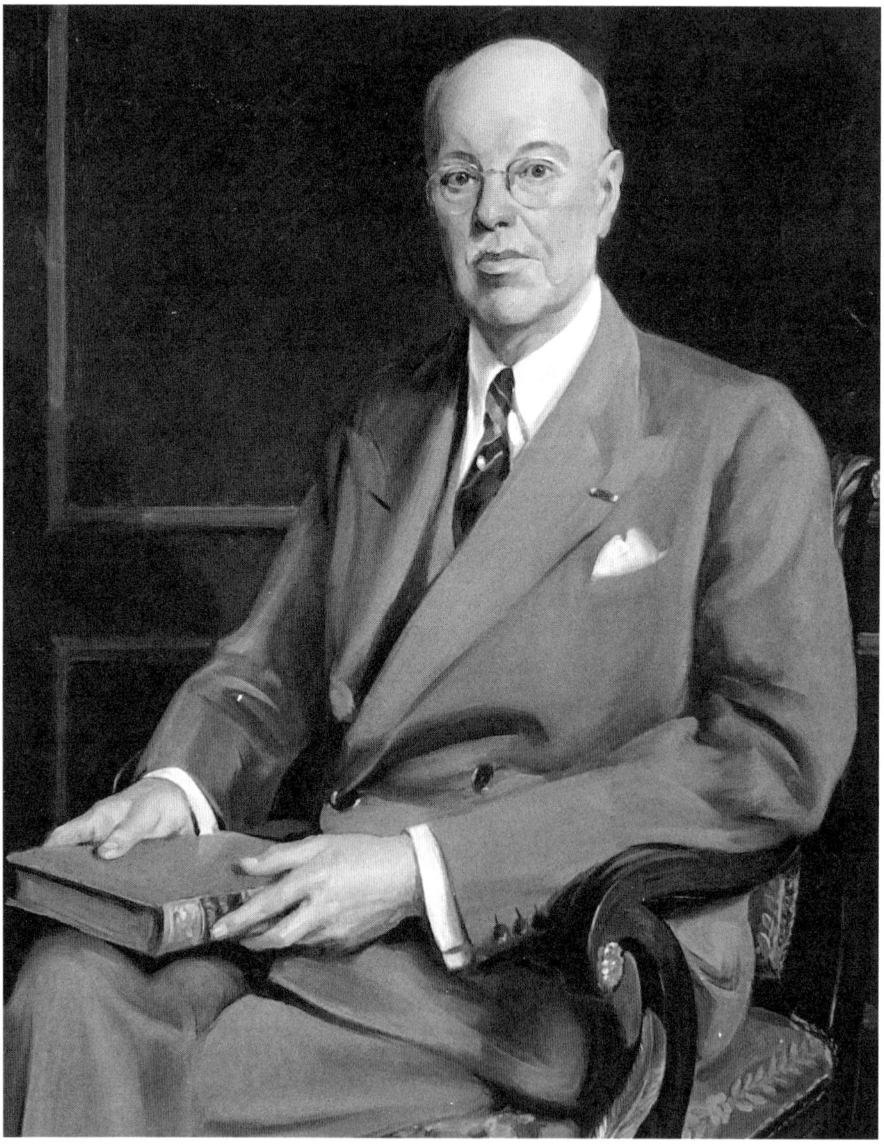

Fig. 10 Fenwick Beekman, MD, was a general surgeon and second in command in the Department of General Surgery at Hospital for the Ruptured and Crippled in 1937. (From Hospital for Special Surgery Archives)

served 21 years under Gibney and the next three surgeons-in-chief, who were most indebted for his devoted assistance. Overseeing a number of expansions of the building during periods of crisis and change, he was succeeded by Edward A. B. Willmer, a civil and mechanical engineer from Labrador.

The history of the first 75 years of the R&C has been meticulously and carefully documented by Fenwick Beekman, MD (1882–1962) (Fig. 10), attending surgeon at R&C. It is the only book published on the history of R&C and was written on the occasion of the hospital's 75th anniversary.[2] Beekman served as the hospital's first chairman of the Library Committee and was president of the New York Historical Society in 1947. A member of the legendary New York Beekman family, for whom Beekman Street was named, he was a founding member of the Board of Surgery and the American Board of Plastic Surgery and Clinical Professor of Surgery at New York University School of Medicine.

REFERENCES

1. Wilson PD Jr., Levine DB. Hospital for Special Surgery. A brief review of its development and current position. *Clin Orthop.* 2000;374:90–105.
2. Beekman F. *Hospital for the Ruptured and Crippled. A historical sketch written on the occasion of the seventy-fifth anniversary of the hospital.* New York, NY: Statistical Press; 1939.
3. Brown RS. Base Hospital No. 9 A.E.F. New York, NY: privately printed; 1920.
4. Comorow A. Best hospitals. In: *Best Hospitals*, 2012 ed. Washington, DC: U.S. News & World Report; 2011:56–102.
5. Pool EH. *Seventy-Second Annual Report of the New York Society for the Relief of the Ruptured and Crippled.* New York, NY: New York Society for the Relief of the Ruptured and Crippled; 1935;7–11.
6. McGowan FJ. Eugene Hillhouse Pool—1874–1949. *Bull NY Acad Med.* 1949;25:467–469.
7. Allen FL. *Since Yesterday: The 1930s in America.* New York, NY: Harper & Bros.; 1940.
8. Lyman SE. *The Story of New York.* New York, NY: Crown; 1975.
9. Caro RA. *The Power Broker.* New York, NY: Vintage Press; 1975.
10. Wilson PD. *Seventy-Fourth Annual Report of the New York Society for the Relief of the Ruptured and Crippled.* New York, NY: New York Society for the Relief of the Ruptured and Crippled; 1937;31–32.
11. Coley BL Jr. Personal communication. 2008.
12. Sherk HH. *Getting it Straight: A History of American Orthopaedics.* Rosemont, IL: American Academy of Orthopaedic Surgery; 2008.

NOTES

a. A celebrated veteran of the Spanish-American and Philippine Wars, Major General John "Black Jack" Pershing led the AEF, which other Allied Commanders tried to push into a subordinate role in troop replacement.

b. J. Lawrence Pool, MD (1906–2004), having interned in medicine at New York Hospital, was eventually appointed professor and chairman of the Department of Neurological Surgery at Columbia University in 1949, retiring in 1972. He and his brother, Beckman, were the amateur squash champions of the world and together wrote more than 13 books on the subject.

c. Those interested in learning more about Robert Moses are encouraged to read Robert A. Caro's critical but masterful biography of Moses, *The Power Broker*.

d. As a result of World War II, there were over 15,000 amputees. In World War I, there were over 2,600 major amputees.

e. I am most indebted to "Pete" Coley for his generous time and assistance in providing me with many original documents, photos, reprints, anecdotes, and other materials from his family collections. His recall of the history of the lives of his grandfather William Bradley Coley, his father Bradley L. Coley, and his aunt Helen Coley Nauts enriched my appreciation of the Coley contributions to orthopaedics and cancer in the first half of the 20th century. The name William B. Coley lives on as a foundation enhancing cancer immunotherapy and through an annual award honoring him. The William B. Coley Award is given each year to an accomplished scientist in the field of cancer immunology at the annual dinner of the Cancer Research Institute in New York, founded by Helen Coley Nauts in 1953.[11]

f. Philip D. Wilson Jr., MD, eventually would become surgeon-in-chief of the Hospital for Special Surgery in 1972.

CHAPTER 8
ENTERING WORLD WAR II (1940–1945)
DAVID B. LEVINE, MD

CELEBRATING ITS 75TH ANNIVERSARY, with an event held at the hospital on 42nd Street from October 31 to November 4, 1939, the Hospital for the Ruptured and Crippled (R&C) was anxious to recapture its leadership in the orthopaedic world. Festivities began on a Tuesday and ended the following Saturday evening with a social event at the Waldorf-Astoria Hotel (Table 1).

Now in his fourth year as surgeon-in-chief, Wilson reorganized the hospital staff and added new laboratory space in the building. He introduced new academic programs, including the annual surgeon-in-chief pro tempore. The first to serve in this position was George E. Bennett, MD, professor of orthopaedic surgery at Johns Hopkins Medical School. Edward Gallie, MD (1882–1959), professor of surgery and dean of the Medical School of Toronto University, served next in 1936 as visiting surgeon-in-chief. (Gallie and Bennett had both been house surgeons at R&C in 1906 and 1909.)[1]

With advancement of modern surgery in orthopaedics and the treatment of hernias, the previous relationship between the ruptured and the crippled—once glued together by the brace-maker's role—was becoming undone. This may have precipitated the decision to rename the hospital, but as well known as the name—Ruptured and Crippled—was at that time, it was never popular and was becoming less acceptable. During the nineteenth century, New York hospitals were often known by a disease, a condition, or affiliation with a religious faith or ethnic group. So when R&C first opened its doors in 1863, the inclusion of "ruptured and crippled" in its name was not unusual.

Lenox Hill Hospital was founded in 1857 as the German Hospital. That same year, Saint Vincent's Hospital was incorporated under the legal title of

Table 1 Program of the R&C 75th Anniversary Commemoration in 1939

Calendar of Events

Tuesday, October 31	
Reception and Inspection of the hospital. All departments of the institution shown in operation. (*Details on pages 4 to 6*) .	3:30-6:00 P.M.
Tea in the Solarium.	4:00-6:00 P.M.
Wednesday, November 1	
Reception and Inspection of the hospital. All departments of the institution shown in operation. (*Details on pages 4 to 6*) .	3:30-6:00 P.M.
Tea in the Solarium.	4:00-6:00 P.M.
Thursday, November 2	
Scientific program and operative clinics at the hospital. (*Details on pages 7 and 8*)	8:30 A.M.-12:00 M. 2:00-5:00 P.M.
Meeting and luncheon of Alumni Association of the Hospital for Ruptured and Crippled at the hospital. . . .	12:15-1:30 P.M.
75th Anniversary Dinner at the University Club.	7:30 P.M.
Friday, November 3	
Scientific program and operative clinics at the hospital. (*Details on pages 9 and 10*)	8:30 A.M.-12:00 M. 2:00-5:00 P.M.
Alumni Luncheon given by the Board of Managers at Woodstock Tower, 320 East 42nd Street	12:00 M.-2:00 P.M.
Saturday, November 4	
Scientific program at the hospital. (*Details on page 11*)	9:00-11:00 A.M.
Golf Tournament. Time and place will be announced at luncheon on Friday.	
*75th Anniversary Dance of the Alumni Association in the Astor Gallery of the Waldorf-Astoria.	10:00 P.M.-3:00 A.M.

the Sisters of Charity of St. Vincent de Paul. Mount Sinai Hospital, founded in 1852, was first known as the Jews' Hospital in New York. Aristocratic German Jews controlled the board, the hospital, and staff. Until the turn of the century, poor patients of Russian Jewish descent were often treated as second-class citizens, whereas non-Jewish patients could only be seen when an emergency existed. Prejudice in class, religions, and ethnic backgrounds prevailed among both hospital staff and patients.

In 1868, James Lenox, a distinguished member of the Presbyterian Church of New York, circulated a letter among his own group, stating that while the Jews, Germans, Roman Catholics, and Episcopalians had established hospitals for themselves, the Presbyterians had done nothing of the kind. The

Presbyterian Hospital in the City of New York was then incorporated in 1868, with Lenox chosen as president of the board.

Hospitals were not restricted to acute and chronic care as they are today. There were "homes" for long-term care, "asylums" for the disabled, "infirmaries" for outdoor care, and "almshouses" for needy immigrants who arrived at port cities early in the nineteenth century.[a] There were institutions in Manhattan and Westchester County often called by descriptive conditions that would likely be unacceptable in our society today (Table 2).[2]

It was not until after the 1870s that hospitals became institutions of medical science rather than social welfare. A few voluntary hospitals, such as Massachusetts General Hospital and the Pennsylvania Hospital, existed and were generally cleaner and better managed than municipally run hospitals but still were not widely used by the middle and upper classes.[3, b] They had close affiliations with university medical schools. Their poorer patients were useful for teaching purposes, while their wealthy patients provided revenues and bequests.

R&C Changes Its Name

On February 13, 1941, Lawrence McK Miller, the secretary of the Board of Managers of the New York Society for the Relief of the Ruptured and Crippled, reported in the 77th annual report that the name of the hospital had been changed in 1940 to the Hospital for Special Surgery (HSS). "For many years objections have been raised at various times regarding this name," he wrote. The incorporated title, The New York Society for the Relief of the Ruptured and Crippled, was retained.[4]

Table 2 Additional Nineteenth-Century New York Institutions and Founding Dates

Bloomingdale Asylum for the Insane—1806
The New York Orphan Asylum—1807
The Stranger's Hospital—1871
The Home for Incurables—1866
The Home for Friendless Women—1865
The House of Rest for Consumptives—1869

In 1969, Wilson wrote in the foreword of the biography of Virgil Gibney, "The adjective orthopedic had been preempted by other Institutions of New York working in this field, and so the board decided to make use of the title devised by the great British pioneer, Sir Robert Jones, to designate the surgical hospitals he organized for the care of the wounded soldiers who had received injuries of the bones and joints in World War I, all of whom were assigned to the division of orthopedics, and so one historic title was exchanged for another."[5, c]

Both Wilson and his predecessor, Eugene H. Pool, had served in Europe in World War I, but now another war was looming to interrupt Wilson's career. On September 1, 1939, Germany invaded Poland. Great Britain and France, having signed a pact to come to Poland's defense, declared war on Germany. President Franklin D. Roosevelt and a great majority of the United States wanted to avoid war at any cost, particularly because the country was rebounding from the Great Depression.

As early as 1939, Wilson had proposed that a representative from the American Orthopaedic Association be appointed to a Joint Committee on Military Affairs set up by the American Academy of Orthopaedic Surgeons. The next year, a committee of five was established and was chaired by Wilson.[6]

American Hospital in Britain

In the summer of 1939, while visiting in England, Wilson met with leading British orthopaedic surgeons and inquired if, in the event of war, the assistance of American surgeons would be desired, as in World War I? The British surgeons were most grateful for the offer.

On May 20, 1940, Wilson telegraphed Harry Platt (1886–1986), professor of orthopaedic surgery at the Royal Infirmary of Manchester, England, offering to set up a hospital unit of orthopaedic facilities in Britain. On May 31, Platt replied, "Officially authorized to say that your offer is gratefully accepted. All facilities will be granted by our Government for entry of members of a unit to Great Britain. Our greatest need is surgeons with orthopaedic training. Grim days are ahead but we are undaunted"[4] (Fig. 1).

Wilson incorporated the hospital under the laws of the State of New York so that it could be registered with the Department of State in Washington under the Neutrality Act. It could then be licensed to raise funds. The Board

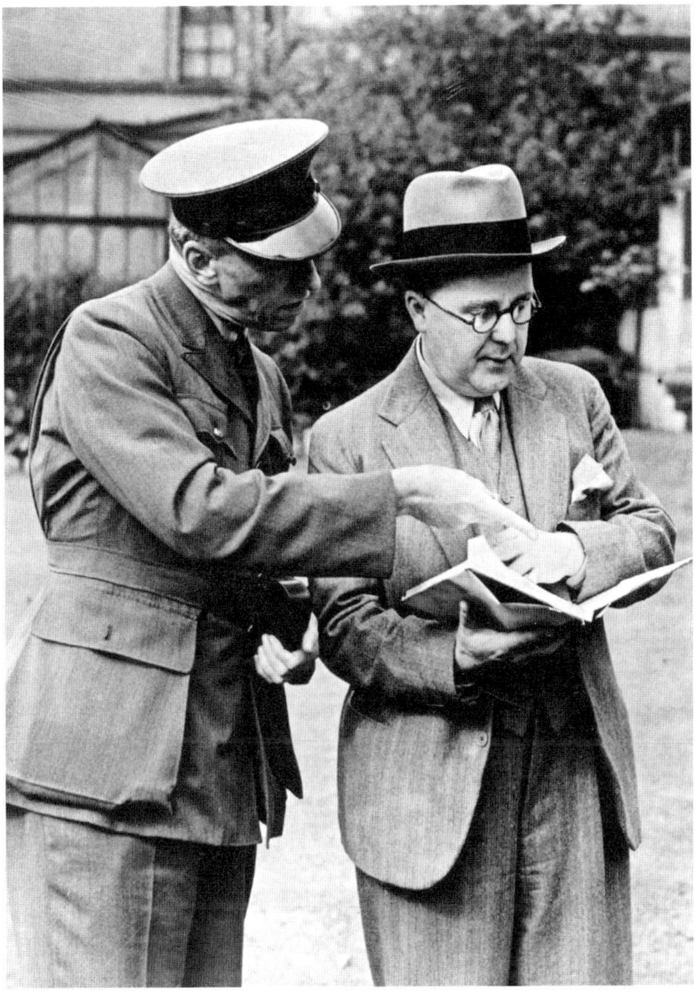

Fig. 1 Philip D. Wilson, MD, conferring with Sir Harry Platt early in the World War II. (From Hospital for Special Surgery Archives)

of Managers of the Society for the Relief of the Ruptured and Crippled was overwhelmingly supportive. William Church Osborn, president of the R&C Board of Managers, was appointed president of the new board. Others from HSS were to serve on the new board. Winthrop Aldrich, president of the Allied Relief Fund (which later merged with the British War Relief Society), arranged financial support.

The last step was to form a staff. A small advance group of 12 individuals, dressed in the light blue uniforms of the American Hospital in Britain, sailed from Brooklyn on the steamship *Western Prince* on August 22, 1940 (Fig. 2).

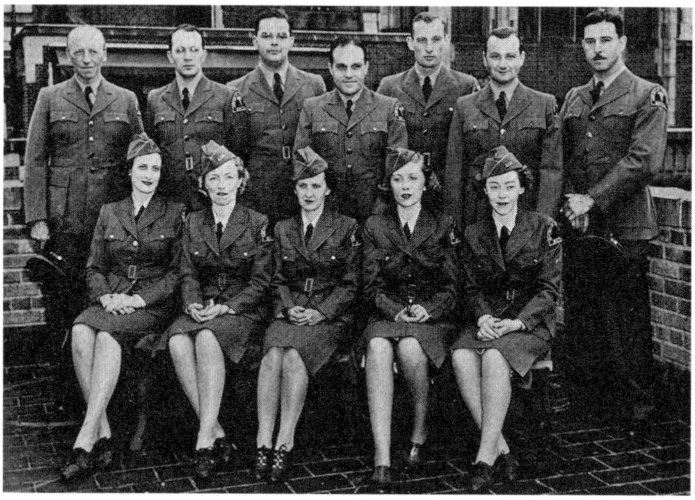

Fig. 2 The first unit of the American Hospital in Britain, Ltd., sailed on August 22, 1940, to Liverpool. Seated (from left): Miriam L. Knight, Adelbert E. Overman, Mildred L. Lewis, Sheila M. Converse, Helen D. Dial. Standing (from left): Philip D. Wilson, MD, Donald E. Dial, MD, Charles H. Bradford, MD, W. Richard Ferguson, MD, Frederick W. Waknitz, MD, John M. Converse, MD, Norman Egel, MD. (From Hospital for Special Surgery Archives)

Their supplies included surgical instruments, orthopaedic appliances, and dressings, sufficient to last 3 months.

After sailing through submarine-infested waters, the ship landed safely at Liverpool on September 1, and the unit was greeted by an outpouring of gratitude from the British people. The Park Prewett Hospital at Basingstoke in Hampshire, a 1,500-bed psychiatric hospital that never actually opened to treat mentally ill patients, had been converted to a general surgical and medical hospital at the beginning of the war. The American Hospital was assigned a block of six wards with 300 beds and a separate operating room. Between then and the end of the year, 254 operations were performed mainly on soldiers, sailors, and members of the Royal Air Force, as well as civilians injured in German air raids. Such raids had intensified just as the Americans had arrived.

The object of creating the American hospital was threefold:

1. To give surgical assistance to the British
2. To provide moral support in time of need
3. To gain experience in the treatment of war casualties

Wilson returned to the United States on January 1, 1941. He was replaced as the director of the American Hospital in Britain by Wallace Cole, MD (1888–1973), professor of orthopaedic surgery of the University of Minnesota. Wilson established an American Hospital headquarters office at the HSS.

Eleven months later, on the morning of December 7, 1941, Japanese attack forces—consisting of 6 aircraft carriers and 423 planes—bombed the U.S. Pacific Fleet at Pearl Harbor, Hawaii. On December 8, the United States and Britain declared war on Japan. President Roosevelt's radio address to the nation on December 7, announcing that the United States was at war with Germany, will never be forgotten by those listening that Sunday morning. His characterization of December 7 as "a day which will live in infamy" still echoes today.[7]

On December 11, Germany and Italy declared war on the United States. These events united the nation behind the President, effectively ending the isolationist sentiments of the American public. The Pearl Harbor attack resulted in the deaths of 2,335 American servicemen and 68 civilians, with 1,178 being wounded.

T. Campbell Thompson, MD (1902–1986), executive assistant to the surgeon-in-chief, presented to the Board of Managers the 78th Annual Report of the Surgeon-in-Chief in place of Wilson, who had been granted a leave of absence to return to England.[8] There, Wilson organized the new Churchill Hospital in Oxford, which was originally designed by the Ministry of Health to care for local air raid casualties (which turned out not to be needed by the British). These facilities were allocated to the U.S. Army for the American Hospital in Britain to be moved from Park Prewett Hospital.[9] On January 1, 1942, the American organization, having grown to a staff of 12 doctors and 140 personnel, moved to Oxford into a 600-bed hospital, where half of the beds were occupied by British war casualties.

After the United States entered the war, it was necessary for the voluntary and private American Hospital in Britain to become part of the U.S. Army Medical Corps. This transfer took place on July 15 and created the 2nd General Hospital, staffed by Presbyterian Hospital from New York. Major Robert Lee Patterson Jr. was appointed director of the Orthopaedic Service.[d]

Patterson had not only been on the Presbyterian staff but also on the R&C staff. During the war, he rose to the rank of colonel and worked in hospitals in both France and England (Fig. 3). Now that the American Hospital in Britain was dissolved, its business office—originally located in HSS—was closed.[10]

The war significantly affected the R&C professional and employee staff, but patient care for a large part proceeded uninterrupted. The orthopaedic resident staff remained at eight, but to cooperate with the Manpower Commission, the length of the residency was reduced from 2 years to 1 year. Although this did not meet the requirements of the American Board of Orthopaedic Surgery, it was felt a greater number of orthopaedic doctors was needed and thus could be trained.

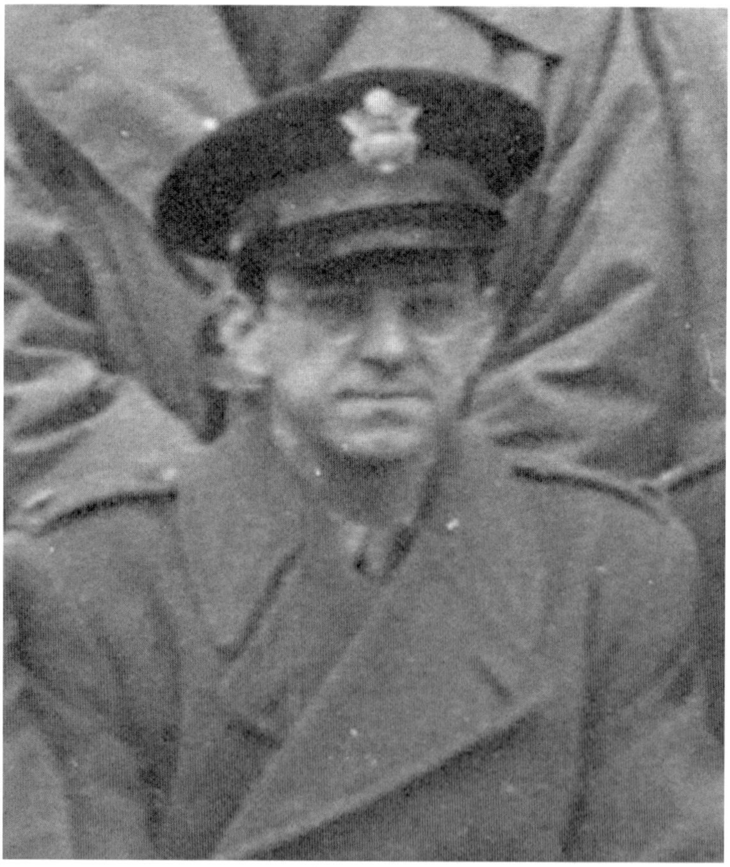

Fig. 3 Colonel Robert Lee Patterson Jr. was attached to the Normandy invasion forces and earned the Legion of Merit. (From Hospital for Special Surgery Archives)

More than 36 attending physicians and surgeons and 11 residents and fellows took leaves of absence to join the military (Table 3). Some of those were key staff, including Charles L. Burstein, MD (1906–1986), director of anesthesia, and Dominic Desanto, MD (1904–2000), director of laboratories. Milton Helpern, MD (1902–1977), temporarily replaced Desanto.

Table 3 Some HSS Staff Physicians on Leave of Absence to the Military During World War II

T. Campbell Thompson, MD, associate attending orthopaedic surgeon
Dominic Desanto, MD, director of laboratory
Francis J. Carr, MD, associate attending orthopaedic surgeon
Robert Lee Patterson Jr., MD, assistant attending orthopaedic surgeon
Peter C. Rizzo, MD, assistant attending orthopaedic surgeon
Henry Lange, MD, assistant attending orthopaedic surgeon
Frederick Waknitz, MD, director of research
John J. Flanagan, MD, orthopaedic surgeon to the Outpatient Department
David Horwich, MD, orthopaedic surgeon to the Outpatient Department
William Cooper, MD, orthopaedic surgeon to the Outpatient Department
Theodore Geiger, MD, assistant orthopaedic surgeon to the Outpatient Department
Robert Mazet, MD, assistant orthopaedic surgeon to the Outpatient Department
Bradley L. Coley, MD, attending surgeon
John E. Sullivan, MD, associate attending surgeon
Norman L. Higginbotham, MD, associate attending surgeon
Joseph Shaeffer, MD, associate attending surgeon
Vansel S. Johnson, MD, associate attending surgeon
W. Ross McCarty, MD, assistant attending surgeon
John M. Converse, MD, attending plastic surgeon
Richard Schorr, MD, assistant attending pediatrics
Edmund Joyner III, MD, pediatric physician to Outpatient Department
Henry Kirkland, MD, cardiologist
Arthur A. Knapp, MD, assistant attending ophthalmologist
Thomas Hoen, MD, attending neurosurgeon
Eugene T. R. Stone, MD, assistant attending gynecologist
Elemer Marjey, MD, assistant attending dermatologist
Clarence A. Dunn, MD, attending oral surgeon
Edward Stroh, MD, associate attending oral surgeon

Table 3 (*continued*)

Sidney Leistner, MD, assistant attending dentist
Charles L. Burstein, MD, attending anesthetists
Residents and fellows
Donald E. Dial, MD
Theodore A. Lynn, MD
Charles F. Kincheloe, MD
William G. Rhorer, MD
Harry Sherman, MD
Lynn R. Callin, MD
Jerome Lawrence, MD
John J. Dorsey, MD
Vincent Turco, MD
Jerome Lawrence, MD
Homer C. Pheasant, MD
Unspecified
William R. Duncan, MD
David Littauer, MD
Joseph Messina, MD
Lowell Thomas, MD
Charles Wohl, MD

Record and Chronicle

Because of the demand of the U.S. Army for physical therapists, a war emergency course for training physical therapy technicians was instituted at the hospital. The R&C staff also did its part in supporting war activities. At the outbreak of war, they promptly organized a unit of the New York City Civilian Defense Corps. In November 1942, F. Wilson Keller (1897–1954), hospital administrator, inaugurated the *Record and Chronicle*, the first hospital newsletter to be published (Fig. 4). The hospital had an outstanding record among greater New York institutions in supporting various war bond campaigns. Individual staff members also generously donated to many voluntary organizations, including the national War Fund and the American Red Cross.

In 1944, there was a major reorganization of the Department of Medicine and Pediatrics at the hospital. Before that time, the departments functioned as

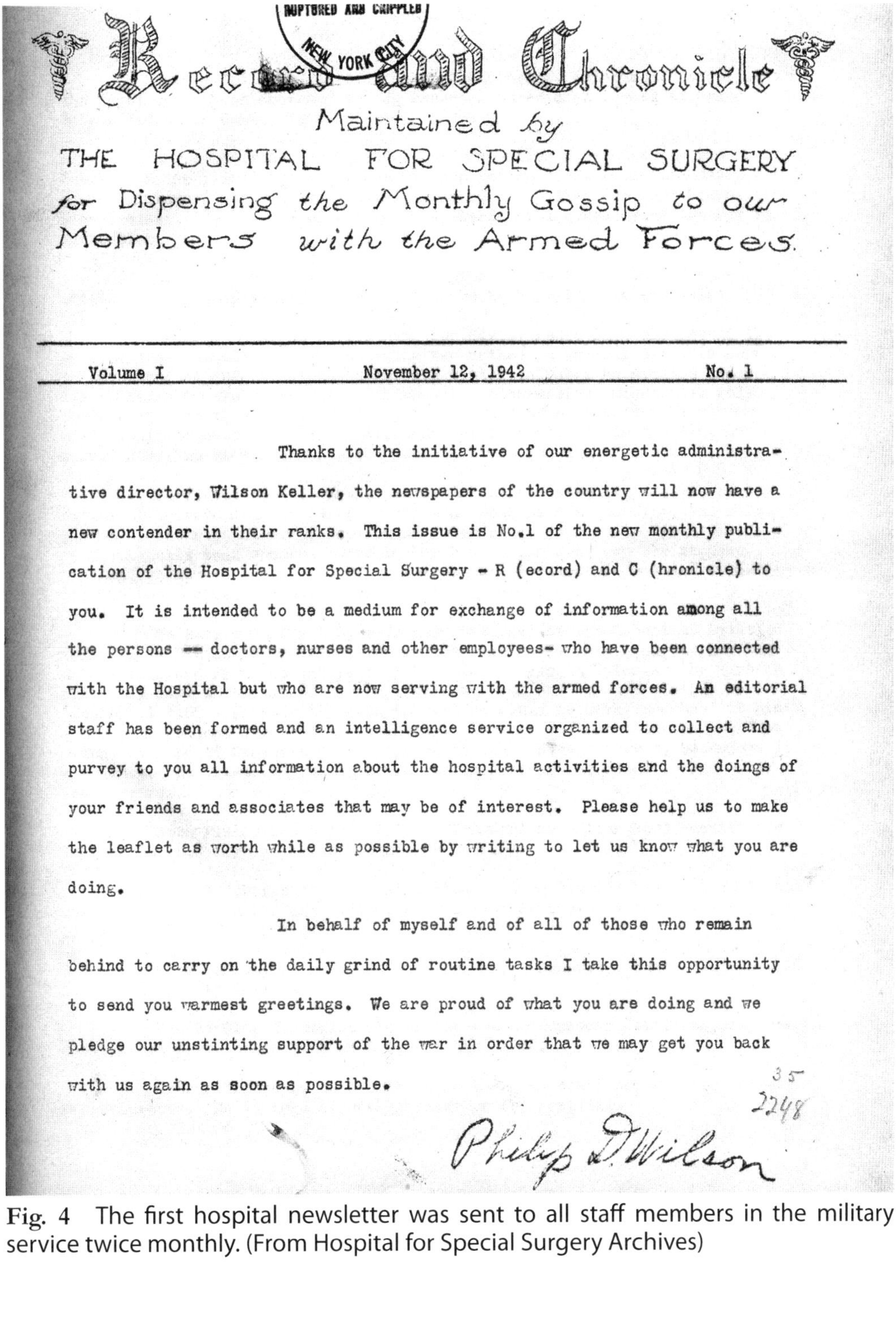
RUPTURED AND CRIPPLED NEW YORK CITY

Record and Chronicle

Maintained by
THE HOSPITAL FOR SPECIAL SURGERY
for Dispensing the Monthly Gossip to our Members with the Armed Forces.

Volume I | November 12, 1942 | No. 1

Thanks to the initiative of our energetic administrative director, Wilson Keller, the newspapers of the country will now have a new contender in their ranks. This issue is No.1 of the new monthly publication of the Hospital for Special Surgery - R (ecord) and C (hronicle) to you. It is intended to be a medium for exchange of information among all the persons — doctors, nurses and other employees- who have been connected with the Hospital but who are now serving with the armed forces. An editorial staff has been formed and an intelligence service organized to collect and purvey to you all information about the hospital activities and the doings of your friends and associates that may be of interest. Please help us to make the leaflet as worth while as possible by writing to let us know what you are doing.

In behalf of myself and of all of those who remain behind to carry on the daily grind of routine tasks I take this opportunity to send you warmest greetings. We are proud of what you are doing and we pledge our unstinting support of the war in order that we may get you back with us again as soon as possible.

35
2248

Philip D. Wilson

Fig. 4 The first hospital newsletter was sent to all staff members in the military service twice monthly. (From Hospital for Special Surgery Archives) separate clinics. Routine pediatric care was provided on the Orthopaedic and Surgical Services. The arthritis clinic was established under R. Garfield Snyder, MD. With the retirement of Carlisle E. Boyd, MD (1881–1971), as chief of the Department of Medicine and Pediatrics, the hospital appointed Richard H. Freyberg, MD (1904–1999), as chief of the Department of Internal Medicine and Pediatrics on September 1, 1944 (Fig. 5). A medical ward of 20 beds was established to study rheumatic diseases. Freyberg had previously held the positions of assistant professor of internal medicine and director of the Rackham

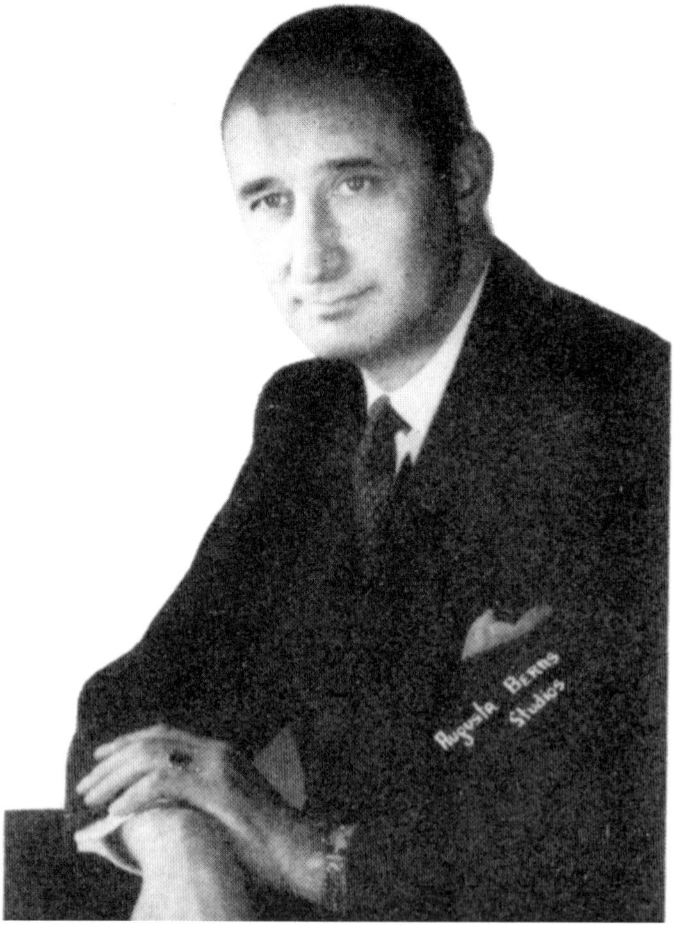

Fig. 5 Richard Freyberg, MD, when he was appointed to head the Department of Medicine and Pediatrics at the Hospital for Special Surgery. (From Hospital for Special Surgery Archives)

Arthritis Research Unit at the Medical School and University Hospital of the University of Michigan.

Meanwhile, the war in Europe was about to escalate. On June 6, 1944, Allied forces launched the Invasion of Normandy. It was the largest seaborne invasion of that time, involving 850,000 troops crossing the English Channel from Great Britain to France (the first successful wartime landing across the English Channel in nine centuries). Allied land forces came from Canada, Free French forces, the United Kingdom, and the United States. There were overnight parachute and glider landings, massive air attacks, and naval bombardments, followed by early morning amphibious landings. The objective was to secure Normandy, which would lead to the downfall of Germany. D-Day was a success, but very costly: over 10,000 allied troops died, were wounded, or were missing in action.[11]

The massive causalities provided a source of advancement in medical care. Nearly 70% had extremity wounds. Major orthopaedic advancements in fracture care, wound management, amputation surgery, and rehabilitation resulted from experiences on the battlefields, in primary battle hospitals, and in major hospital centers. External fixation of fractures, developed during the 1930s, was used in the early war years, but was soon discontinued because of high infection rates.

It was not until after the war in the 1950s that Gavril Ilizarov (1921–1992), a Russian orthopaedic surgeon, introduced his circular external fixation device, significantly reducing infection rates.[12] Gerhard Küntscher (1900–1972), a German surgeon, perfected intramedullary nailing for long bone fractures. The method was first employed in captured Allied airmen in World War II, who were treated while prisoners of war.

About 18,000 members of the U.S. Army lost limbs. Five amputation centers for revision surgery, prosthetic appliance fitting, and rehabilitation physical therapy were established. This was accomplished on the advice of Colonel Norman T. Kirk, MD (1888–1960), who had experienced four wars since 1912. Kirk rose to the rank of major general and became the U.S. Army Surgeon General from 1943 to 1947. He was the first military doctor to become certified by the American Board of Orthopaedic Surgery and become a member of the American Academy of Orthopaedic Surgery.[e] Lt. Colonel T. Campbell Thompson and Major Donald B. Slocum headed the Amputation Center at Walter Reed Army General Hospital.

During 1944, despite 440 persons leaving employment at the HSS (resulting in a 100% labor turnover), the hospital maintained its statistical goals. The inpatient occupancy rate was 77%, with an average daily census of 161, compared with 1943 when there was a 71% occupancy and the average daily census was 174. A few wards had to be closed temporarily because of lack of adequate staff, especially nurses.[13]

That year, there also was an active hospital developing and planning committee to address long-term planning. It met on a number of occasions with academic and municipal leaders in the city, as well as hospital staff, and made the following conclusions:

1. A need for teaching and research makes a close affiliation with a medical school necessary.
2. Such affiliation should be sought, allowing the hospital to retain its own autonomy.
3. Expansion of the physical plant should provide space for 150 beds, private doctors' offices, and a private clinic.

In his 1944 Annual Report, Wilson wrote that the hospital newsletter *Record and Chronicle* had been so favorably received by the military overseas and stateside that the hospital had increased its publication to bimonthly. It provided an important means of communicating hospital news and gossip, so vital for the morale of our service personnel during those challenging war years. An excerpt from the first issue read as follows:

> Phil Wilson has been bouncing around town in a Bantam car. Says it's a cousin to the Austin, and it gets 40 miles to the gallon. The car has been named Archie and rumored to have been garaged in the building of his apartment at 134 East 74th Street on Halloween night to avoid having the ragamuffins carry it away.[14]

The war ended in Europe on May 7, 1945, V-E (Victory in Europe) Day, when Germany surrendered. On August 6, 1945, a B-29 U.S. bomber dropped an atomic bomb on the city of Hiroshima, Japan, killing 75,000 people and injuring over 100,000 in a city of 340,000. Japan hesitated to surrender until three days later, when another atomic bomb was dropped on the city of Nagasaki. The next day, on August 10, 1945, Japan surrendered. The bloodiest war in history was finally over.[15]

The Postwar Era Begins

In 1946, the first year after the war, improvement of nursing services at HSS was critical. Cleanthe Logetheton (1891–1986), director of nurses, resigned in April and was replaced by Bertha Pieraccini. However, the next year, for no known reason, Ms. Pieraccini resigned, and Cleanthe Logotheton resumed the position.

Another important change was the appointment of Milton Helpern, MD, as pathologist and director of laboratories (Fig. 6). He had been serving as

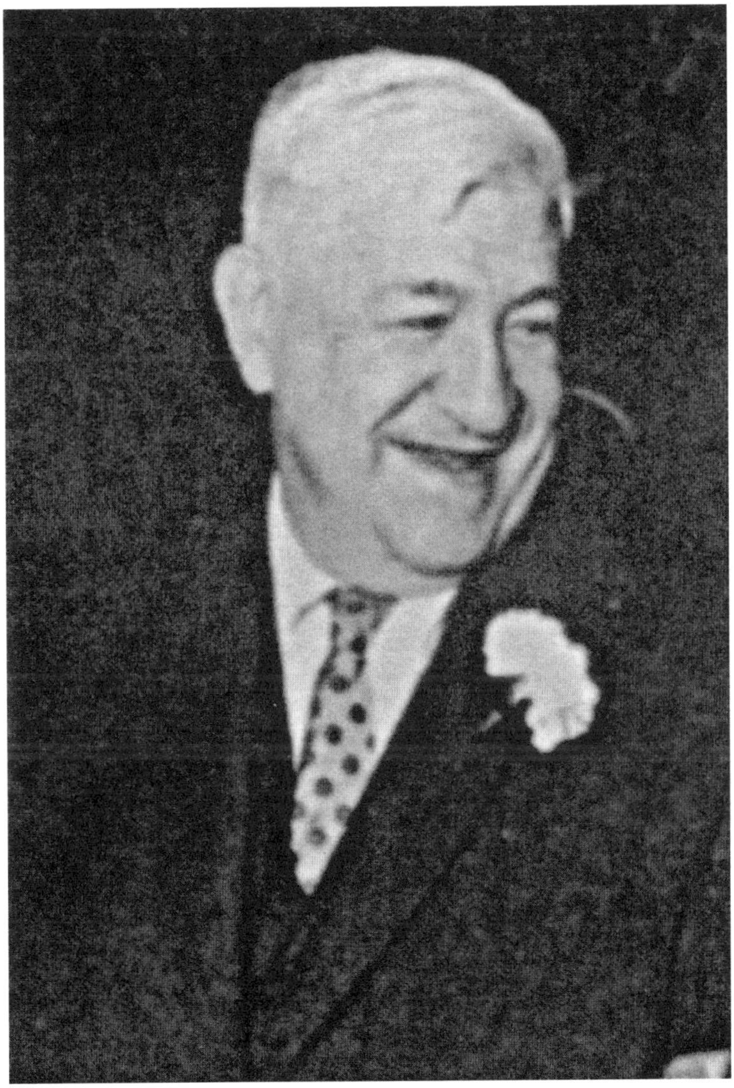

Fig. 6 Milton Helpern, MD, director of laboratories, as published in the hospital's newsletter, the *Record and Chronicle*, July 1966. (From Hospital for Special Surgery Archives)

acting director of laboratories while Dominic DeSanto, MD, the director, was in the military. After the war, DeSanto decided to accept another position in Los Angeles. Helpern's permanent appointment was of great importance because he was considered by the staff to be an excellent diagnostician, very skillful in his field, and always produced excellent reports.[16f]

Wilson, his staff, and a very able and supporting director of the hospital, F. Wilson Keller, courageously led the hospital through very challenging and disruptive years. Looking back, Wilson, a true orthopaedic pioneer, had the foresight and appreciation of long-term goals of the hospital and the ability to make such goals become reality.

In the nineteenth century, Virgil Gibney, surgically trained, possessed the organizational and communicative skills to convert a sleepy orthopaedic hospital, often with a pediatric inpatient length of stay of 2 years, into a true surgical facility. Gibney established the R&C as a leader of orthopaedic surgery at that time. In the twentieth century, Philip D. Wilson restored this distinction.[17]

REFERENCES

1. Beekman F. *Hospital for the Ruptured and Crippled. A Historical Sketch Written on the Occasion of the Seventy-fifth Anniversary of the Hospital.* New York, NY: privately printed; 1939.
2. Richmond JF. *New York and Its Institutions 1609–1872.* New York, NY: EB Treat; 1872.
3. Starr P. *The Social Transformation of American Medicine.* New York, NY: Basic Books; 1982.
4. McK Miller L. *Seventy-Seventh Annual Report of the New York Society for the Relief of the Ruptured and Crippled.* New York, NY: New York Society for the Relief of the Ruptured and Crippled; 1941.
5. Gibney RA. *Gibney of the Ruptured and Crippled.* New York, NY: Meredith Corporation; 1969.
6. Brown T, Brashear RH Jr., Curtiss PH Jr. *The American Orthopaedic Association, A Centennial History.* 1987.
7. Pearl Harbor, Hawaii, Sunday, December 7, 1941. Available at: http://www.historyplace.com/worldwar2/timeline/pearl.htm [accessed June 13, 2008].
8. Thompson TC. *Seventy-Eighth Annual Report of the New York Society for the Relief of the Ruptured and Crippled.* New York, NY: New York Society for the Relief of the Ruptured and Crippled; 1941.
9. Churchill Hospital. Oxford Health Archives. Available at: http://www.oxfordshirehealth-archives.nhs.uk/ [accessed June 14, 2008].

10. Wilson PD. *Seventy-Ninth Annual Report of the New York Society for the Relief of the Ruptured and Crippled.* New York, NY: New York Society for the Relief of the Ruptured and Crippled; 1942.
11. Holderfield R, Varhola M, Varhola MJ. *The Invasion of Normandy, June 6, 1944*, 1st ed. Conshohocken, PA: Savas Publishing; 2000.
12. Dougherty PJ, Carter PR, Seligson D, Benson, D, Purvis JM. Orthopaedic surgery advances resulting from World War II. *J Bone Joint Surg.* 2004;86A:176–181.
13. Keller FW. *Eighty-First Annual Report of the New York Society for the Relief of the Ruptured and Crippled.* New York, NY: New York Society for the Relief of the Ruptured and Crippled; 1944.
14. Keller FW. Record and Chronicle maintained by the Hospital for Special Surgery. 1942;(2):3.
15. Ward GC, Burns K. *The War: An Intimate History 1941–1945.* New York, NY: Alfred A. Knopf; 2007.
16. The Collections of the Milton Helpern Library of Legal Medicine. Available at: http://nyc.gov/html/doh/html/library/lib-helpern.shtml [accessed June 16, 2008].
17. Comorow A. Best hospitals. In: *Best Hospitals*, 2012 ed. Washington, DC: U.S. News & World Report; 2011:56–102.

NOTES

a. Beginning in the colonial era, the City of New York provided almshouses for the poor, sick, homeless, hungry, and destitute.

b. Such hospitals were called "voluntary" because they were supported by voluntary contributions and not taxes.

c. The name "The Hospital for Special Surgery" was later shortened to "Hospital for Special Surgery" in 1996.

d. Robert Lee Patterson Jr. (1907–1994) would eventually serve as surgeon-in-chief of the HSS (1963 1972). Presbyterian Hospital had its own orthopaedic staff until 1945, when New York Orthopaedic Hospital would merge with it.

e. Under General Kirk, the Army Medical Corps was expanded from 1,200 to 47,000 physicians, 15,000 dentists, and 500,000 personnel. President Harry S. Truman chose Kirk as his personal physician during the Potsdam Conference.

f. Eight years later in 1954, Helpern became the chief medical examiner of the City of New York, a post he held until 1973. He was professor and chairman of the Department of Forensic Medicine at New York University's School of Medicine from 1954 to 1974 and was on the faculty of Cornell University Medical College. He was referred to as the "world's greatest detective" and the foremost authority in forensic medicine.

CHAPTER 9

THE NEXT DECADE (1945–1955)

DAVID B. LEVINE, MD

RECALLING THE EARLY HISTORY OF the Hospital for the Ruptured and Crippled (R&C), many staff members had prominent medical school appointments. Besides Gibney's appointment in 1894 as the first professor of orthopaedic surgery at Columbia University College of Physicians and Surgeons, Bull held the professorship and the chair of surgery at the College of Physicians and Surgeons since 1899; William Coley was appointed professor of clinical surgery at Cornell University Medical College in 1911; and Eugene Pool had been appointed professor of clinical surgery at the College of Physicians and Surgeons in 1915. On staff at New York Hospital, Pool assumed the position of chief of the Second Surgical Division at Bellevue Hospital in 1932, when the hospital moved uptown to join Cornell University Medical College (Fig. 1). Simultaneously, he was appointed clinical professor of surgery at Cornell.

Academic Affiliation

When Wilson was selected to be the fifth surgeon-in-chief in 1934, a loose affiliation was arranged with the College of Physicians and Surgeons of Columbia University, of which Pool remarked: "This affiliation affords opportunity for contact with students and at the same time opens the way to cooperative use of the facilities of the two institutions which should prove of mutual benefit." Wilson was given the appointment of clinical professor of orthopaedic surgery in the College of Physicians and Surgeons (1934–1950).

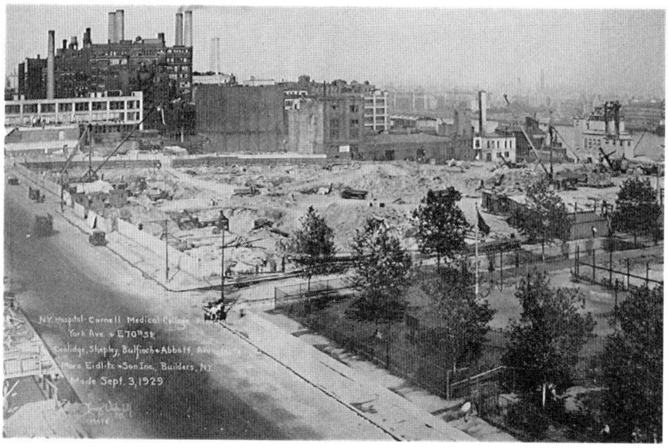

Fig. 1 The site of the future New York Hospital–Cornell Medical College in 1929, as seen looking south on the East River Drive at 70th Street. To the right, where some trees and a flag are pictured, is the future site of the Hospital for Special Surgery. (Courtesy of Medical Center Archives of New York–Presbyterian Hospital/Weill Cornell Medical Center)

This affiliation must have been less than formal, as there was little mention of it recorded in the HSS Annual Reports until 1943, when Wilson wrote:

> An innovation at the Hospital during the year was the assignment to us of medical students from the third year class of the College of Physicians and Surgeons, Columbia University. These men come to us in groups of three for a period of two months under an elective course in surgery. They are assigned in rotation to the Children's and Adult divisions of the Orthopaedic Service and to the Surgical Service. They spend five days a week at the hospital and assist in operations and in the treatment of patients. The course has proved popular and is booked full throughout the year. We enjoy the stimulating influence of these young men.[1]

In 1935, during Wilson's first year as surgeon-in-chief, the hospital's Board of Managers established a developing and planning committee to formulate long-range plans for the hospital. In 1945, at a special session of this committee, a number of prominent New Yorkers were invited to participate in discussing future plans for HSS (Table 1). In addition to patient care, the need for teaching and research led to the conclusion that a close affiliation of a medical school and teaching hospital was vital. Of prime importance was that such an affiliation

Table 1 Planning and Development Committee Members—1945

Willard C. Rappleye, MD—Dean of Columbia University College of Physicians and Surgeons
Alan Gregg, MD—Director of the Medical Division of the Rockefeller Foundation
The Honorable Edwin A. Salmon—Chairman of the Mayor's City Planning Commission
Leverett D. Bristol, MD—Executive director of the Hospital Council of Greater New York
Donald Sheehan, MD—Dean of the Medical College of New York University

must be structured to allow the Hospital for Special Surgery (HSS) to retain its autonomy.[2]

World War II

The hospital would often hold special teaching seminars and classes, and although not closely affiliated with a university, it always proclaimed to be a teaching hospital. At the end of the World War II, the U.S. Navy requested that a course in rehabilitation be held for the benefit of naval personnel. This course was held in cooperation with Hunter College in June and July 1944. One hundred fourteen Waves[a] and medical corpsmen attended lectures by the HSS orthopaedic staff three mornings per week (Fig. 2).

In October of that same year, a program of new developments from war injuries was held in cooperation with the New York Academy of Medicine's Annual Post Graduate Fortnight. Participating from HSS included Cdr. Thomas I. Hoen (1903–1978), Lt. Col. Peter Rizzo (1903–2001), and Lt. Col. T. Campbell Thompson. There were many other educational activities at the hospital, including a program in cooperation with the office of the Coordinator of Inter-American Affairs of the Department of the State, educating orthopaedic physicians from the South American republics.[3]

In 1945, with return of staff from the military, the hospital expanded many departments, including the laboratories, x-ray, and physical therapy. Orthopaedic residents were eligible to take courses in basic medical sciences at the College of Physicians and Surgeons of Columbia University and did so

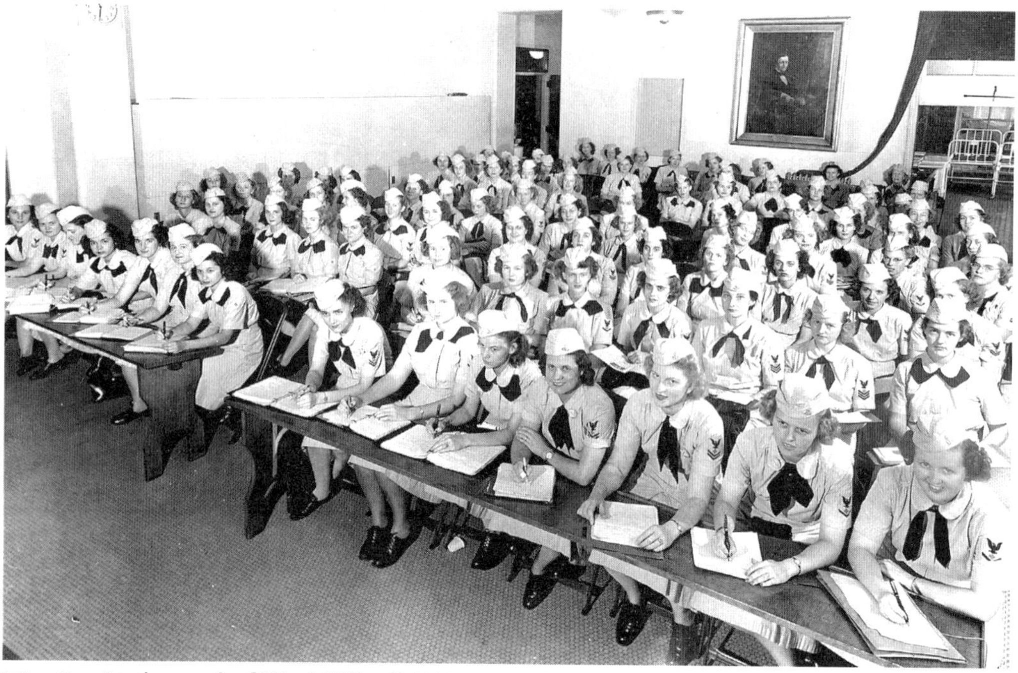

Fig. 2 At the end of World War II, WAVES and medical corpsmen from the U.S. Navy attended a 2-month course on rehabilitation at the Hospital for Special Surgery. Lectures were provided by orthopaedic staff who were already overburdened with work, as many had been deployed to the military. On the back wall hangs the original portrait of James Knight, MD, the founder and first surgeon-in-chief. (From Hospital for Special Surgery Archives)

when time permitted. Opportunities for anatomical dissection were also available to residents and attending staff at the medical school.

Although Wilson and many of the R&C staff had appointments at the medical school of Columbia University, there were obstacles in affiliating with that university. Major among them was that Columbia was not about to allow the HSS to retain its independence.[4]

At about this time, Columbia-Presbyterian Medical Center and the New York Orthopaedic Hospital (NYOH) merged, resulting in NYOH becoming the Orthopaedic Department of the medical center. This merger was ratified in 1945, and NYOH moved into the medical center in 1950, losing its independence.[5]

Negotiations proceeded with New York Hospital–Cornell Medical Center under the careful guidance of Wilson, who had the foresight to promote this affiliation. Fully supporting Wilson, the Planning Committee of the

Board of Managers of the HSS started meeting with members of the Joint Administrative Council of Cornell Medical Center. In order for the two institutions to have a close affiliation, it was decided that HSS would need to construct a new hospital adjacent to the medical center.[6]

During 1948, negotiations between representatives of the HSS Board and representatives of the Society of the New York Hospital progressed and a written agreement was executed in March 1949. The affiliation, which had the approval of the Hospital Council of Greater New York and was to be subject to the approval of the court, called for construction of a new building to house approximately 170 inpatient beds for orthopaedics and arthritis. The land on the East River between 70th and 71st Streets was owned by New York Hospital and was to be given, without monetary exchange, to HSS for its new facility.

Samuel S. Duryee (1893–1979) (Fig. 3), president of the Board of Managers of the New York Society of the Relief of the Ruptured and Crippled, wrote in his 1948 Annual Report:

> Although the hospitals will continue as independent corporations meeting their own operating costs and expenses, each will avail itself of the experience and facilities of the other; general surgery and internal medicine (other than arthritis) will be conducted in New York Hospital, and orthopaedics and arthritis in our Hospital. We believe that we have something to contribute for we are proud of our past and our present work. We know, however, that New York Hospital can help us because more and more it becomes apparent that a voluntary hospital with special interests such as ours must be closely identified with a great center of teaching and research in order to maintain the highest professional standards. For us to try independently to develop a new center would not make sense with a great center in existence a mile or so away. We doubt whether being "closely identified" means being anywhere other than "there"—as part of the center. But we could not move to the New York Hospital–Cornell Medical Center if it were not for what New York Hospital is doing for us. We are intensely interested in the care, treatment and rehabilitation of patients afflicted with crippling conditions including orthopaedics, poliomyelitis, cerebral palsy and arthritis. It's a broad field, but not an isolated one. If we have something to offer New York Hospital and if it has something to contribute to us, this pulling together without a merger but with our becoming in effect the orthopaedic service of New York Hospital while retaining our identity is a hostage to the vitality of voluntary hospitals.[7]

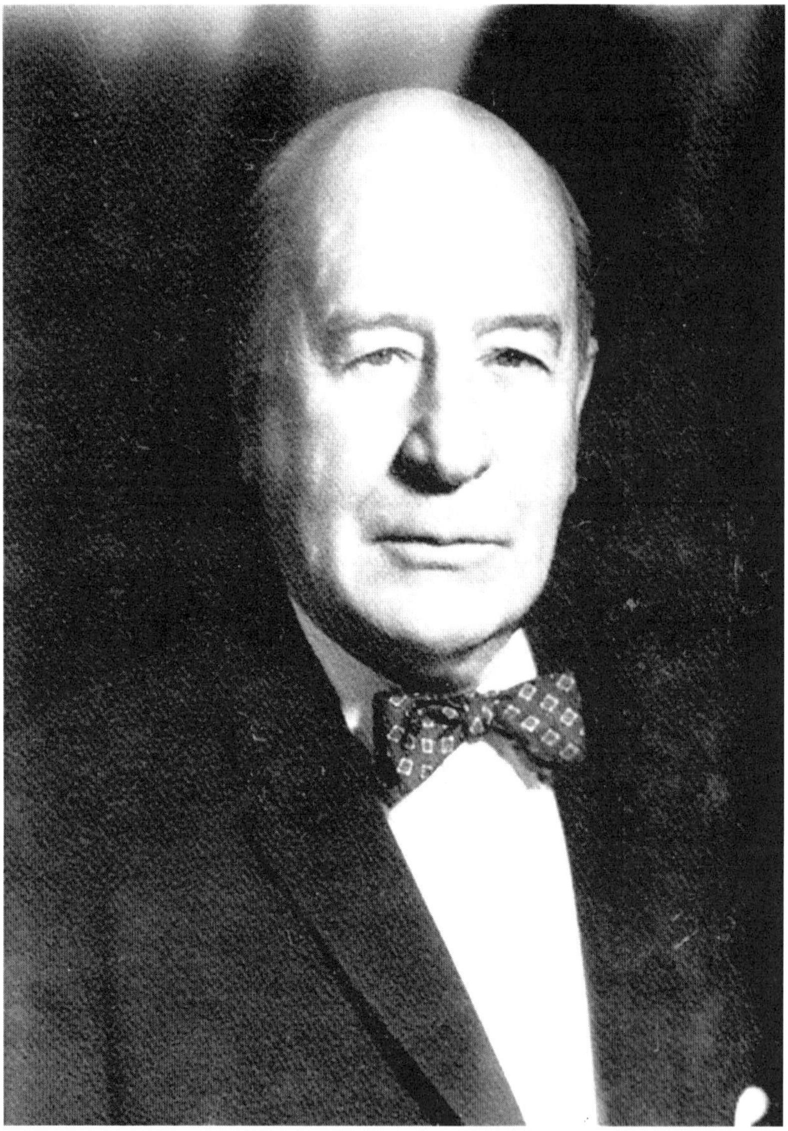

Fig. 3 Samuel S. Duryee (1893–1979), a New York attorney, served as president of the Board of Managers of the Hospital for Special Surgery from 1948 to 1958 and also as a governor of New York Hospital. He successfully led the negotiations of affiliation between the two hospitals. (From Hospital for Special Surgery Archives)

Although the architectural firm of Rogers and Butler was engaged in 1949 to begin designing the new hospital, plans were delayed because of continuous revisions. Expectations to sign the formal agreement were also delayed. Merging the two hospital staffs was complicated, as those on the New York

Hospital staff needed appointments to the HSS staff, and conversely HSS staff required appointments to New York Hospital. Arrangements for exchange of surgical and orthopaedic residents were facilitated by Frank Glenn, MD (1902–1982), chief of surgery at New York Hospital. Staff reciprocity included the Departments of Pediatrics and Medicine at New York Hospital, with the Rheumatology Department to reside in the HSS. The two institutions' Record Committees were confronted with selecting between a uniform record system for both hospitals or continuing independent record rooms.

A Nonproximate Agreement

Finally, on November 1, 1951, a new nonproximate agreement was ratified, and as of that date, the HSS Orthopaedic Department assumed the responsibility of staffing five orthopaedic outpatient clinics at New York Hospital. Weekly orthopaedic lectures for third-year medical students were provided by HSS staff. A 12-bed inpatient orthopaedic service was established at New York Hospital. Since the prior year, surgical residents rotated for four-month periods at HSS, and pediatric residents rotated there for two-month periods. Three senior orthopaedic surgeons from New York Hospital—Frederick Liebolt, MD (1905–1996), Thomas J. Dring, MD, and John T. Croft, MD—were brought on staff at HSS.[8]

In the same year, the Board of Managers of HSS, fully supporting Wilson's vision of a building devoted to research, purchased an additional plot of land on the East River Drive between 71st and 72nd Streets for $400,000. Estimates of the cost of building the new hospital were about $6 million, which were to be funded by the sale of the old building on East 42nd Street for $2.5 million, a legacy of Mrs. Matthew Astor Wilks,[b] other capital funds of $2 million, and by $1.5 million in new money.

Excavation of the land proceeded in September 1953, with pouring of the concrete foundation in February 1954 (Fig. 4). The cornerstone was laid by Governor Thomas E. Dewey, Wilson, and board president Samuel Duryee on May 17, 1954. Erection of the steel framework began in June, and the building was closed in by December 1 (Fig. 5). Completion was in January 1955, and the new hospital opened that May. The final cost of the building and equipment came to what was originally estimated: $6 million in round figures.

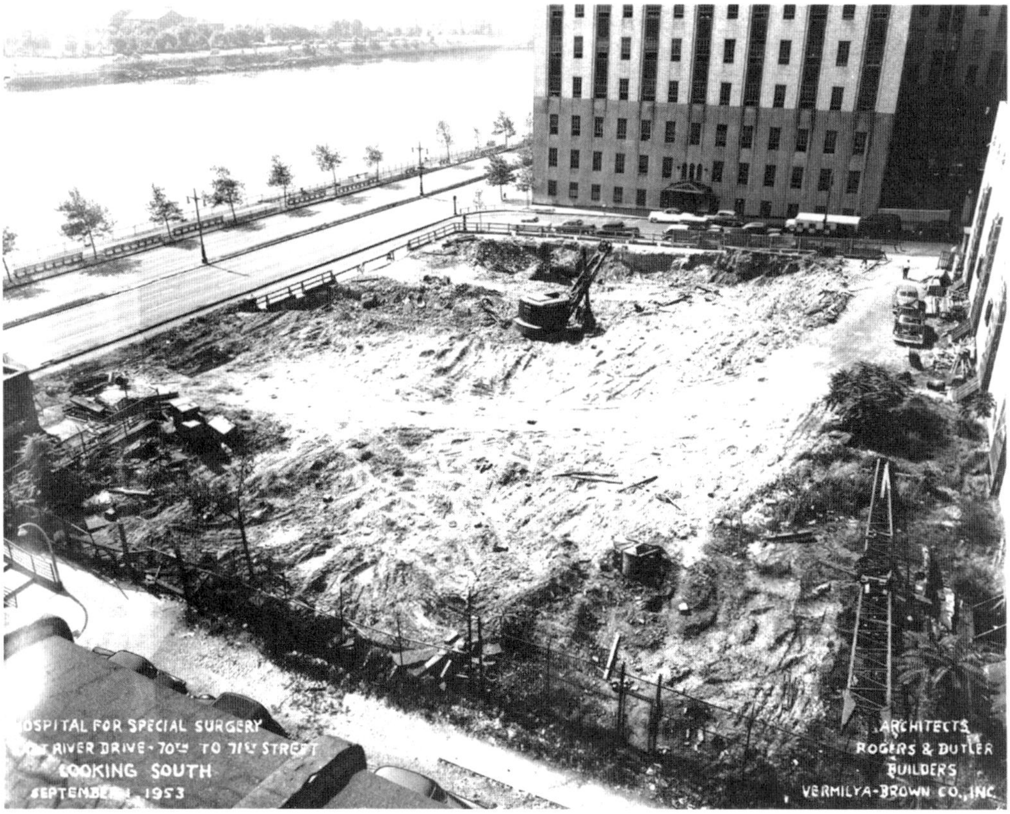

Fig. 4 Excavation for the foundation of Hospital for Special Surgery began in 1953. The site of the new hospital was located between East 70th and 71st Streets and the East River Drive. (From Hospital for Special Surgery Archives)

The "Boss"

Having made remarkable achievements in the first decade (1935–1945) in the office of surgeon-in-chief, Philip D. Wilson continued to restore the hospital to a leading institution in the orthopaedic world. In the latter decade (1945–1955), besides establishing a university affiliation and moving the hospital into a new building, he continued to receive many professional awards and honors, including the King's Medal (England) in 1947; Chevalier, Legion of Honor (France) in 1947; and Honorary Commander, Order of the British Empire in 1948. In 1966, he also garnered the Docteur Honoris Causa from the Sorbonne (Table 2). He was known to have excellent organizational skills and was often asked to serve on many local and national medical committees, lending his expertise in public service to health insurance, children's problems and government agencies at all levels.[9]

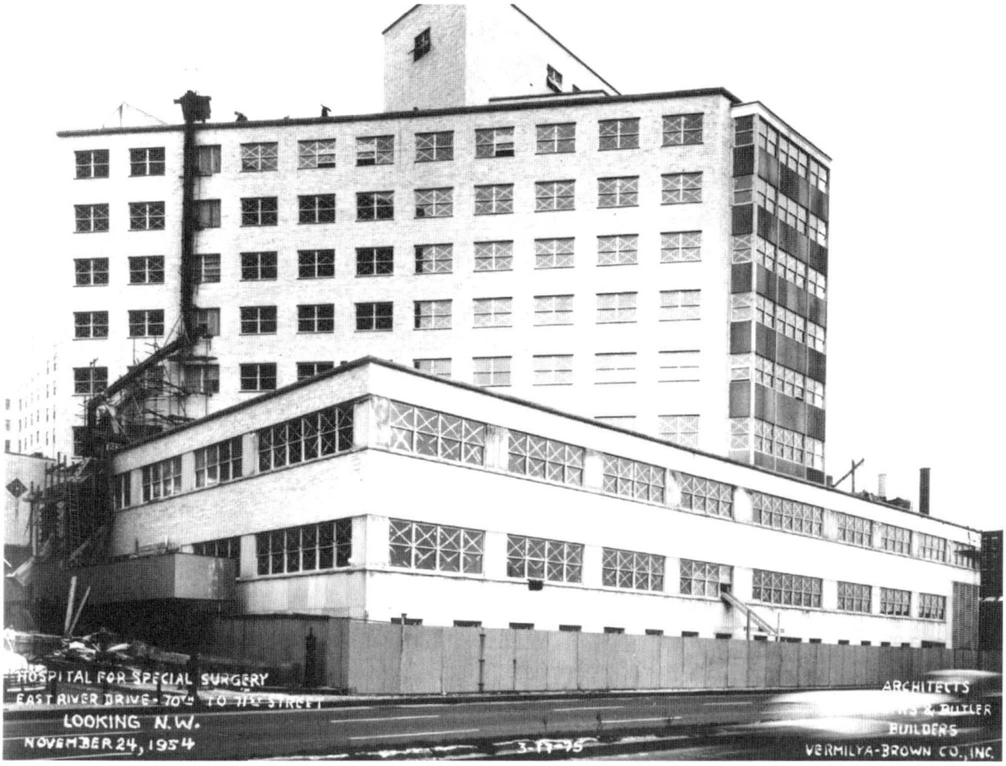

Fig. 5 Looking northwest from the East River Drive in November 1954, the external structure of HSS was nearly completed. The patients' rooms of the upper structure were located in the shape of an "A" so that most of the patients had a view of the East River. (From Hospital for Special Surgery Archives)

He continued to publish orthopaedic and other medical articles, edited or coauthored three books, and participated in numerous professional organizations in various ways. He was a born leader and was known by his colleagues, friends, and those whom he had trained (whom he called "his boys") as the "Boss"; however, his family referred to him as the "Skipper" because of his love for sailing.

Postgraduate training was very important to Wilson, and in 1951, he increased the length of the orthopaedic residency to 3 years by providing two extra 6-month rotations: one at the Kingsbridge Bronx Veterans Administration Hospital and the other on the fracture service of New York Hospital.[10]

A bone bank, one of the earliest in the nation, was established in January 1946. Sterile healthy bone taken at the time of certain orthopaedic operative procedures was stored under refrigeration at temperatures ranging from −10°C to −20°C for extended periods. The staff reported their results at

Table 2 Selected Organizations and Appointments of Philip D. Wilson, MD

Member
Medical Advisory Board of the Nemours Foundation and Alfred I. Dupont Institute
Board of Regents, American College of Surgeons
Board of Orthopaedic Research and Education Foundation (OREF)
Congress of the International Society of Orthopaedic Surgery and Traumatology (SICOT)
Chairman—1960
President—1963
Founding member
American Academy of Orthopaedic Surgeons (AAOS)
President 1935
American Board of Orthopaedic Surgeons (ABOS)
President 1943
Orthopaedic Research Society (ORS)
President 1957
Honorary fellow
Royal College of Surgeons of Edinburgh

scientific meetings and published bone bank results in orthopaedic journals, attracting many visiting physicians to the hospital to review banking methods.

During this era in 1947, the first mention of a scoliosis clinic, directed by John R. Cobb, MD, was reported in the 84th Annual Report. Also noted was the reactivation of the Cerebral Palsy Clinic under William Cooper, MD (1909–1970). At that time, the New York City Board of Education made provisions for a special school for children with cerebral palsy, under the medical supervision of the HSS—the first public school unit in New York City of its kind. A clinic for patients with clubfoot was directed by David Horwich, MD (1901–1975).

In 1951, a hand clinic was established under Lee Ramsay Straub, MD (1913–1994). In 1953, after Cobb was forced to restrict his practice because of illness, Philip D. Wilson Jr., MD, became Chief of the Scoliosis Clinic.

As surgeon-in-chief, Philip D. Wilson was especially recognized for his judgment, sound principles and truthfulness. In addition to these extraordinary qualities, he was compassionate, thoughtful, and considerate. He was also known to have great respect for those around him, whether they were family, friends, peers, students, or office staff.[c]

Famous Patients

Wilson's reputation as one of the most prominent orthopaedic surgeons in the world attracted patients from many parts of the globe. Some were famous; some had unusual conditions; and some could hardly afford to pay any fee for his advice and/or treatment. Frida Kahlo (1907–1954), the well-known Mexican artist, fit into all three categories when she consulted Wilson in 1946. Not only famous in her own right as an artist, she had been through a publicly tumultuous marriage and divorce (1929–1944) to the famous Mexican artist Diego Rivera (1886–1957). She experienced chronic, severe pain due to a fractured spine and multiple injuries resulting from a major bus accident in Mexico City in 1925 and had minimal funds. In June 1946, Wilson performed a four-level lumbar spinal fusion, inserting a steel plate in her back. She was in HSS for 2 months postoperatively. Although her back pain persisted, she considered Wilson to be "marvelous."[11]

President John F. Kennedy (1917–1963) suffered chronic back pain most of his adult life, even until his assassination in 1963. Having had a previous spinal laminectomy in 1944 at the Lahey Clinic, he consulted Wilson in 1954, who recommended a spinal fusion. On October 21, 1955, Kennedy—who at that time was a U.S. Senator from Massachusetts—underwent a posterior spinal fusion with a "Wilson plate" at HSS. His operative management was somewhat challenging, as he had been diagnosed with adrenocortical insufficiency (Addison disease) 7 years earlier. His postoperative course was complicated by a wound infection. Four months later, in February 1955, he underwent removal of the plate, with wound irrigation and open packing.[12,13] Another celebrity consulting Wilson was a well-known cabaret singer and screen star.

During the years 1941 through 1954, the director of the hospital was F. Wilson Keller (1897–1954), who was well respected by the staff and a loyal supporter of Wilson. Keller, a graduate of Ohio State University, had been appointed to this position after having accrued a wealth of experience: first, as an assistant director at Lenox Hill Hospital in New York City, and then as director of the Lawrence Hospital in Bronxville, New York. Wilson described him as a "real genius for organization and hospital leadership."[14]

During the period after the hospital signed the agreement of affiliation with New York Hospital–Cornell Medical Center, Keller immediately undertook a study of the space requirements for the new hospital. He based his conclusions on the current space and volume of departments, and the growth of such, and predicted requirements for assuming expansion of the Orthopaedic Department of New York Hospital. Unfortunately, he acquired an illness, which led to his death at age 57 years on May 7, 1954, before he could witness the completion of the new hospital.

On May 20, the Board of Managers appointed Theodore Gordon Young (1916–2005), who had been a young assistant to Keller, as the new director of HSS. Having received his BS degree from New York University with a major in personnel management, Young came to the HSS in July 1942. Four months

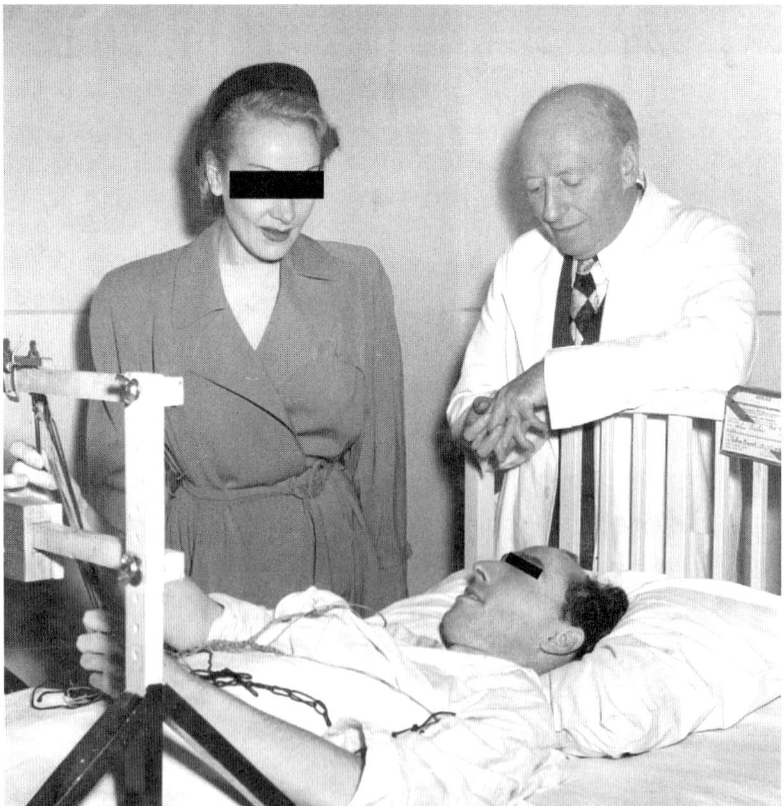

Fig. 6 A well known singer and screen star visited a patient with Philip D. Wilson, MD, at the Hospital for Special Surgery during the 1940s. (From Hospital for Special Surgery Archives)

Table 3 Specialty Clinics and Clinic Chiefs in the Department of Orthopaedics

Cerebral Palsy—William Cooper, MD
Clubfoot Clinic—Alexander Hersh, MD
Scoliosis Clinic—John R. Cobb, MD
Fracture Clinic—Robert Lee Patterson Jr., MD
Hand Clinic—Lee Ramsay Straub, MD
Amputee Clinic—T. Campbell Thompson, MD, and Jerome Lawrence, MD

later, he married Nola Rowland, an obstetric supervisor at Knickerbocker Hospital, who had left the farm life of Canada to come to New York. Later, when the hospital moved up to East 70th Street in 1955, they took up residence in an apartment created for them on the ninth floor of the new building. Young continued as administrator until his retirement in 1977, when Donald S. Broas (1940–2000) replaced him as executive director.

The Annual Report for the year 1953 listed the specialty clinics of the Orthopaedic Department for that year (Table 3).[15] Various other support departments existed prior to the hospital affiliation with New York Hospital (Table 4). The signed agreement in 1949 with New York Hospital–Cornell

Table 4 Supporting Department Chiefs/Attendings—1954

Surgery—John E. Sullivan, MD, chief
Thoracic Surgery—Charles W. Lester, MD, attending
Neurosurgery—Thomas I. Hoen, MD, attending
Otology and Laryngology—Paul H. Breuning, MD, attending
Ophthalmology—David H. Webster, MD, Gordon Cole, MD
Gynecology—George L. Bowen, MD
Urology—Thomas Morrissey, MD
Medicine and Pediatrics—Richard H. Freyberg, MD
Neurology and Psychiatry—Thomas E. Ramford, MD, Joseph Moldaver, MD
Pediatrics—Helen Harrington, MD
Dermatology and Syphilology—Royal Montgomery, MD, attending
Physical Medicine—Kristian G. Hansson, MD, director
Roentgenology—Harold G. Jacobson, MD, director
Laboratory, Pathology, and Research—Milton Helpern, MD, director
Anesthesiology—Charles H. Burstein, MD, chief
Dental—Edward Stroh, DDS, director
Podiatry—Samuel Brezak, Pod.D, director

Medical Center stipulated that the new hospital would be limited to the fields of orthopaedic surgery and rheumatic diseases, unfortunately eliminating the R&C staff of the Department of General Surgery and all surgical specialties. In many cases, some of the staff received privileges at New York Hospital, while others had time to obtain hospital privileges elsewhere. Wilson reported that the loss of a close affiliation with these fine and loyal members of the medical staff of the HSS would cast a shadow for many years to come upon the happiness of the move to the new hospital.

On May 1, 1954, the director of the laboratories, Milton Helpern, was promoted to the position of chief medical examiner of the City of New York by Mayor Robert F. Wagner Jr. (1910–1991). He held the position of professor and chairman of the Department of Forensic Medicine of New York University's School of Medicine from 1954 to 1974 and continued to hold an appointment at Cornell University Medical College.

The Manhattan Transfer

In 1955, the duration of the orthopaedic residency program again was increased to 3.5 years, from the 3-year training program instituted in 1951, with one resident starting every 3 months. The hospital was preparing for its move uptown. Mary Jeanne Clapp, RN, was appointed director of nursing, replacing Cleanthe E. Logotheton, who had been directress of nursing since 1942. Wilson announced his plans to retire.

On May 25, 1955, after 43 years at 321 East 42nd Street, the HSS moved to its new $6 million building at 535 East 70th Street. The move occurred during a time of relative international and domestic tranquility, with low interest rates, low inflation, and plentiful and cheap oil—a period of postbellum prosperity, with life less complicated, and slower moving than at the time of this writing. Dwight D. Eisenhower, the 34th president of the United States, was 2 years into his first term of office. That year, the hospital's average length of stay was 25 days, with 1,500 operative procedures performed annually.

T. Gordon Young, the benevolent administrator who was known for his concern, compassion, and attention to detail, named the moving day the "Manhattan Transfer." Seventy-three patients were relocated without incident before noon, in less than 2.5 hours, in time to have their lunch in the new building. The HSS nurses played a major role in this success story.[16]

On July 1, 1955, Philip D. Wilson, age 69 years, stepped down as surgeon-in-chief to assume the new titles of director of research and emeritus surgeon-in-chief at HSS.

REFERENCES

1. Wilson PD. *Eightieth Annual Report of the New York Society for the Relief of the Ruptured and Crippled.* New York, NY: New York Society for the Relief of the Ruptured and Crippled; 1943.
2. Wilson PD. *Eighty-First Annual Report of the New York Society for the Relief of the Ruptured and Crippled.* New York, NY: New York Society for the Relief of the Ruptured and Crippled; 1944.
3. Keller FW. *Eighty-Second Annual Report of the New York Society for the Relief of the Ruptured and Crippled.* New York, NY: New York Society for the Relief of the Ruptured and Crippled; 1945.
4. Wilson PD Jr. Personal communication. 2009.
5. Shookster L. The role of Theodore Roosevelt's family in the founding of the New York Orthopedic Hospital. *Theodore Roosevelt Assoc J.* 2007;28:8.
6. Wilson PD. *Eighty-Fourth Annual Report of the New York Society for the Relief of the Ruptured and Crippled.* New York, NY: New York Society for the Relief of the Ruptured and Crippled; 1947.
7. Duryee SS. *Eighty-Fifth Annual Report of the New York Society for the Relief of the Ruptured and Crippled.* New York, NY: New York Society for the Relief of the Ruptured and Crippled; 1948.
8. Duryee SS, Wilson PD. *Eighty-Eighth Annual Report of the New York Society for the Relief of the Ruptured and Crippled.* New York, NY: New York Society for the Relief of the Ruptured and Crippled; 1951.
9. Platt H. Philip Duncan Wilson, MD, 1886–1969. *J Bone Joint Surg.* 1969;51A:1445–1450.
10. Wilson PD Jr., Levine DB. Hospital for Special Surgery. A brief review of its development and current position. *Clin Orthop.* 2000;374:90–105.
11. Herrera H. *Frida: A Biography of Frida Kahlo.* New York, NY: Harper & Row Publishers; 1938.
12. Hart RA. Failed spine surgery syndrome in the life and career of John Fitzgerald Kennedy. *J Bone Joint Surg.* 2006;88:1141–1148.
13. Nicholas JA, Burstein CL, Umberger CJ. Management of adrenocortical insufficiency during surgery. *AMA Arch Surg.* 1995;71:737–742.

14. Wilson PD. *Ninety-First Annual Report of the New York Society for the Relief of the Ruptured and Crippled.* New York, NY: New York Society for the Relief of the Ruptured and Crippled; 1954.
15. Wilson PD. *Ninetieth Annual Report of the New York Society for the Relief of the Ruptured and Crippled.* New York, NY: New York Society for the Relief of the Ruptured and Crippled; 1953.
16. Levine DB. The Manhattan Transfer—celebrating our 50th anniversary, 1955–2005. *HSS Alumni News.* Spring 2005.

NOTES

a. The WAVES were a World War II–era division of the U.S. Navy that consisted entirely of women. The name of this group was an acronym for "Women Accepted for Volunteer Emergency Service." Established in 1942, it ceased to exist with the passage of the Women's Armed Services Integration Act (Public Law 625) on June 12, 1948, when women gained permanent status in the armed services.

b. Sylvia Green married Mathew Astor Wilks in 1909. She was the daughter of Hetty Robinson Green, known as the "richest woman in the world." Also known as the "Witch of Wall Street," she was described as being frugal and even a miser, and trusted no one with her money. When Hetty Green died in 1916, she left between $100 and $200 million ($2.4 billion in 2011 dollars). When her daughter, Sylvia Green Wilks, died, her estate left HSS over $1.2 million (equal to over $10 million in 2011 dollars).

c. Near the end of Wilson's career, after I finished my orthopaedic residency at HSS in 1964, I was honored to be asked join the office of Philip D. Wilson, Ramsay Straub, Philip D. Wilson Jr., and Harlan Amstutz. Our office had a number of secretaries who were originally hired by the "Boss" (Wilson) and were so loyal that they rarely left for other employment. On Friday afternoons, after all patients were seen, Wilson invited all of us, including our office staff, for a social hour. In January 1966, when I returned from California after finishing my scoliosis fellowship, the annual meeting of the American Academy of Orthopaedic Surgeons was held in Chicago. Only Wilson and I remained to cover the hospital. A plastic surgeon's wife sustained a transverse fracture of her patella, and I performed the surgery—one of my first operative cases as an attending. It was a great comfort for me to discuss the planned approach with Dr. Wilson. He treated me like a colleague who had been around for years. In fact, during the years in his office, the five of us often took equal night calls.

CHAPTER 10
T. CAMPBELL THOMPSON, MD
SIXTH SURGEON-IN-CHIEF (1955–1963)
ROBERT LEE PATTERSON JR., MD
SEVENTH SURGEON-IN-CHIEF (1963–1972)

DAVID B. LEVINE, MD

THE BOARD OF MANAGERS APPOINTED T. Campbell Thompson, MD (1902–1986), as the sixth surgeon-in-chief of the Hospital for Special Surgery (HSS). He assumed that office on July 1, 1955. During the previous year, Thompson had served as President of the American Academy of Orthopaedic Surgeons.

Thompson was born November 11, 1902 in Ishpeming (an Indian name for "heaven"), a small town in Michigan known as the birthplace of organized skiing in the United States and for its iron ore mines. His father, Henry S. Thompson, was in the mining business, as was his maternal grandfather. His mother, Myrtle T. Thompson, named their son Theodore after her brother and Campbell after his father's brother, Theodore. Growing up, Theodore Campbell Thompson (he never liked either given name) was called "Pete" by his father and brothers. Eventually, he settled for T. Campbell, but he was better known for the rest of his life by his friends and relatives as "Tommy." His initials "TCT" were widely recognized in his later professional life at the hospital.[1]

In his teenage years, he was known to dislike having his picture taken, and once was quoted as saying, "I hate mirrors." In the many sports in which he acquired skills, tennis and swimming were his favorites, and later golf. His love for playing the piano often fostered duets with his younger sister. In later years (September 1934), when Thompson joined the staff at the Hospital for the Ruptured and Crippled (R&C), he rented a one-bedroom apartment in Tudor City[a] and bought his first piece of furniture—a piano.

Educated at the local high school in Ishpemming, he studied at the University of Michigan for 1 year in 1920 and then received his AB degree from Rollins College in 1924. In the summer of 1923, Thompson experienced a serious accident. While working in a steel mill on the night shift, running a planer (set at ¾ inch), his left arm went through the planer up to his elbow. He was able to turn off the machine. No one was near, and because of the usual loud factory clamor, his attempt to call for help went unheeded. So he decided to reverse the machine to extract his arm. Several orthopaedic consultants recommended amputation, but a local surgeon was able to save his arm after multiple tendon and skin graft procedures, allowing him to return to classes in the fall and ultimately pursue a career as a surgeon.[2]

Thompson was accepted at Johns Hopkins Medical School in 1924 and received his MD degree in 1928. Having decided to go into orthopaedics, he completed his residency at Johns Hopkins under George Bennett, MD, professor of orthopaedics.[b] Thompson also spent some time as a resident surgeon at the Wingfield Morris Orthopaedic Hospital in Oxford, England, in 1934. There he published a paper on experimental muscular atrophy while working at the Sir William Dunn School of Pathology.[3] In a rabbit study (10 normal and 2 with miliary tuberculosis), he immobilized the rabbits in plaster, resulting in extensive muscular atrophy, and showed that weight-bearing could lessen any atrophy considerably.

After finishing his training in 1934, Thompson was recruited to the R&C staff by Wilson on recommendation from Bennett, his old friend (Fig. 1). Thompson, with John R. Cobb, MD, and Marvin Stevens, MD, were appointed by Wilson as full-time fellows at the College of Physicians and Surgeons of Columbia University, being awarded a degree in medical science in orthopaedics in 1936.

Having settled in New York as a young attending at R&C, Thompson married Cornelia Tomlin in 1935, whom he had met 9 years earlier. Her father was a judge and her grandfather, Colonel Walter Taylor, was the adjutant to General Robert E. Lee during the Civil War. Their first child, Robert, was born in 1938, and their daughter, Cornelia, followed in 1940. (Robert eventually became an orthopaedic surgeon and set up a practice in Maryland.)

During World War II, Thompson served as a lieutenant colonel in the U.S. Army, heading the Amputation Center at Walter Reed Army General Hospital with Major Donald B. Slocum.

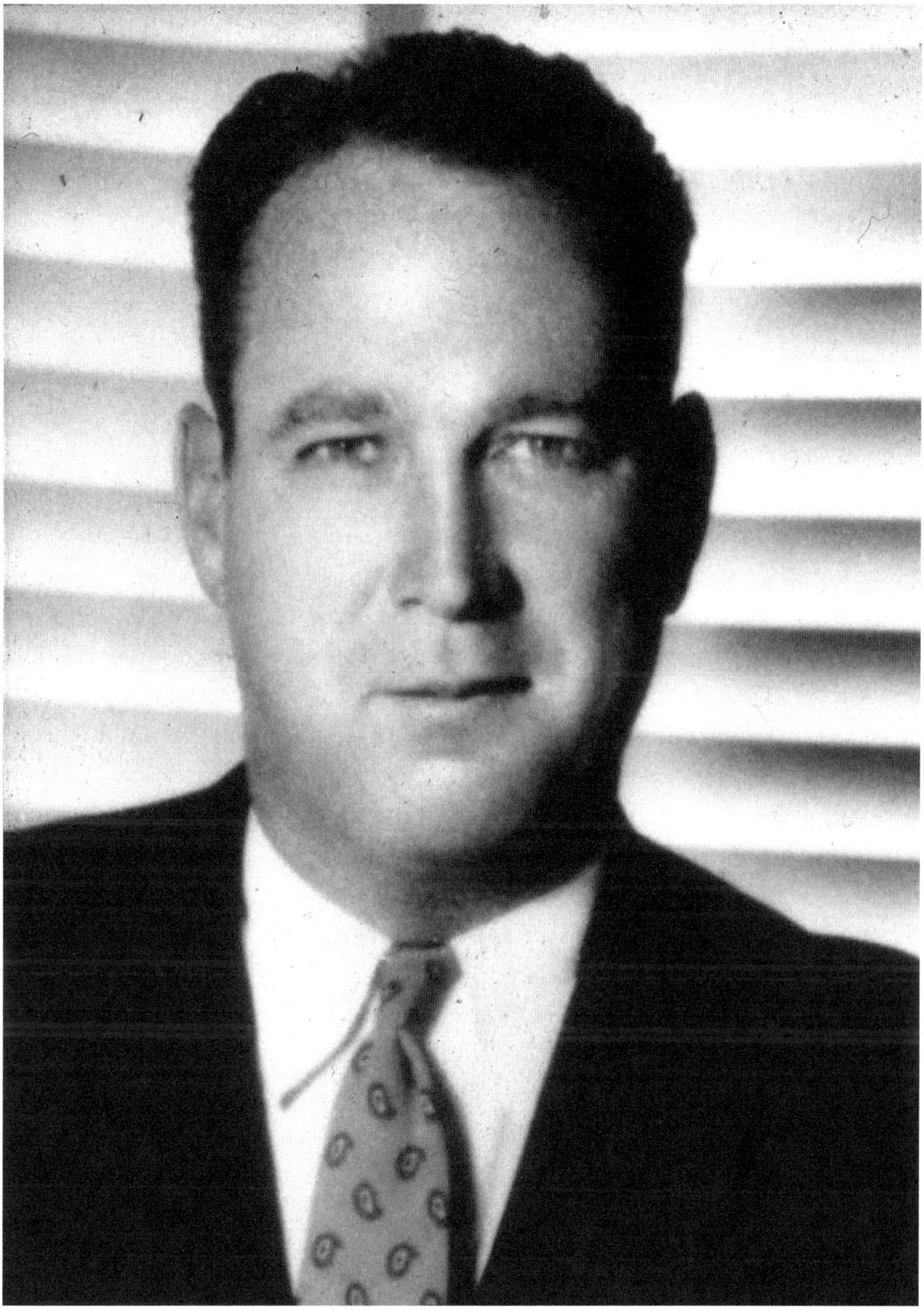

Fig. 1 After 2 years of study at the College of Physicians and Surgeons, T. Campbell Thompson was awarded a degree in medical science (DMSc) from Columbia University. He wrote his thesis on Lambrinudi foot stabilization. (From Hospital for Special Surgery Archives)

Besides being a superb teacher, clinician, and surgeon, Thompson made significant contributions to the field of orthopaedics, many of which are still cited today. In 1944, he published his surgical procedure of quadricepsplasty to improve knee function.[4] This technique was used to release a stiff knee following a fracture or other femoral trauma. Results of this surgery were favorably reported in the literature, particularly in British journals.

Thompson had extensive experience in postpolio deformities. In 1950, with coauthors L. I. Thomas, MD, and Lee Ramsay Straub, MD, he published a technique for transplanting the external oblique muscle for hip abductor paralysis.[5] Thompson performed the first of these procedures in 1941. Their study of 25 patients showed mixed results, with only 3 patients achieving excellent results and none having the abductor limp eliminated; in those days, however, this operative technique was considered to be one of the best.

In 1954, Thompson, Straub, and Rolla D. Campbell, MD (1920–2008), reported on the evaluation of femoral shortening with intramedullary nailing in 22 patients.[6] They concluded that the Kuntscher nail alone does not provide secure internal fixation and recommended oblique osteotomy with screw fixation.

In 1957, Thompson, Straub, and Arnold published a classic study of 25 cases from HSS of congenital absence of the fibula.[7] Thompson and his coauthors described, for the first time, the anatomical characteristics of the fibrous band found in all cases, defined its clinical significance, and recommended surgical treatment.

In a 1959 article published in the *Bulletin of the Hospital for Special Surgery*, Thompson outlined basic principles in selecting an operation or bracing for a paralyzed or artificial extremity.[8] He maintained that with these approaches, a lower extremity with little motor power could be made functional for walking.

One of the classic tests for the clinical diagnosis of a ruptured Achilles tendon is the "Thompson squeeze test," published in two separate journals.[9,10] The test is performed with the patient kneeling to relax the Achilles calf. The examiner squeezes the calf muscles. A normal response is plantar flexion of the foot. If there is a complete tendon rupture, the foot does not move.

The Manhattan Transfer

When the HSS, then 92 years old, made its move from 321 East 42nd Street to its new 6-million-dollar building at 535 East 70th Street on May 25, 1955—on

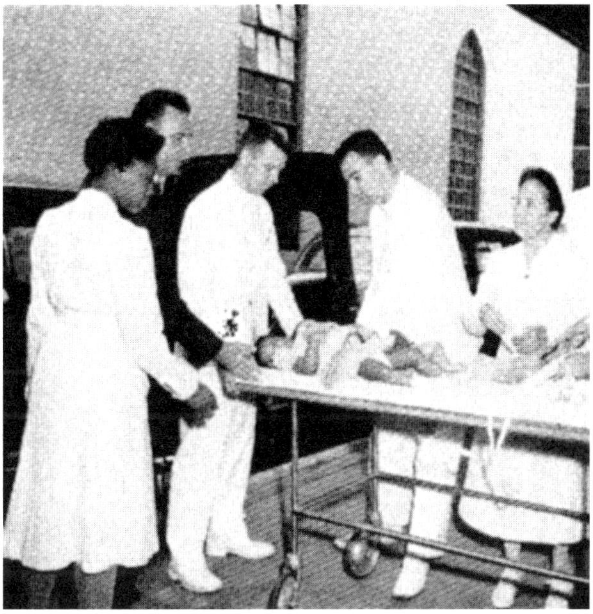

Fig. 2 May 25, 1955: Hospital for Special Surgery director T. Gordon Young (second from left), with two nurses and residents, supervises a patient being transferred from the old Hospital for Special Surgery to the new Hospital for Special Surgery on 70th Street. Young called the relocation the "Manhattan Transfer." (From Hospital for Special Surgery Archives)

the New York Hospital–Cornell Medical Center campus—the formal affiliation with the medical center was finally completed.

T. Gordon Young (1916–2005)—the HSS director who named this flawless move the "Manhattan Transfer"—was born in Long Branch, New Jersey, and received his BS degree in 1942 from New York University (Fig. 2).[11] With 4 years of experience working in hospitals, he was first appointed as an assistant administrator to F. Wilson Keller. As the new administrator, Young founded the Fifteen/Twenty-Five Year Club in April 1955. Membership included regular full-time employees, part-time employees (working 20 hours or more weekly), Board of Trustees, medical staff, and volunteers who have retired after 15 or 25 years of service at HSS in good standing. In 2005, this popular club celebrated its 50th anniversary.

The New 170-Bed Hospital

The eight-story, 170-bed hospital building with a basement and subbasement still had a few unfinished areas when patients were moved into their rooms,

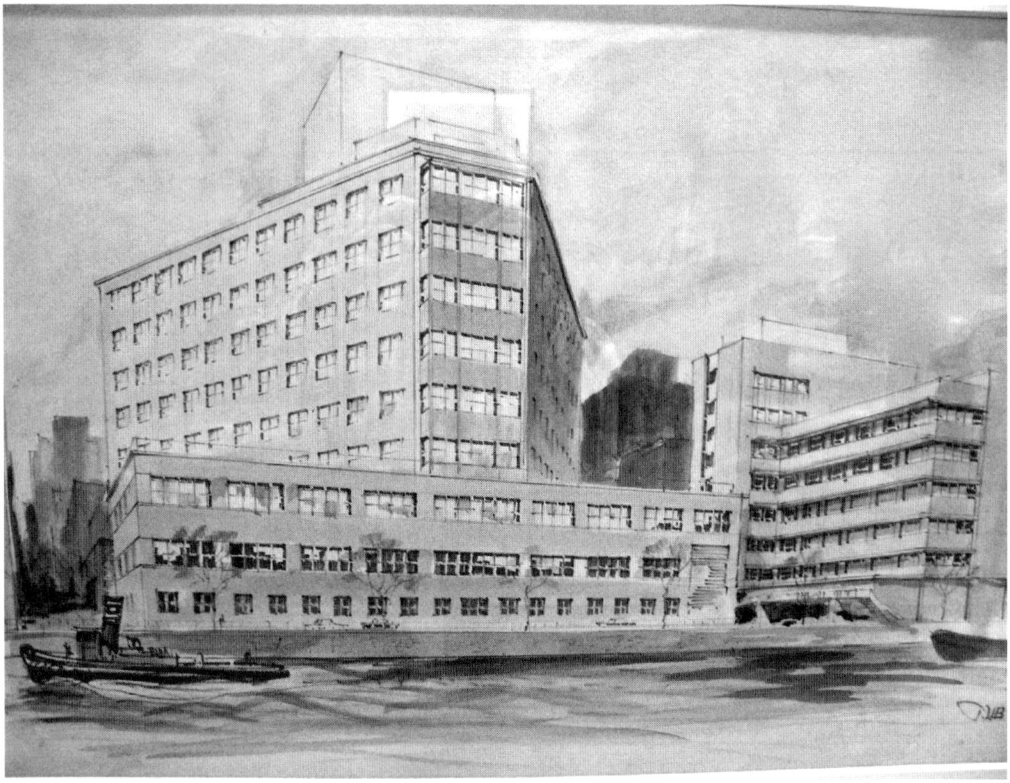

Fig. 3 Architecturally designed with most patient rooms facing the East River, the original eight-story Hospital for Special Surgery building was expanded over the East River Drive and additional floors added on top. The Caspary Research Building (right) was added in 1960. (From Hospital for Special Surgery Archives)

but otherwise provided state-of-the-art hospital amenities. It was connected to New York Hospital by an underground tunnel (with a branch separately connecting to Memorial Hospital). The architects, Rogers and Butler, designed the unique "A"-shaped building so practically all the patient rooms face the East River (Fig. 3). The building site was a gift from New York Hospital to HSS.

The main entrance to the building was located on the front driveway. On the ground floor was the Margaret M. Caspary Outpatient Clinic, with its entrance at the corner of the driveway and East 70th Street (Figs. 4 and 5). Among many gifts willed to the hospital from the Alfred H. Caspary Estate was a fishing lodge on over three acres of wooded land in the Catskill Mountains in upstate New York. It was designated as a vacation haven for HSS residents in training (Fig. 6).[12]

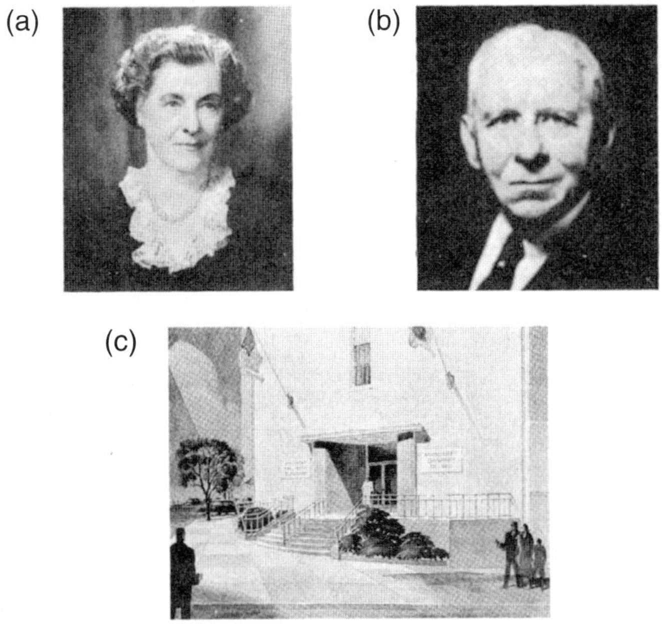

Fig. 4 (a) Margaret Caspary (birth year unknown–1953) was a patient of Philip D. Wilson Sr. (b) Her husband, Alfred H. Caspary (1877–1955), an investment banker, world-renowned philatelist and philanthropist, created one of the greatest stamp collections in philatelic history. He was a founder and member of the Expert Committee of the Philatelic Foundation and advisor to the Expert Committee of the Royal Philatelic Society in London. (c) Looking from East 70th Street: The original entrance to the Margaret M. Caspary Clinic. (From Hospital for Special Surgery Archives)

The Radiology Department, a large cast room overlooking the East River, the lobby with a telephone operator's switchboard, and support offices joined the clinic on the hospital's ground floor.

Facing the front on the second floor was a 48-seat auditorium built for conferences and other teaching rounds. Monday mornings were reserved for the End-Result Orthopaedic Conference, where postoperative patients were examined on stage (Fig. 7). There were two ratings: one by the patient and one by the surgeon. The auditorium was expanded and completely remodeled in 1997, being renamed the Richard L. Menschel Education Center at a dedication ceremony on October 16, 2003, the year Menschel stepped down as chairman of the Board of Trustees, a position he had held since 1991. Laboratories, the pharmacy, a therapeutic swimming pool,[c] and the Physical Therapy Department were also located on this floor.

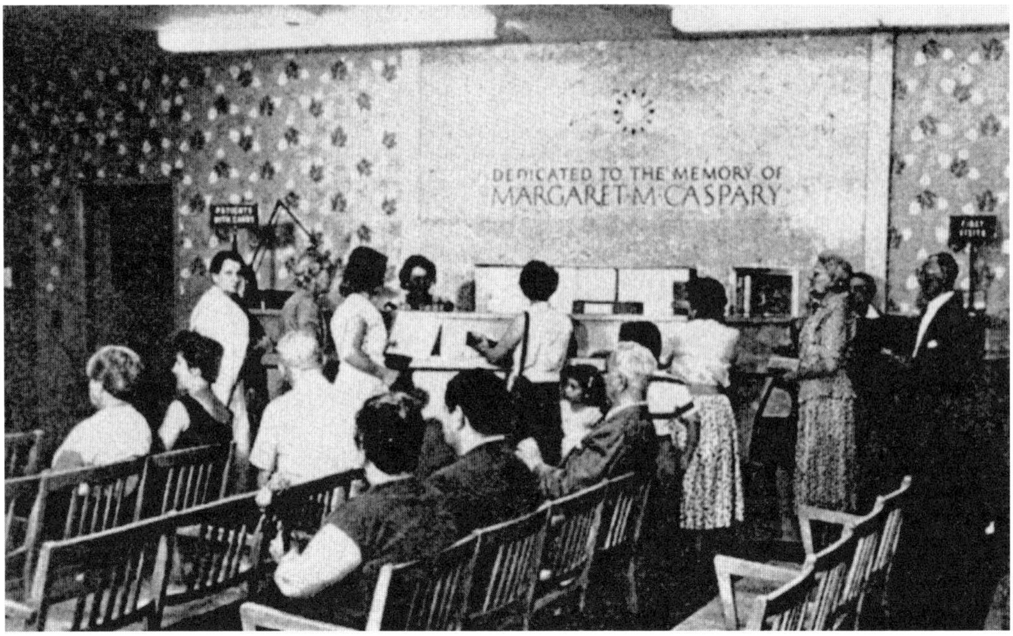

Fig. 5 The outpatient clinic was dedicated to Margaret M. Caspary, supported by a gift of $1.5 million[7] from her husband, Alfred H. Caspary, in 1955. This contribution was just one of many gifts from the Alfred H. Caspary estate to Hospital for Special Surgery, totaling close to $5 million.[16] (From Hospital for Special Surgery Archives)

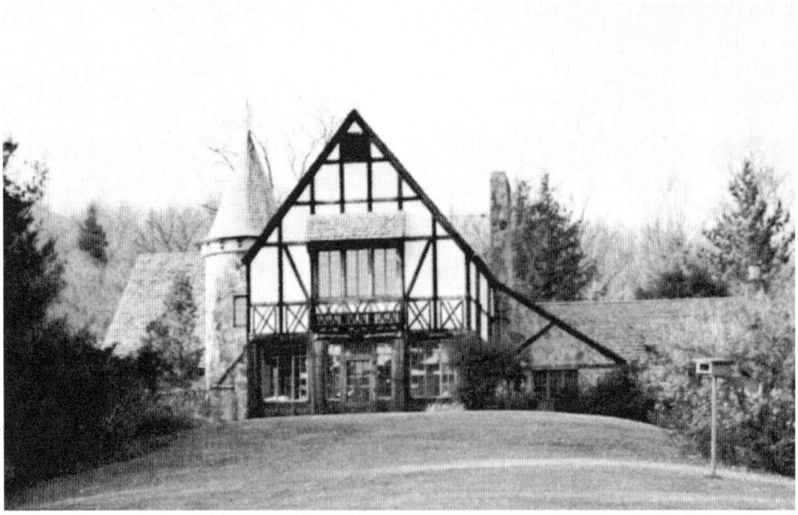

Fig. 6 The main Caspary lodge was built in 1929 with hand-sculptured beams imported from Europe, as a fishing lodge for Alfred Caspary. Funds from the Caspary estate were designated to allow maintenance of the property. (From Hospital for Special Surgery Archives)

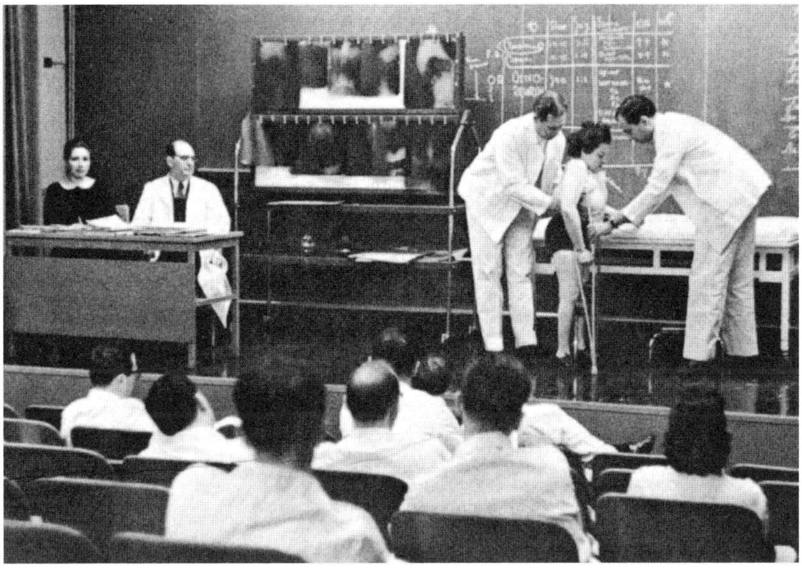

Fig. 7 Two residents present a postoperative patient in the second-floor conference room to John R. Cobb, MD, for rating by the patient and surgeon (circa late 1950s). (From Hospital for Special Surgery Archives)

Above the auditorium on the third floor was the cafeteria, whereas physicians' offices and examining rooms occupied the remainder of the floor (Fig. 8).

Four operating rooms and a five-bed recovery room shared the fourth floor, with on-call facilities for the house staff and a medical library first established by Wilson in 1935. Some 1,500 operative procedures were performed in 1955, with an average length of stay of 25 days.

The upper four floors provided inpatient rooms, with the fifth floor housing a New York City Public School.

The new affiliation expanded graduate education at both New York Hospital and HSS. By the end of 1956, six residents from New York Hospital were assigned to HSS at all times. There were two surgical residents on the Orthopaedic Service, two medical residents on the Rheumatic Disease Service, one pediatric resident, and one radiology resident.

From HSS, two orthopaedic residents were assigned to the fracture service at New York Hospital, where Robert Lee Patterson Jr., MD, and Preston Wade, MD (1901–1982), were co-chiefs. Four orthopaedic residents also rotated on the orthopaedic service at the Kingsbridge Bronx Veterans Administration Hospital. John H. Doherty, MD (1926–1999), who had just finished his HSS

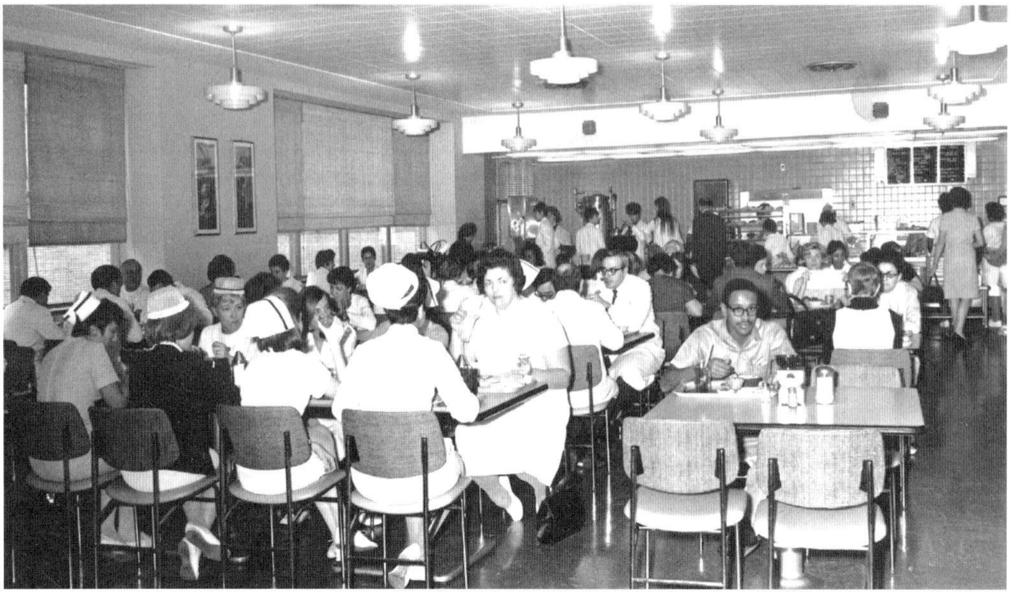

Fig. 8 The cafeteria, mainly for staff, was open daily for three meals. It was the soul of the hospital, where all levels of staff not only could share a meal, but also break up the workday. It was replaced in 1988 by the Belaire Café. (From Hospital for Special Surgery Archives)

orthopaedic residency, was chief of the service. The remaining 18 months were divided in general orthopaedics, for a total of 3 years of resident training. The program was soon expanded to 3.5 years, with the addition of Memorial Hospital rotations on the bone tumor service. Orthopaedic fellows served on various services for different periods and were expected to be involved in research projects, as were the orthopaedic residents.

Nursing at the hospital also witnessed changes after moving to the new building. In addition to the appointment of Mary Jeanne Clapp, RN, as director of nursing (Table 1), a new practical nursing school approved by New York State—the HSS School of Practical Nursing—admitted its first class on January 7, 1955, under the direction of D. Dean Smith, MS, RN, who had been instrumental in organizing the school. The purpose of the school was to train licensed practical nurses (LPNs) to work under physicians and RNs. The school encouraged further nursing education, and 75% of graduates continued their studies for advanced degrees. In the 1960s, nursing education followed new roads in higher education, and in 1996, the HSS practical nursing school was closed.[13]

Table 1 Chief Nursing Officers: The Hospital for the Ruptured and Crippled/ Hospital for Special Surgery

Ella S. Murdock *Matron*	1896–1911
Ella E. Patterson, RN *Matron and directress of nursing*	1912–1916
Jean L. England *Matron and directress of nursing*	1917–1924
Ethel B. Ridley, RN *Directress of nursing*	1924–1942
Cleanthe E. Logotheton *Directress of nursing*	1942–1954
Mary Jeanne Clapp, RN *Director of nursing*	1954–1965
D. Dean Smith, MA, RN *Director of nursing*	1965–1977
Barbara J. Kelly, MA, RN *Director of nursing*	1977–1989
Susan Bowar-Ferres, PhD, RN, CNAA *Vice president for nursing*	1989–1997
Jacqueline Kostic, MS, RN, CNAA *Vice president for nursing*	1997–2005
Stephanie J. Goldberg, MS, RN, NEA-BC Senior vice president for patient care services Chief nursing officer	2005–present

In 1958, Robert H. Freiberger, MD, became the eighth director of roentgenology; Fred H. Albee, MD (1876–1945), had been the first part-time director in 1905. Freiberger established a radiology fellowship, developed a close link with New York Hospital's radiologists and provided daily reading of x-rays taken for the Fracture Department at New York Hospital (Fig. 9). He led the development of arthrography in the United States, which improved the visualization of cartilage and synovial lesions.[14]

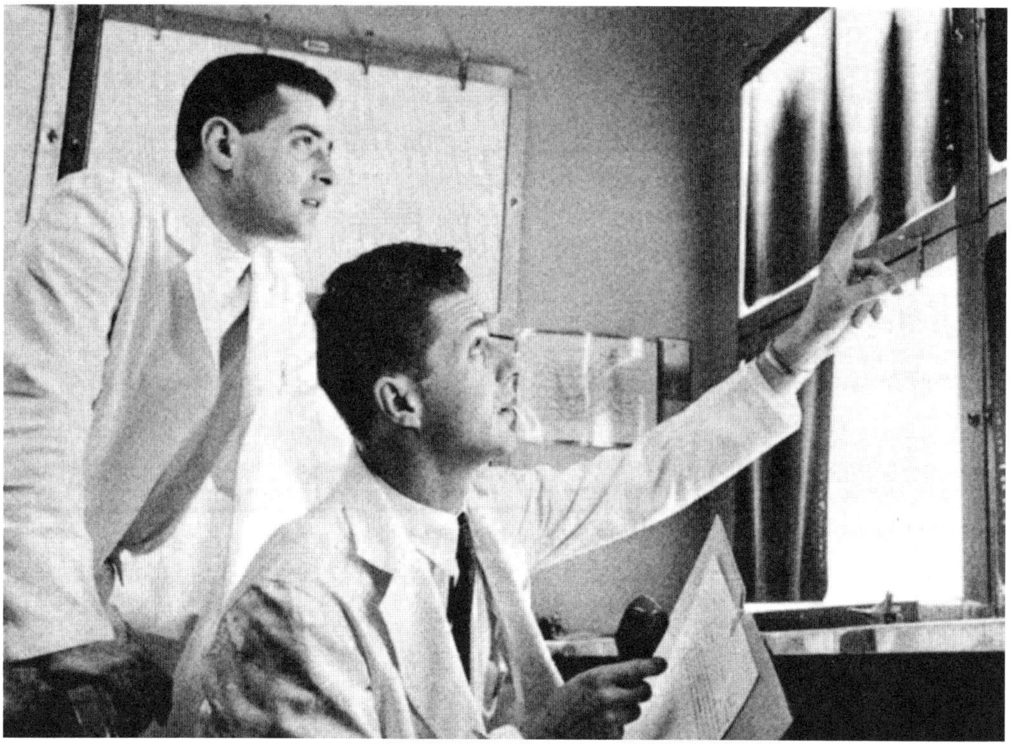

Fig. 9 Richard Freiberger, MD, with a member of the Hospital for Special Surgery house staff, reading an x-ray in 1957. His radiological diagnostic skills were often sought by Hospital for Special Surgery staff, who valued his clinical impressions and expert advice. (From Hospital for Special Surgery Archives)

That same year, groundbreaking began for a new research building on a lot on the corner of 71st Street and the East River Access Drive (Fig. 10). By the end of 1959, the new building was near completion and beginning to become occupied. The first floor contained facilities for animal research, whereas the upper floors included laboratories. The second floor eventually housed the Medical Library and the Medical Education Department, first established in 1961 by Johanna O. Vettoretti, the hospital's first electrocardiograph technician. She served as secretary to Wilson when she became the first coordinator of medical education. Robert C. Mellors, MD, chief of pathology and associate director of research, designed the third floor.

Alfred H. Caspary and other major donors supported the creation of the Philip D. Wilson Research Foundation, the administrative and financial entity overseeing the new building.[15] Wilson's vision of a separate research center at

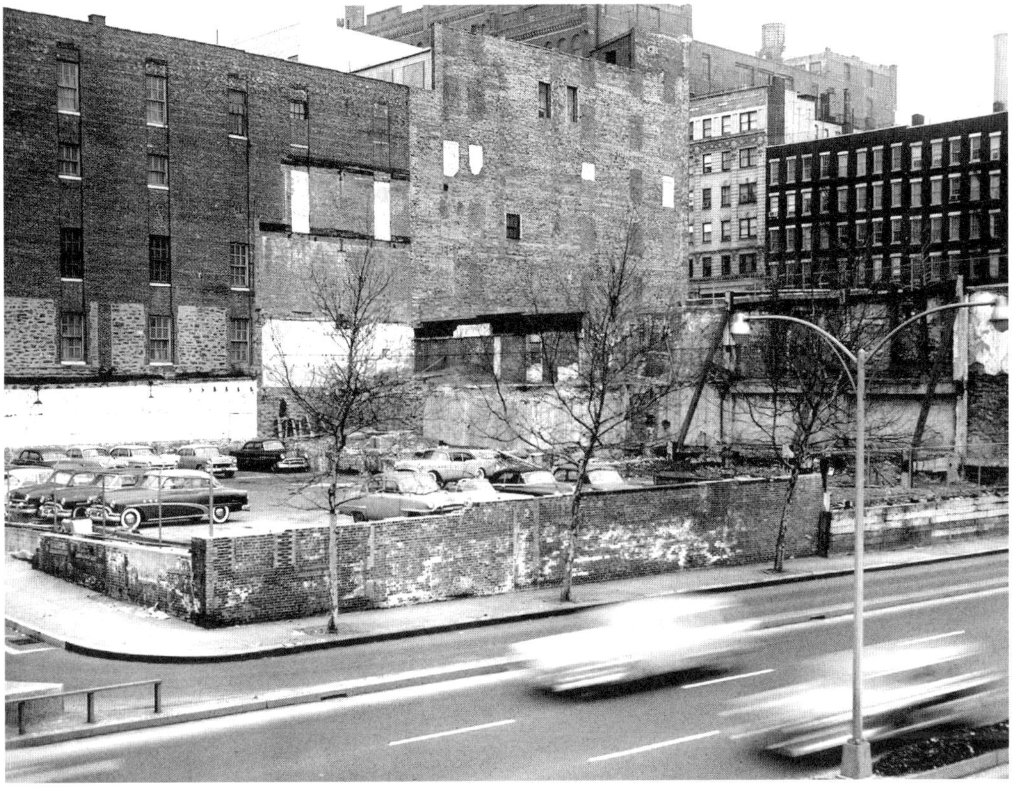

Fig. 10 Looking west from the East River Drive, a building lot between East 71st and 72nd Streets was purchased in 1956 for the future research building. The distant half of the lot, facing 72nd Street, was sold for commercial development. (From Hospital for Special Surgery Archives)

HSS finally came to fruition on November 16, 1960, when a dedication ceremony of the Alfred H. Caspary Research Building was held.

After 8 years as director of research, Wilson retired from that office on June 30, 1963, and was followed by Goran C. H. Bauer, MD (1924–1994), from Malmo, Sweden. At Lund University, Bauer had defended his doctoral thesis on bone mineral kinematics in 1954. After serving as director of research and attending orthopaedic surgeon (and chief of the Knee Clinic) at HSS until 1969, Bauer then returned to Sweden, where he was appointed professor of orthopaedics and chairman of the Department of Orthopaedics at Lund University. He held that post for 20 years until his retirement in 1989. In 1983, Bauer assumed the editorship of *Acta Orthopaedica Scandinavica*, "a commission he conducted with skill and enthusiasm until his death."[16]

R&C still had a limited number of specialty clinics, but one of the earliest, the Scoliosis Clinic, was founded by Cobb in 1947. A graduate of Yale Medical School in 1930, John Cobb had a degree in English literature from Brown University, where he was a member of the swim team. He was born in New York, the second of six children, and attended Stanton Military Institute in Virginia, graduating in 1921.[17]

Cobb became one of the great giants of his time in scoliosis and attracted many foreign fellows, visitors, and interested orthopaedic surgeons from around the world to the hospital. His treatment of scoliosis using the turnbuckle cast method was emulated by many orthopaedic centers (Fig. 11). His measurement of curves, known as the "Cobb angle"—still the benchmark of measuring scoliosis curves—was reproduced in a pocket-sized plastic protractor, called the "Cobb protractor." Whenever a visiting surgeon ended his stay

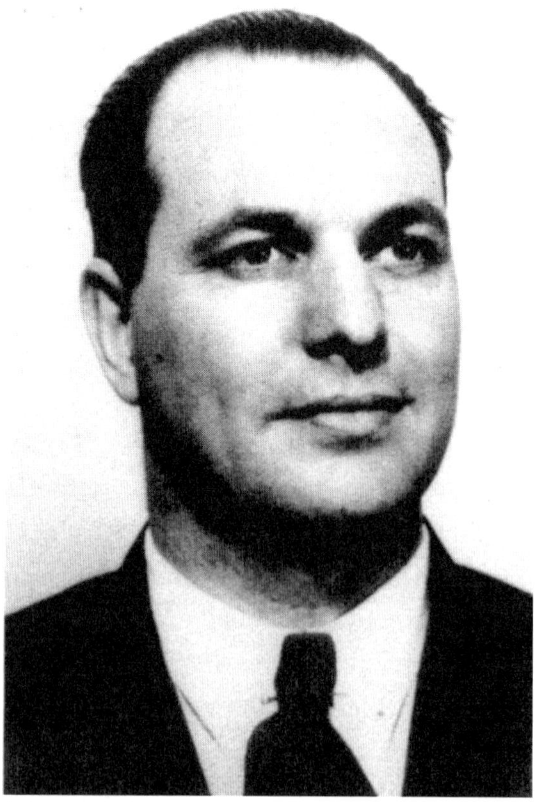

Fig. 11 John Cobb (circa 1940) was a careful and meticulous surgeon who watched over his scoliosis patients with great care and compassion and whose patients, in return, loved him. (From Hospital for Special Surgery Archives)

with Cobb (after weeks to months), he always left with the Cobb protractor, a compass, a set of directions for measuring curves, and a rubber mallet. Cobb believed that the rubber mallet, which he used with his gouges when performing a spine fusion, was less traumatic on the spine than a metal mallet.

His love of language and poetry was often illustrated by his trove of many limericks, which he would recite with a little coaxing.[d] In 1954, he suffered a stroke from which he recovered, returning to full practice 2 years later. Cobb continued to practice until 1965, when he suffered a second stroke. He died in 1967 at the age of 64 years.

The Hand Service, under the direction of Straub, developed into one of the most distinguished hand centers in the United States. A 1-year hand fellowship was very competitive and sought by many young orthopaedic surgeons throughout the world. Straub was a founding member of the American Society for Surgery of the Hand, established after World War II in 1946 by Sterling Bunnell, MD (1882–1957), the world-renowned hand surgeon. Among the many honors received and offices held, Straub was particularly proud of his election as president of the American Orthopaedic Association (AOA) in 1968.

In 1967, Straub's orthopaedic interests expanded when he and Richard Freyberg, MD (1904–1999), director of rheumatology since 1944, formed the Comprehensive Arthritis Program (CAP) for patients with severe arthritis who would benefit from joint surgery. This became the prototype for similar programs in other hospitals around the world.

Lee Ramsay Straub (Fig. 12), the youngest of three brothers and three sisters, traced his roots back to John Ramsay, who sailed in 1776 from Kintire, Scotland, became shipwrecked off the coast of Prince Edward Island and settled there to raise a family. Lee Ramsay (in later years, he preferred to be called Ramsay) was born in Perth Amboy, New Jersey, on December 12, 1913. During his early years, he underwent a number of operations for congenital unilateral hemangiomas, one reason for his interest in pursuing medicine as a profession. Furthermore, his early physical problem of chondromalacia of his knees resulted in multiple knee surgeries.[18] In his later years, he was very disabled, mainly because of his knees and arthritis, but he had great courage and continued to operate and examine patients, with the aid of an electric cart.

After attending the University of California, Berkley, Straub received his medical degree from the Medical School of McGill University. In Montreal,

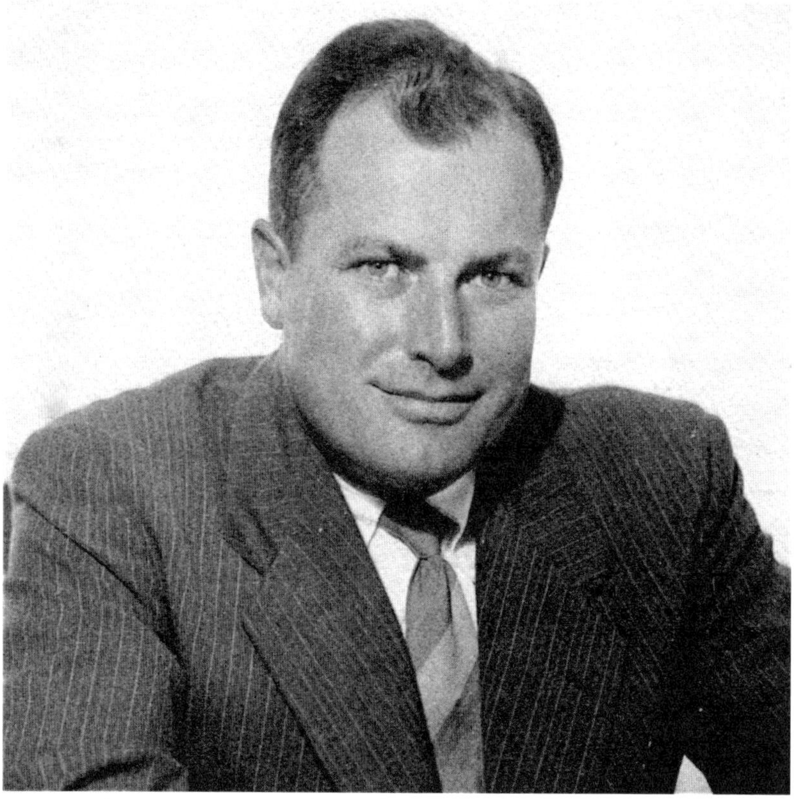

Fig. 12 Lee Ramsay Straub, MD (circa 1950s), was long recognized as one of the country's outstanding hand surgeons. He was executive assistant to the surgeon-in-chief under Philip D. Wilson Sr., MD, and directed the orthopaedic residency program at the hospital for many years. In his later years, he continued to practice orthopaedic surgery from a motorized chair. He was a special mentor to many who trained at Hospital for Special Surgery, including the author. (From Hospital for Special Surgery Archives)

he met his future wife, Mary, who came from Lethbridge, Alberta, and had trained as a physical therapist. They were married in New York in September 1941 and raised three sons—all eventually marrying a Mary (resulting in four Mary Straubs in one family).

Robert Lee Patterson Jr. Becomes Surgeon-in-Chief

In 1962, adverse relations between the HSS and New York Hospital–Cornell Medical Center seriously threatened the affiliation agreement between the two hospitals. Because of difficulties over a faculty and staff appointment, Thompson resigned from the office of surgeon-in-chief. He was replaced in

1963 by Robert Lee Patterson Jr., MD (1907–1994), who had first joined the staff of R&C in 1936 as a visiting surgeon.

T. Campbell Thompson continued to practice orthopaedics and devoted more time to teaching after his retirement as surgeon-in-chief. He was considered to be one of the best clinicians and surgeons in the hospital by his colleagues and an excellent teacher by his students. In conferences, he would often nod off for short periods of light sleep, but should a question be addressed to him, he immediately awakened and responded with a pertinent and knowledgeable answer. He died in 1986.

Robert Lee Patterson Jr., MD, who had been co-chief of the combined New York Hospital–HSS Fracture Service with his good friend and colleague, Preston Wade,[e] a general surgeon, had a number of other close ties with New York Hospital (Fig. 13). Patterson's older brother, Russell H. Patterson, MD (1890–1993), was a senior surgeon at New York Hospital, and his son, Russell H. Patterson Jr. became chief of neurosurgery there in 1971. After Robert Patterson assumed the office of HSS surgeon-in-chief, relations between the two hospitals improved.

The hospital celebrated its centennial anniversary in May 1963 with a 3-day scientific program, chaired by Philip D. Wilson Jr. who had joined the attending staff as an orthopaedic surgeon to the Outpatient Department in 1951. Wilson Jr. had trained as an orthopaedic resident at HSS from 1948 to 1950, and in 1951, he finished his residency at the University of California Hospital Medical Center, San Francisco.

Robert Lee Patterson, born in Athens, Georgia, was the youngest of five children. He graduated in 1928 from the University of Georgia, where he was elected to Phi Beta Kappa. His early intention was to become a minister. Having decided to pursue medicine, he was accepted at Harvard Medical School, receiving his medical degree in 1932. He then interned at Peter Bent Brigham Hospital and stayed in Boston to train as an orthopaedic resident at Children's Hospital and Massachusetts General Hospital. In 1935, he had 6 months of additional training on the Neurosurgical Trauma Service at Boston City Hospital.

Following his Boston experience, he came to New York, where he was an orthopaedic resident on the Fracture Service of Presbyterian Hospital. Completing his training in 1936, he was appointed by Wilson to the attending staff of R&C, where he was assigned to organize the Cerebral Palsy Clinic.

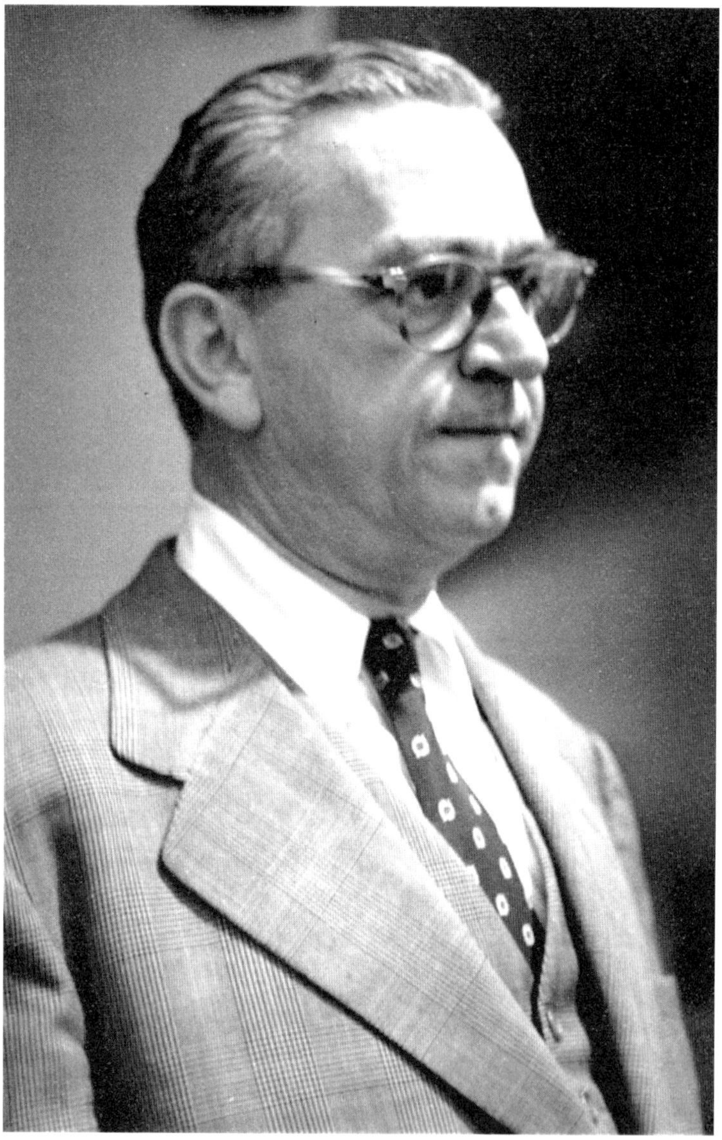

Fig. 13 Robert Lee Patterson Jr., MD (1954), just before he became co-chief of the New York Hospital–Hospital for Special Surgery Combined Fracture Service. As surgeon-in-chief, he took a special interest in all those whom he trained. With a pronounced Southern drawl, he often referred to his roots from Georgia and Harvard. (From Hospital for Special Surgery Archives)

On May 1, 1937, Patterson married Margaret Douglas Sloane, daughter of Mrs. William Sloane and the late William Sloane in a ceremony at the Union Theological Society in New York. Her father was the founder of the famous Sloane Furniture store in 1843 in New York.[f]

During World War II, from 1942 until 1946, Patterson served with the Armed Forces in Europe, being discharged with a rank of lieutenant colonel. He was decorated with three battle stars and the Legion of Merit.

The year Patterson assumed the office of surgeon-in-chief, the hospital celebrated its 100th anniversary.[19] The Department of Rehabilitation, having first been created in 1924 (chapter 12), was now headed by its second director, William Cooper, MD (1909–1970), then chief of the Cerebral Palsy Clinic. Wilson Jr., chief of the Hip Service, favored by his experiences abroad and the laboratory findings of Harlan C. Amstutz, MD, established a protocol for total hip replacement using polymethyl-methacrylate fixation of the components. Insertion of the McKee-Farrar metal-on-metal implant began in 1967 and the Charnley metal–on–ultra-high–molecular weight polyethylene (UHWPE) in 1968.

Amstutz, having finished his orthopaedic residency at HSS in 1960, returned after a tour of military duty to be appointed to the staff in 1964 as orthopaedic surgeon to the Outpatient Department (Fig. 14). That year, he established

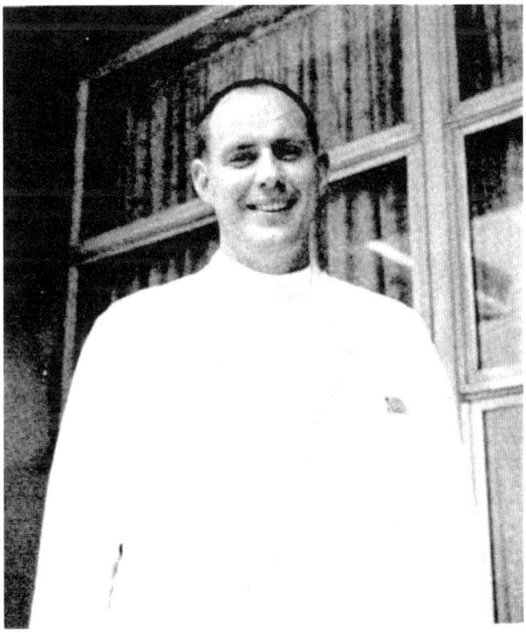

Fig. 14 Harlan Amstutz, MD, as an orthopaedic resident in 1960 at the Hospital for Special Surgery. After returning from the military, he joined the attending staff at Hospital for Special Surgery, leaving in 1970 to become chief of orthopaedics at UCLA. Eventually, he became founding director of the Joint Replacement Institute at St. Vincent Medical Center in Los Angeles. In 2010, he received the Distinguished Alumnus Award of the Hospital for Special Surgery Alumni Association. (From Hospital for Special Surgery Archives)

the Leg Equalization Clinic and soon became chief of the Amputee Clinic. Realizing the coming impact of technology in joint replacement, Patterson established the Biomechanics and Biomaterials Laboratory in 1966 and appointed Amstutz as its director.[20] Amstutz was promoted to director of bioengineering in 1969 and brought Peter S. Walker, PhD, into the department as project engineer that same year (see chapter 17 for more details). Development projects in hip and knee replacement began with the Trapezoidal-28 and the unicondylar and duo-condylar devices. In 1970, Amstutz resigned to become chief of the Orthopaedic Department of the University of California, Los Angeles. Wilson Jr. replaced him as director of applied biomechanics.

Undergraduate education at HSS during this period was directed Allan E. Inglis, MD, who enjoyed a wealth of knowledge in orthopaedics and anatomy and organized classes on both subjects for Cornell University Medical College students. Patterson appointed him executive assistant to the surgeon-in-chief and eventually chief of the CAP Service.

Born in Seattle, Inglis earned his undergraduate, graduate (1951), and medical degrees (1955) from the University of Rochester. He completed his orthopaedic resident training at HSS in 1960 and 2 years of fellowship at Memorial Center for Cancer and Allied Diseases and HSS (1960–1962). In later years, he was appointed professor of clinical surgery (1985) and professor of anatomy in cell biology and anatomy (1986) at Cornell University Medical College (Fig. 15).

The year after Wilson became surgeon-in-chief, Olive Fischer organized the first Photography Department at the hospital. Besides being a photographer, she was an artist who hand-engraved all the diplomas at the hospital and made all the signs, right down to the "no smoking signs." She contributed heavily to the hospital newspaper and wrote informative and hilarious biographies of the staff for the newspaper's "Profiles" column. Every new scoliosis patient was photographed without clothes, and their photos were filed in their charts. Later, in the 1960s, paper bikini bathing suits were provided to "scoli" patients. Fischer retired after 31 years in 1967.

In 1968, John Doherty, MD became chief of the Combined Fracture Service of New York Hospital–Cornell Medical Center, replacing Preston Wade (Fig. 16).

That same year, David B. Levine, MD, was appointed chief of scoliosis at the HSS. Having finished his orthopaedic residency at HSS in 1964, he trained as a scoliosis fellow for 1 year under Jacqueline Perry, MD, at Rancho

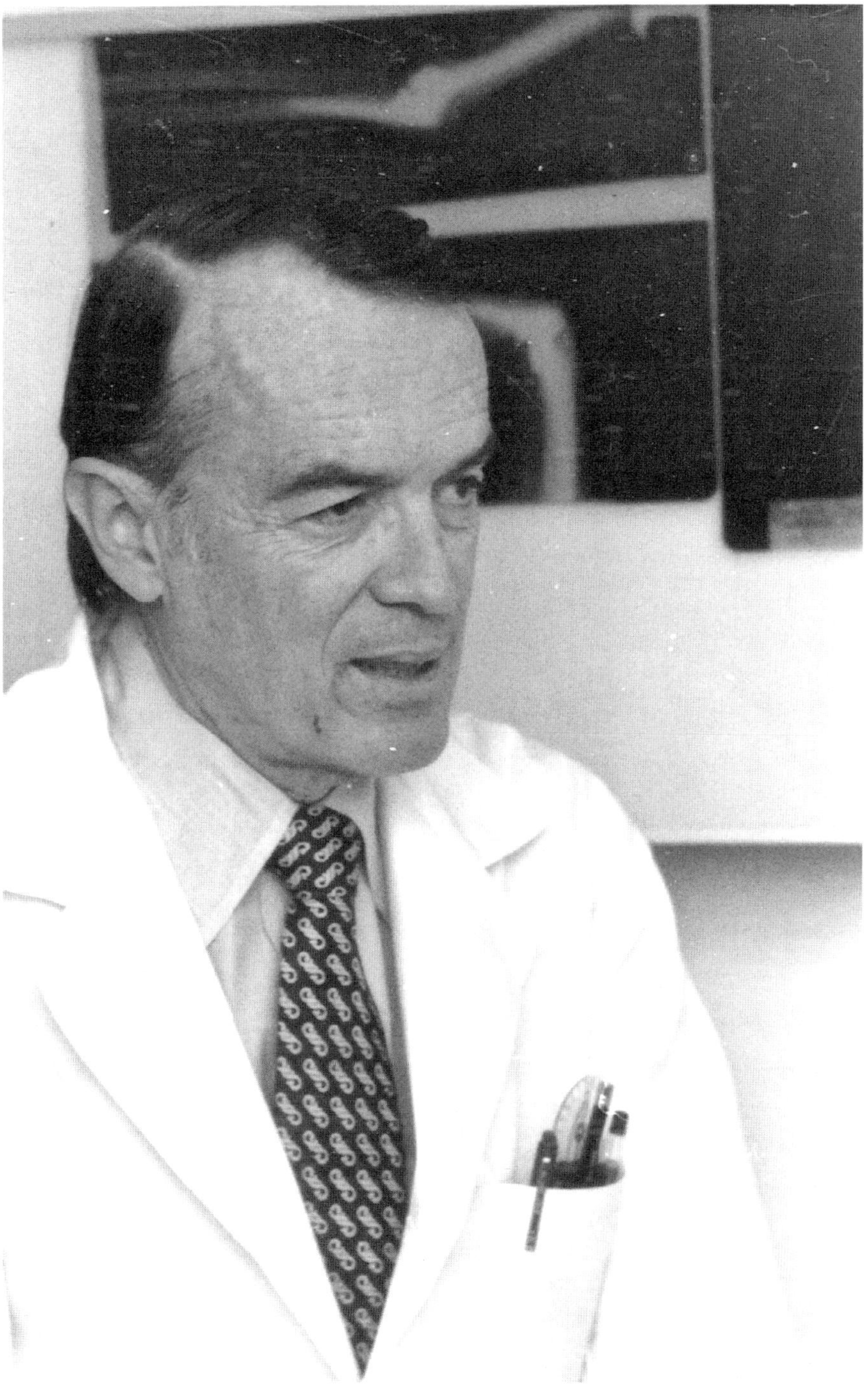

Fig. 15 Allan E. Inglis, MD, executive assistant to the surgeon-in-chief Robert Lee Patterson, circa 1971, was as an expert in hand and arthritis surgery. As attending surgeon at Hospital for Special Surgery, he held a dual appointment at Cornell University Medical College as professor of anatomy and of orthopaedic surgery. (From Hospital for Special Surgery Archives)

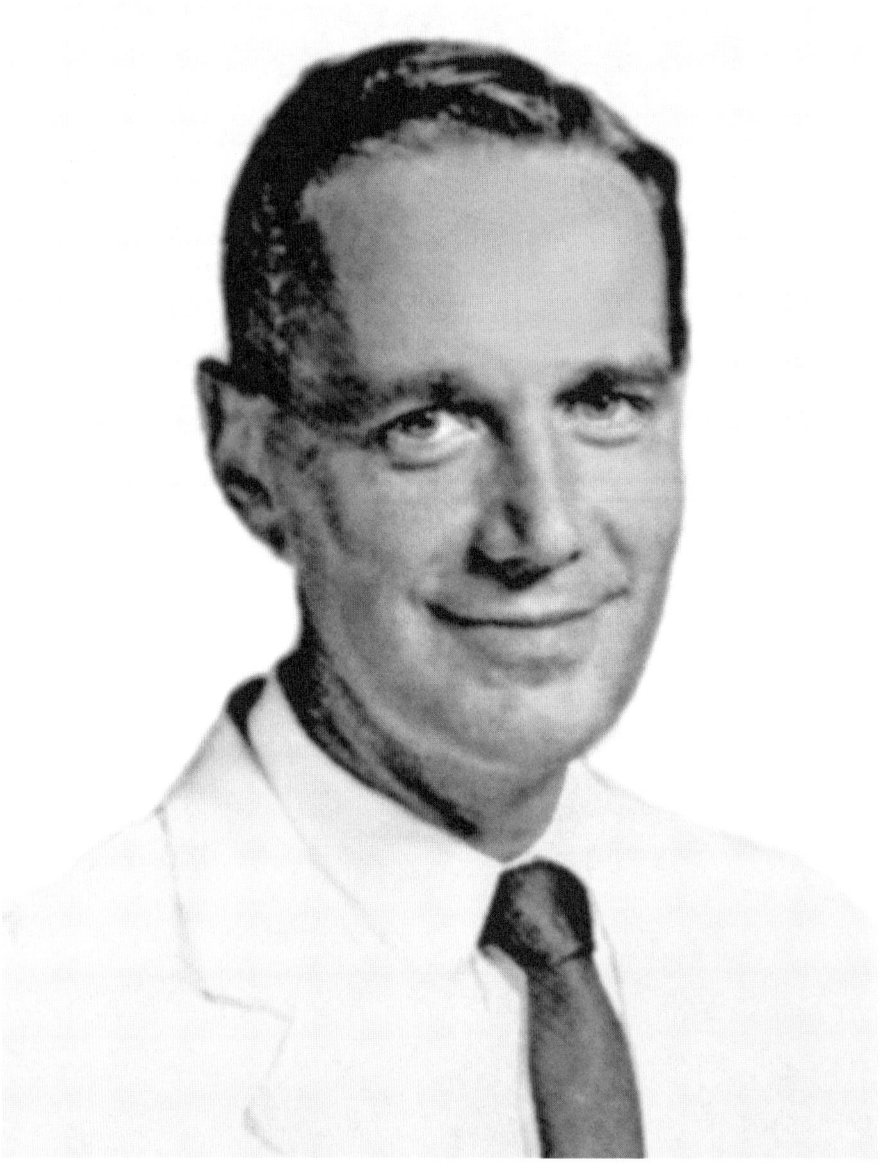

Fig. 16 John Doherty, MD, at age 42 years, became chief of the Fracture Service at New York Hospital in 1968. He served as executive assistant to the surgeon-in-chief Robert Lee Patterson Jr. (From Hospital for Special Surgery Archives)

Los Amigos Hospital in Downey, California, returning to HSS in 1966 as an assistant attending orthopaedic surgeon. He advocated a new approach for treating scoliosis patients, particularly those with cardiopulmonary compromise. Prophylactic tracheostomy, introduction of the halo, adjunct respirators, Cotrel traction, and use of Harrington rod implants were some of the new methods he introduced to HSS—eliminating the cumbersome, restrictive turnbuckle casts of the Cobb era, which necessitated being recumbent in bed for up to a year.[21]

Levine organized a "step-down" pediatric nursing unit on 5 South, where both males and females were in the same room—a first at HSS for mixing male and female inpatients in the same room, except for the Recovery Room. In cooperation with the Anesthesiology Department, he brought routine cardiac monitoring into the operating rooms and arterial blood gas analysis into the hospital.

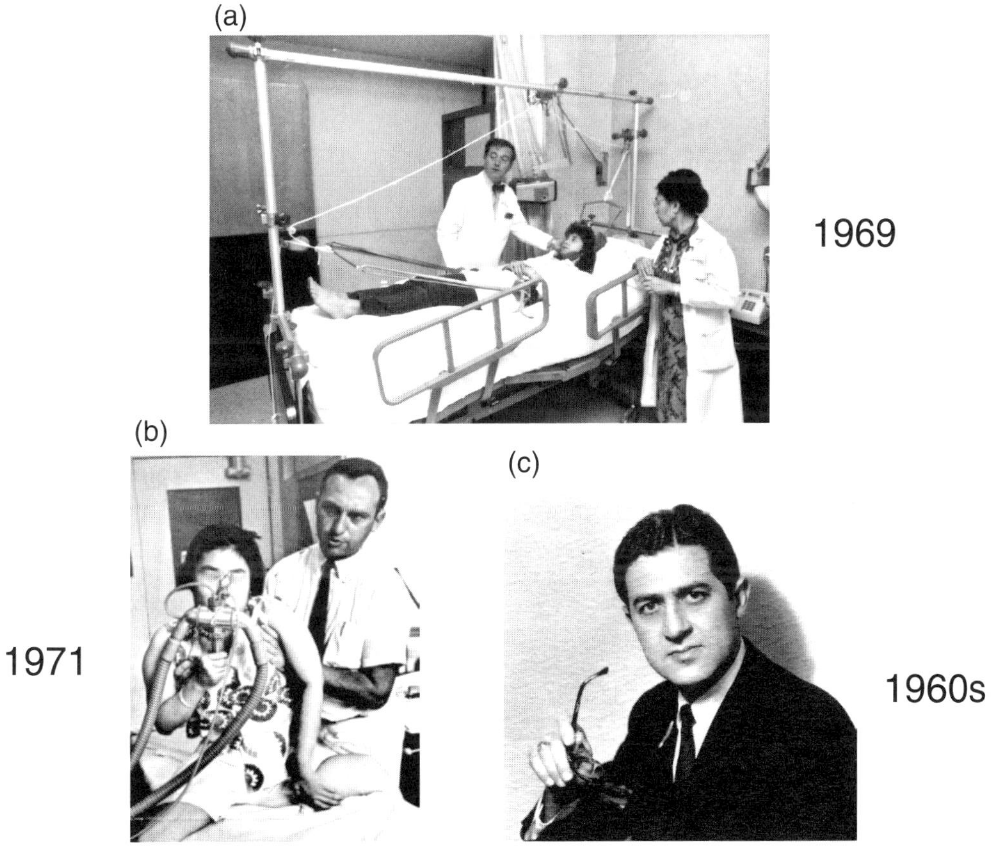

Fig. 17 (a) 1969: David B. Levine, MD, and Wan Ngo Lim, MD, examining a scoliosis patient in preoperative Cotrel traction. (b) 1971: James P. Smith, MD, supporting a postpolio scoliosis patient as she performs her pulmonary function tests. (From Hospital for Special Surgery Archives.) (c) 1960s: Irwin Nydick, MD, cardiologist on Hospital for Special Surgery staff since 1956. (From Brad Hess Photography)

There were four pediatric/medical key players on Levine's scoliosis "multidisciplinary team" (a concept established decades before that term became a buzz phrase) (Fig. 17). Wan Ngo Lim, MD (1920–2004), chief of pediatrics at HSS, attending pediatrician at New York Hospital, and associate professor of pediatrics at Cornell University Medical College, expertly managed pediatric medical complexities and postoperative recovery care. She had complete control of the pediatric floor (5 South), and with her rotating pediatric residents from New York Hospital, she was indispensible to the orthopaedic staff treating children. She also provided a calming influence for the children and their families.

A highly regarded pediatric cardiologist, Lim received her medical degree from Shanghai Medical College in 1945 and trained at Los Angeles Children's Hospital. She served as a pediatric resident at New York Hospital in 1953, followed by a fellowship in pediatric cardiology and cardiac research. With May Wilson, MD (1891–1971), clinical professor of pediatrics at Cornell University Medical College and a renowned pediatric cardiologist, Lim helped to discover the first effective treatment for rheumatic heart disease.

The second key player was James P. Smith, MD, FACP, FCCP, who finished his fellowship in pulmonary disease at New York Hospital in 1967. During his training, he rotated through HSS and was introduced to Levine through his medical school roommate, Bill Bruton, MD, who was an HSS orthopaedic resident (class of 1967).

Smith likes to recount the story of the time Levine came to the New York Hospital pulmonary laboratory and asked him, "What do you know about scoliosis?" To which Smith replied, "You mean kyphoscoliosis?" Levine laughed and said, "You don't know anything." Thus began a long professional collaboration and an enduring friendship between the two men.

Awarded his MD degree from Georgetown University Medical College in 1960, Smith was a medical resident at New York Hospital–Cornell University Medical College from 1960 to 1962 and served as a captain in the U.S. Army Medical Corps from 1962 to 1964. He is currently clinical professor of medicine at Weill Cornell Medical College and attending physician at New York–Presbyterian Hospital and HSS.

In 1967, pulmonary function tests were first performed in scoliosis patients by Sheila Rubinstein, a pulmonary technician, who also read the basic tests. Smith established a one-room scoliosis pulmonary laboratory in 1975 that eventually merged with the EKG Lab to become the hospital's

Cardiopulmonary Laboratory. He continues to read hospital pulmonary function tests to this day.

When asked for his views on working with orthopaedic surgeons, Smith replied, "Orthopaedic surgeons have always struck me as a fine breed whose keen instincts and skills most often produce an overt and desirable functional improvement in their patients. I also suspect that their DNA drives the group to consistently select the most desirable locations on Earth for their tribal meetings."

Number three on Levine's scoliosis team was Thomas K. C. King, MB, BCh, MD, who has been a full-time faculty member of the Division of Pulmonary Medicine and Critical Care at New York–Presbyterian Hospital for many years. King trained in Belfast, Northern Ireland, and was a fellow at the Nuffield Foundation Welsh National Medical School in Cardiff, United Kingdom. He also was a fellow in the Cardiopulmonary Laboratory of Columbia University and the Division of Bellevue Hospital in New York. He has continued to serve as consultant at HSS and now a member of the HSS Complex Case Committee, which is patterned after the multidisciplinary concept and preoperatively reviews high-risk orthopaedic patients with referral to multiple subspecialties for risk reduction and management.

The fourth member of the original multidisciplinary scoliosis team was Irwin Nydick, MD, who started reading EKGs at HSS in 1955 at the request of Henry Kirkland, HSS cardiologist. Nydick joined the HSS staff the following year, soon collaborating in the reading of EKGs with his associate, Frank Perrone, MD, and adding echocardiography readings in 2002. When he left the HSS EKG Lab in 2009, about 12,000 EKGs were being read annually, compared with about 600 tests a year when he started.

When Nydick described how close he felt to the other team players, he said they were "almost like brothers and sisters—without compromise at the learning and performance levels. We learned scoliosis management together as our experiential base increased with these challenging patients. I loved working with the orthopaedists and believed the patients benefitted greatly from our team approach. We were almost always on the same page. It was rare to have divergence."

Nydick received his medical degree from Columbia University's College of Physicians and Surgeons in 1948. He first served as an intern and then as a resident in medicine from 1948 to 1951 at the Cornell Medical Division of Bellevue Hospital. A resident in cardiology at Bellevue's Cornell Division from 1953 to 1954, he pursued additional training as a fellow in cardiology at Memorial Hospital from 1954 to 1955.

Nydick was a medical officer (first lieutenant) in the U.S. Army from 1951 to 1953, serving in Korea and Japan. He was part of a team that performed the original studies of cardiac diagnostic and therapeutic enzymes (transaminase and thrombolytics).

Nydick has since retired from active patient care but still spends much of his time teaching medical residents at Weill Cornell Medical College. In June 2012, at the Annual Residents Graduation dinner at the Roosevelt Hotel Grand Ballroom, an annual award in Nydick's name was presented: "The Irwin Nydick Award for Excellence to the Outstanding Voluntary Staff Practicing Physician." A second award was presented to Nydick from the Department of Medicine Class of 2012, which stated: "Proudly recognizes IRWIN NYDICK, MD 'The Professor.' For his tireless commitment to instilling in each of us a spirit of life-long learning, and inspiring us to be the best clinicians we can be."

There were a number of other consultants—experts in their fields—who were called upon over the years when scoliosis patients presented with unusual diagnoses. Jessica G. Davis, MD, a clinical geneticist, was often consulted when a diagnosis of Marfan syndrome or other connective tissue disorder was suspected. Davis, chief of the Division of Medical Genetics and associate professor of clinical pediatrics at Weill Cornell Medical College, was an Associate Attending Pediatrician at New York–Presbyterian Hospital and HSS.

Patterson assigned Levine as director of the Newborn Hip Examining Service (1966–1976), a new program. With Lim and a team of HSS Hip Fellows and orthopaedic residents, Levine examined over 50,000 newborns at New York Hospital for dislocation of the hip (CDH), preventing the dreaded complications of a missed CDH.[22] Levine retired from active practice of orthopaedic surgery in 1995 (chapter 14).

In 1965, Mary Jeanne Clapp retired as director of nursing and was followed by D. Dean Smith, who held that position until 1975. Another important nursing milestone was the retirement of Hazel Evans, RN, who served as operating room supervisor for 25 years, from 1941 to 1966. She was held in the highest esteem by all of the surgeons. She always scrubbed for Lewis Clark Wagner (Wag), and after her retirement, she ran his office. When she retired, Wilson Jr. wrote, "As a resident, I was fortunate enough to have that rotation that put me on the adult service with Wag, but to this day I do not know whether I learned more surgery from him or Miss Evans. Somehow, Hazel always knew the right instrument for a given situation."

Evans ruled the operating rooms with an iron hand. There were days as a resident when I scrubbed with Wilson Jr. and Hazel would pop her head in the room and blurt out, "Junior, it is 2:30, and we are closing the operating room in a half hour."

Elizabeth Kirsch, RN, held the post of OR supervisor until 1970. Ingrid Andersson, from Malmo, Sweden, followed her.

Another influential Patterson appointment was Peter Bullough, MD, from Oxford, England, who joined the HSS staff as an associate attending pathologist in 1968 under Mellors. Bullough became chief orthopaedic pathologist and attending pathologist in 1980. He succeeded Mellors as director of laboratory medicine in 1984, when Mellors retired (Fig. 18).

After battling peripheral vascular disease, Philip D. Wilson, Sr., died on May 7, 1969 at age 83 years in New York Hospital. A memorial service was held 3 days later at the New York Academy of Medicine. In his obituary, published in the *Journal of Bone and Joint Surgery*, his very close British friend, Sir Harry Platt, wrote in part: "In Great Britain we have long seen Philip Wilson not only

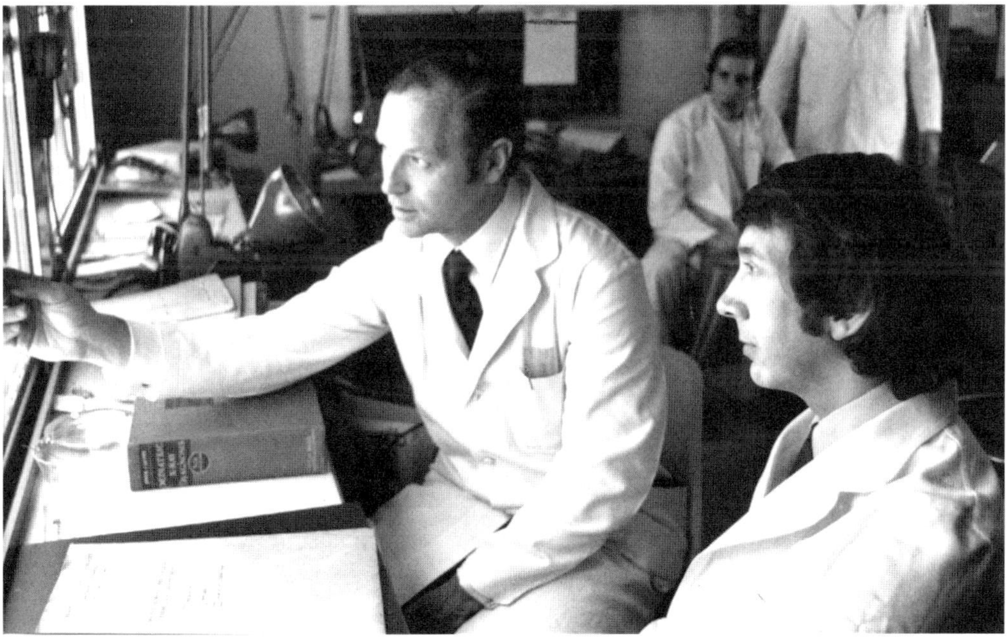

Fig. 18 Leon Root, MD (left), and Peter Bullough, MD, established a clinic in 1970 for patients with osteogenesis imperfecta. (From Hospital for Special Surgery Archives)

as an outstanding surgical leader in the United States, the doyen of orthopaedic surgery, but as a world figure. For us he represented the outward symbol of that *special relationship* between the orthopaedic surgeons of our two countries created in the days of war by Sir Robert Jones and nurtured by Robert Osgood."[23]

In 1969, with the resignation of Goran Bauer, John Insall, MD (1930–2000), became the new chief of the Knee Clinic.[24] Insall, along with Chitranjan Ranawat, MD, Peter Walker, PhD, and Inglis, began an investigation of the design and development of the total knee prosthesis at HSS. In December 1971, Insall, Ranawat, and Joseph I. Hoffman Jr., MD (orthopaedic fellow), performed the first implantation of a duo-condylar knee prosthesis, designed in the laboratory by Walker and Joseph V. Hajek, MD (orthopaedic fellow).[25]

Mildred Hilson

The hospital could never have survived without adequate support from influential donors and board members stemming from its very beginning in the nineteenth century. The original members of the New York Society for the Relief of the Ruptured and Crippled were prominent and influential citizens of New York City, but in later years, one person stood out as the maven of HSS: Mildred Hilson (1898–1994) (Fig. 19).

Mildred Hilson, widow of Edwin I. Hilson, an investment banker who died in 1952, took his seat on the Board of Directors at HSS and 5 years later was named vice president—a title she held until her death. An extraordinarily effective fundraiser, particularly for the Republican Party, she was a patron of the arts, serving on the Boards of the Museum of the City of New York, New York City Cultural Council, and others, as well as Mayor John Lindsay's cultural affairs committee.

Guest lists in her Waldorf Towers suite included the Duke and Duchess of Windsor, the actor Laurence Olivier, President George H. Bush and his wife, Barbara, New York City Mayor Rudolph Giuliani and his former wife, Donna, and numerous ambassadors and other American Presidents. President Dwight D. Eisenhower painted a portrait of her, and in 1988, President Richard Nixon played "Happy Birthday" on the piano at her 90th birthday gala at the St. Regis Hotel.

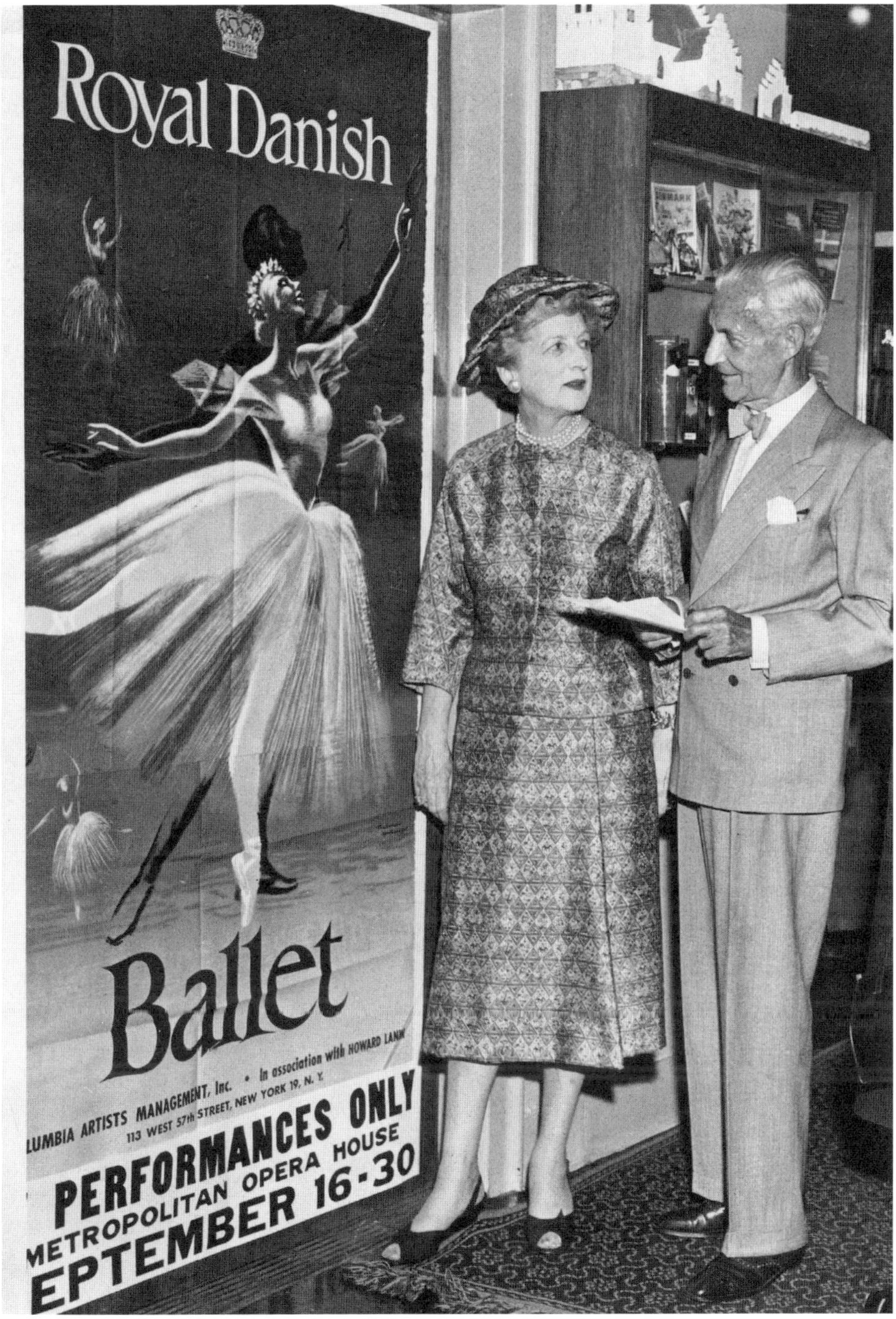

Fig. 19 Mildred Hilson with Henrik Kauffman, Denmark's ambassador to the United States, in front of a poster marking the first annual Hospital for Special Surgery Benefit in 1956. She was a very benevolent and strong supporter of Hospital for Special Surgery. (From Hospital for Special Surgery Archives)

What an extraordinary woman! In 1988, a group of socially prominent men gave a dinner at the 21 Club to honor Mildred Hilson, grand dame of the diamond brigade and New York's charity circuit.

In 1970, with the resignation of Richard Freyberg as director of Rheumatic Diseases, Charles L. Christian, MD, was appointed to that position, becoming physician-in-chief and associate director of research. Christian brought with him from Columbia Presbyterian Hospital Lawrence Kagen, MD, Robert W. Lightfoot Jr., MD, Michael D. Lockshin, MD, and Paul E. Phillips, MD. Among their many investigative studies, Christian and his colleagues were particularly interested in autoimmune disorders such as lupus, erythematosus, and rheumatoid arthritis.

John L. Marshall, DVM, MD (1936–1980), established the first Sports Medicine Clinic at HSS in 1971 and soon became a leading authority in the country in the new subspecialty—sports medicine.

In 1972, Robert Lee Patterson Jr. resigned as surgeon-in-chief. Transformation of technical advancement in joint surgery, major developments in

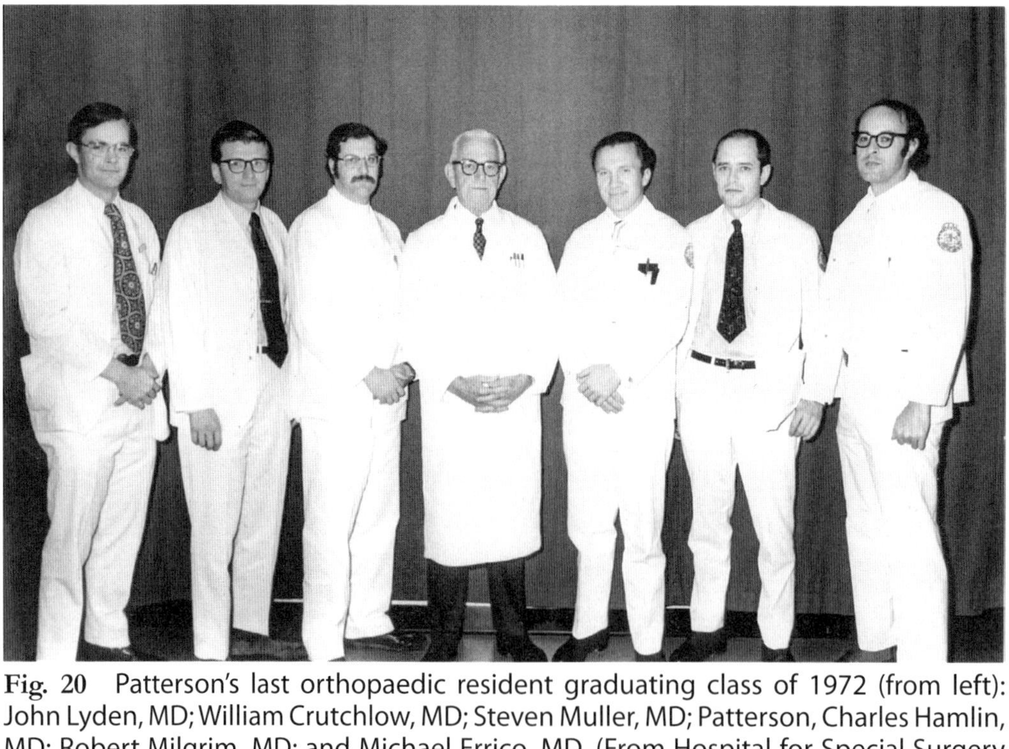

Fig. 20 Patterson's last orthopaedic resident graduating class of 1972 (from left): John Lyden, MD; William Crutchlow, MD; Steven Muller, MD; Patterson, Charles Hamlin, MD; Robert Milgrim, MD; and Michael Errico, MD. (From Hospital for Special Surgery Archives)

arthritis, and establishment of a biomechanics laboratory occurred during his watch. HSS postgraduate education was expanded, with the orthopaedic residency increasing to six residents per year and the introduction of new fellowship opportunities (Fig. 20). One of Robert Lee Patterson's most important accomplishments, however, was bolstering the relationship with New York Hospital–Cornell Medical Center, which saved the affiliation agreement.

REFERENCES

1. Anonymous. Hospital profiles. T. Campbell Thompson, MD. *Record and Chronicle.* 1954;IX:1–5.
2. Anonymous. Hospital profiles. T. Campbell Thompson, MD. *Record and Chronicle.* 1954;IX:1–6.
3. Thompson TC. Experimental muscular atrophy. *J Bone Joint Surg.* 1934;16:564–571.
4. Thompson TC. Quadricepsplasty to improve knee function. *J Bone Joint Surg.* 1944;26:366.
5. Thomas LI, Thompson TC, Straub LR. Transplantation of the external oblique muscle for abductor paralysis. *J Bone Joint Surg.* 1950;32:207–217.
6. Thompson TC, Straub LR, Campbell, RD. An Evaluation of femoral shortening with intramedullary nailing. *J Bone Joint Surg.* 1954;36A:43–56.
7. Thompson TC, Straub LR, Arnold WD. Congenital absence of the fibula. *J Bone Joint Surg.* 1957;39A:1229–1237.
8. Thompson TC. Stabilization of the paralytic lower extremity. *Bulletin of the Hospital for Special Surgery.* 1959;Nov:6–27.
9. Thompson TC, Doherty JH. Spontaneous rupture of tendon of Achilles: a new clinical diagnostic test. *J Trauma.* 1962;2:126–129.
10. Thompson TC. A test for rupture of the tendo Achilles. *Acta Orthop Scand.* 1962;32:461.
11. Levine DB. The Manhattan transfer—celebrating our 50th anniversary 1955–2005. *HSS Alumni News.* 2005;Spring:10.
12. Thompson TC. *Ninety-Third Annual Report of the New York Society for the Relief of the Ruptured and Crippled.* New York, NY: 1956.
13. Kahn BA. The evolution of orthopaedic nursing at the Hospital for Special Surgery. *Orthop Nurs.* 2005;24.
14. Freiberger RH, Kaye JJ, Spiller J. *Arthrography.* New York, NY: Appelton-Century-Crofts; 1979.
15. Wilson PD. *Ninety-Sixth Annual Report of the New York Society for the Relief of the Ruptured and Crippled.* New York, NY: New York Society for the Relief of the Ruptured and Crippled; 1959.
16. Slatis P, Varaart B. Goren Bauer. *Acta Orthop Scand.* 1994:65:19.

17. Sculco TP. John R. *Cobb's outstanding contributions in treating scoliosis.* HSS Horizon. 1984:Summer.
18. Anonymous. The Hospital for Special Surgery. Hospital profiles. Lee Ramsay Straub MD. *Record and Chronicle.* 1960:XIV:1–4.
19. Anonymous. The Hospital for Special Surgery. Dr. Patterson appointed surgeon-in-chief. *Record and Chronicle.* 1963:XVII:1.
20. Wilson PD Jr., Levine DB. Hospital for Special Surgery. A brief review of its development and current position. *Clin Orthop.* 2000:374:90–105.
21. Patterson RL. *One Hundred and Third Annual Report of the New York Society for the Relief of the Ruptured and Crippled.* New York, NY: New York Society for the Relief of the Ruptured and Crippled; 1966.
22. Artz TD, Levine DB, Lim WN, Salvati E, Wilson PD Jr. Neonatal diagnosis, treatment and related factors of congenital dislocation of the hip. *Clin Orthop.* 1975:110, July–Aug.
23. Platt H. Philip Duncan Wilson, MD 1886–1969. *J Bone Joint Surg.* 1969:51A:1445–1450.
24. Patterson RL. *One Hundred and Seventh Annual Report of the Hospital for Special Surgery.* New York, NY: New York Society for the Relief of the Ruptured and Crippled; 1970.
25. Patterson RL. *One Hundred and Eighth Annual Report of the Hospital for Special Surgery.* New York, NY: New York Society for the Relief of the Ruptured and Crippled; 1971.

NOTES

a. Tudor City, an apartment complex on the East Side of Manhattan, is bordered by 40th Street to the south, First Avenue to the east, Second Avenue to the west, and 43rd Street to the north. Many of the R&C staff lived and/or had offices in Tudor City when the hospital was located on East 42nd Street.

b. Bennett had been a house surgeon at R&C in 1909.

c. R&C was the first hospital to have a therapeutic pool in New York City in 1928.

d. Two of John Cobb's famous limericks were

- *In the field of scoliosis, there is one thing to observe—keep your eye on the patient and not on the curve.*
- *You don't have to be crazy to do scoliosis, but it helps.*

e. Preston Wade was brought out of retirement in 1970 to assume the post of interim chief of surgery at New York Hospital.

f. The name was changed to W. & J. Sloane when his brother, John Sloane, joined the store in 1852. For years, it was located on Fifth Avenue at 38th Street. Its staff decorated the homes of the wealthy and famous, created Hollywood movie sets, and even designed furniture for the interior of the White House.

CHAPTER 11

PHILIP D. WILSON JR., MD EIGHTH SURGEON-IN-CHIEF (1972–1989)

DAVID B. LEVINE, MD

THE BOARD OF MANAGERS OF the New York Society for the Relief of the Ruptured and Crippled appointed Philip D. Wilson Jr., MD, as the eighth surgeon-in-chief of the Hospital for Special Surgery (HSS) in 1971.

That same year, Wilson became the president-elect of the American Academy of Orthopaedic Surgeons (AAOS) at its 39th Annual Meeting in San Francisco (Fig. 1). The following year, he assumed both the offices of AAOS president and surgeon-in-chief of the HSS. Recalling the past, his father, Philip D. Wilson, became the third AAOS President in 1934 and at the same time was appointed the fifth surgeon-in-chief of the HSS.

Philip Duncan Wilson Jr. was born on February 14, 1920, in Boston, Massachusetts, to Germaine Porel, the daughter of a famous French actress, and Philip D. Wilson, MD, a well-known young orthopaedic surgeon at Massachusetts General Hospital. Wilson Jr. had an older brother, Paul Wilson, and a younger sister, Marianne Wilson Finkel.

Educated at Harvard College, he received his MD degree in 1944 from the College of Physicians and Surgeons of Columbia University. He was a general surgical intern and resident at Massachusetts General Hospital from 1944 to 1946 and then served in the military at Brooke General Hospital from 1946 to 1948, being discharged as a captain. After training as an orthopaedic resident at HSS from 1948 to 1950, he completed an additional year of orthopaedic training under LeRoy C. Abbott, MD (1890–1965), and pursued biomechanics studies with Verne T. Inman, MD (1905–1980), at the University of California Hospital Medical Center in San Francisco and also in Berkeley.[1]

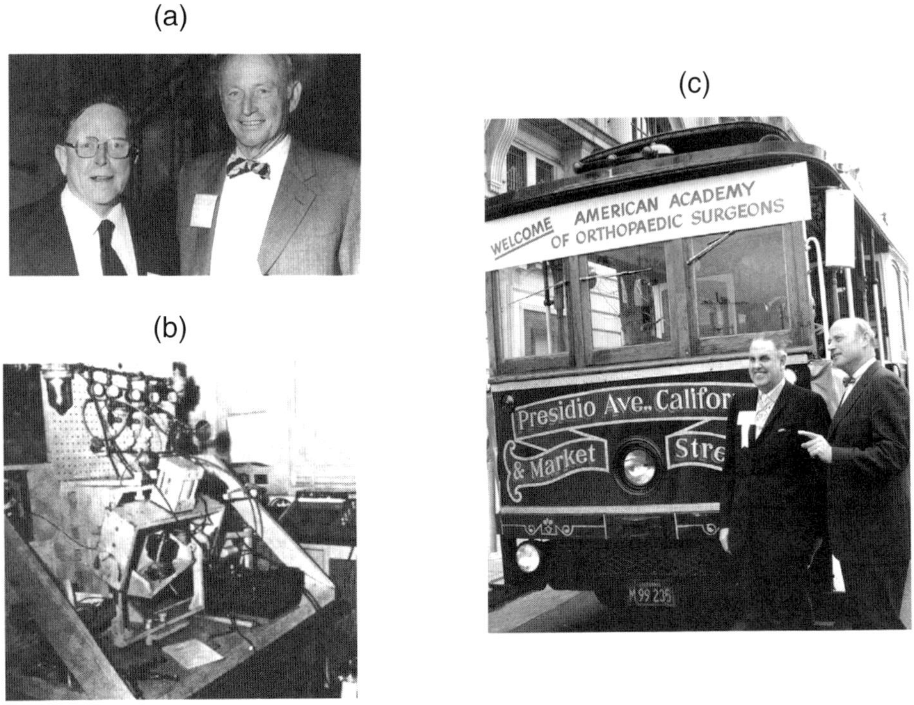

Fig. 1 (a) John Charnley, FRS, and Philip D. Wilson Jr., MD (circa 1972). (b) An early (circa 1970s) joint-simulating machine resembling the loads and motion cycles from walking on artificial hip joints. This device was designed and constructed by Peter Walker, PhD, and B. L. Gold at Hospital for Special Surgery to compare metal-on-metal McKee-Farrar implants with metal-on-polyethylene Charnley implants. (c) John Hinchey, MD, with Wilson Jr., in 1971 at the 39th annual meeting of the American Academy of Orthopaedic Surgeons in San Francisco, when Wilson Jr. became the AAOS president-elect. (From Hospital for Special Surgery Archives and Cristof Studio)

Wilson Jr. joined the HSS staff as an Orthopaedic Surgeon to the Outpatient Department (1951–1954) and quickly rose through the ranks to become an attending orthopaedic surgeon in 1963. During these years, he accumulated wide experience and knowledge in many fields in adult and pediatric orthopaedics, including the spine and scoliosis, disorders of the foot and knee, and fractures, in addition to his focus on the hip.[2–11] He was also very interested in orthopaedic education at the undergraduate and graduate levels, as well as orthopaedic pathology, the application of bioengineering to orthopaedics, and medical history.[12–14]

Wilson Jr. was often consulted by his colleagues for his opinion on the diagnosis of various difficult orthopaedic problems and the choice of the most appropriate treatment. He was considered among the best surgeons in the operating room, with residents and fellows always anxious to scrub in with him.

John Charnley, FRS—Wrightington Hospital

In 1966, Wilson Jr. visited John Charnley, FRS (1911–1982) at Wrightington Hospital in Lancashire, United Kingdom, to learn about a new operation: the total hip replacement. Charnley, professor of orthopaedic surgery at Manchester Royal Infirmary, had introduced a new concept of "low-friction arthroplasty," which was designed to be used as a hip implant. A Fellow of the Royal Society (FRS), Charnley was eventually knighted in 1977 for his achievements (Fig. 1).

In 1967, Wilson Jr., with Harlan Amstutz, introduced this new surgical procedure to HSS. The procedure was quickly adapted by others on the orthopaedic surgical staff and was originally performed under intubation general anesthesia in one of three operating rooms at the hospital. (A fourth operating room was inadequate for hip, knee, and spine surgeries.)

In 1972, the inpatient length of stay for total hip replacement procedures was 19 days.[15, a] A five-bed recovery room was supervised by the director of the Department of Anesthesia, John L. Fox, MD (1917–2001), with his staff of five attending anesthesiologists.

Wilson Jr. recognized how times had changed at the hospital, which originated as an inpatient rehabilitation home for children with musculoskeletal conditions. After the turn of the century, surgical treatment for postpolio deformities evolved, and later, surgical and nonsurgical management of patients with crippling arthritis grew. General orthopaedics was now being reorganized into "supraspecialty" services by condition and anatomy, featuring new specialty clinics and services focusing on the hip, back, foot, knee, metabolic bone disease, osteogenesis imperfecta, familial dysautonomia, and others. These joined the already existing specialty clinics (such as those devoted to the care of scoliosis, clubfoot, hand disorders, cerebral palsy, and amputees). The supraspecialty services soon became known just as "specialty" services and clinics and were organized into outpatient and inpatient treatment programs. Likewise, teaching and research were compartmentalized by specialty.

John Marshall, MD, DVM

When John Marshall organized the first Sports Medicine Clinic in 1971 at HSS—likely the first such clinic in New York City—he was only 31 years old.[16]

Originally trained in veterinary medicine, Marshall eventually obtained his MD degree in 1965 from Albany Medical College. As an orthopaedic resident at HSS in 1967, he worked in the HSS Comparative Orthopaedics Laboratory, directed by Sten-Erik Olsson, DVM (1921–2000)—a Swedish veterinarian who returned to Sweden in 1968.

Marshall was an experienced basic researcher in the laboratory as well as an excellent clinician and surgeon. He quickly rose to the top of his field to become a world-renowned figure in sports medicine. He went on to serve as team physician for the New York Giants football team and as orthopaedic consultant to the New Jersey Nets basketball team, the U.S. Olympic Ski Team, and the New York City Public Schools Athletic League (Fig. 2).

Marshall's career, however, came to a sudden and unexpected end on February 19, 1980, when he was killed at the age of 44 years—along with the pilot and his accountant—in the crash of a light airplane during a snowstorm. He was flying from the annual meeting of the AAOS in Atlanta, Georgia, to consult for the U.S. Ski Team at the Winter Olympics that year in Lake Placid, New York.[17]

(a) (b)

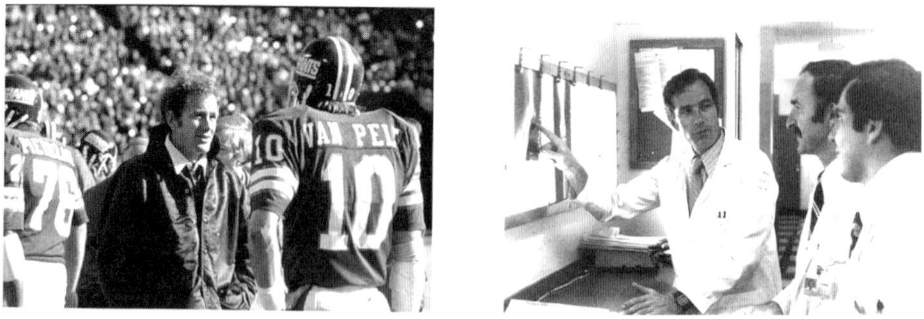

Fig. 2 (a) John Marshall, MD, served as the team doctor for the New York Giants. (b) Marshall, chief of the Sports Medicine Clinic (circa 1977), describing an x-ray of the knee to Russell Warren, MD, and a house officer. (From Hospital for Special Surgery Archives)

To replace Marshall, Russell F. Warren, MD, was appointed chief of sports medicine. Warren had obtained his medical degree from Upstate University of New York at Syracuse, and he finished his orthopaedic residency at HSS in 1973. After a brief trial of private practice followed by a shoulder fellowship with Charles S. Neer II, MD (1917–2011), at the New York Orthopaedic Hospital, Warren joined the HSS attending staff in 1977.

Steven Arnoczsky, DVM, whom Marshall had persuaded before he died to direct the Comparative Orthopaedics Laboratory, continued in that role, working with Warren.

James Nicholas, MD

The physician regarded as the pioneer in the treatment of sports injuries in New York City, however, was James Nicholas, MD (1921–2006), going back to 1960, when he became the team doctor for the fledgling American Football League's New York Titans (the forerunner of the Jets). Nicholas founded one of the earliest hospital-based research and clinical center for the treatment and prevention of sports injuries in 1973 at Lenox Hill Hospital.[18]

Nicholas trained at HSS as an orthopaedic resident under Philip D. Wilson and was part of Wilson's team that managed Senator John F. Kennedy when he had spine surgery at HSS in October 1954.[19] After Nicholas's residency training, he joined the HSS attending staff, eventually dividing his time between HSS and Lenox Hill Hospital (Fig. 3). His expertise in sports injuries stemmed from his early association with Sidney S. Gaynor, MD (1905–1987), the New York Yankees team physician and, in 1956, chief of orthopaedic surgery at Lenox Hill Hospital.

A superb orthopaedic surgeon, Nicholas had an insightful vision of his specialty's future. He was a devoted teacher with enthusiasm for his students and compassion for his patients. (I know, because he was one of my mentors when I was an HSS orthopaedic resident from 1961 to 1964.)

In the sports world, Nicholas was considered the "surgeon to the stars." During that period, Nicholas was the best-known orthopaedic surgeon in the

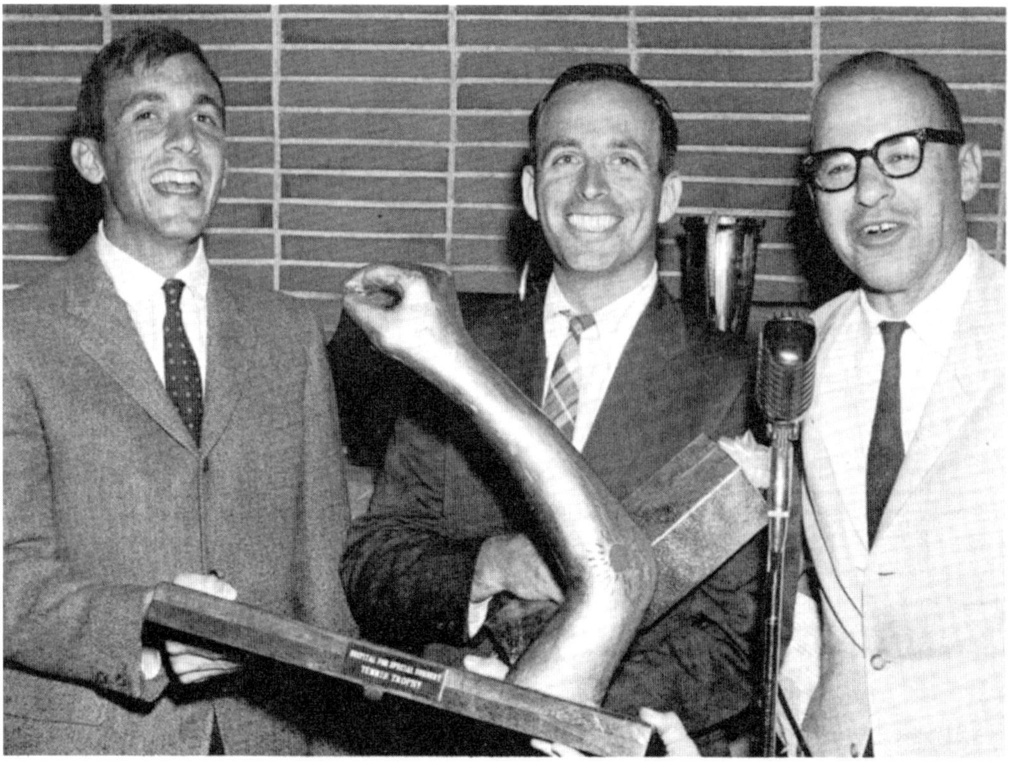

Fig. 3 James Nicholas, MD (right), was the winner of the 1967 HSS Golf Trophy for a second year in a row. HSS resident Clifford W. Colwell Jr., MD, presented the tennis trophy to resident Robert Goldstone, MD. (From Hospital for Special Surgery Archives)

United States for the Jets, the Knicks basketball team, and the Rangers hockey team.

Sports medicine in those days, however, was still in its infancy. Nicholas was a founding member of the American Orthopaedic Society for Sports Medicine (AOSSM), which held its first organizational meeting in 1972 in Washington, DC. The first issue of the *American Journal of Sports Medicine* was published that same year.[20]

Reorganization

In 1973, the orthopaedic staff of HSS included 24 orthopaedic surgeons—some with admitting privileges and others with only outpatient privileges (Table 1). These attendings supervised the residents and fellows in the specialty clinics and general orthopaedic and children's clinics. A senior attending served as chief of the clinics on a daily basis for each of the five weekdays. The

Table 1 HSS Department of Orthopaedics (1973)

THE HOSPITAL FOR SPECIAL SURGERY
MARGARET M. CASPARY CLINIC

July 1, 1973

PROFESSIONAL STAFF

SURGEON-IN-CHIEF........................Philip D. Wilson, Jr., M.D.

PHYSICIAN-IN-CHIEF......................Charles L. Christian, M.D.

DEPARTMENT OF ORTHOPAEDIC SURGERY

DIRECTOR OF ORTHOPAEDIC SURGERY..........Philip D. Wilson, Jr., M.D.

ASSOCIATE DIRECTOR OF ORTHOPAEDIC SURGERY......David B. Levine, M.D.

Attending Orthopaedic Surgeons

William D. Arnold, M.D.
Rolla D. Campbell, M.D.
John H. Doherty, M.D.
Alexander Hersh, M.D.
Allan E. Inglis, M.D.
Bernard Jacobs, M.D.
Peter J. Marchisello, M.D.
James A. Nicholas, M.D.
Lee Ramsay Straub, M.D.

Associate Attending Orthopaedic Surgeons

Sidney Eichenholtz, M.D.
John N. Insall, M.D.
David B. Levine, M.D.
Ralph C. Marcove, M.D.
Victor Mayer, M.D.
Leon Root, M.D.

Assistant Attending Orthopaedic Surgeons

Samuel Avnet, M.D.
Howard Balensweig, M.D.
Walther H. Bohne, M.D.
John P. Lyden, M.D.
John L. Marshall, M.D.
Chitranjan S. Ranawat, M.D.
Eduardo A. Salvati, M.D.
Konstantin P. Velis, M.D.

Orthopaedic Surgeons to Out-Patient Department

Michael Browne, M.D.
William J. Bruton, M.D.
Gary A. Gallo, M.D.
Robert A. Goldstone, M.D.
Joseph V. Hajek, M.D.
David G. Mendes, M.D.
Thomas D. Rizzo, M.D.
Irwin A. S. Spira, M.D.
N. D. Krishne Urs, M.D.
William J. Walsh, Jr., M.D.

Fellows in Orthopaedic Surgery

Paolo Aglietti, M.D.
Tyrone D. Artz, M.D.
James R. Cole, M.D.
Joseph R. Macys, M.D.
Saghir U. Mir, M.D.
Jeanne Pamilla, M.D.
Jon Wang, M.D.
James B. Wessinger, M.D.
Dennis W. Wise, M.D.

"Wednesday Clinic" was led by Peter Cyrus Rizzo II, MD (1903–2001), who was first appointed to the staff of the Hospital for the Ruptured and Crippled in 1936 and was one of the many well-respected teachers and clinicians. If, as a house officer, you had not reported to clinic by 1 PM, you were paged.[b]

At that time, a clinic patient who needed surgery was approved by an attending, admitted at least one day before surgery, and operated on by a member of the house staff (often a different resident/fellow, but a surgeon who was always supervised by an attending orthopaedic surgeon). When the clinics and services were reorganized into specialties, there was much less confusion and better care and follow-up.

Orthopaedic Affiliate Rotations

Over the years, there have been many external clinical rotations for resident training, with the longest standing rotation at the orthopaedic service of the Bronx Veterans Administration (Kingsbridge) Hospital, going back to 1947 (Table 2).

A newer rotation, at North Shore University Hospital on Long Island, was started in 1969 by Richard M. Stark, MD (1932–2007). Stark, an orthopaedic resident at HSS (class of 1963), structured a highly respected program at North Shore, establishing an all-orthopaedic floor. He arranged for Wilson Jr. to make teaching rounds every 6 weeks for the residents. Stark retired as director of orthopaedic surgery in 1990 and died in 2007, at age 75 years (Fig. 4). The North Shore University Hospital rotation was discontinued in 1996; a new rotation at New York Hospital–Queens had been added in 1995.

Education of the house staff was always very important, both within and outside of the operating rooms (Fig. 4). There were daily resident conferences from 7:30 to 8:30 AM during the week, with a surgeon-in-chief's conference on Fridays. A list of journal articles that were required to be read was left in the medical library the night before, and residents prepared themselves to be quizzed the next morning by attendings in conferences. (Computer and Internet technology had not yet arrived.) House staff education depended greatly on a few classic texts, the journals, and teachings by attendings, postgraduate fellows, and senior residents.

Before 1965, four residents were accepted into the HSS orthopaedic program for 3.5 years, to be started after completion of a year of internship and a year of general surgery. A new resident started quarterly. The number of

Table 2 Affiliate Hospitals and Chiefs of Services

Orthopaedic Affiliate Rotations and Year Established Chiefs of Service

Bronx Veterans Administration Hospital (Kingsbridge) Orthopaedic Service (1947)
1947–1956: Sidney Eichenholtz, MD
1956–1962: John Doherty, MD
1962–1973: Bernard Jacobs, MD
1973–1984: William Arnold, MD
1984–1987: Thomas P. Sculco, MD
1987–1990: Norman Johanson, MD
1990–1996: Charles N. Cornell, MD
1989–2000: Patrick McMahon, MD, Co-Chief
1996–2002: Douglas E. Padgett, MD
2002–2005: Michael J. Maynard, MD
2005–2012: Sabrina M. Strickland, MD
2012–Present: Allan E. Inglis Jr., MD

New York Hospital—Queens (1995)
1995–2003: Charles N. Cornell, MD
2003–2005: John D. MacGillivray, MD, acting chief
2005–2008: Michael J. Maynard, MD
2008–present: Jeffrey Rosen, MD, not HSS staff

Memorial Sloan-Kettering Cancer Center Orthopaedic Service (circa 1956)
1915–1933: William Bradley Coley, MD, first chief, Bone Service
1933–1959: Bradley L. Coley, MD, chief, Bone Service
1959–1970: Theodore R. Miller, MD, chief, Bone Service
1970–1976: Ralph Marcove, MD, acting chief, Bone Service
1976–1991: Joseph Lane, MD, chief, Orthopaedic Surgical Service
1991–Present: John Healey, MD, chief, Orthopaedic Surgical Service

New York Hospital Combined Fracture Service (1955)
1955–1968: Preston Wade, MD, and Robert Lee Patterson Jr., MD
1968–1973: John H. Doherty, MD
1973–1984: William Arnold, MD
1984–1991: John Lyden, MD
1991–present: David L. Helfet, MD

North Shore University Hospital Orthopaedics (1969)
1969–1990: Richard Stark, MD
1990–1991: Daniel Rich, MD
1991–1996: David Dines, MD

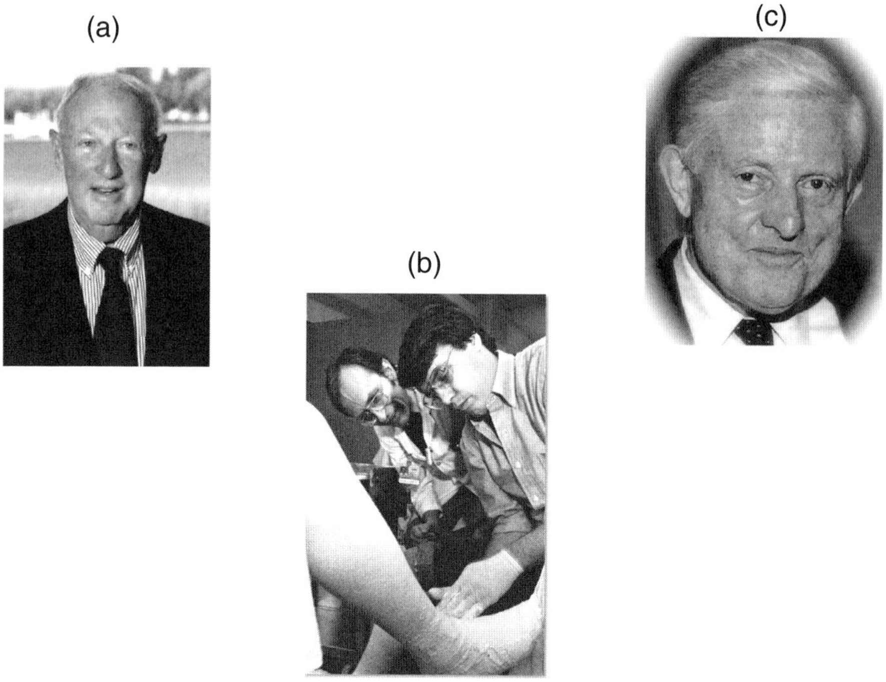

Fig. 4 Resident educators. (a) Richard Stark, MD, director of orthopaedic surgery at North Shore University Hospital, as seen after he retired in 1993. (b) Walther Bohne, MD, teaches HSS resident Norman Johanson, MD (foreground), the fine points of applying a cast in the Foot Clinic. (c) David Clayson, PhD, served as the clinical psychologist at HSS. He not only sat on the Orthopaedic Resident Selection Committee but held monthly meetings with the first-year orthopaedic residents as their advisor. (From Hospital for Special Surgery Archives)

residents increased from four to six per year in 1965; a new rotation system was introduced, with all six residents beginning July 1.

In 1972, residents rotated through the new supraspecialty clinics every 2 months. The next year, at the 40th annual meeting of the AAOS, Wilson Jr. delivered his presidential address, highlighting the pursuit of excellence, education, and supraspecialization.[21]

In 1974, the size of the orthopaedic program increased to eight residents per year, for a total of 32 positions. The length of the orthopaedic residency was extended to 4 years, while 2 years of required prior surgical training were reduced to 1 year.[22] Clinical orthopaedic fellows rotated through four different services for a total of 1 year. Some were assigned to only one service for the year, such as the hand, scoliosis, pediatric, or cerebral palsy service. When the supraspecialty clinics and services were formed, most clinical orthopaedic fellows were assigned to one service.

In 1972, there were also three research orthopaedic fellows—six clinical and research rheumatic disease fellows, and one research fellow in biochemistry. At that time, there were no fellows in anesthesiology, radiology, or other supporting services. By 1999, the number of orthopaedic residents remained constant, but there were increasing numbers of orthopaedic and nonorthopaedic fellows, through 2012 (Table 3).

Resident Selection

A unique orthopaedic resident interviewing system was introduced in 1973. Interviews were held all day Friday and Saturday morning in January. Each candidate was assigned a 10-minute interview, which was usually conducted by two interviewers who were orthopaedic attendings, members of the research staff, orthopaedic residents, or other staff. There were three 2-hour sessions on Fridays and two sessions on Saturday mornings, to which a group of about 80 candidates (selected from some 400 or more applicants) were awarded interviews. Each interviewer scored each candidate, and together they met after the sessions for further discussion to rank each candidate.

The rankings were personally tabulated by Wilson Jr. who was in charge of the entire orthopaedic residency program. At first, he would chalk the results on a blackboard. Later, with introduction of the computer, Tim Wright, PhD, who joined the staff in 1977 as an assistant scientist in the Research Division, was able to computerize the data instantaneously, so that the results from the Friday morning interviews were available by lunchtime for discussion. By Saturday noon, all scores were finalized. For the next few days, a few members of the committee analyzed resulting scores to submit their rankings. Eight ranked applicants (of the top 20) were offered positions. When the resident match system evolved, this list was submitted to the match.

This detailed process was a far cry from the previous less-organized selection system, and was the only such resident selection system in academic orthopaedics. It remains the basis of the current HSS Resident Selection System. One of the interviewers of resident candidates was David Clayson, PhD (1934–2001), associate clinical psychologist on the HSS Psychiatry Service. Clayson, who served as head of psychology in the Department of Psychiatry at New

Table 3 Summary of the House Staff at the Hospital for the Ruptured and Crippled and the Hospital for Special Surgery

First Orthopaedic Residents at R&C

1887: W. Travis Gibb
1887: Eli E. Josselyn
1888: J. M. Johnston
1888: Samuel E. Milliken
1888: Howard G. Myers
The designation of the term resident, indicating a young physician/surgeon in-training, was first used in the United States at R&C by Virgil Gibney, MD, in 1887.

	House staff	
Years	*Orthopaedic residents*	*Fellows*
1933–1959	61	62
1960–1969	39	71
1970–1979	67	59
1980–1989	79	122
1990–1999	83	143
2000–2012	108	550
Total	**437**	**1,007**

	Orthopaedic fellows, by specialty: a comparison	
Service	*1999*	*2012*
Adult Reconstruction/Joint Replacement	5	8
Foot and Ankle	2	3
Hand	3	4
Hip Preservation	0	1
Limb Lengthening/Complex Reconstruction	0	2
Irving and Sally Lipstock Fellowship	0	1
Metabolic Bone Disease/Oncology	0	2
Niarchos Foundation International	0	1
Orthopaedic Trauma	0	3
Pediatric Orthopaedic	2	1
Spine	3	6
Scoliosis	0	1
Sports Medicine/Shoulder	5	9
Trauma	3	0
Total	**23**	**42**

Table 3 *(continued)*

Service	Number of nonorthopaedic fellows *1999*	*2012*
Anesthesiology	4	9
Biomechanics	2	4
Neurology	1	3
Pediatric Rheumatology	2	4
Physiatry	2	4
Primary Care Sports Medicine	0	1
Radiology and Imaging	2	8
Rheumatology	6	10
Total	**19**	**43**

York Hospital/Cornell Medical Center from 1968 to 1993, was brought onto the HSS staff in 1967 by David B. Levine, MD, chief of the Scoliosis Service. Levine sought his expertise in managing adolescent and adult scoliosis patients who presented challenges, particularly with regard to their body image.[23] Clayson was initially introduced to orthopaedics when he subjected a dozen senior HSS orthopaedic staff members to psychological tests, which apparently had never been done before. After all the orthopaedists returned their questionnaires, Clayson reviewed them and reported the results anonymously (Fig. 4).

Clayson's role in the resident interview program was to quiz every candidate alone for 10 minutes to uncover any possible psychological issues. In later years, he became so adept at this that he could identify a potentially "problematic" candidate in 3 minutes.

He also met with the first-year residents monthly for counseling, had yearly dinners with residents and their spouses, and scheduled weekend retreats with residents and their families at the Caspary Estate in the Catskill Mountains of New York—a property left to the HSS house staff for vacation time by Alfred H. Caspary.[1] As far as was known, no other orthopaedic residency/fellowship program in the country enjoyed such a perk, which at the time of writing still exists.

Department of Medicine and Rheumatology

By 1972, Charles L. Christian, MD, was 2 years into his position as director of rheumatic diseases and physician-in-chief (refer to chapter 18). In his 1972

Annual Report, he stated that "the mission of the department is to gain new information regarding the cause of common rheumatic diseases, such as rheumatoid arthritis, systemic lupus erythematosus, arteritis syndromes, polymyositis, etc."[22] (Table 4). In addition to his role in clinical medicine, he also held the position of associate director of the Department of Research (Fig. 5). In 1978, the hospital received its first Multipurpose Arthritis Center grant from the National Institutes of Health and received its second grant 10 years later (see Chapter 18 for more information).

Infectious Diseases Organized

Until 1976, infectious disease consultations were performed by members of the Infectious Diseases Division at Cornell University Medical College on a monthly rotational basis. This changed in 1976, when Barry Brause, MD, and Henry Mazur, MD, approached Wilson Jr. with a clinical research protocol to determine the proper duration of antibiotic therapy to cure uncomplicated osteomyelitis. Wilson was supportive of the proposal but noted that at HSS, bone infections were most often very complex and involved large, indwelling foreign bodies. He asked that a new protocol be designed to effectively treat these patients, most of whom had infected prosthetic joints.

Etiologic microorganisms had become remarkably diverse, and included anaerobes (such as *Propionibacterium acnes*), mycobacteria (both tuberculosis and atypical types), and fungi. The treatment regimen they designed employed a two-stage removal and reimplantation approach to eradicate joint prosthesis infections and used antibiotics on the basis of their quantitative potency for the patient's specific microbe strain. The initial orthopaedic surgeons participating in this new protocol included Wilson Jr., Insall, and Eduardo Salvati, MD. This approach was extraordinarily successful and became the standard of care for treating prosthetic joint infections. It remains, with modifications, the definitive protocol 36 years after its creation.

Brause received his medical degree at the University of Pittsburgh. He was then a medical intern at Boston City Hospital and completed his medical residency and an infectious diseases fellowship at New York Hospital–Cornell University Medical College. Applying the microbiological and pharmacological elements of the infectious diseases discipline, Brause and the orthopaedic

Table 4 HSS Department of Medicine (1973)

DEPARTMENT OF MEDICINE

DIRECTOR OF RHEUMATIC DISEASES..............Charles L. Christian, M.D.

Attending Epidemiologist

Leon J. Kutner, M.D., Ph.D.

Attending Physicians

William H. Kammerer, M.D.
Irwin Nydick, M.D. (Cardiology)

Associate Attending Physicians

Carl A. Berntsen, Jr., M.D.
Abraham S. Jacobson, M.D.
Lawrence J. Kagen, M.D.
William C. Robbins, M.D.
Bernard Rogoff, M.D.
Emmanuel Rudd, M.D.

Assistant Attending Physicians

Harry Bienenstock, M.D.
Edgar J. Desser, M.D.
Martin Gardy, M.D.
Jose Luis Granda, M.D., Ph.D.
Herbert Koteen, M.D.
Robert W. Lightfoot, Jr., M.D.
Michael D. Lockshin, M.D.
Francis Perrone, M.D. (Cardiology)
Paul E. Phillips, M.D.
Marcos Rivelis, M.D.
Robert Thoburn, M.D.

Physicians to Out-Patient Department

Richard L. Danehower, M.D.
Leroy H. Hunninghake, M.D.
Bento Mascarenhas, M.D.
Bruce Nitsberg, M.D.
Milton A. Wald, M.D.

Assistant Physician to Out-Patient Department

Robert Winchester, M.D.

Fellows in Rheumatic Disease

Sidney R. Block, M.D.
Teresita Go, M.D.
William Gough, M.D.
J. Steven McDougal, M.D.
Ronald Saykaly, M.D.
John Sergent, M.D.

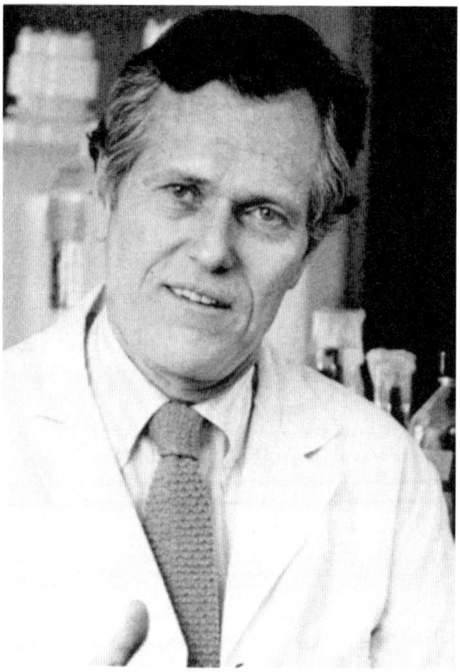

Fig. 5 Besides being HSS physician-in-chief, Charles Christian, MD, also held an interim role as acting physician-in-chief at the New York Hospital and Acting Chairman of the Department of Medicine at Cornell University Medical College. (From Hospital for Special Surgery Archives)

surgeons at HSS fostered a close collaboration, and Brause became the first infectious diseases consultant dedicated to the care of patients at HSS. In 1978, Wilson and Christian arranged for Brause to have a full staff appointment at HSS and to serve on the HSS Infection Control Committee under the leadership of Salvati, who had followed (David B.) Levine as chairman.

Brause subsequently collaborated with Russell Warren and Riley Williams III, MD, to design a successful protocol for the treatment of infected anterior cruciate ligament reconstructions. This protocol has also remained the most successful approach to salvage these complicated reconstructions.

A major concern going into the twenty-first century was the battle against the rising incidence of antibiotic-resistant staphylococci infections. Because quantitative antibiotic potency for each patient's specific bacterial isolate was an essential component in antibiotic therapy design at HSS, cure rates have remained in the 91% to 100% range at the hospital for both methicillin-sensitive and methicillin-resistant staphylococcal infections.

Research

Robert C. Mellors, MD, PhD (1916–2007), was appointed director of research in 1969 and pathologist-in-chief of the Department of the Laboratories (refer to chapter 17). There were over 40 scientists listed in the Research Department in 1973, with offices and laboratories in the Caspary Research Building, across the street from the hospital on East 71st Street (Table 5). As the first free-standing orthopaedic research unit in this country, the building opened with a formal ceremony in 1960. It was the product of a vision of Philip D. Wilson, who realized that a close interaction between research and clinical orthopaedics was essential for new developments in the musculoskeletal field to occur.

To advance the field, Wilson Jr. recruited young engineers, particularly to expand and formalize the design and development of joint replacement implants. HSS was already at the forefront in the development of a total knee implant system, with a team of surgeons and engineers led by Chitranjan S. Ranawat, MD, John Insall, MD (1930–2000), Peter Walker, PhD, and Allan E. Inglis, MD, who produced the first duocondylar and unicondylar prosthesis in 1971.[24, c] A more stable prosthesis led to the development of the total condylar knee by Walker, Ranawat, and Insall in 1974. The total condylar knee became the first successful and widely utilized total knee replacement in the world.[25] Continued development of this implant at the hospital led to the introduction of the Insall-Burstein Total Condylar III in 1976 and the Insall-Burstein posterior stabilized knee prosthesis in 1978 (Fig. 6).

In 1975, Walker resigned as director of the Department of Applied Biomechanics and chief of the Biomechanics Laboratory. He was replaced in May 1976 by Albert H. Burstein, PhD, from Case Western Reserve University in Cleveland, Ohio.

A formal program developed between the hospital and the Sibley School of Mechanical and Aerospace Engineering at the main Cornell University campus in Ithaca, New York to promote collaborative research, teaching, and patient care projects. This program served as a model for linkage programs between engineering faculty and students in Ithaca and HSS clinical and research staff in New York City.

Beginning in 1976, custom implants for difficult cases were fabricated from computer-assisted designs in the hospital's biomechanics department,

Table 5 HSS Research Department 1973

RESEARCH DEPARTMENT

July 1, 1973

ADMINISTRATIVE STAFF

Robert C. Mellors, M.D., Ph.D....................Director of Research

Charles L. Christian, M.D..............Associate Director of Research

Aaron S. Posner, Ph.D..................Associate Director of Research

Walter J. Schulz, B.A...................................Administrator

PROFESSIONAL STAFF

Senior Scientists

Charles L. Christian, M.D.......................Professor of Medicine
Allan E. Inglis, M.D...................Clinical Professor of Surgery (Orthopaedics) and of Anatomy
Leonhard Korngold, Ph.D.................Associate Professor of Microbiology
Klaus Mayer, M.D.........................Clinical Associate Professor of Medicine
Robert C. Mellors, M.D., Ph.D..................Professor of Pathology
Aaron S. Posner, Ph.D......................Professor of Biochemistry
Robert F. Watson, M.D..................Clinical Professor of Medicine

Associate Scientists

Lawrence M. Blau, Ph.D................Assistant Professor of Radiology (Physics)
Walther H. Bohne, M.D.........Clinical Assistant Professor of Surgery (Orthopaedics)
Peter G. Bullough, M.D...............Associate Professor of Pathology
Jose Luis Granda, M.D., Ph.D..........Assistant Professor of Medicine
Lawrence J. Kagen, M.D.................Associate Professor of Medicine
Leon J. Kutner, M.D., Ph.D........Assistant Professor of Microbiology in Surgery (Orthopaedics)
Robert W. Lightfoot, Jr., M.D.........Assistant Professor of Medicine
Michael Lockshin, M.D.................Assistant Professor of Medicine
John L. Marshall, M.D.........Clinical Assistant Professor of Surgery (Orthopaedics) and of Anatomy
Paul E. Phillips, M.D.................Assistant Professor of Medicine
Peter S. Walker, Ph.D...........Assistant Professor of Bioengineering in Surgery (Orthopaedics)

Table 5 *(continued)*

Assistant Scientists

Foster Betts, Ph.D.	Research Associate in Biochemistry
Norman Blumenthal, Ph.D.	Research Associate in Biochemistry
Jane W. Mellors, Ph.D.	Assistant Professor of Biochemistry in Surgery (Orthopaedics)
Takashi Yoshiki, M.D.	Fellow in Pathology

Research Associate

Paul Tannenbaum, D.D.S.	Research Associate in Biochemistry

Visiting Scientist

Chen-Ya Huang, Ph.D.

Research Fellows

Enrique Blazquez, M.D.	Orthopaedics
Sidney R. Block, M.D.	Rheumatic Diseases
Adele Boskey, Ph.D.	Biochemistry
Teresita Go, M.D.	Rheumatic Diseases
William Gough, M.D.	Rheumatic Diseases
J. Steven McDougal, M.D.	Rheumatic Diseases
Harry Robinson, Jr., M.D.	Orthopaedics
Roy Rubin, M.D.	Orthopaedics
Ronald Saykaly, M.D.	Rheumatic Diseases
John Sergent, M.D.	Rheumatic Diseases

Visiting Research Fellow

Hiroshi Saito, M.D.	Immunopathology

Special Consultants

Fakhry G. Girgis, M.D., Ph.D.	Comparative Orthopaedics
Sten-Erik Olsson, D.V.M., M.D., Ph.D.	Comparative Orthopaedics

in collaboration with device manufacturers. Initially located in the Caspary Research Building, the facilities moved in 1982 to the new Dana Center on East 73rd Street.[d]

In November 1976, G. Dean MacEwen, MD, medical director of the Alfred I. duPont Institute (1969–1986), served as the "surgeon-in-chief Pro Tempore," a program started in 1935 by Wilson Sr. As an honorary alumnus, MacEwen has continued to return to HSS functions over the years, attending many HSS annual alumni meetings (Fig. 7).

In that same year, Joseph M. Lane, MD, was recruited from the University of Pennsylvania Hospital to lead a metabolic bone disease service. The next

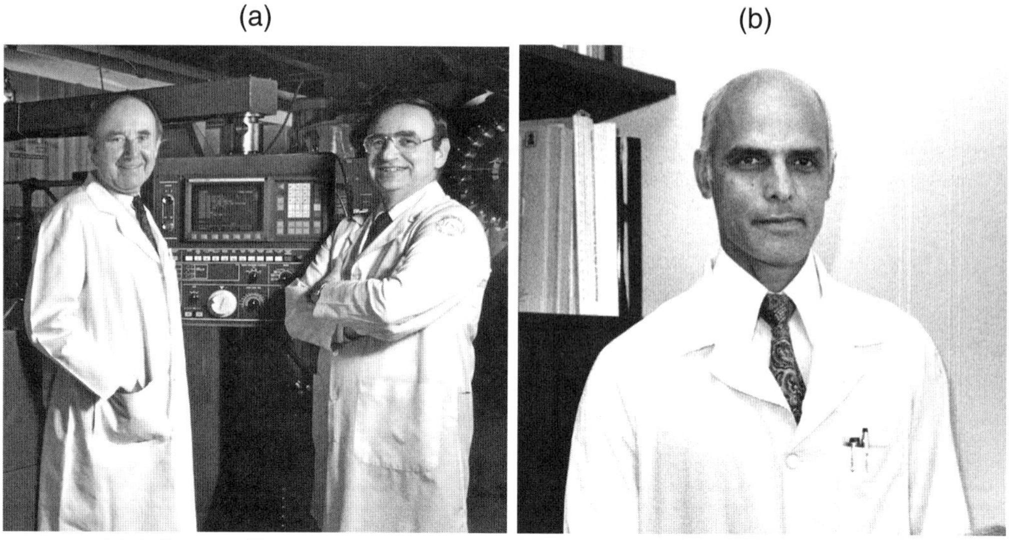

Fig. 6 (a) John Insall, MD, appointed chief of the Knee Service in 1969, discusses a knee implant with Albert Burstein, PhD (right), appointed director of biomechanics in 1976. (b) Chitranjan Ranawat, MD, Together, these three principal investigators pioneered many knee implants designed at HSS.

year, Lane was appointed chief of the Bone Tumor Service at Memorial Sloan-Kettering Cancer Center (Fig. 8).[22] He worked closely with Herbert Kramer, CPO, director of the HSS Orthotics and Prosthetics Department (originally known as a brace shop in the days of James Knight's hospital in the latter part of the nineteenth century) in overseeing the fabrication of

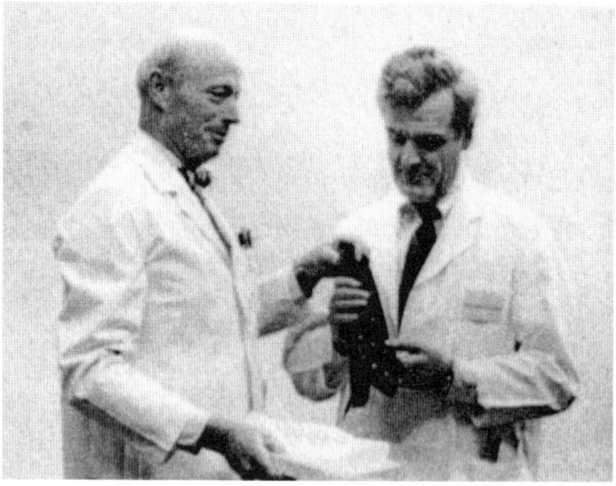

Fig. 7 G. Dean MacEwen, MD (right), the surgeon-in-chief pro tempore at HSS in 1976, receives his HSS tie at the end of the 58th HSS Alumni Association Meeting, where he was made an Honorary Member of the HSS Alumni Association. (From Hospital for Special Surgery Archives)

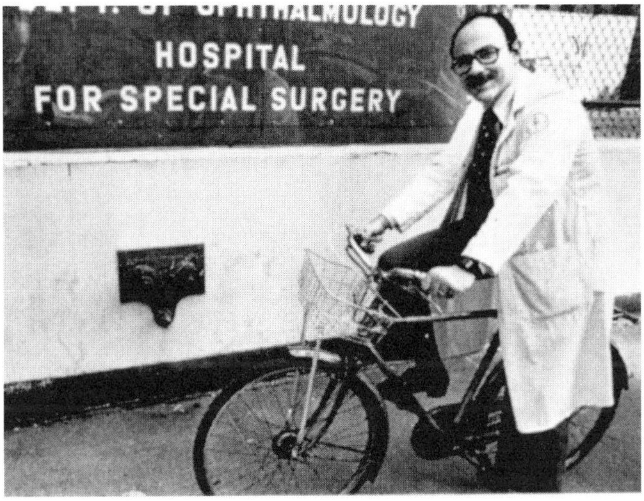

Fig. 8 Joseph Lane, MD (circa 1976), held dual appointments at HSS and Memorial Sloan-Kettering Cancer Center, where he eventually was chief of the Bone Tumor Service. (From Hospital for Special Surgery Archives)

prostheses for amputees. In 1985, Lane started an Osteoporosis Prevention Center and was assisted by Theresa Galsworthy, RN, who managed the program's daily operations.

Expansion and Change

In 1977, a new hospital administrator, Donald S. Broas, was appointed HSS vice president and executive director, when T. Gordon Young retired after 24 years of serving in that role (Fig. 9). That same year saw the retirement of D. Dean Smith, MA, RN, director of nursing from 1965 to 1977. She was succeeded by Barbara J. Kelly, MA, RN, as vice president for nursing, who continued in that role until 1989, when she retired.

The HSS Board of Managers, chaired by Henry U. Harris (1926–2008), made a major commitment in 1977 to expand and relocate the surgical suites and to modernize and add new physician office spaces and private accommodations for ambulatory patients. The board proposed adding three floors over the front driveway from East 70th Street to near 71st Street. The third floor would house a cafeteria, examining areas, and physician offices. The fourth floor would include a modern operating suite of six operating rooms,

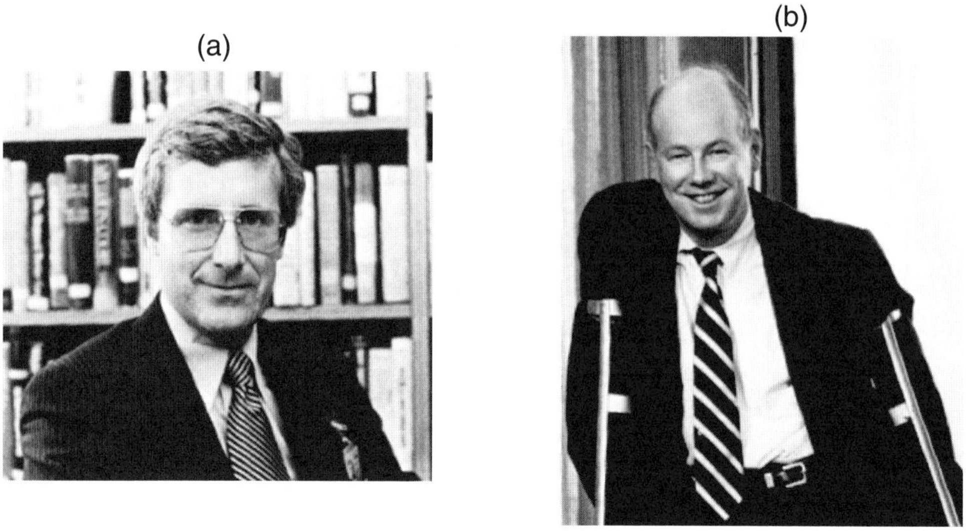

Fig. 9 (a) As HSS executive director, Donald S. Broas orchestrated a large hospital expansion program that gained city, state, and federal approval in 1978 and was completed in 1980. (b) Henry U. Harris, an investment banker[e] who had been on the HSS Board of Managers since 1961, was elected chairman of the board in 1972 at the same time that Philip D. Wilson Jr., became surgeon-in-chief. He led major HSS expansion efforts for nearly two decades until he resigned as chairman in 1989. He was a very effective leader, a good friend of the professional staff, and a close and respected colleague of Wilson Jr. (From Hospital for Special Surgery Archives)

a 15-bed recovery room, and facilities for the Radiology Department, including one room for computed tomography scans. A holding area of six beds would be located on the fifth floor. Funding came from a major campaign named "The New Horizon Fund," chaired by HSS board member Charles H. Theriot of Kidder, Peabody and Company. The projected goal of $8 million was reached by December 1980, and the goal was then extended to $12 million to cover actual increased costs.

The new addition included space for sports medicine services. Interest in sports medicine grew significantly under Warren, and the Sports Medicine Service became very popular with patients and staff. Because of the demand of treating an increasing number of sports-related orthopaedic injuries, an Orthopaedic Sports Medicine Research and Performance Center opened in 1983, with trainers and therapists as part of the staff.

Further renovation and expansion of space on the third floor proceeded in 1986 to provide physician facilities for outpatient services, and construction of the Belaire Building on East 71st Street began. The first 13 floors were for HSS use, while the remaining floors, with a dedicated entrance on East 72nd Street, housed private residential condominiums. A hospital café was located on the ground level, and the cafeteria in the main building was closed. The newly created Sports Center moved into the area opposite the café in 1988, when the Belaire Building was completed.

In 1985, Mellors retired and Aaron S. Posner, PhD, associate director of research, was appointed as director of research. Peter Bullough, MD, on staff as chief orthopaedic pathologist since 1968 and attending pathologist since 1980, was appointed director of laboratory medicine. Posner retired in 1987 and was replaced by Wilson Jr.

One of the many specialty clinics and services was the Back Service, whose chief was Bernard Jacobs, MD (1924–1992). He specialized in low back pain, and managed complex cases in patients who came from around the world to seek his expert orthopaedic advice (Fig. 10). Jacobs, known affectionately as "Jake," was a special mentor to many of the orthopaedic

(a)

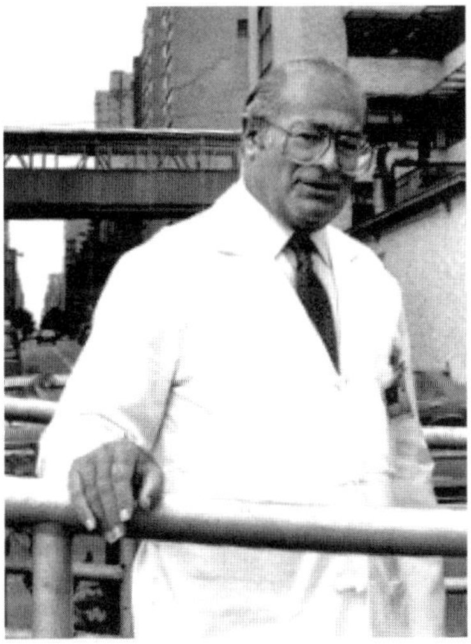

(b)

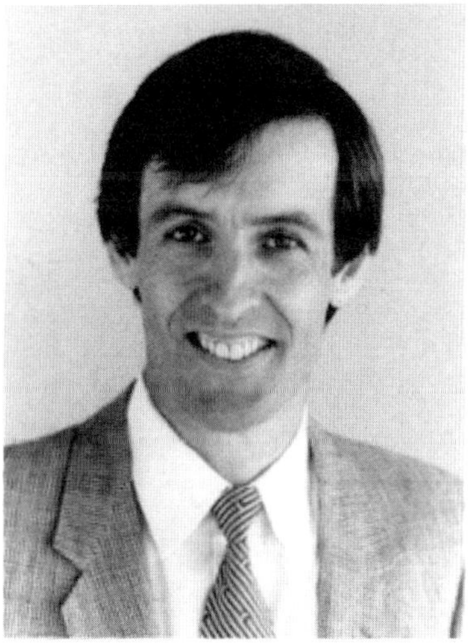

Fig. 10 (a) Bernard Jacobs, MD, on the East 71st Street ramp next to the Caspary Research Building in 1988. Born in London, he graduated from the University College Hospital Medical School in 1948 and became an American citizen in 1950. (b) Nigel Sharrock, MB, ChB appointed chief of anesthesia in 1986, investigated patients undergoing total joint replacement and assessed their cardiopulmonary and vascular status postoperatively. He introduced epidural pain control at HSS and quickly became a leading authority, addressing orthopaedic meetings across the nation. (From Hospital for Special Surgery Archives)

residents who learned the techniques of neck and back surgery, particularly when they rotated under him at the Bronx Veterans Hospital. He never shied away from a patient with a "redo" back operation, particularly if it was his, and he could gracefully gain the confidence of any challenging case. For his patients who were disabled with severe pain, he would even make a house call to a New York apartment.

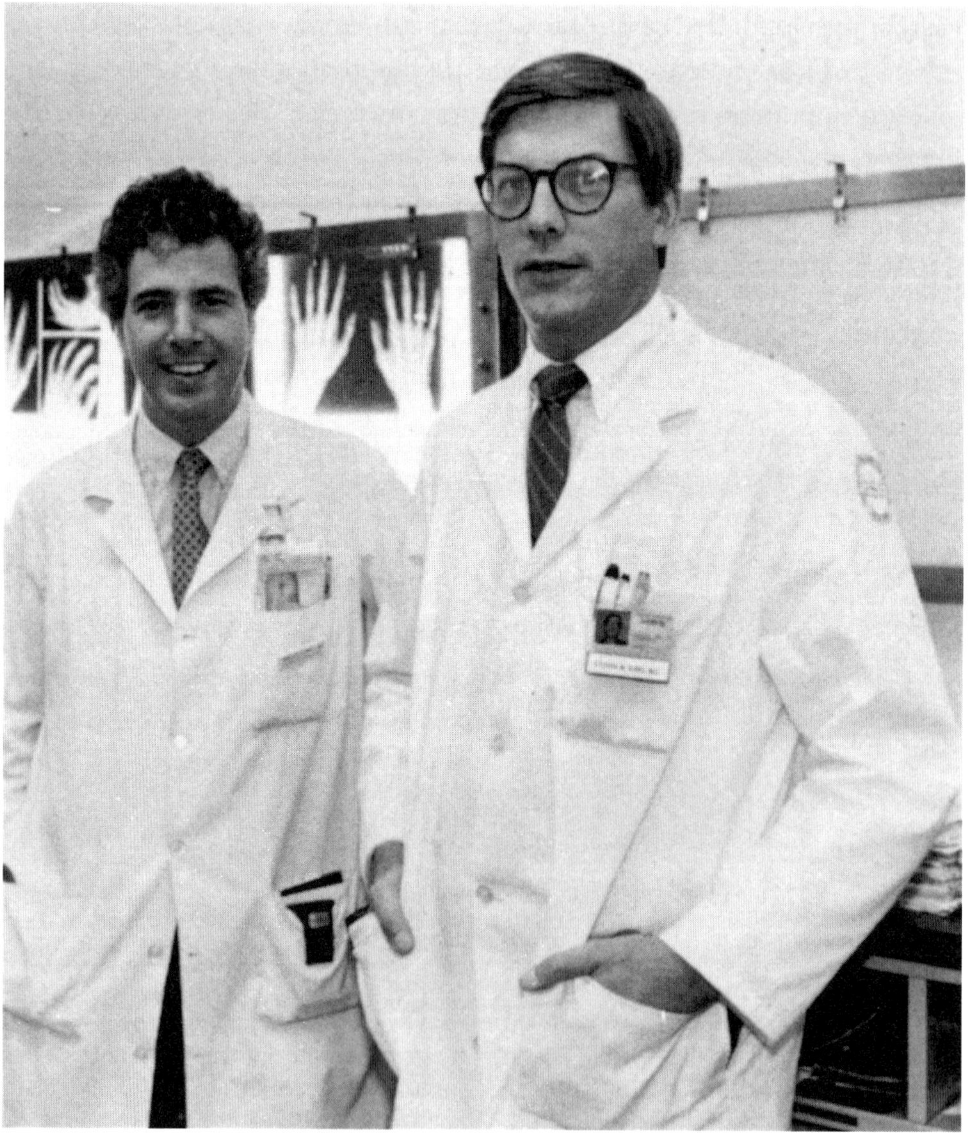

Fig. 11 Charles Cornell, MD (left), who joined the HSS staff in 1986, became chief of the Bronx Veterans Hospital Orthopaedic Section in 1990. Stephen Burke, MD, joined the HSS orthopaedic pediatric staff, becoming its chief. (From Hospital for Special Surgery Archives)

With the retirement of Fox, Nigel E. Sharrock, MB, ChB, was appointed director of the Department of Anesthesia in July 1986 (Fig. 10). Sharrock brought new staff physicians to the department, introduced regional anesthesia techniques, implemented a pain service, and explored hypotensive anesthesia methods and sophisticated monitoring systems.

Two other new orthopaedic staff appointments in 1986 were Stephen W. Burke, MD, and Charles N. Cornell, MD. A 1971 graduate of Cornell Medical College, Burke was an associate professor of pediatric orthopaedics at Louisiana State University Medical School and had been on staff at Tulane Medical Center, Children's Hospital and Touro Infirmary, all in New Orleans.

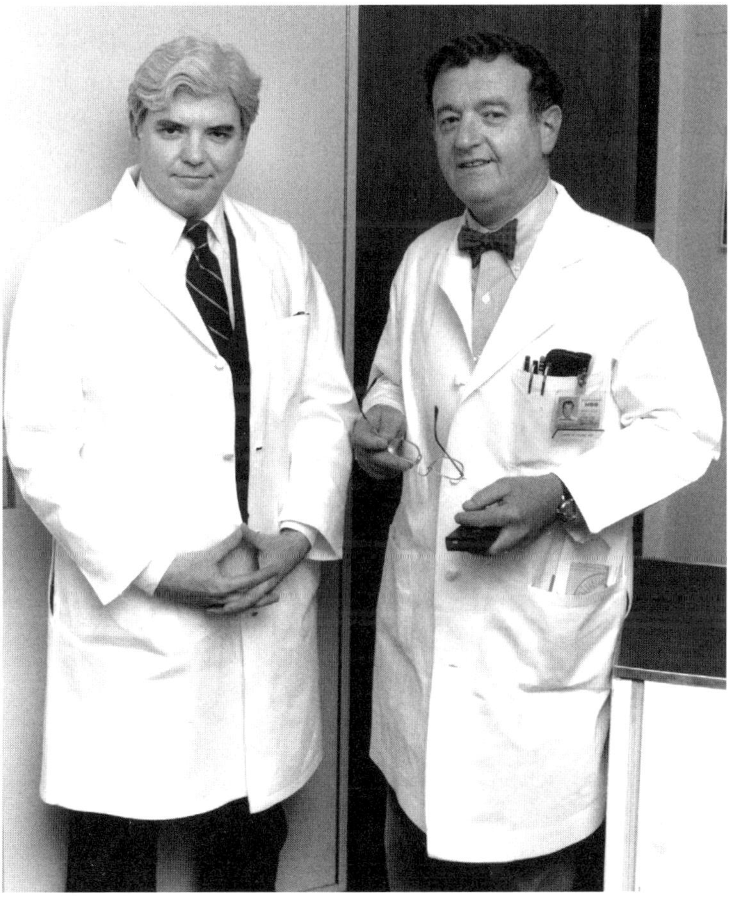

Fig. 12 David B. Levine, MD (right), appointed the new director of orthopaedic surgery in 1987 under Philip D. Wilson Jr., MD, was assisted by Thomas P. Sculco, MD, as associate director. Levine graduated as an orthopaedic resident from HSS in the class of 1964. Sculco graduated in the HSS resident class of 1972. (From Hospital for Special Surgery Archives)

Cornell, an HSS orthopaedic resident from 1982 to 1985, received his medical degree from Cornell University Medical College in 1980. Following his orthopaedic residency, he was the recipient of the Hoar Fellowship in Orthopaedic Trauma, granted by the New York Academy of Medicine. He pursued an additional trauma fellowship at the Harborview Medical Center in Seattle, Washington (Fig. 11).

David B. Levine, MD, having been the associate director of orthopaedic surgery (1973–1986), was appointed director of orthopaedic surgery in July 1987, a position previously held by Wilson Jr. (Fig. 12).

With the hospital running into progressive operative deficits by the end of the 1980s, Levine initiated a total hospital Cost Containment Program. He called a number of meetings of interdisciplinary hospital staff to address widespread waste, calling for heightened awareness of problems, education, and communication among all members of the HSS staff. The initial focus was on operating room performance and specifically addressed the control,

(a) (b)

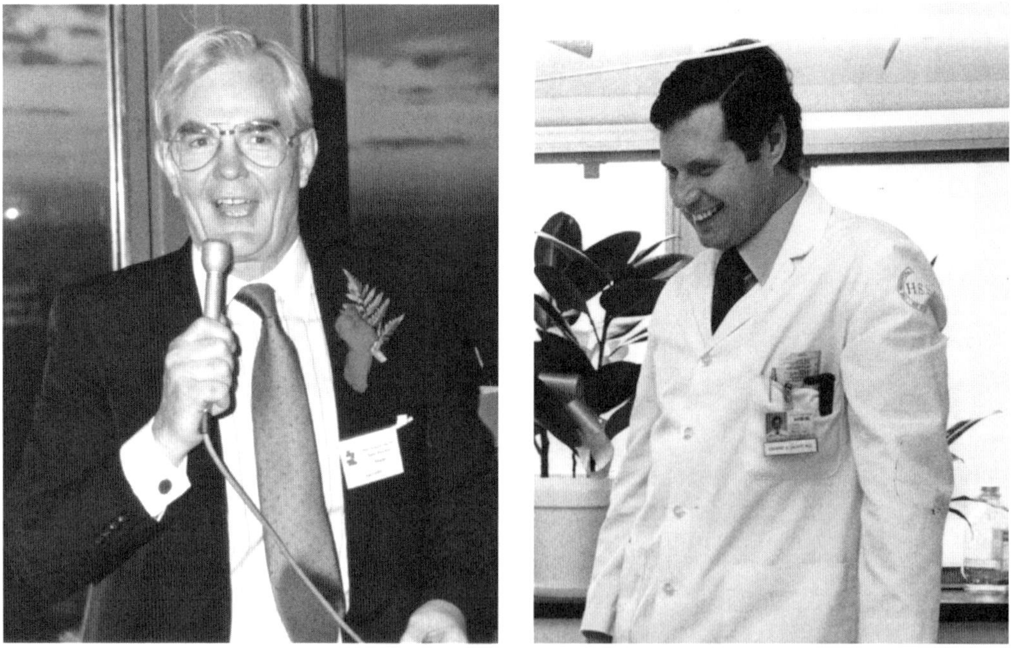

Fig. 13 (a) John Lyden, MD, being inducted as a 25-year member of the 15–25 Year Club; he started his HSS orthopaedic residency in 1969. (b) Eduardo Salvati, MD, who had received his medical degree in Buenos Aires, Argentina, was an orthopaedic resident in Florence, Italy, and Buenos Aires before becoming a hip and knee fellow at HSS. (From Hospital for Special Surgery Archives)

use, and costs of joint implants. Attention to reimbursement became a significant issue, particularly the knowledge, performance, and responsibility of the coders in the Record Room. The bottom line was education of all staff, particularly the professional staff.[26, 27] Moreover, it was occurring at a time when HSS was experiencing hospital staff layoffs. Throughout the hospital, posters were displayed with the following message: *Reduce waste—help save a job—that job that may be yours* (refer to chapter 12).

Straub retired in 1987, having established a Hand Clinic in 1953 and the Comprehensive Arthritis Service (CAP) in 1967 with Richard H. Freyberg, MD (1905–1999), then director of rheumatic diseases. Following Straub's retirement, Allan E. Inglis was appointed as chief of the Hand Service, and Chitranjan Ranawat as chief of the CAP Service. In 1984, John Lyden, MD, was appointed chief of the Combined Fracture Service at New York Hospital—a post he held until 1991 (Fig. 13).

In 1989, Robert Freiberger, MD, resigned as director of radiology and nuclear medicine. He was followed in that position by Jeremy Kaye, MD.

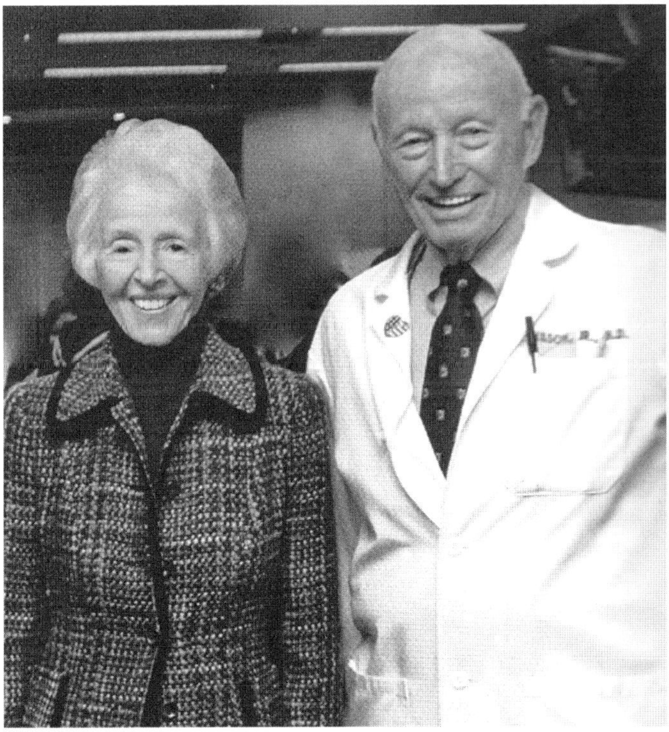

Fig. 14 Katherine Wilson, and Philip D. Wilson Jr., attending the 50th anniversary (2005) of the HSS move from East 42nd Street to East 70th Street. (From Hospital for Special Surgery Archives)

About that time, Wilson Jr. announced his intent to retire as surgeon-in-chief, and a search committee for his replacement was formed. For more than two decades, Wilson Jr. led the development and advancement of and investigative research in total hip replacement surgery at HSS. When he first became surgeon-in-chief in 1972, he appointed Eduardo Salvati, MD, who had just completed a fellowship in hip and knee surgery at the hospital, to become chief of the Hip Service (Fig. 13).

With Salvati as a coauthor, Wilson Jr. published a number of studies on successful results and complications of total hip replacement, particularly analyzing postoperative infections and methods of prevention.[28–31] He reported a long-term follow-up of Charnley total hip replacements and revision hip surgery in the early 1980s.[32, 36] Wilson Jr. selectively studied mechanical failures of hip replacements, the histology of the bone-cement interface, and the role of polymethylmethacrylate in total hip arthroplasty.

On December 31, 1989, Philip D. Wilson Jr. retired from the office of the surgeon-in-chief, after more than 17 years in that position. He continued to treat patients, gradually giving up surgery. As of 2012, he continued to consult new patients and followed many of his old patients. His longstanding secretaries, Mary Birnbaum (who has been with his office since 1956) and Leslee Wong (since 1979), faithfully assist him. In 2005, his devoted wife, Katherine (Kit) Wilson, passed away after battling cancer (Fig. 14).

REFERENCES

1. O'Brasky M. *Reflections on and celebrations of Dr. Philip D. Wilson Jr.* HSS Alumni News. 2009;Fall.
2. Wilson PD Jr. *Paralytic foot deformities.* Pediatr Clin North Am. 1955;2:987–1001.
3. Wilson PD Jr., Levine DB. *Internal derangements of the knee joint.* In: Comroe's Arthritis and Allied Conditions, edited by J Hollander. Philadelphia, PA: Lea & Febiger; 1972:1411–1421.
4. Wilson PD Jr. *Fracture dislocations of the shoulder girdle.* In: Surgical Treatment of Trauma, edited by PA Wade. New York, NY: Grune & Stratton. 1960;405–411.
5. Wilson PD Jr., Amstutz HA, Czerniecki A, Salvati EA, Mendes DG. *Total hip replacement with fixation by acrylic cement: a preliminary study of 100 consecutive McKee-Farrar prosthetic replacements.* J Bone Joint Surg. 1972;54A:207–236.

6. Wilson PD Jr. Ritter MA. *Colonna capsular arthroplasty—a long term follow-up of forty hips.* J Bone Joint Surg. 1968;50A:1305–1327.
7. Wilson PD Jr., Levine DB. *Compensatory pelvic osteotomy for ankylosing spondylitis.* J Bone Joint Surg. 1969;51A:142–148.
8. Amstutz HC, Wilson PD Jr. *Dysgenesis of the proximal femur (coxa vara) and its surgical management.* J Bone Joint Surg Am. 1962;44A:1–24.
9. Wilson PD Jr., Dangelmajer RC. *The problems of atlanto-axial dislocation in rheumatoid arthritis.* J Bone Joint Surg. 1963;49A:1780.
10. Wilson PD Jr., Levine DB. *Low back pain and sciatica.* In: Comroe's Arthritis and Allied Conditions, edited by J Hollander. Philadelphia, PA: Lea & Febiger; 1972.
11. Wilson PD Jr. *Low back pain—a problem for industry.* Arch Environ Health. 1962;5: 505–510.
12. Wilson PD Jr. *Nationally organized courses and symposia in orthopaedic education.* Clin Orthop. 1971;75:129–134.
13. Wilson PD Jr. *A clinical study of the biomechanical behavior of massive bone transplants used to reconstruct large bone defects.* Clin Orthop. 1972;87:81–109.
14. Wilson PD Jr. *James Knight (1810–1887) of the Hospital for the Ruptured and Crippled.* Clin Orthop. 1958;11:1–8.
15. Wilson PD Jr. *The Hospital for Special Surgery Annual Report*, New York, NY; 1973.
16. Patterson RL. *The Hospital for Special Surgery Annual Report*, New York, NY; 1971.
17. Gross J. Marshall, *sports-medicine expert, killed in air crash.* New York Times. 1980; Feb. 14.
18. Goldstein R. James Nicholas, *85, leader in treating sports injuries, dies.* New York Times. July 17, 2006.
19. Nicholas JA, Burstein CL, Umberger CJ. *Management of adrenocortical insufficiency during surgery.* AMA Arch Surg. 1995;71:737–742.
20. Jackson DW. *The history of sports medicine.* Part 2. Am J Sports Med. 1984;12:255–257.
21. Wilson PD Jr. *One for all; all for one.* J Bone Joint Surg. 1973;55A:859–865.
22. Wilson PD Jr. Levine DB. *Hospital for Special Surgery; a brief review of its development and current position.* Clin Orthop. 2000;374:90–106.
23. Clayson D, Levine DB. *Adolescent scoliosis patients' personality patterns and effects of corrective surgery.* Clin Orthop. 1976;116:99–102.
24. Ranawat CS. *History of total knee replacement.* J South Orthop Assoc. 2002;11:218–26.
25. RDS. John N. Insall, MD, *1930–2000.* J Bone Joint Surg. 2001;83A:635.
26. Levine DB, Kille A, Keenam M, Carr J, Wright T, Burstein A. *Cost awareness and containment for the 1990s; recycling orthopaedic implants.* Contemp Orthop. 1992;25:376–381.
27. Levine DB, Cole BJ, Rodeo SA. *Cost awareness and cost containment at the Hospital for Special Surgery.* Clin Orthop. 1995;311:117–124.
28. Wilson PD Jr., Salvati EA, Aglietti P, Kutner LJ. *The problem of infection in endoprosthetic surgery of the hip joint.* Clin Orthop. 1973;96:213–221.

29. Aglietti P, Salvati EA, Wilson PD Jr., Kutner L. *Effect of a surgical horizontal unidirectional filtered air flow unit on wound bacterial contamination and wound healing.* Clin Orthop. 1974;101:99–104.
30. Wilson PD Jr., Aglietti P, Salvati EA. *Subacute sepsis of the hip treated by antibiotic and cemented prosthesis.* J Bone Joint Surg. 1974;56A:879–898.
31. Salvati EA, Wilson PD Jr., Jolley MN, Vakili F, Aglietti P, Brown GC. *A ten-year follow-up study of our first one hundred consecutive Charnley total hip replacements.* J Bone Joint Surg. 1981;63A:753–67.
32. Pellicci PM, Wilson PD Jr., Sledge CB, Salvati EA, Ranawat CS, Poss R. *Revision total hip arthroplasty.* Clin Orthop. 1982;170:34–41.
33. Pellicci PM, Wilson PD Jr., Sledge CB, Salvati EA, Ranawat CS, Poss R., Callaghan JJ. *Long-term results of revision total hip replacement; a follow-up report.* J Bone Joint Surg. 1985;67A:513–516.
34. Callaghan JJ, Salvati EA, Pellicci PM, Wilson PD Jr., Ranawat CS. *Results of revision of mechanical failure after cemented total hip replacement.* J Bone Joint Surg. 1985;67A: 1074–1085.
35. Johanson NA, Bullough PG, Wilson PD Jr., Salvati EA, Ranawat CS. *The microscopic anatomy of the bone-cement interface in failed total hip arthroplasties.* Clin Orthop. 1987;218:123–135.
36. Wilson PD Jr. *Revision total hip arthroplasty: current role of polymethylmethacrylate.* Clin Orthop. 1987;225:218–229.

NOTES

a. In 1989, the last year that Wilson Jr. was surgeon-in-chief, the average length of the hospital stay had been reduced to fewer than 9 days, with ambulatory surgery increasing to 1,129 procedures (up from only 74 in 1980). Four operating rooms in 1972 doubled to eight by 1989.

b. Rizzo had twin sons—Peter Rizzo III, MD, and Thomas Rizzo, MD—who both trained as orthopaedic residents at HSS. The Rizzo legacy was carried on by Tom's son, Peter F. Rizzo, MD, who also trained as an orthopaedic resident at HSS. At the time of this writing, Peter F. Rizzo—who had previously taken over his father's and grandfather's practice in Bronxville, New York—explained that many of the practice's long-time patients still thought they were under the care of his grandfather, Peter Cyrus Rizzo II.

c. HSS surgical records indicated that 103 knee replacements were performed in 1972, increasing to 836 in 1989.

d. The Dana Center moved back to the Caspary Research Building in January 2004.

e. Henry U. Harris, grandson of John F. Harris—the founder of Harris, Upham & Co. and the grandson of Edwin S. Webster, the founder of Stone & Webster, Inc.—was president and CEO of Harris, Upham & Co. As a second lieutenant in the Army, just after marching in front of General Douglas MacArthur in the Philippines on July 4, 1946 (the day the Philippines became independent), Harris contracted polio. He was medically transported to Hot Springs, Arkansas, and then later to Warm Springs, Georgia, to convalesce.

CHAPTER 12
ANDREW J. WEILAND, MD NINTH SURGEON-IN-CHIEF (1990–1993)

DAVID B. LEVINE, MD

ON JANUARY 1, 1990, AFTER an 18-month nationwide search, the Board of Trustees of the Hospital for Special Surgery (HSS) announced the appointment of Andrew J. Weiland, MD, as the ninth surgeon-in-chief. It was only the second time in the history of the hospital that an outside staff member assumed professional leadership of HSS, the other being Philip D. Wilson Sr. in 1934. Weiland acknowledged that he had a hard act to follow after Philip D. Wilson Jr., who was so highly regarded by HSS staff and had served as surgeon-in-chief for 17 years.

The year 1990 ushered in an unsettled decade. Just 7 weeks before on November 9, 1989, in East Berlin, the guards at the wall separating the "Free World" from the "Communist World" abandoned their posts. Within weeks, the wall was torn down, and with the collapse of the Soviet Union, an end came to the 40-year-old Cold War. The United States, truly the superpower of the world, was now about to be confronted with a new war—the Gulf War, when Iraq invaded Kuwait in August 1990.

Back in New York City, the city's first black mayor, David Dinkins, was inaugurated, having defeated incumbent Ed Koch. The subway fare rose from $1 to $1.15 on January 1, the same day 567,000 gallons of oil spilled from an Exxon pipeline into the Arthur Kill in New York Harbor. The bond market collapsed, with Drexel Burnham Lambert going bankrupt. The names of Ivan Boesky and Michael Milken suddenly became front-page headlines in newspapers across the nation.[1]

Postgraduate Training

Disorder in the world prevailed when Weiland arrived at HSS from the Johns Hopkins University School of Medicine. He was particularly distinguished in the fields of hand, upper extremity, and microsurgery surgery.

Weiland earned his MD degree in 1968 from Bowman Gray School of Medicine of Wake Forest University in Winston-Salem, North Carolina (Fig. 1). He then spent a year as a surgical intern, followed by a second year as a surgical resident at the University of Michigan. His training was interrupted in 1970 by a 2-year assignment in the U.S. Army Medical Corps at Fort Jackson Army Hospital in Columbia, South Carolina, being discharged with the rank of major. After finishing a 4-year orthopaedic residency training program at Johns Hopkins, he was an ASIF fellow in internal fixation of fractures under Professor Hans Willenegger in Leistal, Switzerland, for 3 months. In July 1975, he trained as a Christine Kleinert Fellow in hand surgery for 6 months at the University of Louisville.

Returning to Hopkins in 1976, he rose through the ranks, being appointed professor of orthopaedic surgery and professor of emergency medicine in

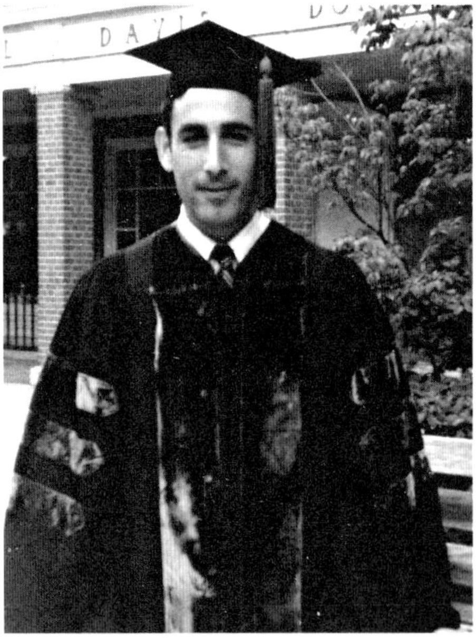

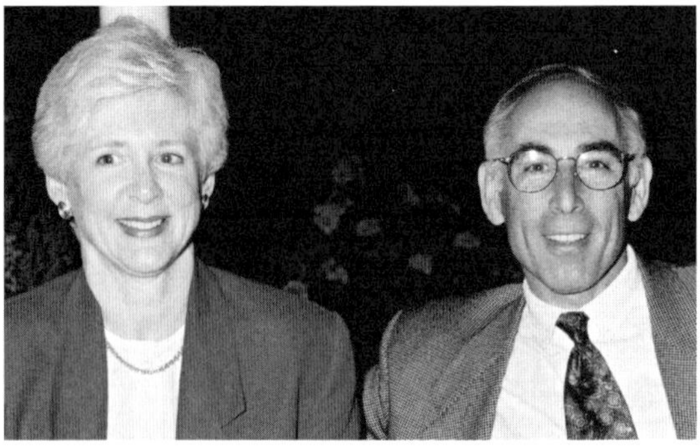

Fig. 1 (Right) Married to Nancy Greer in 1963, here are Andrew and Nancy Weiland in later years. In 1968, Weiland received his medical degree from Bowman Gray School of Medicine. (From A. Weiland)

1983 at the medical school. Two years later, he was appointed professor of plastic surgery.

Family Life

Born in 1942 and raised in New York City, Weiland met his future wife, Nancy Greer, at Colby College in Waterville, Maine, where he received his BA degree in 1964. She received her bachelor's degree the next year. They were married in the spring of 1965. Nancy Weiland was awarded a master's degree in 1967 from Bowman Gray School of Medicine and, in 1984, a PhD in physiology from the University of Maryland School of Medicine. She published over 50 papers in scientific journals and served as an assistant professor in neuroendocrinology at the Rockefeller University from 1990 to 1999.

The Weilands raised two children: Sarah Weiland Holland, MD, a plastic surgeon, and Daniel E. Weiland, MD, an orthopaedic surgeon who trained as an orthopaedic resident at HSS. Both obtained their medical degrees from Cornell University Medical College.

1990–1991 Hospital and Staff Expansion

Expansion of the hospital's physical plant, technological services, and professional staff while promoting new trends in ambulatory surgery and reduction of the average length of stay of inpatients earmarked the beginning of the 1990s. After 6 years, a Certificate of Need for building an East Wing of the hospital was finally approved by state and federal authorities. The Dana Center, a new engineering facility for the design and manufacture of implants, was completed on East 73rd Street.

In 1991, a ninth operating room was added to the fourth-floor surgical suites. Two new ambulatory operating rooms, a holding area, and a 10-bed postoperative care unit were added on the first floor that October. As the length of stay was declining, 32 beds were decertified, leaving an inpatient bed capacity of 160. Plans were being made to expand the first floor ambulatory operating suite to four operating rooms.

In 1991, Weiland appointed Richard Laskin, MD (1940–2008), and Russell Windsor, MD as co-chiefs of the Knee Service (Fig. 2); Laskin eventually became chief of the Division of Arthroplasty in 2006. This division was

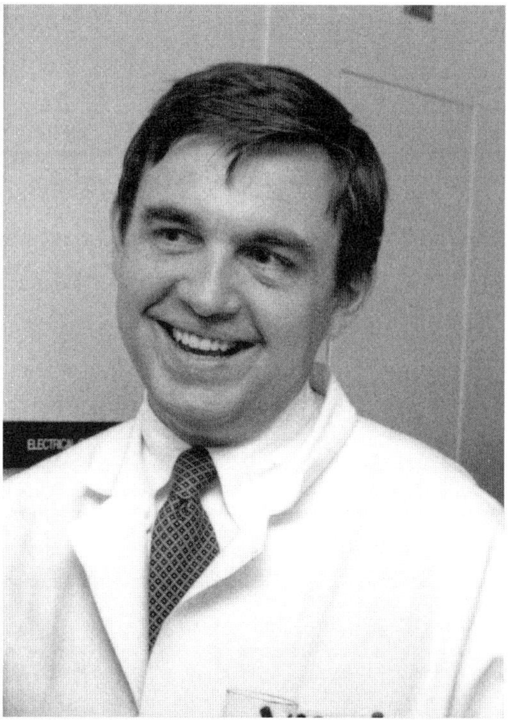

Fig. 2 Russell E. Windsor, MD, received his medical education at the Georgetown, Thomas Jefferson, and Cornell Universities. He completed his orthopaedic training at the University of Pennsylvania and did a fellowship in knee reconstructive surgery at the Hospital for Special Surgery under John Insall, MD. Windsor was President of the American Knee Society in 2005.

reorganized as the Adult Reconstruction and Joint Replacement Division in 2008 (see chapter 11 for more information). Laskin came from Long Island Jewish Medical Center, where he had served as chief of orthopaedic surgery. He received his MD degree from New York University School of Medicine in 1964 and trained in orthopaedic surgery at Albert Einstein College of Medicine. Serving in the U.S. Army in Vietnam, he received the Purple Heart for injuries resulting from a grenade.

Laskin was active in the Knee Society, serving on its Board of Directors and acting as program director a number of times. He was known for his investigational research, expertise in technical surgical procedures, and teaching in the field of total knee reconstruction. He had many talents as a brilliant writer and engaging speaker, often giving presentations in Spanish, Italian, Japanese, and Chinese in foreign countries.

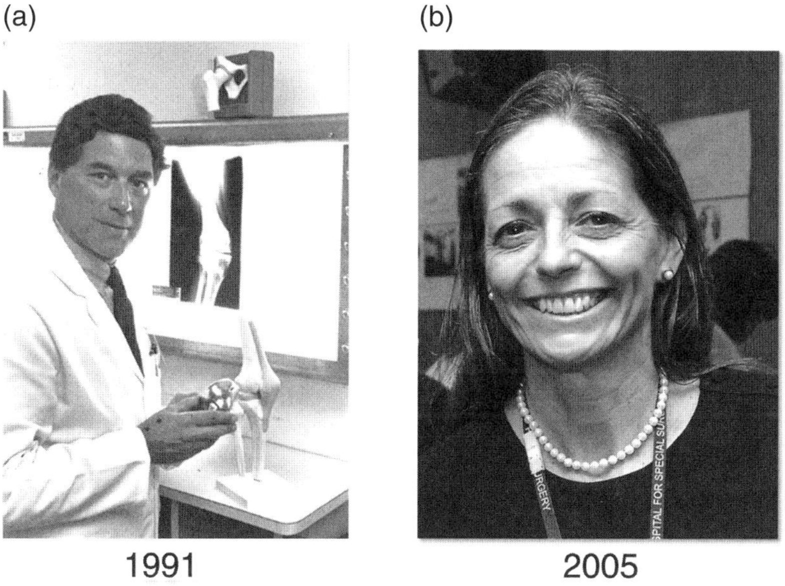

Fig. 3 (a) Richard Laskin, MD, studying a knee implant in 1991. In 2005, (b) Laura Robbins collaborated with Laskin to launch the *HSS Journal.* (From Hospital for Special Surgery Archives)

In 2005, the 11th surgeon-in-chief, Thomas P. Sculco, appointed Laskin as editor-in-chief of the newly created *HSS Journal* with Laura Robbins, DSW, senior vice president of Education & Academic Affairs, as executive editor. The first issue was published in September of that year (Fig. 3). Historically, this marked the fourth scientific journal published at HSS since 1958 (Table 1).

Two and a half years later, on March 1, 2008, Laskin passed away after a long battle with cancer. Charles N. Cornell, MD, replaced him as editor-in-chief of the *HSS Journal.* By 2012, the *HSS Journal* was publishing three issues annually. The aims and scope of the publication have been to promote cutting-edge research, clinical pathways, and state-of-the-art techniques to educate the orthopaedic and musculoskeletal communities. Cornell and Robbins were assisted by an editorial board of over 35 physicians, scientists, and support staff.

Other new appointments in 1991 included Jonathan T. Deland, MD, as co-chief of the Foot and Ankle Service, David L. Helfet, MD, as chief of the Trauma Service, and Robert N. Hotchkiss, MD, as chief of the Hand Service (Fig. 4). Paul M. Pellicci, MD, had been appointed chief of the Hip Service in 1990, a position he held until 2005. Reorganization of the Hip and Knee Services continued through the next two surgeons-in-chief (Table 2).

Table 1 Scientific Journals Published at the Hospital for Special Surgery

The Bulletin of the Hospital for Special Surgery—published from 1958 to 1962, when its editor, J. Paul Harvey, MD, resigned from the Hospital for Special Surgery staff
The Review of the Hospital for Special Surgery—published from 1971 to 1972 by editor Allan E. Inglis, MD
The Journal of the Hospital for Special Surgery—published one issue in November 1975 (editor and staff unlisted)
HSS Journal—published in 2005–present. Richard Laskin, MD, died in 2008 and was replaced with Charles Cornell, MD, as editor-in-chief

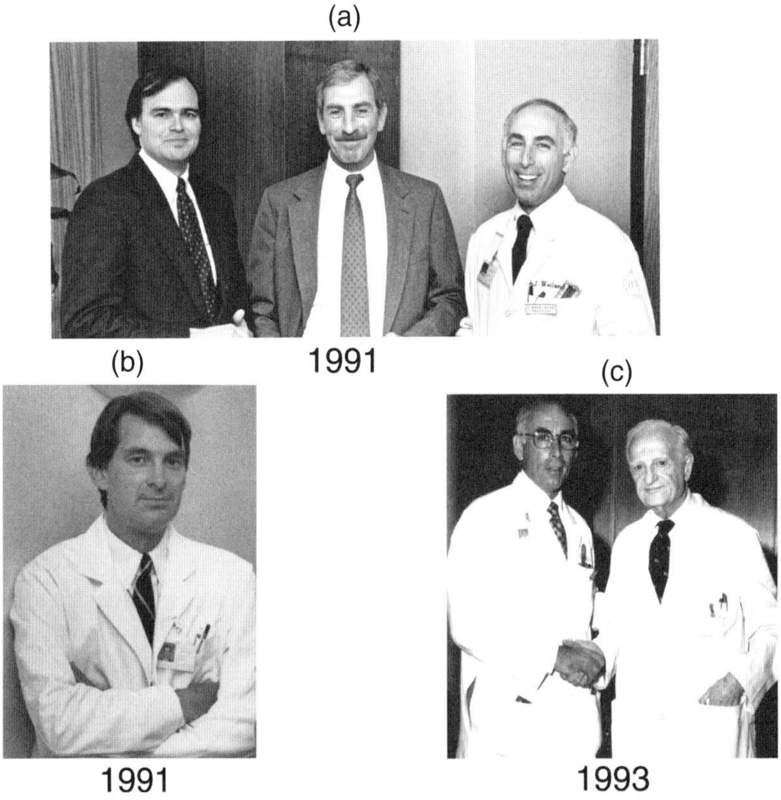

Fig. 4 (a, from left) Robert N. Hotchkiss, MD, David L. Helfet, MD, and Andrew Weiland in the second year of Weiland's administration as surgeon-in-chief. (b) Jonathan T. Deland, MD, joined the staff, coming from Boston. (c) Weiland honored Alexander Hersh, MD (1909–2005), on his 50th anniversary of beginning his orthopaedic residency at R&C. (From Hospital for Special Surgery Archives)

Table 2 Organization of Hip and Knee Services (1990–2012)

Hip Service
Eduardo A. Salvati, MD
Chief: 1972–1990
Hip and Knee Service (1990)
Eduardo A. Salvati, MD
Director: 1990–2005
Paul M. Pellicci, MD
Chief, Hip Service: 1990–2005
Richard S. Laskin, MD
Co-Chief, Knee Service: 1991–2005
Russell E. Windsor, MD
Co-Chief, Knee Service: 1991–2005
Division of Arthroplasty (2006–2008)
(Reorganized into)
Adult Reconstruction
and
Joint Replacement Division (ARJR): 2008–present
Richard S. Laskin, MD
Chief: 2006–2008
Douglas E. Padgett, MD
Chief, ARJR: 2008–present
Chief, Hip Service: 2006–present
Steven B. Haas, MD
Chief, Knee Service: 2006–present
Mark P. Figgie, MD
Chief, Surgical Arthritis Service: 2006–present

Cost Containment Program

As noted in chapter 11, Levine started a Cost Awareness & Containment Program at the hospital in January 1990. About that time, the price tag on the delivery of health care in our country was predicted to exceed $800 billion.[a] It was then estimated that costs attributable to misuse, abuse, and duplication totaled more than $200 billion nationally. HSS operating costs included $22 million for supplies, with a $4 million revenue deficit.

A multidisciplinary team—including orthopaedic attending physicians, operating room administrators, senior financial staff, nursing staff, cost center representatives, and orthopaedic residents and fellows—met regularly to discuss ways to contain costs. Cost-awareness initiatives were established to achieve substantial savings while improving the delivery of health care.

Using alternatives to disposable supplies and negotiating with vendors resulted in an immediate savings of $200,000. The regulation of medical wastes in 1992 shaved $127,000 off the original annual costs of $300,000 in 1 year alone. Levine and his collaborators presented an exhibit about the cost-

Table 3 Handout at the 60th Annual Meeting of the American Academy of Orthopaedic Surgeons in 1990

COST AWARENESS & COST CONTAINMENT

A Necessity in the Delivery of Orthopaedic Care for the 1990's.

RECYCLE

Brian J. Cole, M.D.
Scott A. Rodeo, M.D.
David B. Levine, M.D.
James Carr, B.A.

535 E 70th Street, New York, NY 10021 — The Hospital for Special Surgery

containment initiatives at the 60th Annual Meeting of the American Academy of Orthopaedic Surgeons in 1993, held in San Francisco (Table 3).

Early Medical Education

Before 1961, there was no formal Medical Education Department at HSS, but by the time of Weiland's arrival, an established department was in place. In the early 1940s, Lee Ramsay Straub, MD, the executive assistant to Philip D. Wilson Sr., surgeon-in-chief, was in charge of orthopaedic resident recruitment. Straub's secretary, Dolores Mattia, arranged interview appointments for candidates applying to the resident program (Fig. 5). She was the only executive secretary to Straub for over 50 years, and at the time of this writing, she was doing well in retirement, approaching age 90 years.

The first coordinator of medical education was Johanna O. Vettoretti, previously a secretary to Wilson Sr.; she served in that position from 1961 to 1965. From 1965 to 1967, Joan Cook was coordinator of medical education. When Cook left, Jean McDaniel became coordinator of medical education, and she served in that capacity until she retired in 1989. She was then voted into the Alumni Association as an honorary member (Fig. 5).

After her death in 1995, the HSS Alumni Association created the Jean C. McDaniel Award. It was her wish that the Jean C. McDaniel Memorial Fund, established in her memory, be used to benefit the residents. The award was to be given to the chief resident who most embodied the principles that McDaniel would herself have endorsed. These include, but are not limited to, a chief resident who serves as a role model to other residents by her/his high moral standards, professional skill, and dedication to the HSS community and resident education.

At the end of 1989, Nancy Kane Bischoff was appointed head of medical education. Soon after, in 1991, Maureen Bogle, who had been secretary to John Doherty, executive assistant to surgeon-in-chief Robert Patterson Jr. joined Bischoff as her assistant. At about that time, after Weiland arrived, there was a shift in offices, and Bischoff assumed additional responsibilities as director of Medical Staff Services. From 1991 to 2000, Bogle also served as the administrator of the HSS Alumni Association. Her role was to organize the annual alumni meetings in November, including the evening social events and the alumni receptions at the annual meeting of the American Academy of

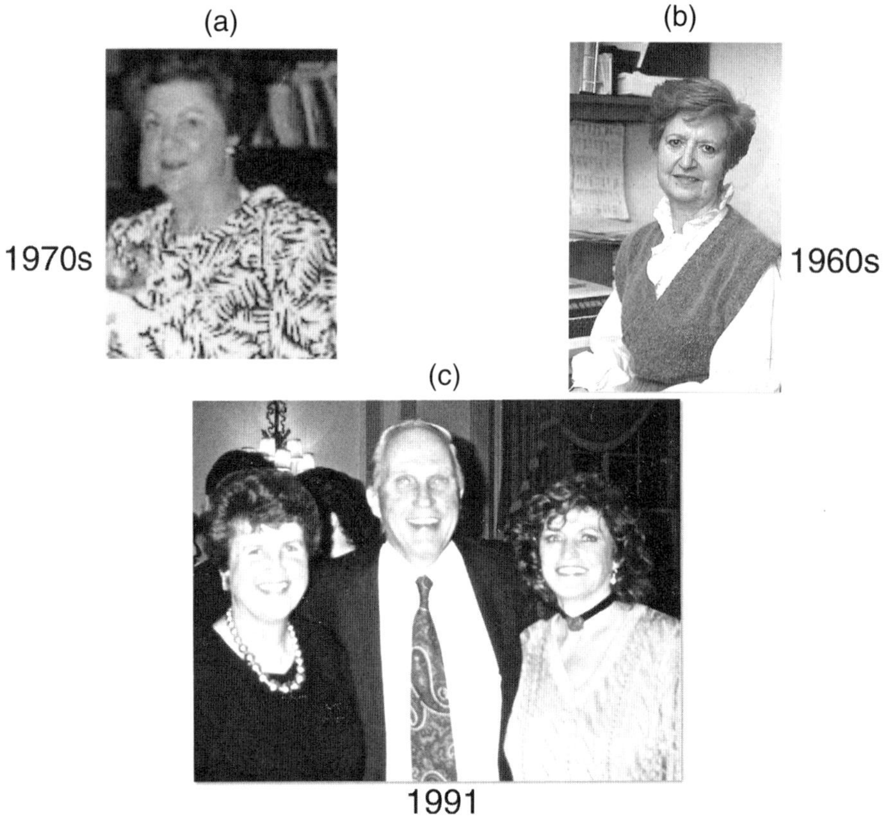

Fig. 5 (a) Jean McDaniel was coordinator of medical education from 1967 to 1989. (b) Dolores Mattia acted as a secretary of medical education before a formal department was established. (c) Lou Jordan, MD, orthopaedic resident, 1971, with Nancy Kane Bischoff, director of medical education from 1989 to 2000 (left), and her assistant, Maureen Bogle. (From Hospital for Special Surgery Archives)

Orthopaedic Surgeons. At the 2007 Annual Meeting of the Alumni Association, Bogle was voted in as an honorary member.

Bischoff retired in 1999, and in recognition of her dedication to graduate education, she also became an honorary member of the Alumni Association. In 2000, the Nancy Kane Bischoff Award was established by the association, to be "presented to the individual who has been a trusted guide and mentor, demonstrating consistent concern for the interests and welfare of the residents." Following Bischoff's retirement, the Medical Education, Graduate Education, and the Alumni Association office all became part of the Education Division, under the leadership of Laura Robbins, DSW.

In 1999, the Medical Staff Services (MSS) became a department under Marion Hare, Vice-President for Administration, and Maureen Bogle became its first administrator. Bogle's main responsibility was credentialing members of the HSS Medical Staff and Allied Health Professional Staff at the time of initial and biennial appointments, in accordance with the Joint Commission, Center for Medicare, and Medicaid Services, and New York State Department of Health standards and regulations. Additionally, this department prepared documentation and recorded minutes for the monthly Credentials Committee, Medical Board meetings, and medical staff conferences. From 1991 to 2012, the medical staff grew over 400% (Table 4). Bogle also became the administrator for the Department of Orthopaedic Surgery, a role she still maintains. Her responsibilities have included overseeing initial and biennial appointments to the New York–Presbyterian Hospital medical staff and initial academic appointments and promotions at Weill Cornell Medical College for all members of the Department of Orthopaedic Surgery. She is also administrator for the HSS Orthopaedic Promotions Committee.

Birth of the Physician Assistant

With the rapid growth of the hospital over the past 50 years, there was one part of the staff that was so regulated by outside agencies that it not only failed to expand but was forced to shrink in labor-hours units. The orthopaedic resident physicians, first appointed in 1888, reached a maximum number of eight graduating per year in 1974, and to date has never changed. Orthopaedic residents have been expected to be involved in research and teaching. However, the hospital also greatly depended on them for daily patient services that have varied over the years.[h] Enter the physician assistant (PA), whose numbers began to grow during Weiland's leadership. When New York State passed a law in 1989 limiting the number of weekly hours a resident could work to 80, PAs and other healthcare professionals were hired in hospitals to meet patient care demands. (The Accreditation Council for Graduate Medical Education eventually followed suit, adopting a similar regulation nationally.)

The first PA was Dawn Cannon, who was hired in September 1989. Pamela Katkin, director of the Department of Physician Assistants since 1994, was hired in April 1993. By 2000, 11 more PAs were added to the staff. As of February 2012, the hospital had a staff of 115 physician assistants (Table 4). They are an indispensable part of the healthcare team.

Table 4 Hospital for Special Surgery Medical Staff Statistics (1991–2012)

	July 1, 1991	February 29, 2012
Department attending physicians		
Orthopaedic surgery	26	109
Medicine	22	67
Primary care sports medicine	0	6
Anesthesiology	12	48
Laboratory medicine	3	6
Neurology	2	13
Pediatrics	3	12
Physiatry	0	14
Radiology	4	14
Podiatrists	0	3
Total	**72**	**292**
Allied health professional staff		
Physician assistants (PAs)	1	115
Certified registered nurse anesthetists (CRNAs)	0	10
Nurse practitioners	0	21
Total	**1**	**146**

The Growth of Rehabilitation

Two years into Weiland's tenure, in March 1992, JeMe Cioppa-Mosca, MBA, PT, became director of the Rehabilitation Department, having first joined the department 4 years prior and later becoming an HSS vice president in 2008 (Fig. 6). The hospital had always placed a major emphasis on rehabilitation, ever since the early twentieth century at the Hospital for the Ruptured and Crippled (R&C). When a Medical Board was first created in 1923, one of its first acts was to recommend a "Complete Department of Physiotherapy." The prime mover on the Medical Board was Royal Whitman, who recognized the importance of physiotherapy as part of a dual approach with surgery to achieve the best results.

With this background, the Board of Managers sought the very best physician who specialized in physiotherapy to become director of the department.

Kristian Gosta Hansson, MD, was chosen (see chapters 6 and 18 for more information). As a young man in Sweden, he spent much of his time rehabilitating casualties of World War I. After he came to America, he obtained his medical degree from Cornell University Medical College in 1923.

In the decades to follow, R&C would open a "posture clinic," become the first and only hospital in the country to offer an internship in physical therapy, open the first pool in a hospital in New York City (for underwater exercises), develop the first program in New York State for physiotherapy technicians, and establish an Occupational Therapy Department. A brace shop dating back to the days of James Knight in the late nineteenth century occupied a significant section of the early hospital, with braces constructed for orthopaedic patients and for those with hernias (Fig. 7).

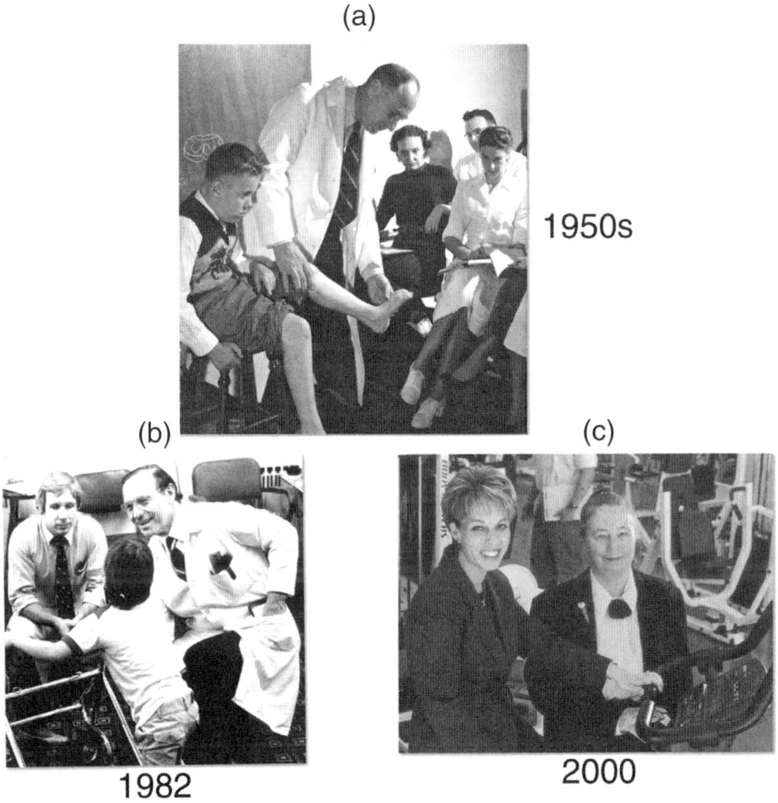

Fig. 6 (a) William Cooper, MD, second director of rehabilitation, examining a child with cerebral palsy. (b) Leon Root, MD (right), examining a child with Sean Hanley, MD, Hospital for Special Surgery resident. (c) JeMe Cioppa-Mosca, MBA, PT, and Margaret G.E. Peterson, PhD, often collaborated on clinical studies. Peterson joined the staff in 1990 to provide biostatistical and analytical skills support. (From Hospital for Special Surgery Archives)

With the arrival of Wilson Sr. as the fifth surgeon-in-chief in 1935, William Cooper, MD, joined the staff. He soon headed a Cerebral Palsy Clinic and became the second chief of the Rehabilitation Department. An orthopaedic surgeon, Cooper trained at the University of Iowa, and had a unique ability to deal with severely disabled patients with cerebral palsy. He was revered by his patients and their families, was a true mentor to all those whom he trained, and was an excellent surgeon. He was an attending orthopaedic surgeon on staff for over 30 years and served as the Susan Greenwall Director of Rehabilitation Medicine. In 1970, Cooper passed away and was replaced by one of his previous fellows, Leon Root, MD, who trained under him in 1962.

In December 1949, tragedy struck the assistant director of physiotherapy under Hansson, Jack Lovelock, MD. While suffering from the flu, Lovelock became dizzy and fell in front of a subway car at the Church Street Station in Brooklyn, killing him instantly. Born in New Zealand, Lovelock had a Rhodes Scholarship to Oxford University. He later obtained his medical degree from St. Mary's Medical School in London. Setting many track records over the years, in the 1936 Olympic Games in Berlin, he set a world record, winning the 1500-meter race, and earning New Zealand its first Olympic Gold Medal.

Virginia F. and William R. Salomon Rehabilitation Department

In March 1988, thanks to a generous donation, the rehabilitation department became known as the Virginia F. and William R. Salomon Rehabilitation Department. There were 58 staff members in the Rehabilitation Department by that time. By 2012, there were over 230 rehabilitation staff members, including more than 130 clinicians, researchers, and engineers on a multidisciplinary team.

The Rehabilitation Department was restructured in the early 1990s and expanded in the following years. On the main campus, the department was organized into separate sections corresponding to specialty orthopaedic services. These sections include Acute Care Orthopaedics (formerly Inpatient Rehabilitation), a dedicated Hand Therapy Center (which opened in March 1992), a Joint Mobility Center for arthritis and arthroplasty patients (in 2005), the state-of-the-art Leon Root, MD, Motion Analysis Laboratory (established in 2006, one of only 40 such facilities nationwide), Pediatric Rehabilitation,

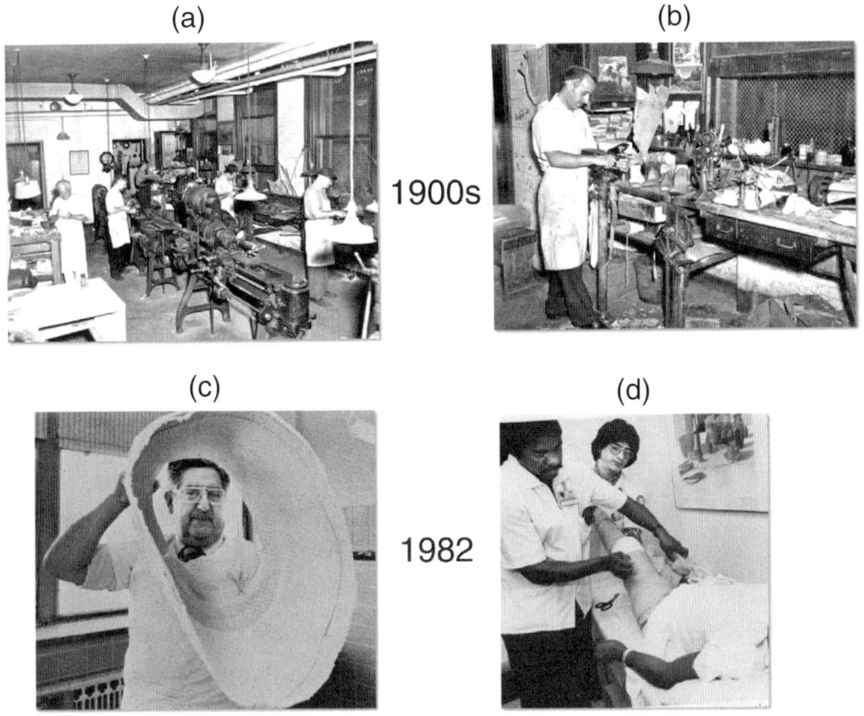

Fig. 7 (a) The brace shop at the East 42nd Street hospital. (b) Bill Locascio specializes in shoe corrections. (c) Sol Houtkin prepares a mold for a body brace. (d) Andrew Jenkins and Mario Orsagna prepare a fracture cast brace for a patient. (From Hospital for Special Surgery Archives)

and the Sports Rehabilitation and Performance Center (which became part of Rehabilitation in 1991). The brace shop, which became the Prosthetics and Orthotics Service, moved under the Rehabilitation umbrella in 1990.

The Rehabilitation Department continued to expand therapy to off-site locations, such as the Integrative Care Center (ICC) affiliated with the hospital, which opened in May 2001. The ICC offers traditional medical and therapeutic approaches along with complementary therapies to promote wellness and enhance the mobility and health of patients with musculoskeletal diseases. HSS Spine and Sport in Jupiter, Florida, opened in September 2011. This site marked the first HSS expansion outside of the New York metropolitan area.

In 1994, the Rehabilitation Department launched the HSS Rehabilitation Network, a community-focused, hospital-based network of preferred rehabilitation providers. There are currently over 130 member sites in the New York tri-state and Palm Beach County, Florida, areas. In addition to physical, occupational, and speech therapy, the Rehabilitation Department offers numerous services to promote patient function, mobility, and quality of life. Additional services include massage therapy, sports-specific analysis, performance training, ergonomics, and an Osteoporosis Prevention Center.

With the establishment of Rehabilitation Grand Rounds in 2011, the Rehabilitation Department has been a leader in the clinical education of colleagues in all disciplines. HSS was the first facility in New York City to be designated as a New York Education Department Office of the Professions–approved provider for continuing education in physical therapy education.

Department of Volunteers

In 1991, Wendy Yondorf was appointed director of volunteers at HSS, a position she currently holds. The two previous directors were Richard Elefante and (before him) Virginia Roberts. The concept of volunteers began at R&C with James Knight, who described the crucial role of volunteers by stating that the hospital's success was rooted in "the kindest sympathy and patronage of all classes of citizens." The role of volunteers grew during the war years, from 1913 into the 1950s.

Jane Bannerman, having celebrated her 100th birthday and a hospital volunteer for 52 years, noted, "Mrs. Wilson was probably the most instrumental person in the development of this department." During World War II, Germaine Wilson (wife of the fifth surgeon-in-chief, Philip D. Wilson) was a director of American Aid to France and was named a Chévalier of the Legion of Honor in 1946. Upon returning to the hospital after the war, she devoted her organizational skills to the Volunteer Department, and continued to do so until her death in 1973. In 1974, Yvonne Andre Estel was the first recipient of the Germaine B. Wilson Award. The 38th Award was given out in 2012 (Fig. 8).

When Yondorf came aboard in 1991, there were 85 volunteers, a number that would grow to more than 350 by 2012. There were 42 hospital areas in 2012 where volunteers were assigned, ranging from Social Work to the Motion Analysis Lab, the Patients' Library to Public Relations. In addition to the Germaine B. Wilson Award, the Volunteer Department annually recognizes two outstanding individuals with the Mary Ryan Student Award, which includes scholarship money.[c]

In 2012, the American Hospital Association gave HSS the national Hospital Award for Volunteer Excellence in Washington, DC, to recognize the HSS Community Outreach Program called "Charla de Lupus" (Lupus Chat). HSS was the only hospital to achieve this award in the category of community outreach. Just three other hospitals across the country were recognized.

Board Leadership Changes

As HSS entered the 1990s, it established a co-chairmanship of the Board of Trustees for the first time to deal with an increasing complexity of issues facing the hospital. Richard L. Menschel, a senior director of Goldman Sachs, and Winfield P. Jones, a principal in the law firm of Jones Hirsch Connors & Bull, shared the position of co-chairs of the board. Jones continued in that role until 1998, and Menschel stepped down in 2003. They led the hospital into the 1990s in a new direction, with a record-breaking year for hospital fundraising in 1991, surpassing $7.4 million. Very much appreciated by the professional and hospital staff, both have continued to be active members of the board and continue to provide major support to the hospital (Fig. 9).

The hospital lost an important member of its physician staff when Lee Ramsay Straub died on January 6, 1994. Straub was the first chief of the Hand Service and co-founder and co-chief with Richard Freyberg of the Comprehensive Arthritis Program. He had been on staff for 46 years and was 80 years old.

In December 1991, after serving 14 years, Donald Broas resigned as president of the hospital. John Ahearn, vice president and executive director, was appointed acting president. Six months later, in July 1992, after a national search, the board appointed Ahearn as president of HSS (Fig. 10).

Resignation

Weiland resigned as surgeon-in-chief on July 1, 1993. He continued to practice orthopaedic and hand surgery at the HSS, specializing in upper extremity and hand reconstructive surgery. He has won numerous awards, including the prestigious Kappa Delta Award from the American Academy of Orthopaedic surgeons twice (1986 and 1991). Weiland received the Distinguished Clinical

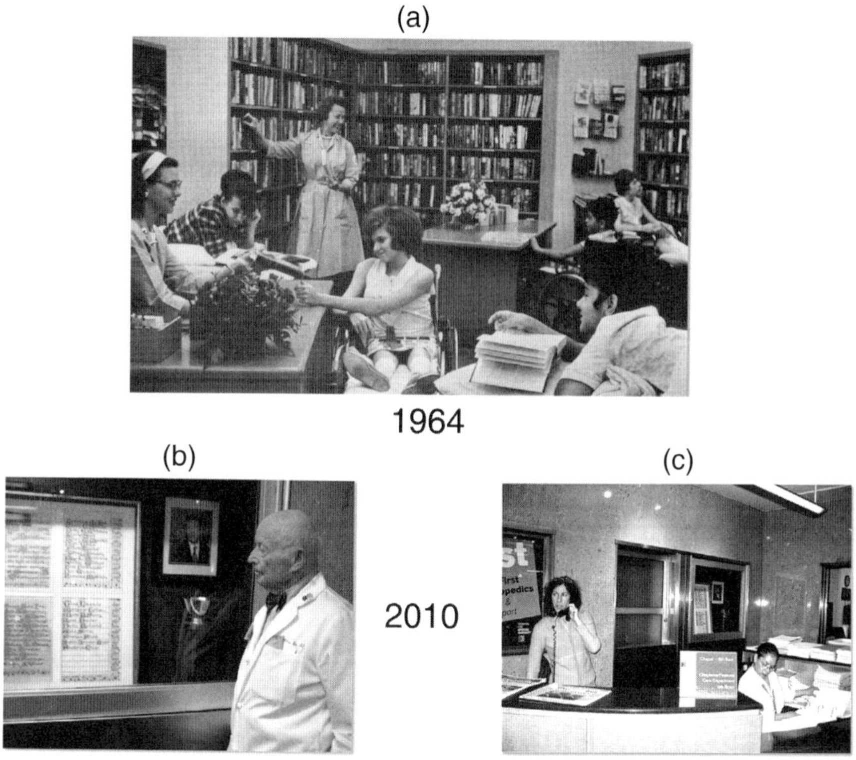

Fig. 8 (a) The Arents Library for Children was founded by Mrs. George Arents in memory of Mary Arents Averell in 1905. This was combined with the Alker Memorial Library, founded in 1926 by Henry A. Alker in memory of his parents to provide books for patients in the hospital. In the background is the Germaine B. Wilson Award Showcase that Germaine Wilson's son, Philip D. Wilson Jr., MD (b), is studying. (c) In the front lobby are Wendy Yondorf (left), director of volunteers, and Lillian D. Arroyo, information desk clerk, who first joined the Hospital for Special Surgery Staff in 1971. (From Hospital for Special Surgery Archives)

Educator Award from the American Orthopaedic Association in 2010 and was honored by the American Society for Surgery of the Hand with an award for outstanding research named in his honor.

He has also been president of numerous organizations, including the American Society for Reconstructive Microsurgery (1991), American Society for Surgery of the Hand (1995), American Orthopaedic Association (1998), and American Board of Orthopaedic Surgeons (1998), and he served as Treasurer of the American Academy of Orthopaedic Surgeons (2000).

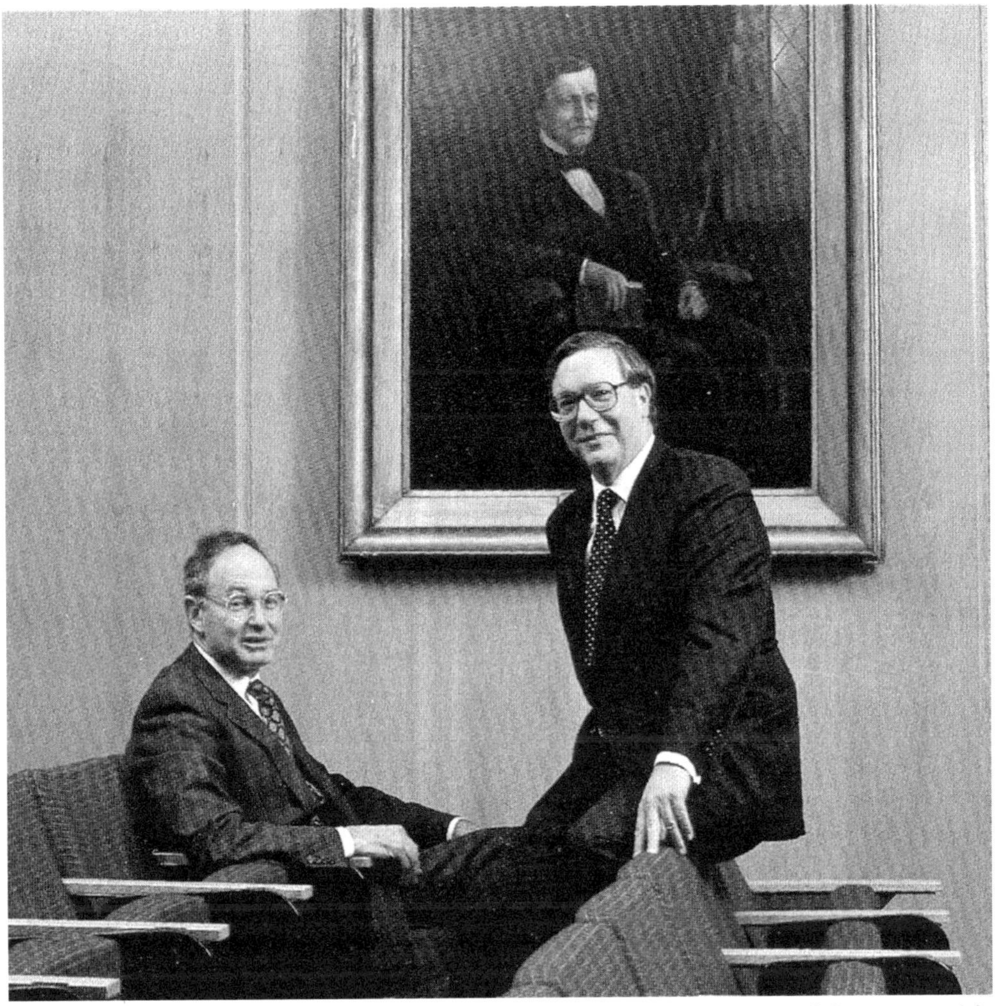

Fig. 9 Richard L. Menschel (left) and Winfield Jones, co-chairmen of the Hospital for Special Surgery Board of Directors, seated in 1991 in front of the original portrait of James Knight, MD, founder and first surgeon-in-chief at the Hospital for the Ruptured and Crippled. (From Hospital for Special Surgery Archives)

Weiland has continued to be very active in teaching at HSS and has been chosen four times by the resident staff to receive the Nancy Kane Bischoff Annual Award for Mentoring (in 2001, 2003, 2007, and 2010). He also received the American Orthopaedic Association Distinguished Clinician Award in 2010. In 2012, he was appointed to the Board of Trustees of the *Journal of Bone and Joint Surgery* (Fig. 10). Through these roles, he continues to contribute significantly to the field of orthopaedic surgery.

(a) (b)

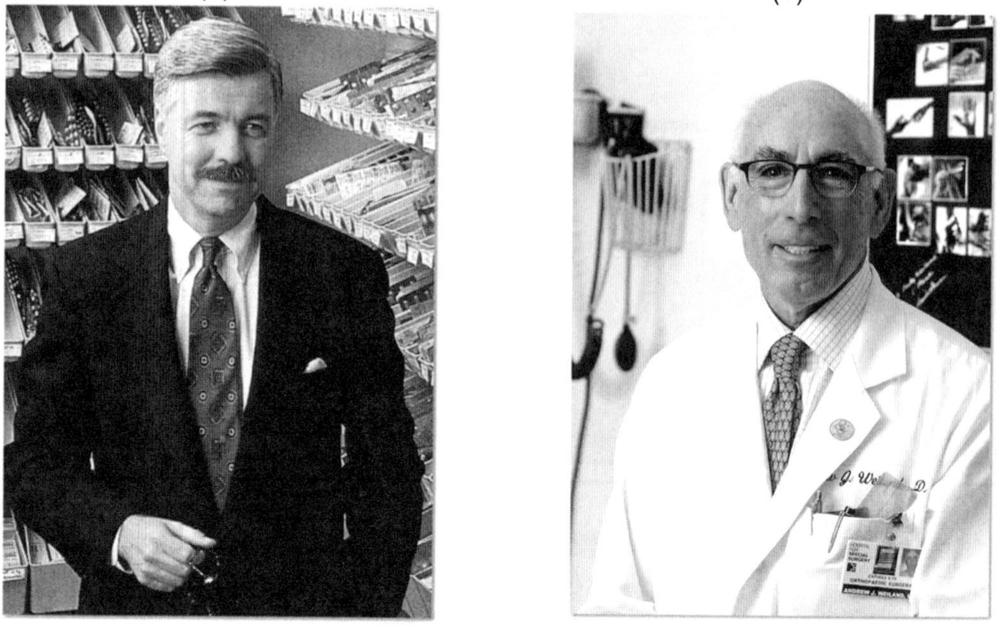

1992 2011

Fig. 10 (a) John Ahearn became president of Hospital for Special Surgery in July 1992. On staff at the Hospital for Special Surgery since 1978, he served as chief operating officer before becoming acting president in December 1991. (b) After resigning as surgeon-in-chief in 1993, Andrew Weiland continued to practice orthopaedic and hand surgery at the Hospital for Special Surgery. He continued to win many awards and to serve as president of a number of national professional organizations. (From Hospital for Special Surgery Archives)

REFERENCE

1. Kroessler JA. *New York Year by Year.* New York, NY: New York University Press; 2002.

NOTES

a. In 2011, that figure was $2 trillion.

b. As an HSS orthopaedic resident from 1961 to 1964, I performed such hospital functions as taking a chest x-ray on new weekend admissions, drawing routine bloods, performing a urinalysis, performing admission histories and physical examinations, starting routine IVs, and a number of other functions.

c. Mary Ryan was the executive assistant to the former director of development, Richard Kearns, and for over 30 years, she was the informal historian of HSS. She worked next to the Volunteer Department, and if the students were rowdy or loud, she was the first person to call them on their behavior. She was stern, yet she was very interested in seeing these young men and woman make their way in the world. After her death, the hospital deemed it fitting that an award for student volunteers be named in her honor.

CHAPTER 13

RUSSELL F. WARREN, MD TENTH SURGEON-IN-CHIEF (1993–2003)

DAVID B. LEVINE, MD

IN THE SPRING OF 1993, at age 46 years, newly elected President William Clinton launched his first mission: to reform the country's healthcare system. He assigned First Lady Hillary Rodham Clinton to lead a team to accomplish this purpose. Unfortunately, because of numerous flaws—including lack of transparency and lack of experience—the mission failed. Two decades later, healthcare reform continued to be a political football, with the Healthcare Law eventually enacted on March 23, 2010, during the administration of President Barack Obama. (In May 2012, the United States Supreme Court, in a five-to-four vote, upheld the Affordable Care Act).

With a national cloud hovering over our healthcare system and an unexpected change in medical leadership at HSS, Russell F. Warren, MD, became the tenth surgeon-in-chief of the Hospital for Special Surgery (HSS), taking office on September 1, 1993. He also assumed an important role as president-elect of the American Orthopaedic Society for Sports Medicine. He immediately appointed Thomas P. Sculco, MD, to assist him as director of orthopaedic surgery.

Professional Training and Societies

Receiving his BA degree from Columbia College and his medical degree from the State University of New York Upstate Medical University in 1966, Warren served on active duty in the U.S. Naval Reserve in Vietnam for 2 years. He was discharged as a lieutenant commander in 1969 and received the U.S. Navy

Medal of Commendation that year. Before his military service, he had been an intern and surgical resident at St. Luke's Hospital for 2 years.

After completing an orthopaedic residency at HSS from 1970 to 1973, Warren joined an orthopaedic group of former HSS alumni, Paul Fitzgerald, MD, and Terry Miller, MD, in Lynchburg, Virginia. Seeking more of an academic career, he returned to New York in 1976 as a shoulder fellow with Charles Neer, MD, the world's foremost shoulder surgeon, at Columbia Presbyterian Hospital. Warren had always been interested in the shoulder. He was Neer's second fellow and followed him closely, examining patients and assisting him in the operating room.

In 1981, when John Marshall died in an airplane crash (see Chapter 11), Warren became chief of the Sports Medicine and Shoulder Service, and in 1984, he was appointed head team physician for the New York Giants football team, a post originally held by Marshall. Warren has continued in his post with the Giants and was present for all five of the New York Giants Super Bowl appearances, with victories over the Denver Broncos after the 1986 season, the Buffalo Bills after the 1990 season, and the New England Patriots after the 2007 and 2011 seasons (Fig. 1). In 1984, with Neer and others, Warren helped to found the American Shoulder and Elbow Society, of which he was president in 1994.

Having served on over 10 committees of the American Orthopaedic Society for Sports Medicine, he became secretary in 1991, vice president in 1993, and president in 1994. He has experienced a long and illustrious career as a National Football League team physician and internationally recognized sports medicine specialist.

Personal Life

Born in 1939 in Burlington, Vermont, Warren was always interested in sports. While attending Columbia College, he was named All-East in football, won the Smyth Cup for the Most Valuable Player in Football and the Roker Prize, and was named All Ivy in football. As center fielder for the Columbia Lions baseball team, he batted over .300 (Fig. 2). After college, Warren had a try-out with the New York Giants in 1962 and then played semiprofessional football for the Providence Steamrollers.

While at Columbia College, Warren met his future wife, Laurie Adams, who grew up in Tenafly, New Jersey. They were married during Warren's

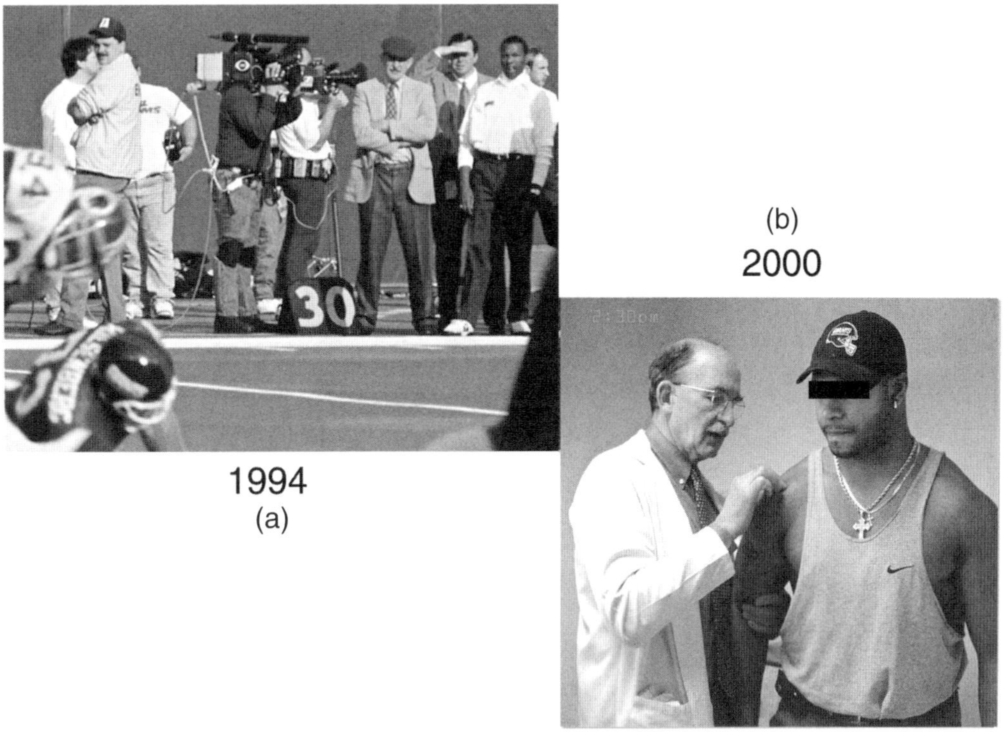

(b)
2000

1994
(a)

Fig. 1 (a) Russell Warren, MD (with tie and cap), New York Giants team physician, and HSS associate Stephen O'Brien, MD (shading eyes), joined head athletic trainer Ronnie Barnes (white shirt) on the side lines of the Giants in action. (b) Warren examines a member of the Giants.

sophomore year in medical school. Laurie Warren received her BA degree in 1963 from Barnard College. She was an avid tennis player, often defeating her husband and was particularly interested in interior decorating and American Impressionism (along with Warren). They had two children, Lisa and Rusty, who are now both married with families.

Academic Interests

After returning to HSS in 1977, Warren worked closely with Marshall, whose prime interest was in the knee. Being a veterinarian, Marshall had many years of experience with the anatomy and pathology of the animal knee, particularly the anterior cruciate ligament. Warren's expertise and interest in the shoulder complemented Marshall's focus on the knee. Together, they published papers on the diagnosis and treatment of both joints.

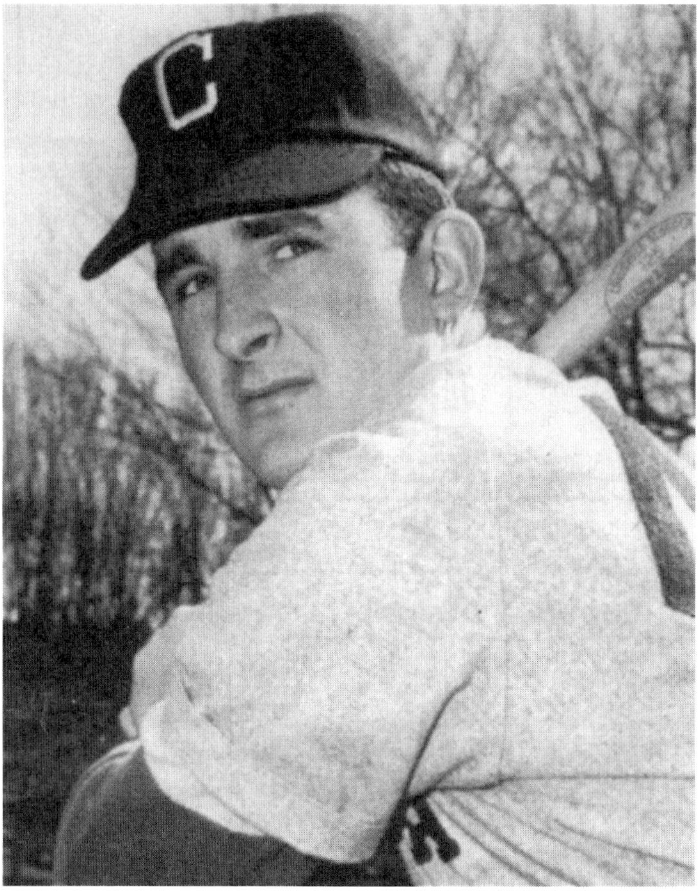

Fig. 2 Warren batted over .300 playing for the Columbia College Lions. (From Hospital for Special Surgery Archives)

Warren became involved in the laboratory, working closely on shoulder research with Peter Torzilli, PhD, from the Biomechanics Department and Steve Arnoczky (see Chapter 17), the veterinarian brought to the hospital by Marshall. From the 1980s to the early 1990s, residents, fellows, and junior/senior HSS staff members who collaborated with Warren included Thomas Wickiewicz, MD, Bruce Reider, MD, Helene Pavlov, MD, Dom Sisto, MD, Bill Donaldson, MD, Steve O'Brien, MD, Bernard Bach, MD, Mark Sherman, MD, David Altchek, MD, Scott Rodeo, MD, David Dines, MD, Dan Buss, MD, George Paletta, MD, Bruce Moeckel, MD, Michael Pagnani, MD, Chit Ranawat, MD, and Allan E. Inglis, MD. The cast of Warren's co-investigators was certainly impressive and demonstrated the vast attraction that colleagues had for Warren, who served as a true mentor.

New Chief, Sports Medicine

When Warren became surgeon-in-chief, he appointed Wickiewicz as chief of the Sports Medicine and Shoulder Service (Fig. 3). Wickiewicz had come to HSS as an orthopaedic fellow in Sports Medicine in 1977 and was an HSS orthopaedic resident from 1978 to 1981. During those years, he experienced a unique training not only with Warren, but also Marshall and Arnoczky. In 1982, he completed a Biomechanics Laboratory Fellowship at California

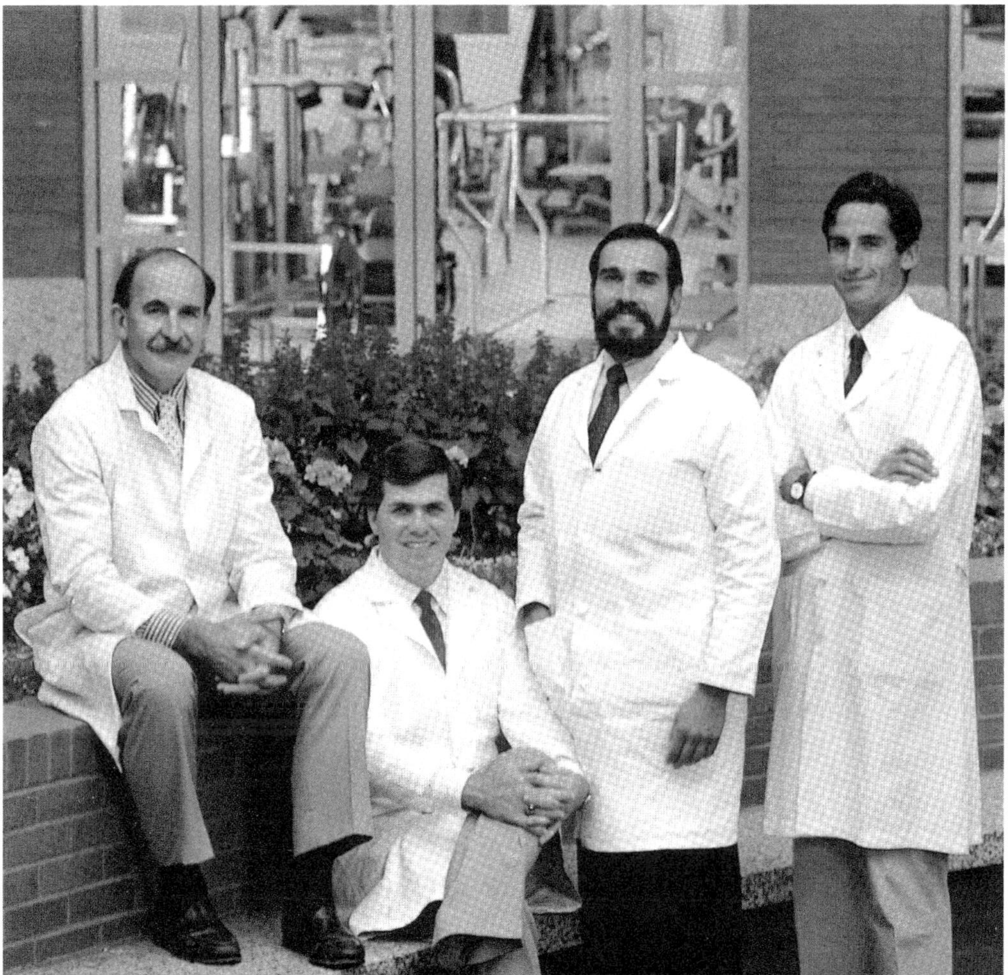

Fig. 3 Leading the Sports Medicine and Shoulder Service in 1989 were (from left) Warren as chief, Stephen O'Brien, MD, MBA, Thomas Wickiewicz, MD, and David Altchek, MD. (From Hospital for Special Surgery Archives)

Southwest Orthopaedic Group and a Sports Medicine Traveling Fellowship in the Department of Kinesiology at UCLA.

Teaching was a passion of Wickiewicz, and he helped build a strong Sports Medicine and Shoulder Service, which had nine fellows in training by 2012. Over the past 20 years at the forefront of his specialty, he pioneered minimally invasive surgical techniques for knee and soft-tissue injuries.

During his years as chief, Wickiewicz supported a Women's Sports Medicine Center at HSS, started in 1996 by Lisa Callahan, MD, a primary care physician, and Jo A. Hannafin, MD, PhD, an orthopaedic surgeon. The first of its kind in the United States, the Women's Sports Medicine Center at HSS is a nationally recognized health resource for active women of all ages and abilities, from professional athletes to eager novices. Its physician staff has expanded to include Marci A. Goolsby, MD, primary care physician; Beth E. Shubin Stein, MD, orthopaedic surgeon; Sabrina M. Strickland, MD, orthopaedic surgeon; and Terry Karl, MD, RD, CDN, assistant director of Food and Nutritional Services. The supporting staff includes a physical therapist, exercise physiologist, and sports nutritionist.

Having served as president of the American Orthopaedic Society for Sports Medicine (AOSSM), Wickiewicz has been a three-time winner of the O'Donoghue Research Award from that society and a three-time winner of the Neer Award from the American Shoulder and Elbow Society. In 2006, after 13 years building one of the strongest sports medicine departments in the country, Wickiewicz stepped down as chief, becoming emeritus chief of the Sports Medicine and Shoulder Service.

The Marketing of HSS

Consumer research in 1992 revealed that the hospital's name had limited brand recognition to the public. Under the leadership of Board Trustee Aldo Papone, a marketing campaign to generate awareness of the name HSS was created (Fig. 4). The campaign has been continuous and has grown each year. Papone has been outstanding in developing awareness of HSS locally and nationally, resulting in a significant increase in the number of patients.

In 1998, Papone became co-chair of the HSS Board of Directors with Menschel, after Winfield Jones resigned from the co-chair position. Papone

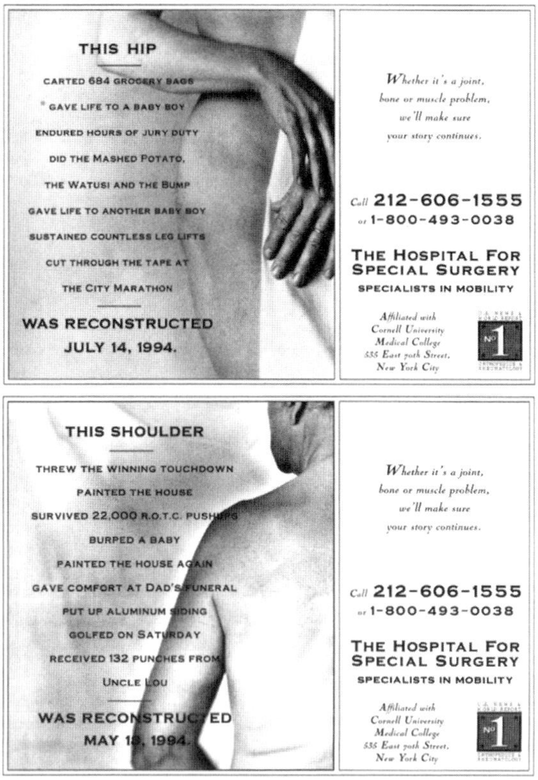

Fig. 4 Print advertisements had such a great response in various newspapers that they were expanded to the *New York Times* and *New York Magazine* and accompanied by a radio commercial, supplemented by Beverly Sills and Frank Gifford. The results were impressive: a 26% increase in calls to the HSS Physician Referral Service. (From Hospital for Special Surgery Archives)

had come to HSS from American Express, where he had served as chairman and CEO of American Express Travel Related Services until 1991.[a]

Menschel made a major donation to the hospital to renovate the second floor auditorium, which was renamed the Richard L. Menschel Conference Center (now the Richard L. Menschel Education Center). He stepped down as co-chair in 2003 and was replaced by Dean R. O'Hare, who had retired as CEO of the Chubb Corporation in 2002.[b]

The Growth of Physiatry

Realizing the need for nonsurgeons to manage patients with musculoskeletal conditions, Warren created a Physiatry (Physical Medicine and Rehabilitation)

Service in 1993 and recruited Gregory Lutz, MD, as its director. Under Lutz's leadership, the service became an independent department in 2002 and had grown to a staff of 13 physicians by 2012. Clinical services included the treatment of patients with spine, sports-related, and general musculoskeletal disorders. Physiatrists, who are specially trained in the field of musculoskeletal disease, performed minimally invasive spine procedures such as fluoroscopic spinal injections, ultrasound-guided joint and soft-tissue injections, and electrodiagnostic studies for patients with suspected nerve injuries.

The department has grown to more than 50,000 patient visits annually and is one of the largest outpatient physiatry treatment centers in the area. Research has led to publications primarily in the area of spine medicine and peripheral nerve/brachial plexus disorders. Resident physicians from the New York–Presbyterian Hospital Physiatry Residency Program rotate through the HSS department on a regular basis as part of their core curriculum. An HSS Physiatry Spine and Sports Medicine Fellowship was established in 1997 and expanded to four fellowship positions a year in 2011.

In 2011, Lutz stepped down as physiatrist-in-chief, and Joseph Feinberg, MD, assumed the leadership of the department. Feinberg, formerly the director of sports medicine at the Kessler Institute in West Orange, New Jersey, first joined HSS in 1996. A specialist in electrodiagnostics, he is also co-medical director of the Center for Brachial and Traumatic Nerve Injury and team physician for St. Peters College in New Jersey.

PSEL/BSEL

The Fracture Service and Trauma Service were merged under the leadership of Helfet. David S. Levine, MD (not related to the author, David B. Levine, MD), who had finished his orthopaedic residency at HSS in 1997 followed by a fellowship in foot, ankle, and trauma in Seattle, Washington, was assigned to the Trauma Service to develop foot and ankle trauma programs. Helfet realized the need for an anatomical teaching facility.

Warren also felt strongly that a surgical dissection laboratory should be implemented for the orthopaedic residents. A surgical skills laboratory was created, which quickly became very popular with the resident staff. Warren asked Laura Robbins to carry the concept further, under the umbrella of the Education Division. A psychomotor skills laboratory, with Helfet developing saw-bones skills and Warren a "wet" laboratory in arthroscopy skills, was created. The official name was the Psychomotor Skills Education Laboratory (PSEL), which eventually became known as the Bioskills Education Laboratory (BSEL) in 2009.

The first coordinator was Emily Mallin, followed by six more coordinators. In 2010, Jennifer Hammann, CST, became the seventh and current coordinator. Under her direction, the BSEL has expanded to encompass anatomical and surgical approaches in hand, spine, and other joints, and anesthesia, rheumatology, basic surgery, and physiatry. In addition to orthopaedic residents, students include orthopaedic and nonorthopaedic fellows, attending staff, physician assistants, and research staff. More recently, product development sessions have been scheduled.

In 2011, there were 371 core sessions with over 2,000 participants (Table 1). Eight corporate sponsors participated in other programs where company representatives educated attending and house staff about their products. Sixteen companies participated with HSS staff to develop new products. Additionally, 14 residents/fellows utilized the laboratory for their individual research projects. Mathias P. Bostrom, MD, is currently the academic director of the BSEL Laboratory, and Andrew A. Sama, MD, is chair of the BSEL Advisory Committee. Every week for an hour and a half, residents and fellows on the sports rotation hone their arthroscopic skills.

In the mid-1990s, Warren instituted the *Sign Your Site* program in conjunction with the AAOS. Every surgeon was required to personally verify the site of proposed surgery and sign off on the patient. It was one of the first such programs in the country.

The year 1997 continued to be a very productive year for the HSS staff, led by Warren. Surgical admissions were up 10% to 6,521, and ambulatory surgery continued to leap 20%, to 5,701. The average length of stay continued to fall to 5.64 days, resulting in a low occupancy rate of 63%.

Stephen Burke, MD, replaced Leon Root as head of the Pediatric Orthopaedic Service in 1997. Root had been chief for over 25 years and built a strong service. His leadership in cerebral palsy was respected worldwide.

A Cartilage Repair Registry was first established in 1998 by Warren in collaboration with Robert Marx, MD. This was to be the benchmark of HSS registries to follow later. Subsequently, Riley J Williams III, MD, directed the group, resulting in the publication of a number of papers related to prospective

Table 1 BSEL Core Sessions 2011 (in part)

	Number of sessions	Number of participants
Anesthesiology	8	76
Foot and ankle	7	46
Hand (weekly)	47	325
Independent study	94	315
Limb lengthening	1	5
PA core (monthly)	2	26
PA sports	1	9
PA suturing (weekly)	23	140
Pediatric	15	93
Physiatry	1	10
Rheumatology	16	121
SAS (fellow)	15	155
SAS (monthly)	14	91
Spine (monthly)	15	135
Sports (weekly)	47	251
Summer anatomy	9	18
Trauma (monthly)	5	46

research. The Metabolic Bone Disease Service, headed by Joseph Lane, continued to grow, with the Osteoporosis Prevention Center directed by Theresa Galsworthy, RN, ONC. Seventy percent of patients were referred by outside primary care and obstetrician/gynecologists.

The Foot Service under the leadership of Jonathan T. Deland, MD, grew stronger with the help of Walther H. O. Bohne, MD, and Martin J. O'Malley, MD. Bohne, a long-time attending staff member, had been an HSS Foot Fellow in 1969, while O'Malley—who had taken his orthopaedic residency at Tufts University Affiliated Hospitals in Boston—was a Foot Fellow at HSS in 1993. David S. Levine joined the Foot Service in 1998, having been an HSS orthopaedic resident who then completed a fellowship in Seattle, Washington.

Other appointments in the Orthopaedic Department that occurred about this time included Daniel Green, MD, to the Pediatric Service; Frank Cordasco, MD, MS, John MacGillivray, MD, and Robert G. Marx, MD to the Sports Service; and Scott W. Wolfe, MD, and Pamela Sherman, MD, to the Hand Service.

In 2001, Richard R. McCormack, Jr., MD, who was an HSS orthopaedic resident (class of 1980), resigned from his active practice of hand surgery and orthopaedic surgery to retire to upstate New York. McCormack was a dedicated teacher and gave special care to his patients. Wolfe was appointed as director of the Hand Service, a position held by Hotchkiss since 1990. Dean G. Lorich, MD, was appointed associate director of the Orthopaedic Trauma Service at New York Hospital.

Nursing

From the founding of the hospital in 1863 to the twenty-first century, nursing has always played a strong role in patient care. The evolution of chief nursing officers from Ella S. Murdock (matron from 1896 to 1911) to the current senior vice president for Patient Care Services and chief nursing officer (2005–2012) Stephanie J. Goldberg, MS, RN, NEA-C, has been critical to the success of HSS (see Chapter 5).

In 2002, HSS was awarded its first Magnet Recognition by the American Nurses Credentialing Center (ANCC)—the nation's highest honor for nursing excellence. Since then, the ANCC awarded a second designation in 2007 and a third redesignation in 2011. This rigorous application process demonstrated nursing's commitment to transformational leadership, structural empowerment, exemplary of professional practice, and new knowledge and innovation—all hallmarks of a Magnet organization. Established in the 1990s, the Magnet Recognition Program promotes high-quality care, identifies excellence in the care by nurses, and provides a way to highlight the best nursing practices in the country.

While the applicant pool for new nurses continued to expand significantly, there was always a core of long-time nurses, with deep roots extending many years back (Fig. 5). Satisfaction of the HSS nursing staff was reflected in a turnover rate of RNs in 2003 of only 7%, compared with a national average of 15.5%.[2] In 2012, the turnover rate was reduced significantly to just 2%.

In 2004, under the leadership of Jacqueline Kostic, MS, RN, CNAA, senior vice president of Patient Care Services and Chief Nursing Office, who first came to HSS in 1990, there has been an increase in the percentage of baccalaureate-level nurses to greater than 65% (Fig. 6). It was already realized

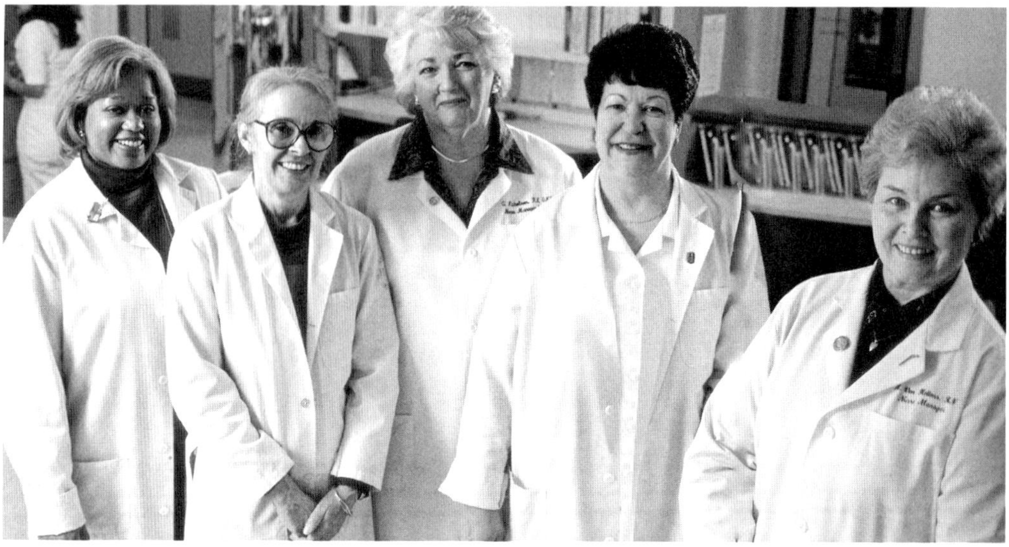

Fig. 5 In 2000, five of the most highly respected nurses together made up a total of 167 years of nursing service to HSS. (From left) Doreen L. Johnson, MS, RN, ONC, came to HSS in 1968 to attend the LPN nursing school and rose to become the hospital's nurse educator. Marjorie Pangas, MSN, RN, also started in 1968 as head nurse in the outpatient clinics and eventually became nurse manager for rheumatology, presurgical screening, and infusion therapy. Geri Nicholson, RN, ONC, came to HSS in 1959 and held a number of administrative nursing roles, finishing as nurse manager of a combined pediatric-adult unit. Marguerite Palmieri, RN, joined HSS as a staff nurse and eventually became nurse manager for ambulatory care (32 specialty clinics, the cast room, and 65 physician offices). Anita von Hellens, MBA, RN, ONC, came to HSS in 1974 after graduating from Cornell University School of Nursing and became nurse manager of the adult orthopaedic surgical unit. (From Hospital for Special Surgery Archives)

at that time that the changing role of the nurse toward one centering on critical thinking and planning was just around the corner.

Mary McDermott, MSN, RN, ANP, NE-C, having joined the HSS staff in 1991 as nurse manager of 7 South, was promoted to assistant vice president of nursing in 2008. McDermott contributed to the hospital's expansion and growth, including its move to the East Wing in 1996, the subsequent opening of the Nursing Station on 8 East in 2007, and the successful opening of a step-down unit in July 2007. She has played an important role in the hospital's Magnet applications since 2002. In 2012, she assumed responsibility for all Nursing Department business functions, recruitment, payroll, and nursing practice and was involved in the planning, selection, and implementation and enhancements of CliniCIS, the hospital's electronic medical record program.

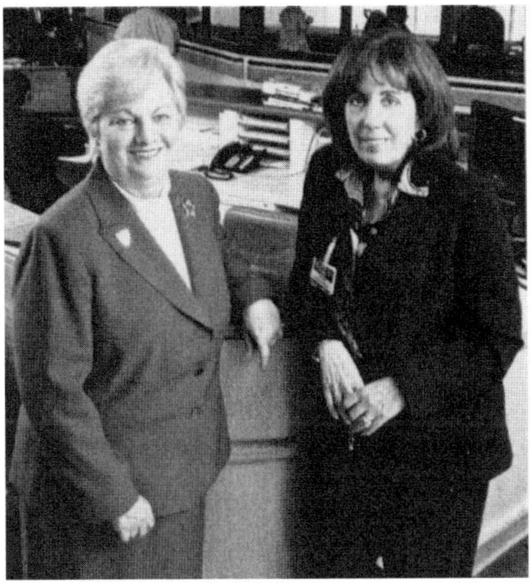

Fig. 6 In 2006, Jacqueline Kostic, vice president for nursing (left), turned over the leadership of HSS nursing to Stephanie Goldberg. (From Hospital for Special Surgery Archives)

In 2012, Ronald Perez, RN, JD, CNOR, was promoted to vice president of Perioperative Services, having served as assistant vice president. Perez first joined HSS in 1994 as an operating staff nurse, and rose through the ranks to become director of the Main Operating Room. Perioperative Services has overseen an expansion from 13 operating rooms in 1994 to 33 operating rooms and three procedure rooms in 2012.

There has always been mutual respect and camaraderie among HSS nurses, attending staff, and house staff. This relationship initially existed with RNs and LPNs. With the addition of the role of the physician assistant in 1989, this new staff element grew and was easily integrated. Most recently, the advanced practice registered nurse role (in the form of nurse practitioners and certified registered nurse anesthetists) has also provided key nursing practice incentives.

"Simply stated, HSS nurses are the best of the best, and centrally important and key reasons why HSS is number one," declared Stephen Paget, MD, physician-in-chief, in 2008. "That is because, while on the front line of care 24/7, they deliver sensitive and thoughtful care that is world class."[3]

Case Management and Social Work Programs

The establishment of a social service department at R&C dates back to the late nineteenth century, when Gibney established a follow-up system for discharged patients—one of the first of its kind. He engaged social workers and visiting nurses to investigate the home conditions of patients (mostly children at that time). This important part of medical care had been almost completely neglected.

HSS recognized that the concept of a social service department had changed significantly since the early years of R&C, as relationships among patients, acute and chronic medical facilities, and diagnostic and therapeutic tools became more complex. What has not changed is that social work is rooted in the understanding of patients, families, and communities in the context of a biological and psychosocial model of the impact of illness. Interventions have been designed, in collaboration with the healthcare team, to help patients achieve optimal health outcomes in an ever-changing environment.

Over the years, two separate but complementary departments have been developed to address the specific needs of the inpatient and outpatient/community experience: the Departments of Case Management and Social Work Programs. The Department of Case Management serves as the advocate of the patient before and during the hospital stay. Offering the highest quality patient services and utilizing appropriate resources to maximize patient recovery and foster a sense of well-being, social work case managers collaborate with the patient and the healthcare team to develop and implement an appropriate discharge plan. They assess all patients admitted to the hospital to ensure they receive the appropriate care across the continuum and provide supportive counseling to patients and their families to help them navigate the healthcare system and cope with their illnesses.

Some of the needs of adult and pediatric patients addressed by the professional staff in this department are listed in Table 2. Since 2007, Rachelle Schwartz MA, RN-BC, CCM, has directed this department.

The mission of the Department of Social Work Programs is to support, empower, and enhance quality of life for adults and children with musculoskeletal conditions and their loved ones. The programs are outpatient-focused, provide needed resources, and reduce barriers to access in culturally diverse communities. Social workers assess patient/family concerns related to the understanding and impact of illness and treatment options, provide emotional support, and facilitate access to many community and government resources.

The Department of Social Work Programs has more support and educational programs than any other hospital in the country with designated

Table 2 Case Management Services

• Preadmission evaluation
• Preoperative counseling
• Insurance company communications
• Durable medical equipment
• Discharge planning
• Transportation
• Child life program

specialties, such as HSS. Roberta Horton, LCSW, ACSW, who came to HSS in 1977, has been its director since 2006. Consistent with the outstanding leadership of HSS in musculoskeletal health, social work leaders serve on national task forces, publish peer-reviewed research, present at professional conferences, and are an integral part of Community Service Plan of HSS, which is submitted to the New York State Department of Health.

Since 2001, given the wide breadth of services provided, these departments have reported to Susan Flics, MA, MBA, RN, assistant vice president, Operations of the Executive Office. Before this role, Flics had managed Quality and Utilization Review at HSS at a director level since 1992.

1990s: Leg Lengthening Returns to HSS

The decade of the 1990s marked a return to HSS of leg-lengthening services, which originated at the hospital in the 1960s (when Harlan Amstutz, MD, performed the first such procedures) but which were later abandoned. In 1964, when Amstutz returned to HSS in a faculty role and was asked to participate in the Child Amputee Clinic, the clinic name was changed to the Child Amputee and Leg Equalization Clinic, at his suggestion. Many of the patients had either postpolio leg shortening or a variety of congenital anomalies, such as absence of the fibula and proximal femoral deficiencies, including congenital coxa vara, which had been a special interest of Amstutz during his residency.

During his fellowship year (1963–1964) in the United Kingdom at the Royal National Orthopaedic Hospital and at the Hospital for Sick Children in London, Amstutz continued to focus on these conditions. In addition, he visited other hospitals where there were many patients with deformities caused by thalidomide, some similar to those he was studying. He also visited Edinburgh and Birmingham to view various leg-lengthening techniques.

All of the patients in the HSS clinics completed standardized data collection forms. Skeletal age was used to estimate the final amount of leg length inequality. Up until that time, limb equalization at HSS was accomplished by contralateral tibial or femoral epiphyseal arrest or femoral shortening with varying prosthetic devices or shoe raises, most of which were made in the hospital's basement brace shop. At first, tibial and femoral lengthening were performed with the Anderson device (from Edinburgh), mostly for postpolio patients, while the Wagner device was later used for femoral lengthening in cases of posttraumatic or congenitally short femurs. Amstutz visited Wagner several times at the Altdorf Hospital outside of Nuremberg in Germany and made many modifications of his devices.

Later, a modification of the open Cauchoix technique of one-stage femoral lengthening was employed. Winches were attached to two walls in Operating Room 2 in HSS and lengthened up to 15% of the femoral length by using a Z-step osteotomy of 10 to 15 centimeters in length. Then, after monitored lengthening, modified Wagner plates were applied.[4]

In 1969, Amstutz's classification of proximal femoral focal deficiencies was published in the *Proceedings of National Academy of Sciences* (Fig. 7).[5] Although Amstutz continued to use these techniques at UCLA when he became Chairman there in 1970, the first one-stage femoral lengthening results were not published until 1975.[4] Leg-lengthening services at HSS had ceased completely after Amstutz had moved to California in 1970.

S. Robert Rozbruch, MD, who completed his HSS orthopedic residency in 1995, was initially enamored by orthopedic trauma, and pursued the AO/ASIF Orthopaedic Trauma Fellowship at the University of Bern, in Switzerland. In the late 1990s, he approached Warren with the idea of re-establishing leg-lengthening services at HSS.

Warren encouraged Rozbruch to pursue a fellowship in 1999 with Dror Paley, MD, and John Herzenberg, MD, at the Maryland Center for Limb Lengthening & Reconstruction in Baltimore (currently known as the International Center for Limb Lengthening at the Robin Institute of Sinai Hospital). This led to a major career shift for Rozbruch.

Rozbruch reintroduced leg lengthening at HSS upon his return in 1999. He used the Ilizarov method—"distraction osteogenesis"—which achieved

(a) (b)

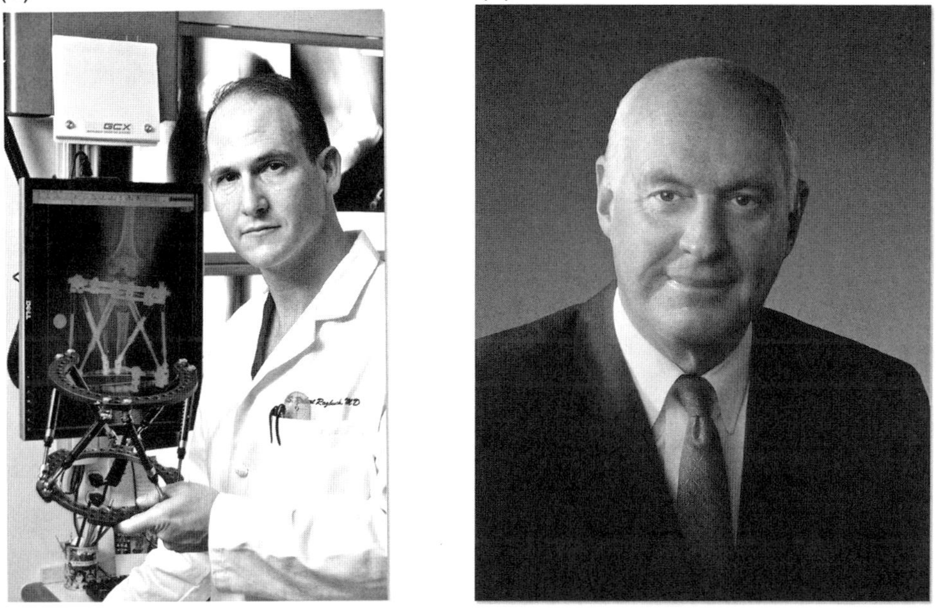

2012 1989

Fig. 7 (a) S. Robert Rozbruch, MD, displaying a Taylor spatial frame (Smith & Nephew, Memphis, Tennessee) designed in the mid-1990s by J. Charles Taylor, MD. (b) Harlan Amstutz, MD, when he was professor and chief of the Division of Orthopaedic Surgery at UCLA. (From Hospital for Special Surgery Archives and H. Amstutz)

gradual lengthening with external fixation pioneered earlier by Professor Gavril Ilizarov. Joined by Svetlana Ilizarov, MD, daughter of the professor, and then later by his first fellow, Austin T. Fragomen, MD, the limb-lengthening program was underway.

It was later named the Limb Lengthening and Complex Reconstruction Service (LLCRS) in 2005, with Rozbruch serving as the first service chief, under the leadership and vision of the 11th surgeon-in-chief, Thomas Sculco.

By 2012, the LLCRS trained two clinical fellows each year. Considered one of the top programs in this country, it is the only limb-lengthening program at a major academic teaching hospital. The service runs a very active clinical program for adults and children, with 689 surgical cases and 3,471 outpatient visits in 2011. With education and research a major focus of the LLCRS, the Pediatric Orthopedic Service at HSS has also been involved in limb-lengthening surgery.

In addition to many peer-reviewed publications, Rozbruch and Ilizarov published *Limb Lengthening and Reconstruction Surgery*, a comprehensive textbook on the subject, in 2006.[6] The service was active at the national level in 2012, with Rozbruch as the president-elect and Fragomen as the treasurer of the Limb Lengthening and Reconstruction Society. Having already developed a circular external fixator for ankle distraction surgery, Rozbruch and Fragomen moved on to design an internal lengthening intramedullary rod.

MRI at HSS

The Magnetic Resonance Imaging (MRI) section was developed by Hollis G. Potter, MD, who graduated as an HSS/New York Hospital musculoskeletal radiology fellow in 1991 and joined the HSS Radiology Department (see Chapter 16). This section grew out of HSS sports medicine meetings with Warren, when he and his staff presented cases to Potter, comparing photos taken of pathology at the time of surgery to MRI images.

Warren had personally invited Raymond V. Damadian, MD, to talk with the HSS staff about his invention—then known as the "nuclear magnetic resonance (NMR) device."[c] There was little enthusiasm from the HSS staff at that time. In the mid-1990s, Warren asked Potter to draft a proposal to expand the MRI program. The proposal was presented to Richard Menschel, co-chairman of the HSS Board of Trustees, who arranged for financing. Expansion of the MRI program led to a significant increase in MRI applications at HSS, resulting in a productive service and many clinical and research publications. General Electric was very supportive of the research position, enabling the MRI group to increase its innovations greatly.[8]

Education

In 2000, Laura Robbins was appointed to lead the hospital residents' and fellows' educational program. The 80-hour workweek for residents and fellows had been created and needed supervision. Robbins set up a monitoring system. At Warren's request, she was subsequently appointed to become vice president of education. It seemed that education at HSS, while important, had not had the full administrative support to align it with the demanding interests of clinical care and research. Robbins became outstanding in building an educational program for patients, residents, and staff, which has exploded in the past decade.[9]

Changes in Administration

The president and chief executive officer, John R. Reynolds, who replaced John Ahearn in 1998, was assisted in the Executive Office by Lisa A. Goldstein, executive vice president and chief operating officer, and eight other vice presidents (Fig. 8). During the early 1990s, there was a great deal of financial pressure on HSS. Each year, the projected budget had a dismal forecast. About that time, there was an anticipated deficit of $15 million or more, as HSS was in the process of expanding by adding operating rooms and rebuilding part of the hospital. Much of the problems related to high fixed costs that the volume would not support. Warren thus proposed a plan with Reynolds and Ahearn (then co-administrators) to meet the obstacles by having the professional staff cover 50% of the deficit with volume, while the hospital covered the other 50% by efficiency. For several years this system worked, as younger staff was

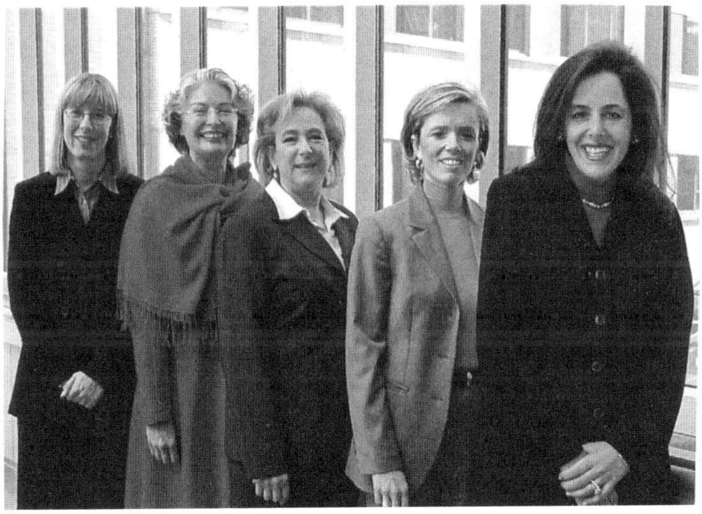

Fig. 8 (From left, circa 2002) Lisa A. Goldstein, executive vice president and chief operating officer; Deborah Sale, executive vice president for external affairs; Constance B. Margolin, Esq., executive vice president for legal affairs; Paddy C. Mullen, executive vice president for business services; and Stacey L. Malakoff, executive vice president and chief financial officer. Four vice presidents missing from this photo are Jacqueline Kostic, vice president for nursing; Marion Hare, vice president for operations; Ralph J. Bianco, vice president for operations; and Stephen A. Reday, vice president for human resources. (From Hospital for Special Surgery Archives)

added and they grew in their practices. In 1993, there were 6,000 operative cases, which increased to about 20,000 in 2003. Eventually, financial controls led to a stable corporate structure that could increase its research efforts.[9]

In 2003, Warren stepped down from the office of surgeon-in-chief but continued to practice sports medicine and orthopaedic surgery, teach, participate in research, and maintain his role as team physician for the New York Giants. In 2008, Warren received the Columbia University Hall of Fame Award. In 2010, he was chosen by the HSS resident staff to receive the Philip D. Wilson, Jr. Resident Teaching Award, and in 2011, he won the Distinguished Clinician Educator Award of the American Orthopaedic Association.

"My experience at HSS has been something that I have greatly enjoyed, particularly the involvement with our residents, colleagues and staff. The hospital has allowed me to perform research in various ways and participate at a high level nationally," said Russell Warren when summing up his experiences as surgeon-in-chief. "The staff and hospital have grown a great deal since the early 90s, and its reputation has increased. Our Board has been outstanding, and I found it a true privilege to work with them. Richard Menschel and Donald Stone always kept me on my toes. I felt that I learned a great deal from all the Board members on how to guide an organization."

REFERENCES

1. Papone A. The Power of the Obvious: Notes from 50 Years in Corporate America. Palo Alto, CA: Palo Alto Press; 2005.
2. Kahn BA. The evolution of orthopaedic nursing at the Hospital for Special Surgery. *Orthop Nurs*. 2005;24:343–348.
3. Goldberg SJ. HSS Nursing Annual Report. New York: 2008.
4. Amstutz HC. One-stage femoral lengthening. J Hosp for Spec Surg. 1975;1:57–64.
5. Amstutz HC. The morphology, natural history and treatment of proximal femoral focal deficiencies. In: Proximal Femoral Focal Deficiency. A Congenital Anomaly, edited by GT Aitken. Washington, DC: National Academy of Sciences; 1969;1734:50–57.
6. Rozbruch SR, Ilizarov S. Limb Lengthening and Reconstructive Surgery. New York, NY: Informa Healthcare; 2006.
7. Available at: http://en.wikipedia.org/wiki/Raymond_Vahan_Damadian
8. Damadian, R. Tumor Detection by Nuclear Magnetic Resonance. *Science 171*, 1151–1153 (1971).
9. Warren RW. Personal communication. 2012.

NOTES

a. Educated in Europe, Papone came to the United States as a young man and began his career with Macy's in 1956. He served as a president of two other American Express divisions. In 2005, he authored a book, *The Power of the Obvious: Notes from 50 Years in Corporate America.*[1]

b. O'Hare, who has sat on a number of boards, has been a leading voice on international trade issues. In 2012, he continued to serve with Aldo Papone as co-chair of the board.

c. Raymond Vahan Damadian, MD, professor at the State University of New York Health Science Center in Brooklyn and the inventor of the MRI scanner, was the first to perform a full-body scan of a human being in 1977 to diagnose cancer.[7]

CHAPTER 14
THOMAS P. SCULCO, MD ELEVENTH SURGEON-IN-CHIEF (2003–2013)

DAVID B. LEVINE, MD

IN FEBRUARY 2003, AFTER AN extensive search, the Board of Trustees of Hospital for Special Surgery (HSS) announced the appointment of Thomas P. Sculco, MD, as the 11th surgeon-in-chief. That May, Sculco assumed the office of surgeon-in-chief and medical director of HSS from Warren, who had stepped down after 10 years. At the same time, HSS marked this new era with the election of Dean R. Hare as co-chair of the Board of Trustees.[a] O'Hare joined Aldo Papone, who continued to serve as co-chair.

On May 1, 2003, 42 days after the United States and three other countries invaded Iraq, President George W. Bush—landing on the deck of the *USS Abraham Lincoln*, which was returning from a mission in Iraq, off the coast of San Diego—stood in front of a banner reading "Mission Accomplished" and declared in a primetime speech that the major combat operations were over. The nation, still in mourning over 9/11, thought this was the bright light they had been waiting for at the end of the tunnel. But unfortunately, that light soon flickered and dimmed.

Back in New York City, Mayor Michael Bloomberg (Republican at that time) introduced a $3 billion tax increase in the middle of the 2003 fiscal year. The move, unpopular with New York citizens, would be credited for stabilizing the city's financial crisis. Five months later, on August 14, the lights of New York went out in a sudden unexplained blackout of the northeast that presented Bloomberg with yet another crisis. Stranded by a shutdown of the subways, traffic gridlock and a crippled Amtrak rail system, New Yorkers coped with the challenges, as they looked unfavorably on their mayor. With its emergency generator, however, HSS was able to continue to function on a normal weekday schedule.

Early Education

Thomas Sculco earned his AB degree in classics from Brown University in 1965 and his MD degree from the College of Physicians and Surgeons of Columbia University in 1969. He served as an intern and resident in surgery at Roosevelt Hospital from 1969 to 1971, at which time he was appointed an HSS orthopaedic resident, graduating in 1974. The following year, he served as a lecturer and senior registrar at the London Hospital, having won the New York Academy of Medicine Bowen-Brooks Scholarship for Study Abroad.

From 1975 to 1977, Sculco served in the U.S. Air Force Medical Corps as a major and was stationed at Malcolm Grow Medical Center in Washington, DC, where he was awarded the USAF Commendation Medal for meritorious service. He performed the first total knee replacement in a hemophiliac patient in the military.

He returned to New York in 1977 and was appointed an assistant attending orthopaedic surgeon at HSS, New York Hospital and Memorial Hospital for Cancer and Allied Diseases. Also appointed assistant professor of surgery (orthopaedics) at Cornell University Medical College in 1977, he rose through the ranks, becoming professor of orthopaedic surgery in 2002.

A member of over 30 medical associations, Sculco has served on the Board of Directors of the American Academy of Orthopaedic Surgeons and was either chair or a member of over a dozen of its committees. In 1983, he helped found the Knee Society and was its treasurer from 2005 to 2009. He also founded the Association of Veterans Administration Orthopaedic Surgeons in 1986. Among his many honors and awards were the Gold Medal Award for Clinical Medicine from Columbia University College of Physicians and Surgeons in 2005 and the Lifetime Achievement Award from the Arthritis Foundation. He has published over 285 papers in peer-reviewed journals and has been an author of more than 70 books and chapters.

More recently, in 2006, Sculco founded the International Society of Orthopaedic Centers (ISOC). Its ultimate goal is to facilitate the exchange of ideas and best practices among the premier specialty orthopaedic centers in the world and to collaborate on patient care, education, and research-based programs, thus affecting improvement in patient care on a global scale. Membership was set at a maximum of 75 registrants. The first ISOC meeting was held in New York in May 2007 at HSS. By 2012, there were 16 international member organizations on four continents.

The Early Years

Raised in Westerly, Rhode Island, Sculco was born in New York City at Columbia Presbyterian Hospital on February 20, 1944. At that time, his father was playing trumpet with the Tommy Dorsey Band in New York.[b] His father also played with two other popular big bands—those led by Benny Goodman and Harry James. Sculco's mother had emigrated from Ireland at age 16 years and was an aspiring actress.

In junior high school in Westerly, he met his future wife, Cynthia. They were married in 1966, a year after she obtained her BSN degree at the University of Rhode Island. She went on to receive her MEd in medical-surgical nursing in 1971 and her EdD in curriculum and instruction in 1975 from Columbia University Teachers College (Fig. 1).

Cynthia Sculco has been an adjunct associate professor of nursing at New York University School of Nursing since 1998 and was president and CEO of Nurse Ed Communications, Inc., from 1996 to 2002. She had foreign experience as a visiting nurse instructor and professor from 1968 to 1975 and has authored a number of publications.

The Sculcos have maintained a passionate interest in opera and classical music, which originated from his uncle, an opera fanatic. They have two children: a married daughter who teaches high school and a son, who currently is an HSS orthopaedic resident.

Opening the Lines of Communication

Recognizing he needed to act responsively when national and local issues might adversely affect the quality of daily HSS medical practice and hospital operations, Sculco found himself very busy reorganizing the internal structure of the Orthopaedic Department in his first year as surgeon-in-chief, supporting divisions and subspecialty services and their relations with the Hospital Board and Administration. From the time board co-chairman Aldo Papone

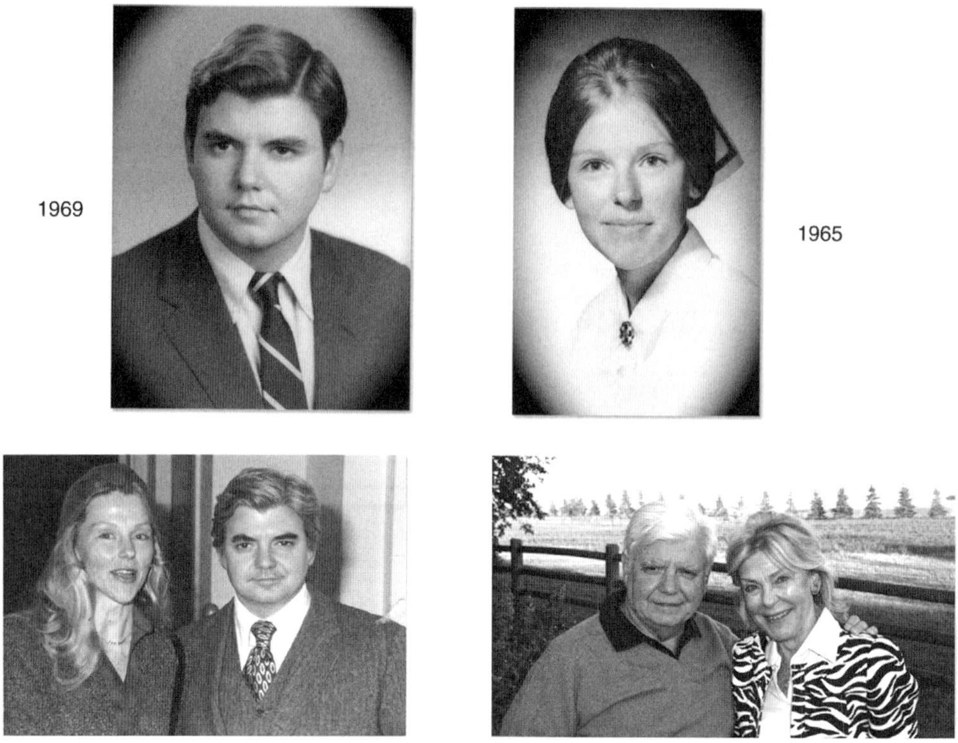

Fig. 1 In 1969, Thomas Sculco, MD, graduated medical school, and in 1965, Cynthia Sculco graduated nursing school. They celebrated their 25th anniversary in 1981. 2011: The Sculcos in the Tetons. (From Hospital for Special Surgery Archives)

called to offer him this appointment, until 2 months later, when he actually assumed command, Sculco conceptualized a new reorganizational plan (Table 1). He felt that during the prior decade of Warren as surgeon-in-chief and Sculco as director of clinical orthopaedics, the HSS system—although ranked at the top in its field—was growing more complex. Regulatory healthcare agencies were multiplying with expanding jurisdictions, requiring a closer interrelationship among clinicians, teachers, researchers, administrating body, and governing body, as well as their close interactions with the medical center and national medical societies and healthcare agencies.

Working with the administration and the board, Sculco proposed the following:

- An increase in the number of beds
- An increase in the number of operating rooms
- Expansion of private and clinic patient facilities

Table 1 Orthopaedic Department Reorganization 2003: Executive Committee of the Surgeon-in-Chief

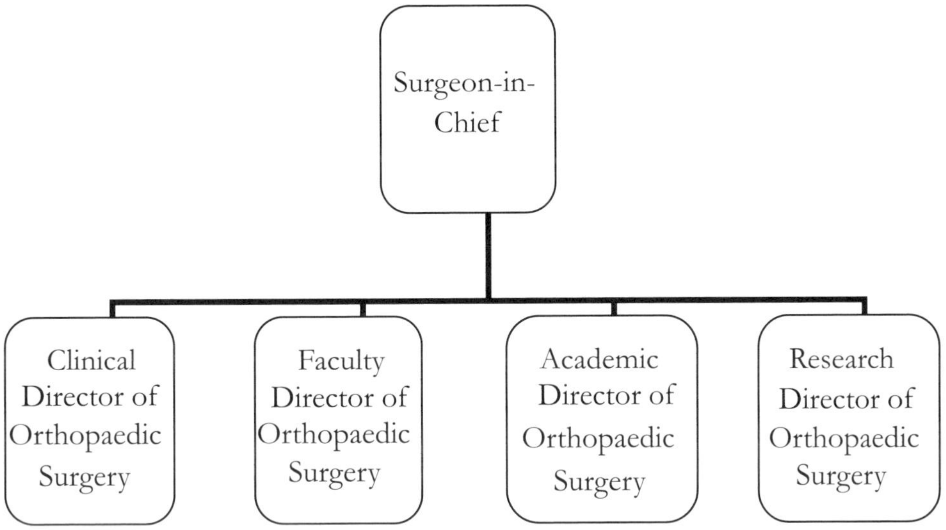

- Creation of a children's hospital within the hospital building
- Renovation of the Leon Root Motion Analysis Laboratory

Orthopaedic Department Restructuring

Realizing that the surgeon-in-chief serves as medical director of the hospital, an executive committee was established to provide leadership for clinical operations, faculty development, academics, and research (Table 1).

Each surgeon was a member of one of 10 service lines. These service lines would be responsible for the development of service-based research and education plans, quality initiatives, and service-based recruitment and growth plans (Table 2).

Sculco's next step was to create a service chief's council. Services had been in place, but their chiefs had never sat in a room and met. In 2012, this council met monthly with Sculco, Shapiro, and various invited key administrators. Discussion included current and future activities of the hospital and individual service issues. Service chiefs reported on activities of their services, and the chief made a presentation about every 2 years describing patient care,

Table 2 Orthopaedic Services: August 2012

Service	*Chief*
Hip	Douglas E. Padgett, MD
Knee	Steven B. Haas, MD
Surgical Arthritis	Mark P. Figgie, MD
Foot and Ankle	Jonathan T. Deland, MD
Hand and Upper Extremity	Edward A. Athanasian, MD
Limb Lengthening and Complex Reconstruction	S. Robert Rozbruch, MD
Metabolic Bone Disease/ Musculoskeletal Oncology	Joseph M. Lane, MD
Orthopaedic Trauma	David L. Helfet, MD
Pediatric Orthopaedics	Roger F. Widmann, MD
Scoliosis	Oheneba Boachie-Adjei, MD
Spine	Frank P. Cammisa Jr., MD
Sports Medicine and Shoulder	David W. Altchek, MD, and Scott A. Rodeo, MD (co-chiefs)

educational activities, and research programs to the entire council. This allowed cross-fertilization of ideas. In 2006, Sculco created a new publication, the *Annual Report of the Department of Orthopaedic Surgery* (Fig. 2).

Sculco created the Departmental Directors' Council, composed of orthopaedics and eight other departments (Table 3). Directors met, with Sculco and Shapiro, every 2 months.

The Research Division had undergone a change of leadership in 2002, with Francesco Ramirez, PhD, assuming the position as chief scientific officer (see chapter 17 for more information) (Fig. 3). The Institutional Review Board (IRB) had been reorganized under the leadership of Edward C. Jones, MD, MA. Clinical volumes had driven the need for additional beds, operating rooms, office space, and program expansion. Close collaboration with administration and the Board of Trustees resulted in many of these changes being approved and then moved forward. Plans proceeded to build a new inpatient operating room on the fourth floor and an eight-bed "swing unit" on top of the East Wing of the building, over the FDR Drive.

Additional reorganization activities included a major review and revamping of the Academic Training Program led by Mathias P. Bostrom, MD, executive

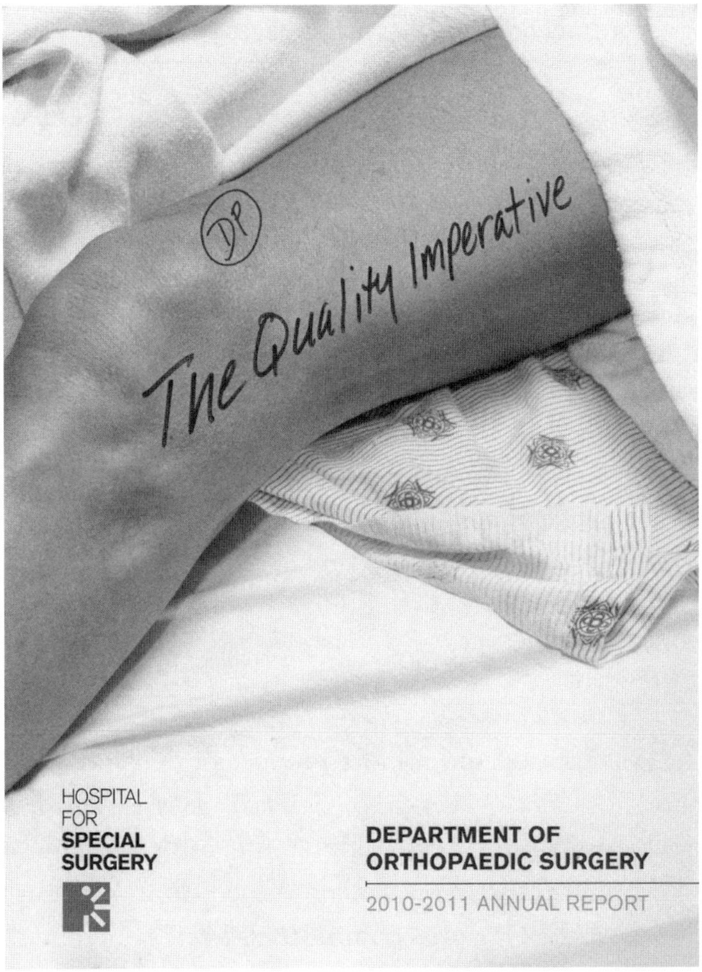

Fig. 2 In 2006, Thomas Sculco created a new publication, the *Annual Report of the Department of Orthopaedic Surgery*.

assistant to the surgeon-in-chief, in collaboration with Laura Robbins, DSW, senior vice president for Education and Academic Affairs.

Establishment of the HSS Alumni Association

On February 23, 2003, Sculco made his first appointment as surgeon-in-chief when he asked (David B.) Levine to assume a newly created position as director of alumni affairs (HSS Alumni Association). Retiring from the attending staff in 1995 after 34 years at HSS and 28 years as chief of the Scoliosis

Table 3 Departmental Directors' Council: August 2012

Department	*Director*
Medicine	Mary K. Crow, MD
Anesthesiology	Gregory A. Liguori, MD
Neurology	Dale J. Lange, MD
Pathology and Laboratory Medicine	Michael J. Klein, MD
Physiatry	Joseph H. Feinberg, MD
Radiology and Imaging	Helene Pavlov, MD
Rehabilitation Medicine	Leon Root, MD
Services	
Pediatrics	Lisa S. Ipp, MD
Primary Care Sports Medicine	Bryan C. Halpern, MD
Psychiatry	John W. Barnhill, MD
Research Division	
Chief Scientific Officer	Steven R. Goldring, MD
Applied Biomechanics in Orthopaedic Surgery	Timothy M. Wright, PhD
Education and Academic Affairs Division	
Senior Vice President	Laura Robbins, DSW

Service, Levine was pleased and honored to accept this appointment. He had great admiration for Sculco ever since Sculco's days as an HSS resident in 1971. Levine was also deeply devoted, grateful, and committed to HSS during the years before his retirement, having served on four committees of the Board of Trustees and 22 hospital committees, 14 of which he had chaired.[c]

Over the next 9 years, Levine created the Alumni Affairs Committee to oversee expansion and reorganization of the HSS Alumni Association, whose membership had increased to about 1,500 worldwide. The once-annual *Alumni News* was expanded to twice yearly, with a new cover and layout in 2009 featuring many photos and expansion of content. The revamped magazine garnered numerous publication and communication awards, including the Apex Award of Excellence, honoring excellence in medical marketing in the category of the Most Improved Newsletter.

A Distinguished Alumnus Award was created and at the annual meeting in November 2004, Charles Christian, MD, became the first recipient. A Thursday evening social reception was held at the Rockefeller University, often dedicated to honor one of the alumni receiving the Distinguished Alumnus Award. Poster exhibits were displayed at annual alumni meetings and at the HSS Alumni receptions held in conjunction with the annual meeting of the American Academy of Orthopaedic Surgeons.

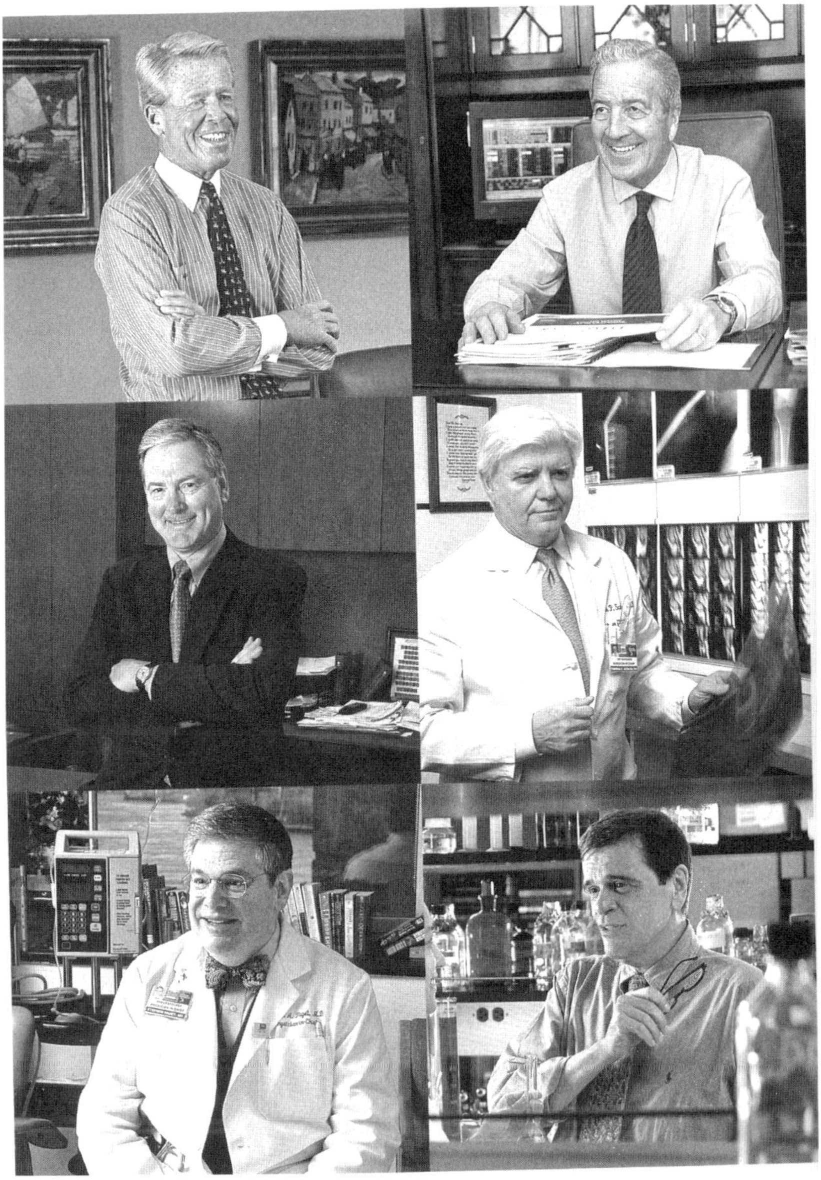

Fig. 3 (Clockwise from top left) Dean O'Hare, board co-chair; Aldo Papone, board co-chair; Thomas Sculco, MD, surgeon-in-chief; Francesco Ramirez, PhD, chief scientific officer; Stephen Paget, MD, physician-in-chief; John R. Reynolds, president and chief executive officer. (From Hospital for Special Surgery Archives)

Holiday greeting cards were created using images of the "old hospital" and sent to alumni starting in 2005, and the Alumni e-News was reinvented.

In 2006, Daniel S. Rich, MD, an HSS orthopaedic resident in the class of 1982 and the 2012 president-elect of the Alumni Association, was named associate director of the Alumni Affairs Committee and the Alumni Association (Fig. 4). Gary M. Gartsman, MD, an orthopaedic resident of the class of 1980 and 2006 president of the Alumni Association, pledged a major donation of $50,000 in 2006 to establish the Alumni President's Fund, which supported travel expenses for the sitting president to attend the HSS annual meeting.

Alumni stationery was created. A new Finance Subcommittee of the Alumni Affairs Committee, with Levine as chair, and later an Editorial Committee for *Alumni News* were established. A tribute to Lewis Clark Wagner, MD, was held at the 2008 alumni meeting and another to Philip D. Wilson Jr., MD, at the 2009

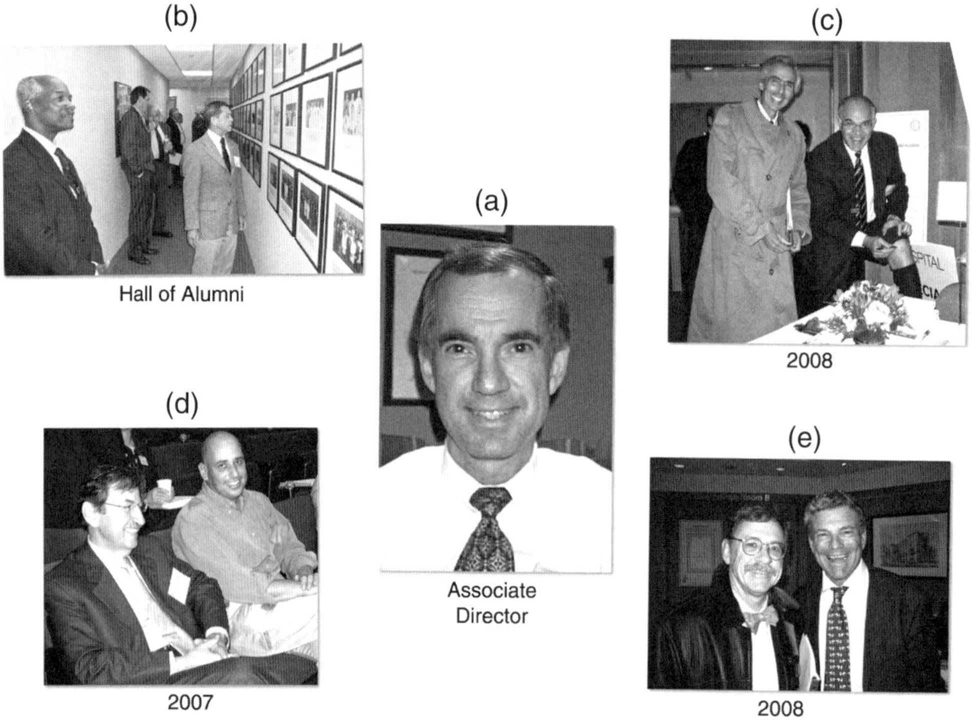

Fig. 4 (a) Daniel Rich, MD, 2013 alumni association president, became the first associate director of the Alumni Association in 2006. (b) 1983 scoliosis fellow Roger Antoine, MD, and 2011 alumni president Jon Wang, MD, study previous HSS graduates in the eighth floor Hall of Alumni. (c) At the 2008 alumni meeting, standing is 2012 alumni president Dominick Sisto, MD, learning a few tips about a knee incision from Bernard Bach, MD, director of sports medicine at Rush Medical Center. (d) At the 2007 alumni meeting, class representative (resident 1988) Robert Klapper, MD, listens intensely to presentations with Eugene Krauss, MD (resident 1987), on his right. (e) At the 2008 meeting, resident 1978 and scoliosis fellow 1979 John Morrison, MD (in bow tie), with David Fleiss, MD, resident 1979. (From Hospital for Special Surgery Archives)

meeting, honoring his approaching 90th birthday. The procedure for collecting dues was restructured, and the opportunity for alumni to make additional donations to alumni projects was encouraged with the implementation of the HSS alumni fund. A class representative program for resident and fellow graduates was inaugurated by Rich, Martha O'Brasky, MPA, assistant vice president of Education and Academic Affairs and administrative director of the Alumni Association, and Colleen O'Shea, MPA, manager, Office of Alumni Affairs.

In June 2009, Laura Robbins launched the Georgette "Gigi" Viellion, RN, ONC, Orthopaedic Nursing Education Scholarship Award Fund in memory of Viellion, a member of the HSS Nursing staff for over 25 years. This fund established an Orthopaedic Nursing Education Endowed Scholarship, to be awarded annually to a deserving nursing candidate.

Other new alumni funds followed, including The Leon Root, MD Pediatric Outreach Program; being a sponsor of the Bioskills Education Laboratory; Medical Education Scholarships; Charles L. Christian, MD, Musculoskeletal Research Award; Andrew N. Swanson, MD, Memorial Spine Award; the Sam Delgado, CST, Teaching Award; Pier Giorgio Marchetti, MD, Award for International Achievement; and the Lance Peters, MD, Memorial Biomechanics Award, created in his memory by members of his resident class of 1999.

From 2000 to 2013, the Alumni Association and supporting administrative staff came under the Division of Education headed by Robbins. Daily operations of the Alumni Office were conducted by O'Shea. Marcia Ennis, director of education publications and communications in the division of Education & Academic Affairs, and her staff produced award-winning publications. Both Ennis and O'Shea reported to O'Brasky (Fig. 5a).

In 2013, the HSS Alumni Association, which holds its annual meetings each November, celebrates its centennial birthday, the same year that the hospital celebrates its 150th anniversary. In recent years, the alumni meetings included a successful fundraising benefit, skillfully organized and chaired by Cynthia Sculco and the Autumn Benefit Committee. It supplemented financial support for the *HSS Journal*, along with other important HSS medical education initiatives. In 2011, over $800,000 was raised.

Growth of the Medical Library

By 2013, the HSS medical library had witnessed significant growth and advances since it was first created in April 1935 by Philip D. Wilson Sr. in his first

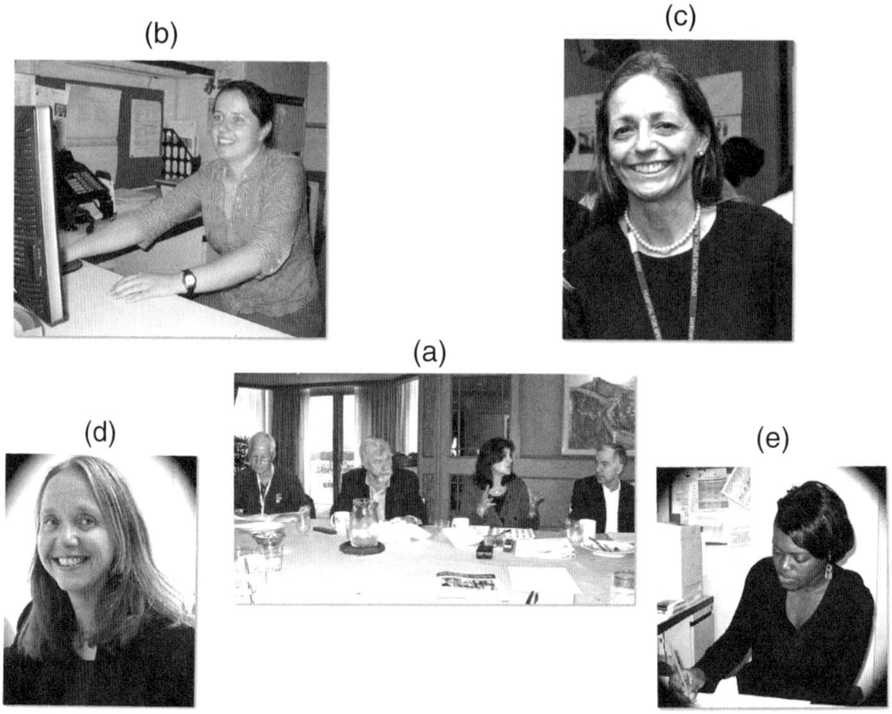

Fig. 5 (a) Annual class representatives breakfast meetings held at the time and place of the AAOS annual meetings were popular. (Seated from left) Thomas Nordstrom, MD, resident 1983; Patrick McMahon, MD, 2010 alumni president; Martha O'Brasky; and Dan Rich, MD, committee chair. (b) Colleen O'Shea is invaluable as alumni office manager. (c) Laura Robbins, DSW, senior vice president of Education and Academic Affairs, where the Alumni Association is located. (d) Marcia Ennis, editor of *Alumni News*, directs all publications and communications in the division. (e) Natanya Gayle, MPH, is managing editor for the *HSS Journal.* (From Hospital for Special Surgery Archives)

year as the fifth surgeon-in-chief at Hospital for the Ruptured and Crippled (R&C) (see chapter 7). It proved to be a great success.[1] Initially, a secretary was assigned to the library, but a medical librarian named Miss Wiederhold (first mentioned by Wilson in his 1939 Annual Report) soon followed.[2]

In 1941, Kim Barrett (1911–1976) became the second medical librarian, a position she held for 35 years until just before her death on July 25, 1976.[3] She made weekly rounds to all the physicians' offices, unannounced, collecting the "borrowed" library books (she called them "her children") and quietly returning them to the shelves of her library. Extremely knowledgeable in orthopaedics, Barrett could always find a reference instantaneously in a world without computers. She was devoted and moved her library with the institution in 1955 when the hospital relocated from East 42nd Street to East 70th Street. She guarded her books carefully so that the library could be easily reestablished in its new home.

After the death of her husband, Chester, in the Normandy Invasion in World War II, Barrett developed a passion for flowers and nurtured her potted plants on the library's windowsills. A quiet, knowledgeable, and warm person, she was adored by the entire staff.

Just before her death, Barrett helped complete a grant application to the National Library of Medicine to establish a consortium of libraries, including HSS, for the purpose of making common use of audiovisual materials. In 1977, the Alumni Association commemorated her by naming the library the Kim Barrett Memorial Library (Fig. 6).

Following Kim Barrett, there were four full-time librarians until the arrival of Tim Roberts, MLS, AHIP, who was appointed the medical librarian in 2006 (Table 4). During these years, the library—always a very popular meeting ground for house staff, nursing, and other hospital staff—grew, relocated, expanded, and was transformed with the arrival of the computer age by Roberts (Fig. 7).

Mathew Roberts, MD (no relation), who was appointed the Library Committee Chair in 2005, had worked to strategically position the library to become a premier resource for musculoskeletal information for the entire HSS Community. He was able to orchestrate a major library renovation, which was completed at the end of 2007. The changes included relocating shelving and creating a quiet study space, moving computer workstations to the area of the library with windows, and relocating the copiers.

The library's collection has included over 2,000 print monographs and 300 electronic textbooks in the areas of orthopaedics, rheumatology, sports medicine, and related disciplines. The library also maintained an archival collection of monographs that are significant to the history of orthopaedics and the history of HSS. There are over 450 active journal subscriptions, both electronic and print. In 2012, Tim Roberts became director of academic training at HSS.

Creation of the HSS Archives

In 2003, realizing that a rich history of original patient records dating back to 1863, photographs over 100 years old, bound hospital annual reports from the days of the Civil War and various other saved documents and archival press releases were lying unfilled and had not been catalogued, Levine—with

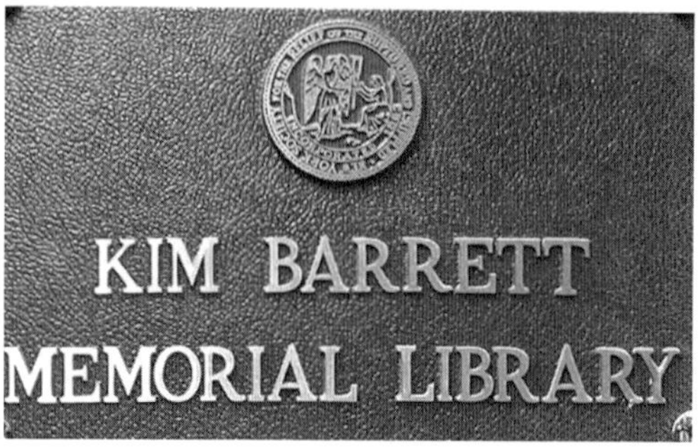

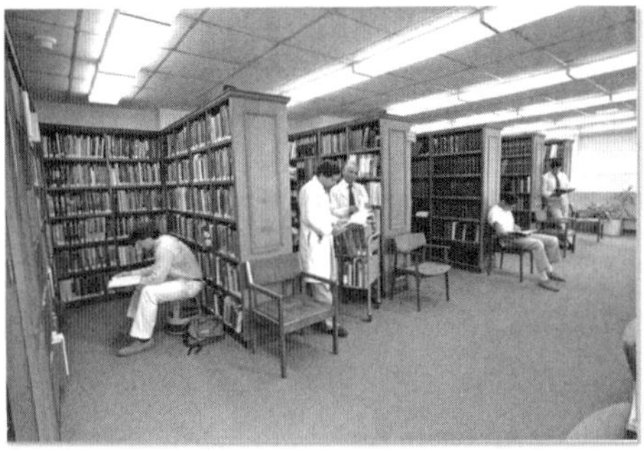
1960s – 2nd Floor Caspary Research

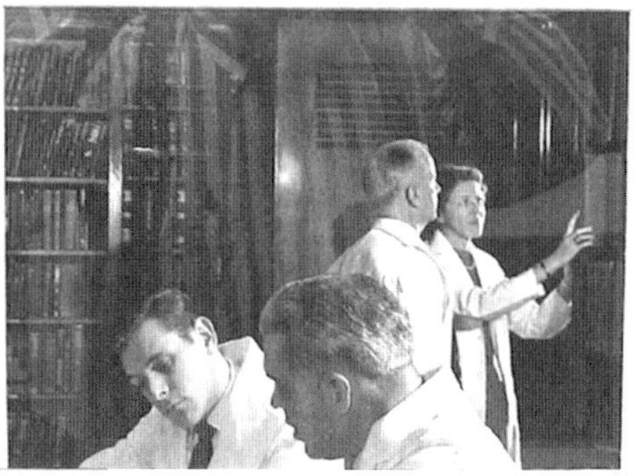
1950s – 42nd Street

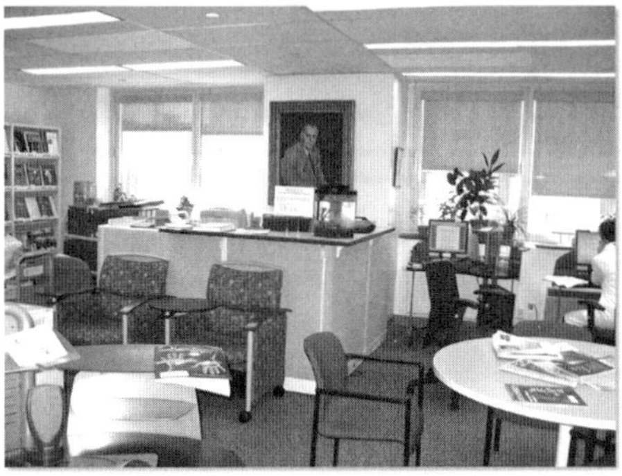
2007 – 8th Floor

Fig. 6 In 1977, the HSS Alumni Association dedicated the medical library to Kim Barrett (upper left) who died the year before after serving 35 years as librarian. Moving to the new building in 1955, the library was located on the fourth floor but was soon moved to the second floor of the research building and eventually to the eighth floor, where it remains. (From Hospital for Special Surgery Archives)

financial support from Sculco and Shapiro—ordered cabinets and supplies to start organizing this collection. If these collections had not been saved by Barrett from a fire in the medical library on August 3, 1974, there would be no archives today as we know it. After volumes were saved, she had them

Table 4 Medical Librarians, R&C and HSS: 1935–2012

1935–1939	Secretary (no librarian)
1939–1941	Miss Wiederhold
1941–1976	Kim Barrett
1976–1994	Munir Din
1994–1996	Laura Match
1996–2005	Inga Zhygalo
2006–2012	Tim Roberts

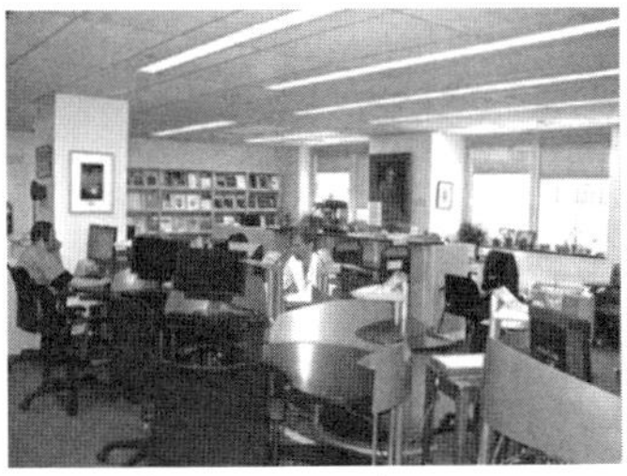

Computers arrive

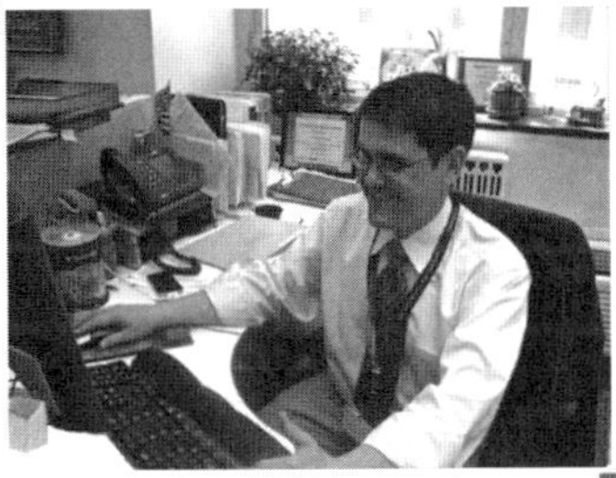

2012

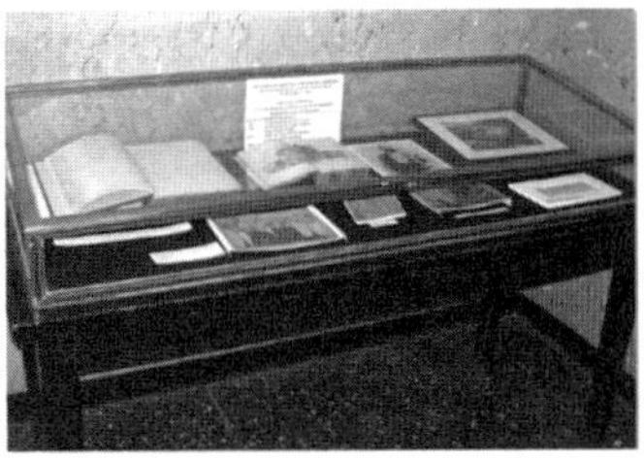

2004 Lobby Exhibit

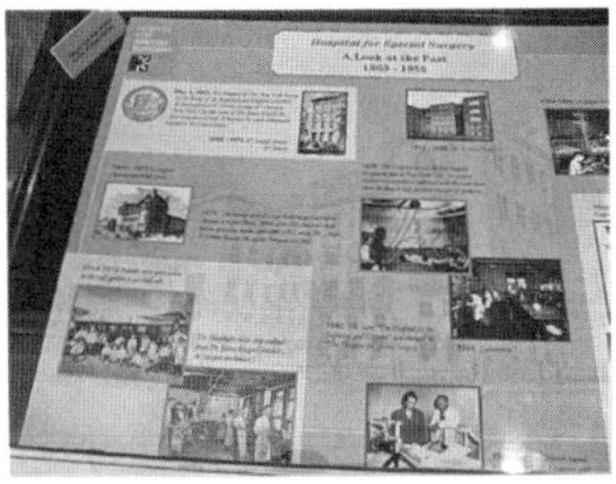

2004

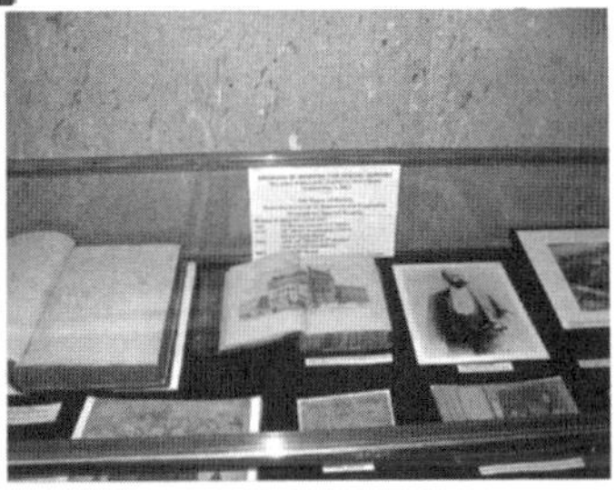

2004

Fig. 7 Medical librarian Tim Roberts, MLS, AHIP, introduced additional computers and work stations to the library after he arrived. The HSS archives was created in 2004 and at first was displayed periodically in an antique showcase in the hospital lobby. (From Hospital for Special Surgery Archives)

bound, preserving much valuable memorabilia from the mid-19th century. At the time of the fire, one of the orthopaedic staff surgeons, Alexander Hersh, MD, was in the hospital and helped Barrett save these memorable collections.

By 2004, with the addition of four filing cabinets and members of a recently formed Archives Committee that met three times a year, Levine started to curate homemade exhibits on his computer at his farm located 2 hours north of New York City. He used foam core that was cut to fit the 5-foot-long, heavy antique brass, and steel showcase that had been donated by New York Hospital. In January 2004, he launched his first exhibit: the *Founding of the Hospital for the Ruptured and Crippled.* It was on display until April 2004, when his second exhibit, *The Board of Trustees of R&C*, was displayed until September 2004. This exhibit was then moved up to the fourth-floor family atrium, where a modern maple display case had been custom-built. Its first display was installed in October 2004, and it remained there until February 2005 (Fig. 8).

The HSS patients and staff received the exhibits very favorably, with many of the hospital employees, and professional staff noting they had never been aware of the rich history of their institution. As external marketing of the hospital expanded after 1996, so did the internal marketing of our own institutional heritage.

There were seven "homemade" lobby exhibits until they were replaced at the end of 2009 with a commercial exhibit, still in use by the HSS

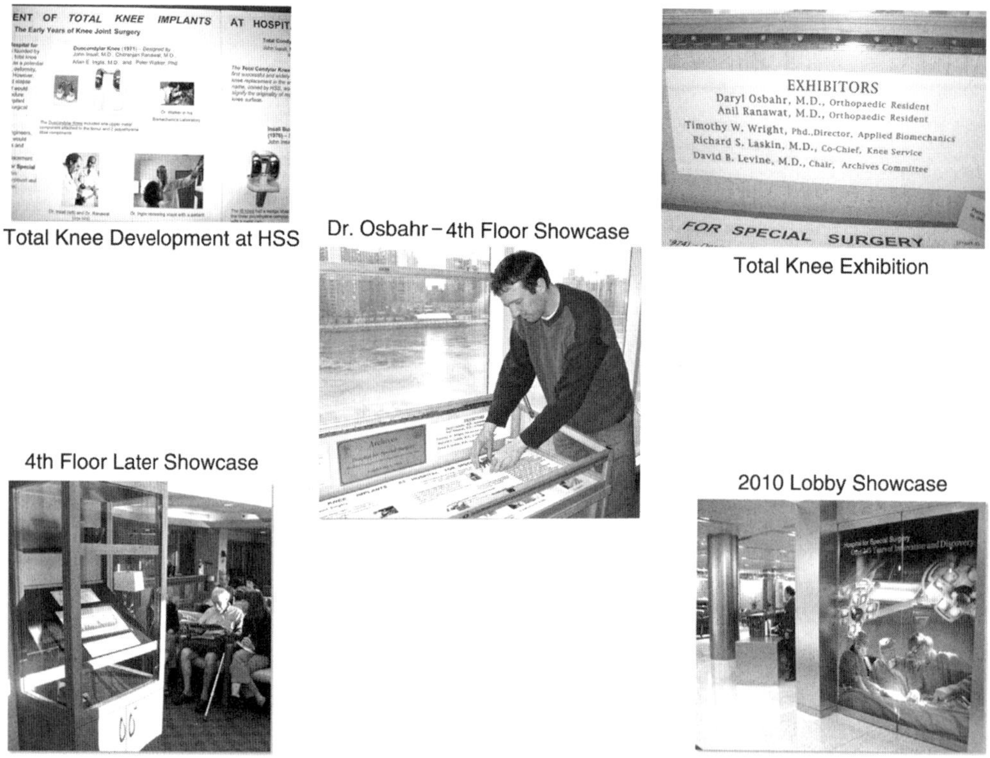

Fig. 8 One of the early major archives exhibits (above) was the development of the total knee implant in the hospital, being arranged here by one of the exhibitors, Daryl Osbahr, MD, an orthopaedic resident. This exhibit was originally placed in the custom maple showcase in the fourth-floor atrium, in front of the windows facing the East River. Later, because of the need for floor space for seating, another smaller maple showcase was designed and installed (lower left), and the first maple showcase was moved up to the eighth floor, near the West elevators. When the lobby was totally renovated in October 2010, a newly installed commercial showcase replaced the antique showcase. It was retired to the Caspary Estate main house, where a permanent archives exhibit may be viewed. (From Hospital for Special Surgery Archives)

Archives staff. After 2007, exhibits in the fourth-floor atrium and on the eighth floor were also stepped-up and curated by creative professional talent from the Education and Academic Affairs Division. From November 2009 to June 2010, an exhibit called *Philip D. Wilson, MD—World War II American Hospital in Britain—1940* was produced by Tim Roberts and installed on the eighth floor.

Andrew Sama, MD, agreed to become the first associate director of the HSS Archives in 2004 and has been an important contributor of articles on HSS history, including a history of Margaret and Alfred Caspary. Articles on the history of the hospital have also been serially published in the monthly hospital newsletter *Echo* and in *Alumni News*. On the annual HSS Education Day, HSS history is made available; it was first displayed in 2005 in the Richard L. Menschel Education Center as a major 100-foot canvas timeline.

Sculco felt there was also a need to disseminate HSS research and clinical practice intermittently, and the *HSS Journal* was created in 2005. Sculco appointed Richard Laskin, MD as the first editor-in-chief, with Robbins as executive editor.

The HSS Archives staff has been fortunate to have the advice and counsel of James L. Gehrlich, head, Medical Center Archives, New York–Presbyterian/Weill Cornell Medical Center. Since his retirement in 2011, his successor, Lisa Mix, continues to provide professional guidance and attends the HSS Archives Committee meetings.

The existence of the HSS Archives has generated limitless historical resources of the hospital since its founding in 1863 and has provided rich materials to promote and market the Sesquicentennial Anniversary of HSS, scheduled for May 2013. Furthermore, in the first issue, it provided the lead article on the history of the hospital, the first of a series of 11 articles written by Levine and covering the years 1863 through 1989. The first eleven chapters of this book have been based on these articles. The *HSS Journal* published two issues annually until 2012, when it increased to three a year (see chapter 12).

Currently, a designated archives staff includes a part-time archivist with an Advanced Certificate of Archival Management, Pamela A. Kerns, MLS, MPA, and a volunteer, Lynne Calman Erlanger, BA, MA. Further support is provided by a full-time medical library coordinator, Indira Garcia, and a part-time medical librarian, Tom Garnica, MLS, all reporting to Tim Roberts. In October 2012, a new full-time librarian, Rie Smethurst, MSLIS, was appointed to replace Tim Roberts, who became Director, Academic Training.

Center for Skeletal Dysplasias

The Kathryn O. and Alan C. Greenberg Center for Skeletal Dysplasias was established in 2003 and is dedicated to the comprehensive medical care of people of all ages with skeletal dysplasias. The first of its kind in New York City, the center brings together a multidisciplinary team of healthcare professionals committed to improving the quality of life for people with skeletal dysplasias through clinical care, research, and education. The center's co-directors are Jessica G. Davis, MD, and Cathleen Raggio, MD, who collaborate with radiology consultant Bernard Ghelman, MD.

Neurology Department

One of the earliest neurologists on the HSS medical staff was Joseph Moldaver, MD (1899–1982), who was part-time and was listed as an attending neurologist as far back as 1954, in the Division of Medicine and Pediatrics. A clinical professor of neurology at Columbia's College of Physicians and Surgeons, Moldaver retired in 1969, but remained at HSS for a short time. In 1971, Peter Tsairis, MD, PhD, replaced him at HSS as chief of the neurology service and attending neurologist. During these years, the neurology staff included Hart deC. Peterson, MD; Paul J. Maccabee, MD; and Richard Schoenfeldt, MD, as attending neurologists at various times.

Tsairis retired as director of neurology in 1995 and was replaced by Abe M. Chutorian, MD—professor of neurology and pediatrics at Cornell University Medical College—as chief of the Neurology Service until 2000. Paget acted as chief of neurology from 2000 to 2003, followed by Moris Jak Danon, MD (2004–2009). Following Danon, Dale J. Lange, MD, was appointed neurologist-in-chief and director of the Department of Neurology, as well as professor of neurology at Weill Medical College of Cornell University.

Department of Pathology and Laboratory Medicine

When Peter Bullough retired as director of the Department of Pathology and Laboratory Medicine in 2008, Michael J. Klein, MD, was appointed as pathologist-in-chief and director of pathology and laboratory medicine, as well as professor of pathology and laboratory medicine at Weill Cornell Medical

College. Klein became the sixth full-time pathologist at R&C and HSS (see chapters 6, 8, 10, and 11 for more information). Prior to that time, R&C had a part-time pathologist and head of the laboratories, F. M. Jeffries, MD (1865–1943), who served from 1914 to 1929 (see chapter 5 for more information).

Klein had served as associate director of pathology and laboratory medicine at Hospital for Joint Diseases Orthopedic Institute from 1980 to 1987, professor of pathology and orthopaedics at the Mount Sinai School of Medicine from 1987 to 2003, and professor of pathology at the University of Alabama (Birmingham) School of Medicine from 2003 to 2008.

Klein's primary expertise was in surgical and clinical orthopaedic pathology. His textbook, the *Atlas of Non-Neoplastic Diseases of Bone and Joints*, published by the American Registry of Pathology, was the only published peer-reviewed volume of its kind. He chairs the members' meeting of the International Skeletal Society and is a member of the World Health Organization consensus committee on the classification of bone and soft-tissue tumors, in addition to being active in several national and international pathology societies.

The department was staffed with four other specialists in their fields of medicine. Manjula Bansal, MD, received her medical degree in India and took a pathology residency at Mount Sinai School of Medicine and an immunopathology fellowship at Columbia Presbyterian University Hospital. She joined the HSS staff in 1983 and is now attending pathologist and chief of clinical pathology at HSS and associate professor of clinical pathology at the Weill Cornell Medical College.

Edward F. DiCarlo, MD, was appointed assistant pathologist at HSS in 1985, after completing his residency in anatomic pathology at New York Hospital, followed by a fellowship in orthopaedic pathology at HSS. He is currently associate pathologist and chief of surgical pathology as well as associate professor of clinical pathology at Weill Cornell Medical College. After joining HSS, DiCarlo quickly introduced PC-type computer functions to the department, starting with computer-assisted histomorphometry of bone, followed by the introduction of a diagnostic pathology reporting system based on the then-new concept of multiple related database tables.

Giorgio Perino, MD, joined the HSS staff in 2002, having trained as an anatomic pathology resident at the Mount Sinai School of Medicine and serving as a fellow in bone pathology at Hospital for Joint Diseases, and soft-tissue tumors at Memorial Sloan-Kettering Cancer Center. His interests lie in the body's reactions to implants, especially metal-on-metal devices, osteonecrosis secondary to corticosteroid therapy, and inflammatory diseases of the synovia.

The final staff pathologist, a transfusion medicine specialist and director of the Blood Bank at HSS, is David L. Wuest, MD. He is a transfusion medicine specialist and director of the Blood Bank, Donor Room, and Cytotherapy Laboratory Service at Memorial Sloan-Kettering Cancer Center. Having completed his residency training at New York Hospital and a blood banking fellowship at Cedars-Sinai Medical Center, Los Angeles, California, Wuest was appointed director of the HSS Blood Bank in 2005 and is also a professor of clinical medicine at Weill Cornell Medical College.[d]

Fifty Years at East 70th Street: 1955–2005

A celebration marking the 50th anniversary of the hospital's move from East 42nd Street to its present location on East 70th Street was held on May 25, 2005 in the Richard L. Menschel Education Center. Attending the afternoon festivities were some "old-timers" who worked at the 42nd Street hospital and recalled memories of the 1950s. Among them were orthopaedic staff members Wilson Jr., James Nicholas, MD, Peter Marchisello, MD, and secretaries Dolores Mattia (who worked for Straub) and Mary Birnbaum (who worked for Wilson Jr.). Ron Gilates, of Information Technology, recounted his memories of treatment as a pediatric patient at the old R&C (Fig. 9).

The year 2005 marked the 15th consecutive year that HSS ranked No. 1 in the northeast in both orthopaedics and rheumatology in the *U.S. News and World Report* "America's Best Hospitals" survey. New patient programs in 2005 included the Children and Adolescent and Arm (CHArm) Center, directed by Michele Carlson, MD. Dedicated to patient care, research, and education, the CHArm Center excels in providing quality care through both surgical and nonsurgical interventions and is committed to increasing awareness about treatment options available to families of children affected by hand and arm conditions. It provides educational programs on injury prevention to area schools, parents, athletic coaches, and healthcare workers. Additionally, the center is dedicated to research to improve the quality of patient care.

Other notable programs include the Joint Mobility Center, which focuses on the rehabilitation of patients who have had total joint replacement and

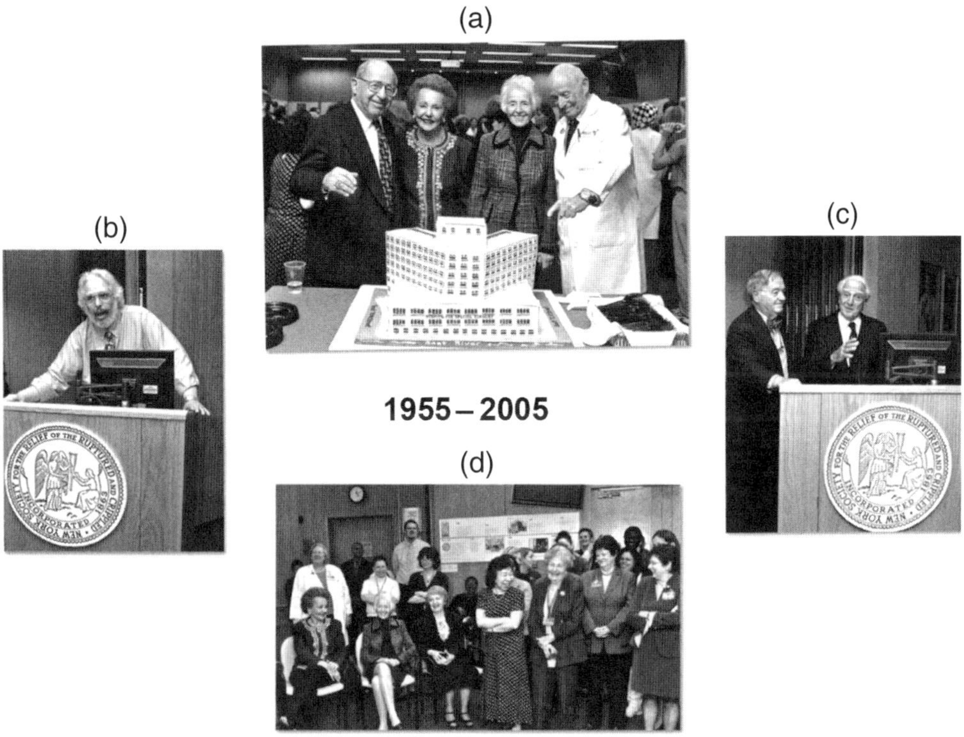

Fig. 9 On May 25, 2005, HSS staff celebrated the move from East 42 Street 50 years before. (a) Dr. and Mrs. Nicholas (left) and Dr. and Mrs. Wilson Jr., with a cake made as a replica of HSS. (b) Ron Gilates, Information Technology, recalls his time as a patient at the old hospital. (c) David B. Levine, MD (left), with Peter Marchisello, MD. (d, seated from left) Kiki Nicholas, Katherine Wilson, and Dolores Mattia. (Standing) Leslee Wong, Mary Birnbaum, Anne Tarpey (director of Organizational Learning and Development), and Marion Hare (vice president for administration). (From Hospital for Special Surgery Archives)

wellness initiatives that encompass both education and exercise programs. The HSS wellness platform features collaborative efforts with the HSS Public and Patient Education Department, the Rehabilitation Department, Nursing, and medical staff at the main HSS Campus, as well as the Integrative Care Center on Madison Avenue.

Advances in technology included the hospital's filmless Picture Archiving and Communication System (PACS) and the new Eclypsis Clinical Information System (CIS). Sparked by a landmark issue of *Discovery to Recovery* (published under the leadership of Deborah Sale, executive vice president, External Affairs), the Campaign for Research, chaired by Richard L. Menschel, drew to a close in 2005, having raised $115.7 million—more than $5.7 million over its goal. The Starr Foundation contributed $19 million, the largest aggregate gift the hospital had ever received at that time and helped to establish 21 endowed chairs (Table 5).

The year 2005 was a banner year on several fronts. The premiere issue of the *HSS Journal* was mailed to 10,000 orthopaedic surgeons, 3,500

Table 5 Endowed Chairs, Professorships, and Fellowships

Franchellie M. Cadwell Chair	Sergio Schwartzman, MD
Chase and Stephanie Coleman Chair in Magnetic Resonance Imaging Research	Hollis G. Potter, MD
Joel and Anne Bick Ehrenkranz Research Chair	
John N. Insall Chair in Knee Surgery	Steven B. Haas, MD
Collette Kean Research Chair	Jane E. Salmon, MD
F. M. Kirby Chair in Orthopaedic Biomechanics	Timothy M. Wright, PhD
David H. Koch Chair for Arthritis and Tissue Degeneration Research	Lionel B. Ivashkiv, MD
Korein-Wilson Professorship in Orthopaedic Surgery	Thomas P. Sculco, MD
Richard S. Laskin, MD Chair in Musculoskeletal Education	Charles N. Cornell, MD
David B. Levine, MD Chair in Scoliosis	Oheneba Boachie-Adjei, MD
C. Ronald MacKenzie, MD Chair in Ethics and Medicine	C. Ronald MacKenzie MD
Richard L. Menschel Research Chair	Steven R. Goldring, MD
Stephen A. Paget, MD Chair in Rheumatology	Stephen A. Paget, MD
Leon Root, MD Chair in Pediatric Orthopaedics	Leon Root, MD
Benjamin M. Rosen Chair in Immunology and Inflammation Research	Mary K. Crow, MD
Joseph P. Roth Professor of Rheumatic Diseases in Medicine	Mary K. Crow, MD
Virginia F. and William R. Salomon Chair in Musculoskeletal Research	Carl Blobel, MD, PhD
Eduardo A. Salvati, MD Chair in Hip Arthroplasty	
St. Giles Research Chair	Theresa Lu, MD, PhD
Starr Chair in Mineralized Tissue Research	Adele L. Boskey, PhD
Starr Chair in Tissue Engineering Research	
Russell F. Warren Research Chair	

rheumatologists, and 1,500 radiologists, physiatrists, and rehabilitation specialists. HSS orthopaedic residents scored the highest ever on the Orthopaedic In-Training Examinations, and the hospital received more than 450 applicants for eight highly sought-after orthopaedic residency positions.

There was also a change in nursing leadership. In spring 2005, Jacqueline Kostic, RN, who was vice president of nursing for the previous 8 years, retired and handed the leadership to Stephanie Goldberg, MSN, RN, CNA. Kostic had overseen the process that led HSS to become the first Manhattan hospital to receive the prestigious Magnet Recognition for Excellence in Nursing Services (see chapter 13).

President and CEO

In October 2006, Louis A. Shapiro joined HSS as president and chief executive officer. Shapiro, who came to HSS from the Geisinger Health System, a highly respected healthcare system in northeastern and central Pennsylvania, had begun his career at Allegheny General Hospital. He had earned his BA and MHA degrees at the University of Pittsburgh.

In fall 2006, under the leadership of Lisa Goldstein, chief operating officer, the first phase of the hospital's expansion project resulted in a new Ambulatory Surgery Center on the ninth floor, the opening of two operating rooms on the first floor for hand and foot surgery, 30 new inpatient beds on the eighth floor, and a new 8,000-square-foot Central Sterile Supply Center.

Steven R. Goldring, MD, an internationally recognized expert in orthopaedic and rheumatology research, was named chief scientific officer (see chapter 17). Other new orthopaedic appointments for 2006 are listed in Table 6.

In 2008, the hospital lost two key members. On January 15, Henry U. Harris, a Board of Trustees member for over 45 years and chairman from 1972 until

Table 6 Clinical Orthopaedic Service Appointments: 2006

Sports Medicine Service Co-Chiefs	David W. Altchek, MD, and Scott A. Rodeo, MD
Clinical Director, Orthopaedic Surgery	Charles N. Cornell, MD
Orthopaedic Residency Director	Edward V. Craig, MD, MPH
Knee Service Chief	Steven B. Haas, MD
Hip Service Chief	Douglas E. Padgett, MD
Orthopaedic Faculty Development Director	Scott W. Wolfe, MD

1988, passed away at the age of 81 years (see chapter 11). No one surpassed Harris as an involved Board Chairman, devoted supporter of HSS, and a true friend to all staff physicians. Laskin, editor-in-chief of the *HSS Journal*, passed away on March 1. The Richard Laskin Chair in Medical Education was established with significant funding.

The hospital lost another devoted member of the Board of Trustees when Patricia Mossbacher passed away in 2009. She had been a member of the board since 1987 and played a pivotal role in raising funds for the hospital as Vice Chair Emerita of the Board of Trustees and Chair of the HSS Benefits Committee. Among her legacies was the annual Patricia Mosbacher Honorary Lecture in Orthopaedic Trauma and the Patricia Mosbacher Flower Fund to provide, with board support, daily fresh flowers for the front lobby. She will be long remembered for her grace and wit and for being a most elegant, kind, and dedicated woman and a special friend to HSS.

Center for Hip Preservation

The Center for Hip Preservation was established in 2009, with Bryan Kelly, MD as its Director. Ernest L. Sink, MD, was recruited in 2011 from Denver Children's Hospital to be co-director. The center uses a multidisciplinary approach to treat a broad range of hip conditions by combining the expertise of a wide variety of healthcare professionals, including orthopaedic surgeons, radiologists, physiatrists, rheumatologists, physical therapists, and researchers. The goal of the center is to provide joint-preserving treatment options to young, active adult patients suffering from hip pain in order to restore a high level of function. In May 2010, the center's new location on the ground floor of the Belaire Building was inaugurated with a ribbon-cutting ceremony.

2010 Physician-in-Chief

On April 1, 2010, Mary K. Crow, MD, assumed the office as fifth physician-in-chief and director of medicine at HSS. Stephen A. Paget, MD, who had expanded and enriched that office since 1995, became physician-in-chief, emeritus, and focused on the next phase of his career in education, training, research, and international outreach.

Receiving her MD degree from Cornell University Medical College in 1978, Crow took an internship and residency in medicine at New York Hospital–Cornell Medical Center (1978–1981) and became a postdoctoral fellow at the Rockefeller University under Henry G. Kunkel, MD (1916–1983), from 1981 to 1984. A world leader in applying the principles of immunology to clinical medicine in the 1940s, Kunkel was especially known for his dedication to teaching and was remembered by his students as a special mentor. He concentrated on training MDs, many of whom became world leaders in the field of immunology and emerged from their training carrying the Henry Kunkel imprint. Crow served as president of the distinguished Henry Kunkel Society from 2007 to 2009.

Introduced to HSS as a medical student, Crow first joined the staff in 1981 as a fellow in rheumatic disease and research. In 1983, she was appointed assistant attending physician at HSS and rose through the ranks, holding the titles of associate chief of rheumatology and director of rheumatology research, just prior to her new appointment. Her major interests have been research in rheumatic immunology, focusing on clinical and research programs in systemic lupus erythematosus and osteoarthritis.

Having won over 25 awards and honors, Crow occupies the Benjamin M. Rosen Chair in Immunology and Inflammation Research at HSS. She has been president of the American College of Rheumatology, associate editor of the *Journal of Immunology*, and associate editor of the *Annals of the Rheumatic Diseases*, in addition to being a member of many national and medical center committees.

As physician-in-chief at HSS, she assumed the helm of a department of over 85 medical attending physicians, 11 fellows in rheumatic diseases, and 4 fellows in pediatric rheumatology (Fig. 10).

New Facilities

Phased modernization of the hospital's main entry was completed with new lighting, driveway improvements, and an enlarged and handsome lobby—with its new archives showcase in front of the west elevators—in 2010–2011. The East Wing expansion project was completed in September 2011 with the opening of three additional floors. Floors 10 and 11 housed inpatient beds, including an all-private room unit on the north side of the 11th floor.

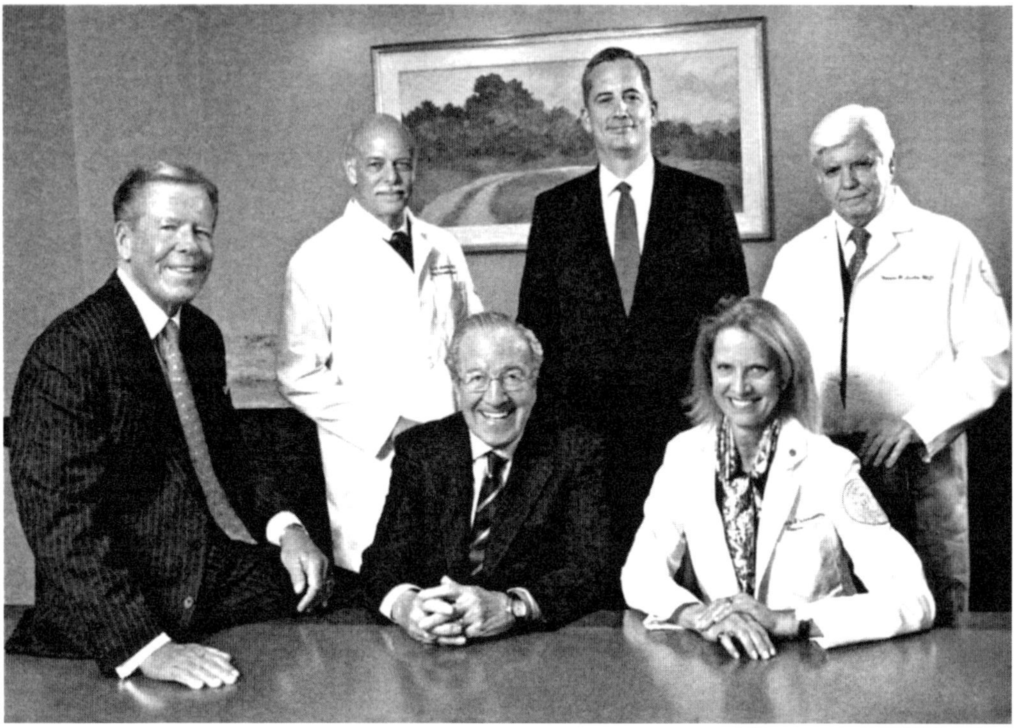

Fig. 10 (Seated from left) Dean R. O'Hare, co-chair, Board of Trustees; Aldo Papone, co-chair, Board of Trustees; Mary K. Crow, MD, physician-in-chief. (Standing from left) Steven R. Goldring, MD, chief scientific officer; Louis A. Shapiro, president and CEO; and Thomas P. Sculco, MD, surgeon-in-chief. (From Hospital for Special Surgery Archives)

The Pharmacy Department moved into its new, expanded space on the ninth floor.

The hospital also opened the doors to the new home of the Ambulatory Care Center, located on East 72nd Street, in August 2011. At the end of the year, it opened a new 30,000-square-foot facility on East 75th Street, housing physiatry, pain management, imaging facilities, and procedure rooms.

In October 2011, the first phase of the new Lerner Children's Pavilion opened on the ninth floor as the CA Technologies Rehabilitation Center, while the fifth floor, under construction at the time of this writing, will house 10 new private rooms designed for parents to stay overnight with their children. A support system was designed to provide unparalleled health care in this "children's hospital within a hospital."

Also in October 2011, Steve K. Lee, MD, joined the medical staff as a member of the Hand and Upper Extremity Service and the director of research for the hospital's Center for Brachial Plexus and Traumatic Nerve Injury, which was launched in 2012. Scott Wolfe, MD, transitioned from his role as Chief of the Hand and Upper Extremity Service to assume a new role as the Center's Director.

Allan E. Inglis Jr., MD, rejoined the HSS staff on the Surgical Arthritis Service as an assistant attending orthopaedic surgeon and clinical assistant professor of orthopaedic surgery at Weill Cornell Medical College. Awarded his MD degree from Weill Cornell Medical College in 1983, Inglis was a member of the HSS orthopaedic residency class of 1988. Following his residency, he completed fellowship training in London, Hamburg, and Los Angeles.

HSS continued to grow in physical plant, professional and hospital staff, employing innovative management and new technology with strong board and external support (Table 6).

Quality

Chasing and attaining "zero" preventable complications while fulfilling the hospital's mission to its patients has been a continuous process. Building on a retrospective study introduced by Andrew Sama, MD, of the Spine Service and Quality Research Center, a project applying the use of computer modeling was developed to identify changes in the environment (such as traffic flow in the operating rooms) and differences in patient characteristics (such as weight or diabetic control) that could help lower infection rates. This innovative approach produced results that may have otherwise taken many years to generate using traditional research methods.

Information Technology

In 2011, the Information Technology Department completed over 50 project implementations, including application upgrades to new versions, replacements of older applications, and the introduction of new and expanded functionality. A number of strategic projects also advanced in 2011. The hospital selected a practice management and electronic medical record system, known as Care Tracker, for physician offices. The goal of the system was to allow for increased alignment of physician offices with the hospital, to improve efficiency in physician offices through automation, and to facilitate the exchange of automated patient information between the hospital and physician practices. The system was up and running by 2012.

In early 2012, Jamie Nelson joined HSS as the new vice president for information technology and chief information officer (CIO). Receiving undergraduate and graduate degrees at the University of Pennsylvania and Cornell University, Nelson came to HSS from Norwalk Hospital in Connecticut, where she was CIO. She succeeded John Cox as CIO. On September 12, 2012, John Cox passed away unexpectedly.

Food Services

Over a span of four decades, food service operations have undergone several major changes. Nutrition care, in contrast, has grown and diversified with evolving demands and the hospital's expansion.

Up until the 1970s, patient and cafeteria food was prepared from scratch in the main kitchen, a fully equipped cooking facility located in the basement of the hospital. Food in bulk was transported by dumbwaiter to the cafeteria and four small pantries located on the inpatient care units, where meal trays were assembled and served. The cafeteria was a gathering place for HSS staff and was located on the third floor of the hospital (see chapter 10).

During the 1980s, the food service pantries were converted into physical therapy satellites, and assembly of patients' meal trays was relocated to the main kitchen. In the 1990s, food preparation in the main kitchen changed radically. The kitchen was scaled down for cold food production only; hot food was requisitioned from NewYork–Presbyterian Hospital's newly renovated "cook-chill" kitchen. Reheating/chilling units were purchased to hold and process meal trays for inpatient meal service.

In 1989, the cafeteria moved to the ground floor of the Belaire Building, its present location, and named the Belaire Café, where services branch out from this location. A coffee service kiosk was opened in the hospital lobby. A satellite food cart on the fourth floor, for lunch service, was made available to the operating room staff.

In the 2000s, the department enhanced the existing inpatient meal service system by adding two new programs: a continental breakfast cart service for the inpatient units, offering food and service near the patient's bedside, and a menu program that allows patients to choose their meals close to the time of service (versus 48 hours in advance).

In the 2010s, the inpatient meal service of the 1990s/2000s continued. With the expansion of the hospital and the addition of a new unit of private room suites, the meal service was enhanced, featuring room service trays, full china service, a stocked refrigerator, snacks on demand, a help-yourself-coffee-station, and a dedicated meal coordinator.

Eden Kalman MA, RD, CDN, the current food services director, first came to HSS in 1974, while her assistant director, Terry Karl, MS, RN, CDN, has been at HSS since 1984 (Table 7). In 1994, there were 108,364 meals served, increasing to 148,567 meals in 2011.

Foundation of Orthopedics and Complex Spine

In 2011, the dream of a very distinguished HSS orthopaedic surgeon, Oheneba Boachie-Adjei, MD, to create an orthopaedic hospital in his native country of Ghana in Africa was coming to fruition. With the support of HSS, a grant of $1.5 million from the government of Ghana and over $10 million from more than 1,800 private donors, the doors of a 50-bed orthopaedic hospital opened in May 2012.

Foundation of Orthopedics and Complex Spine (FOCOS) was the brain-child of Boachie, who was born in Kumasi, Ghana, and immigrated to the United States in 1972 at age 22 years. After completing undergraduate studies at Brooklyn College, where he received a BS degree (summa cum laude) in 1976, he received his doctor of medicine degree from Columbia University's College of Physicians and Surgeons in 1980.

Interning at St. Vincent's Hospital in New York (1980–1982), Boachie took a 1-year fellowship in pathology at HSS under Bullough, followed by his orthopaedic residency at HSS, graduating in 1986. He went on for further fellowship training in Minneapolis and returned to New York in 1995. He was

Table 7 Directors of Food Services

Roseleen Goldstone, RD	Supervising Dietician	1953–1972
Peggy Webb, MBA, RD	Director	1972–1995
Eden Kalman, MA, RD, CDN	Assistant Director	1982–1995
	Director	1996–Present
Terry Karl, MS, RD, CDN	Assistant Director	1996–Present

appointed Chief of the Scoliosis Service, following in the footsteps of Levine, who retired from that position. In addition, Boachie was appointed attending orthopaedic surgeon at HSS and professor of orthopaedic surgery at Weill Cornell Medical College.

In 2004, he was awarded the Humanitarian Award by the American Academy of Orthopaedic Surgeons, and in the same year, he received the Wholeness of Life Award at HSS from the HealthCare Chaplaincy, New York (Fig. 11). He was elected president of the Scoliosis Research Society for the 2008–2009 year and was featured in the Discovery Channel documentary entitled *Surgery Saved My Life.*

Louis A. Shapiro, president and CEO of HSS, commented on the continued international involvement of HSS: "As a world leader in musculoskeletal medicine, HSS is committed to national as well as international outreach. We are proud to support Dr. Boachie in his efforts to make FOCOS Orthopedic Hospital a reality."

Summing Up

Although HSS plans to celebrate its 150th year in May 2013 and is the oldest existing orthopaedic hospital in the United States, its name recognition has been wanting. Even after its name was changed to the Hospital for Special Surgery from the Hospital for the Ruptured and Crippled in 1940, recognition of the hospital was buried in a maze of New York City hospitals.

In fact, the R&C was better known in Europe, especially in Great Britain, where Philip D. Wilson Sr. made inroads in the orthopaedic world by aiding the British during World War I and by organizing the American Hospital in Britain during World War II (see chapters 7 and 8 for more information).

According to Wilson Sr., the origin of the name The Hospital for Special Surgery was derived from the legendary British pioneer, Sir Robert Jones, who designated "surgical" hospitals he organized for the care of wounded soldiers with injuries to bones and joints in World War I (Table 8). These casualties were assigned to the Division of Orthopaedics, and so one historic title was exchanged for another. Even after the 1940 name change, Ruptured and Crippled still remained as the dominant name when referring to the hospital.

The turning point came in 1995, when Board Member Aldo Papone introduced a new marketing strategy for the hospital. That year, "The"

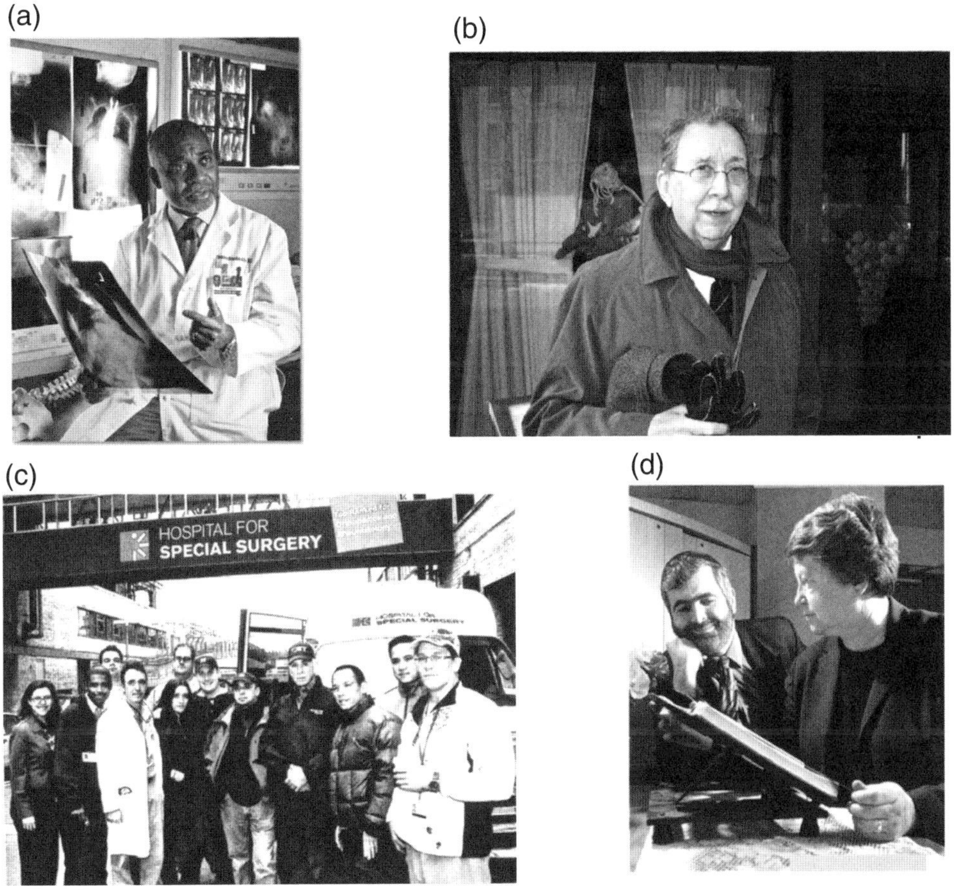

Fig. 11 (a) Oheneba Boachie-Adjei, MD, reading a scoliosis x-ray. (b) Peter Bullough, MD, retired in 2008. (c) HSS emergency team, headed by David Helfet, MD (tallest, wearing cap), traveled to Haiti after the catastrophic earthquake of 2010. (d) Sr. Margaret Oettinger, OP, director of Pastoral Care and head of the HSS chaplains for over 20 years, with Rabbi Ralph Kreger, HSS chaplain. (From Hospital for Special Surgery Archives)

was dropped from the official name, which became Hospital for Special Surgery. A new logo replaced the old Ruptured and Crippled logo[a], although the board retained the governing body title Society for the Relief of the Ruptured and Crippled (see chapter 13). In celebration of 150 years since the founding of the hospital, a third logo has been adopted for 2013 (Fig. 12).

Over a dozen years later, in 2013, HSS, which had risen to the number one rank in this country in orthopaedics, has remained in that position, with a close second in rheumatology (Table 9). These placements were well earned because of the leading medical, surgical, and nursing staff of HSS, experts

Table 8 Changing the Name in 1940

GIBNEY
of the Ruptured & Crippled

Edited by
Alfred R. Shands, Jr., M.D.
Medical Director Emeritus
Alfred I. DuPont Institute
of The Nemours Foundation

Foreword

As the years went by the ties of kinship between the Ruptured and the Crippled began to loosen. At their closest they existed because the brace-maker made a truss for the ruptured and a brace for the crippled and both types of patients depended on him. With the development of modern surgical methods for the treatment of both hernia and crippling conditions, this connection ceased to exist. The patients began to object, the ruptured pointed out that they were not crippled and the crippled that they were not ruptured. Although the name was a famous one, it had become unpopular. In 1940 the Board of Managers voted to change the name to Hospital for Special Surgery while itself retaining the title of Society for the Relief of the Ruptured and Crippled. The adjective orthopedic had been preempted by other Institutions of New York working in this field and so the Board decided to make use of the title devised by the great British pioneer, Sir Robert Jones to designate the surgical hospitals he organized for the care of the wounded soldiers who had received injuries of the bones and joints in World War I, all of whom were assigned to the division of orthopedics and so one historic title was exchanged for another.

I remember meeting Doctor Gibney at the Hospital in the early 1920's when he was still vigorous. There was no special event but I was impressed by his cordiality, simplicity, and charm. He was a man whose kindness radiated to others; he could not easily be forgotten and I treasure that memory.

March, 1969 Philip D. Wilson, M.D.

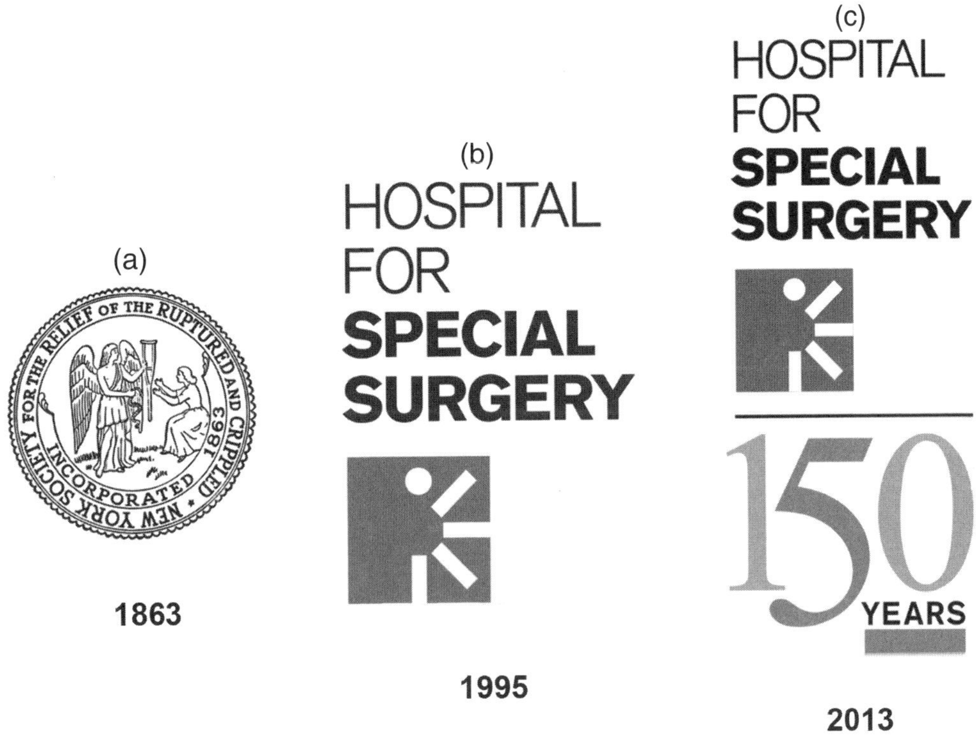

Fig. 12 (a) The original R&C logo in 1863. (b) A new hospital logo was created in 1995. (c) The latest logo was created to celebrate the 150th anniversary of HSS in 2013.

in their fields who are devoted to patient care, research, and teaching. Our achievements could only have been successful with the team efforts of an informed administration and the strong support of a cooperative Board of Trustees. It was the marketing strategy led by Papone that brought the name HSS to the attention of the rest of the world.

Papone submitted his resignation as Board of Trustees co-chair effective at the end of 2012. He was replaced by the vice-chair, Kendrick Wilson. Papone's words of wisdom from his book *The Power of the Obvious*[5] continue to ring true throughout the floors, halls, laboratories, and offices of HSS:

- It all comes down to winning.
- Brands are a preeminent business asset.
- Staying at the top takes leadership with staying power.
- Relationships matter most of all.

Lessons like these will carry HSS as a leader in orthopaedic and musculoskeletal care through the next 150 years.

Table 9 Hospital Facts: 2011

Number of beds	205
Active medical staff	292
Full-time orthopaedic surgeons	89
Scientists	93
Orthopaedic residents	42
Total fellows (2012)	85
Full-time employees (July 2012)	3,638
Operating rooms	35*
Number of surgeries	25,804
Total hips operated	4,385
Total knees operated	4,415
HSS operating expenses (actual)	
Hospital expenses	
2011	$618,326, 000
2010	$567,242,000
Research expenses	
2011	$33,443,000
2010	$32,889,000

See Table 4 of chapter 12.
*Including those under construction.

REFERENCES

1. Beekman F. *Hospital for the Ruptured and Crippled. A Historical Sketch Written on the Occasion of the Seventy-Fifth Anniversary of the Hospital.* New York, NY: privately printed; 1939.
2. Wilson, PD. *Seventy-Sixth Annual Report of the New York Society for the Ruptured and Crippled.* New York, NY: New York Society for the Ruptured and Crippled; 1939:38.
3. Meyerhoff M. Kim Barrett, 1911–1976. Bull. Med Libr Assoc. 1977;65:86.
4. Wilson, PD. Forward. *Gibney of the Ruptured and Crippled.* New York, NY: Meredith Corporation; 1969.
5. Papone A. *The Power of the Obvious: Notes from 50 Years in Corporate America.* Palo Alto, CA: Palo Alto Press; 2005.

NOTES

a. Dean O'Hare served as chairman and chief executive officer of the Chubb Corporation from 1988 until his retirement in 2002. He first joined Chubb, one of the world's leading property and casualty insurance companies, in 1963, and since then has been a director of a number of corporations as well as a trustee of the University of Dublin and the Intrepid Museum in New York. A leading voice in international trade issues, he served as a member of the President's Advisory Committee on Trade Policy and Negotiations. He received his BS degree from New York University and MBA from Pace University Graduate School of Business Administration.

b. Tommy Dorsey hired singer Frank Sinatra from Harry James in 1940. It was during the "Swing Era," also known as the "Big Band Era" (1935–1946), when big band music was the rave in the United States. Sinatra attributed his success in breath control to watching Dorsey play the trombone. Dorsey was known to be volatile and raided other bands for talent, hiring and firing at will. After recording 80 songs with Dorsey from 1940 to 1942, they eventually had a falling out.

c. In 1964, as a senior resident attending a scoliosis instructional course at the University of Minnesota, Levine proposed establishing a Scoliosis Research Society (SRS) and drafted the first by-laws of the society. He had the longest tenure (10 years) of any member of the SRS Board of Directors of the society and served as secretary-treasurer (1970–1972), secretary (1972–1974), and president (1978–1979). Besides winning the first-prize Walter P. Blount Award with Laura B. Flawn, MD (1953–2001), in 1983, Levine received the 2009 SRS Lifetime Achievement Award at the 44th annual meeting of the Scoliosis Research Society in San Antonio, Texas, on September 26, 2009. When Levine returned from retirement to accept the new position as director of HSS Alumni Affairs, he established the HSS archives, pursuing his previous interests in publishing the medical history of the hospital. He was then asked to chair the Caspary Estate Committee, a position he held from 1967 to 1994.

d. Wuest was directing the blood bank before the arrival of Michael J. Klein, MD, making Klein the newest pathologist on staff at the time of this writing.

e. Designed in 1995 by Arnold Saks Associates, the Hospital for Special Surgery logo combines the hospital's name, set in a specially designed typeface, with a graphic symbol. The symbol represents an active, mobile human figure, highlighting HSS care and expertise in orthopaedics and rheumatology in treating patients from all over the world. The logo is the brand of Hospital for Special Surgery.

PART II

ASSOCIATED SPECIALTIES

We can draw lessons from the past,
but we cannot live in it.

—Lyndon B. Johnson (1908–1973)

CHAPTER 15

ANESTHESIOLOGY (1897–2012)

GREGORY A. LIGUORI, MD

MARY J. HARGETT

THE DISCOVERY OF ANESTHESIA CAN be traced back to Crawford W. Long, MD, a medical practitioner in Georgia who first administered ether by inhalation for surgical anesthesia in 1842. Since this event was not well publicized, credit for the earliest anesthetic has traditionally gone to William T. Morton, a dentist from Hartford, Connecticut, who administered ether at Massachusetts General Hospital in 1846.

This highly successful and well-publicized event marked the beginning of one of the most important contributions to the history of medicine. In 2007, the *British Journal of Medicine* surveyed physicians to elicit their opinion regarding the greatest medical advances of the past 150 years. The development of anesthesia ranked third behind sanitation development and vaccines. Future advances in the field of surgery were thought to take place only following the introduction of the art and science of anesthesia.

The first operating room at the Hospital for the Ruptured and Crippled (R&C) was built in the winter of 1887; and in 1898, when R&C expanded to an adjacent building on 43rd Street and Lexington Avenue, the new site included both inpatient and outpatient operating suites. This transformation solidified the future importance of anesthesiology to the institution.

Coincidentally, at the same time R&C started its journey to become the premier orthopaedic surgical facility in the world, regional anesthesia was introduced into clinical practice. Carl Koller, MD, William Halstead, MD, and Leonard Corning, MD, introduced topical anesthesia, nerve blocks, and epidural blockade, respectively. On August 16, 1898, August Bier, MD, performed the first spinal anesthetic procedure in Kiel, Germany, painlessly resecting an ankle joint that was infected with tuberculosis. This is considered the first major regional anesthetic in history and earned Bier the moniker "the father of spinal anesthesia." Surgical treatment at R&C therefore coincided with the advent of regional anesthesia, and the two would be linked, on and off, throughout the next century.

Anesthesiology at R&C: The Early Years

During the first quarter century at R&C, anesthetics were administered very sparingly, and not often beyond the primary stage.[1] The training of the anesthetists was somewhat lacking, and their interest in the profession was suspect. Anesthetists were usually junior assistants who recently graduated from medical school or nurses with an interest in the field. "The anesthetist ... was unable to give his entire time and attention to the site of operation," wrote Virgil Gibney.[1] A few hundred operations were performed in the decade following 1887, including hernia repairs, abscess drainage and a few orthopaedic procedures. The duration of cases was usually 6 to 20 minutes, and on rare occasions lasted up to 90 minutes. Anesthetic techniques included inhalational methods using nitrous oxide, ether, ethyl chloride, somnoform, and (rarely) chloroform.

Anesthetic safety during those years was also being monitored. The 1900 Annual Report of R&C, written by Gibney, referred to hernia surgery as follows: "From an operation that twelve or fifteen years ago, led many surgeons to hesitate in commending, your hospital has furnished the testimony which makes it a surgical procedure without mortality."[2] During his early years as surgeon-in-chief, Gibney recognized the importance of anesthesia to the success of surgical outcomes and patient well-being. At a meeting of the New York Academy of Medicine on May 21, 1908, the program was devoted to a symposium on anesthesia. Gibney presented anesthetic mortality data from R&C, showing that two deaths were likely due to anesthesia at R&C.

The first death involved a male child during a hernia repair in 1894. The anesthetic was ether, and the cause of death was likely aspiration pneumonia. In 1899, the second fatality was a 4-year-old girl who suffered respiratory arrest following a 10-minute stretching for congenital dislocation of the hip under nitrous oxide. Gibney reported, "We have, during the last decade or two, appreciated the value of having an anesthetist, properly trained, at the head of the patient." He continued, "Among the first in the city to employ one skilled in the administration of anesthetics was the Hospital for Ruptured and Crippled, and among the first of the operating rooms to give Dr. Bennett an opportunity of demonstrating the value of such service."[1]

Thomas Linwood Bennett, MD (Fig. 1) was born in 1869 and graduated from Western Ohio Medical College in 1889.[3] In 1891, Bennett moved to Kansas City, Missouri, and developed an interest in anesthesia. Considered to be the first American physician to limit his practice solely to the practice of anesthesia, Bennett arrived in New York City and became one of the first anesthetists at several New York City hospitals, including Roosevelt, Presbyterian, New York Hospital, and R&C.[4] He maintained a private office at 7 East 87th Street in Manhattan. Based on his interests and skills, as well as Gibney's appreciation for the importance of a dedicated anesthetist, Bennett was appointed the first anesthetist and instructor in anesthesia at R&C in 1897. He held this title for the next 3 years.

Bennett is widely known for his development of the Bennett inhaler, which he introduced at R&C in 1899.[5] This device allowed for the "safe" administration of nitrous oxide, ether, and other inhaled agents, and it became the industry standard for anesthetic practice in New York City during the first decade of the 20th century. The apparatus consisted of a facemask with rubber cushion, a gas cylinder, and two bags. It sold for $40.00. The Bennett inhaler was the precursor to many future anesthetic inhalers.

In addition to his contributions to anesthetic equipment, Bennett was one of the first anesthetists to introduce the concept of the nitrous oxide–ether sequence. This method, developed by Clover in England in 1876, involved patients inhaling nitrous oxide until they were unconscious, then slowly introducing ether.[6] This anesthetic technique is described in detail in a review of the operative treatment of hernia at R&C by William T. Bull and William B. Coley in 1899.[7]

Bennett was an authority and published extensively on anesthetic techniques and safety issues around the turn of the century. In an article in the *Journal of the American Medical Association*, he wrote, "I am convinced that the smallest amount of the anesthetic compatible with quiet, relaxation and freedom from reflex manifestations during the operation, will give the patient the least possible after-disturbance attributable to the anesthetic."[8]

Bennett continued to consult and practice anesthesia in New York City for the next decade, during which time he became chief of anesthesia at Presbyterian Hospital.[9] After his death in 1932, friends from the New York

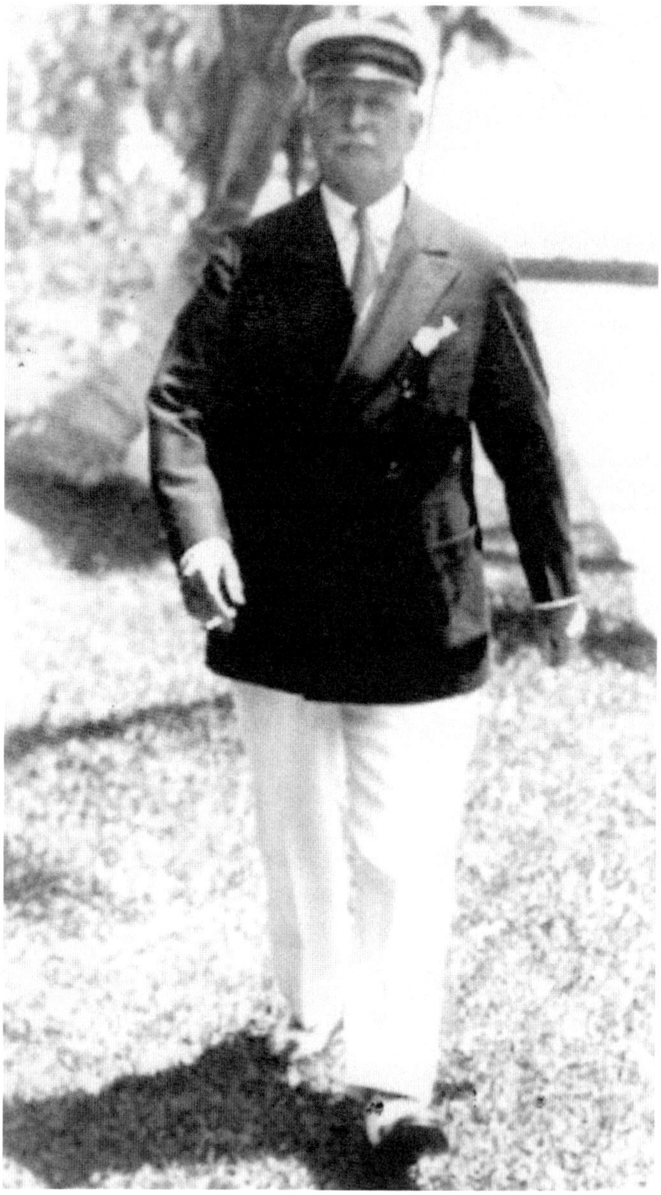

Fig. 1 Thomas Bennett, MD, the first physician to provide anesthesia for the Hospital of the Ruptured and the Crippled, in 1897. (Courtesy of the Wood Library-Museum of Anesthesiology)

Academy of Medicine chartered the Thomas L. Bennett Memorial Fund. In initiating this fund, the *New York Medical Week* reported, "It was pointed out that since this life, devoted as it was to the wise and conservative practice of anesthesia, had resulted in the frequent prevention of death, that a memorial may take the form of a 'fund' for the prevention of asphyxial death."[10]

20th Century Anesthesiology: Preston Satterwhite, MD

Bennett's dedication and skill, combined with Gibney's appreciation for the importance of anesthesia, clearly proved to R&C leadership that a formal role for the specialty was warranted. In 1901, Preston Pope Satterwhite, MD, was appointed anesthetist and instructor in anesthesia at R&C.

Born in Louisville, Kentucky, on September 28, 1868, Satterwhite graduated from Bellevue Hospital Medical College in 1898. He was a member of the final graduating class from Bellevue prior to its merger with the University Medical College to ultimately form the Medical School of New York University. Following graduation, Satterwhite accepted an appointment as an assistant surgeon in the Hernia Department at R&C, as well as surgical appointments at Roosevelt Hospital and the New York Polyclinic Hospital. As was the case with most of his contemporaries, he practiced as a surgeon and had no formal training in anesthesiology. Postgraduate training programs in anesthesiology would not develop for another 20 years.

Satterwhite's private office was located at 27 West 34th Street, and he practiced in the outpatient department at both Roosevelt Hospital and R&C. Over the next decade, serving as anesthetist and instructor in anesthetics at R&C, his duty was to "instruct the members of the house-staff, and particularly the resident junior in the principles of anesthesia, to stand by him, and give real clinical instruction."[1]

During that time, operations were performed 2 days per week at R&C: one day allotted to orthopaedics and one day reserved for hernia repairs. Ten to 20 operations were performed each week, and Satterwhite dedicated approximately 5 to 6 hours per week to the practice of anesthesia. He often supervised two surgical residents simultaneously. Although there were several candidates for the position of anesthetist, it was not considered a major part of Satterwhite's practice, as a "salary was found to be a necessary incentive."[1]

Satterwhite moved his office to Great Neck, Long Island, in 1908, when he married Gladys R. Martin, the wealthy widow of a former U.S. Steel executive, James E. Martin. The couple resided in Ms. Martin's estate in Great Neck, while Satterwhite continued to practice surgery and anesthesia in both New York City and Long Island. He left R&C in 1910 as his practice slowly migrated away from New York City. After his wife's death in 1927, Satterwhite continued to reside at the Great Neck estate until the home was destroyed in 1932, likely from an electrical fire that started in a pipe organ.

Shortly after Satterwhite left R&C, he was replaced as the anesthetist by Carleton I. Dederer, MD. Born in 1880, Dederer completed his undergraduate education at Cornell University in 1904 and medical training at Columbia University College of Physicians and Surgeons in 1907. In 1910, he joined the staff at R&C and was appointed anesthetist and instructor in Anesthesia. Dederer also held an appointment as a surgeon at the dispensary of the J. Hood Wright Hospital in Manhattan. He remained in this role at R&C from 1910 to 1913 and then moved to California to practice as an anesthetist and surgeon at the University of California Medical College in Los Angeles.

Interestingly, he published one of the earliest papers on "The Induction of Anesthesia and Ethyl Chloride," printed in the *California State Journal of Medicine* in 1914. Dederer moved to Michigan in 1919, and based on his published work, his interest in anesthesia seemed to fade. He wrote several articles in surgical journals on topics such as hernia repair and organ transplantation.

Upon Dederer's departure from R&C, William Lent Sneed, MD, took over the anesthesia supervisory duties. Born in 1881, he earned his medical degree in 1910 from Vanderbilt University School of Medicine in Nashville. He became licensed to practice medicine in 1912 and joined R&C as an anesthetist and instructor in anesthesia. Sneed served in that capacity until 1915. He also practiced as a surgeon in the Hernia Department and published several articles on surgical topics, again indicating that his interest in anesthesia was secondary to his surgical practice. Sneed remained on staff at R&C as a surgeon until 1931.

World War I and Beyond

During the next 15 to 20 years, a series of surgeons performed anesthesia and supervised nurses and residents in administering anesthesia at R&C. H. S. Marcley, MD, was an anesthetist from 1916 to 1918 until his death in World War I. Eva Locke, MD, a surgeon in the Hernia Department, supervised anesthesia from 1918 to 1919, thus becoming the first female anesthetist at R&C. A. C. Brown, MD, also performed anesthetist duties in 1919. Around this time, orthopaedic cases began to dominate the surgical schedule. Arthroplasties, fracture repairs, abscess drainage, and a few tenotomies and osteotomies were performed, in addition to the hernia repairs.

In 1920, John O'Dowd, MD, joined the staff at R&C. O'Dowd graduated in 1918 from Columbia University College of Physicians and Surgeons, and after receiving his license to practice medicine in 1919, he became an anesthetist at R&C in 1920. Similar to his predecessors, he received no formal training in anesthesia and likely had minimal experience in the craft. O'Dowd remained on the staff of R&C for 22 years, supervising anesthesia care to the growing surgical population.

In the early 1920s, he was joined briefly by James Stewart, MD, Hector McNeil, MD, and Maud Maltaner, MD, who also provided and supervised anesthesia care. O'Dowd, however, was the constant presence and often the sole physician anesthetist for 11 years at R&C. It is therefore likely he became skilled and interested in the profession. After his departure from the institution in 1942, he continued to practice anesthesia at the Veterans Administration Hospital in New York for several more years. O'Dowd died of heart disease at Doctor's Hospital on November 20, 1956.

In 1931, Earl Calvin Wagner, MD, joined the staff at R&C. He was the first physician since Bennett to be recruited to R&C specifically based on his skill as an anesthetist. In fact, unlike many of his predecessors, he was never trained as a surgeon at all. Born on December 23, 1886, he graduated from the Medical Department of Syracuse University in 1908. Following an internship at St. Joseph's Hospital in Syracuse, Wagner practiced general medicine and pediatrics in Asbury Park and also anesthesia at Spring Lakes Hospital in New Jersey. He enlisted in the Army, served in World War I, and was eventually promoted to the rank of Captain. After the war, he returned to New Jersey and practiced anesthesia more regularly.

Wagner was active in both the American Medical Association and New Jersey Medical Association, and by 1929, he specialized solely in anesthesia. In 1931, having moved to New York City the year prior, he was appointed to the staff at R&C as an anesthetist. Presumably, due to his extensive experience in the field, he was bestowed the title "supervisor of anesthetics" at R&C in 1934, making him officially the first chief of the service. The service was quite small, with the entire group consisting of John O'Dowd and several nurses.

The history of nurse anesthetists dates back to the origins of R&C. Nurses were often called upon to provide anesthesia while caring for wounded soldiers during the Civil War. During the early 1900s, Alice Magaw at the Mayo

Clinic was widely credited as one of the first specialists in nurse-provided anesthesia. In the early years at R&C, it is likely that, while supervised by anesthetists, some nurses—along with junior house staff—provided anesthesia care for most procedures. The first nurse anesthetists identified on staff at R&C were Dorothy McKinstry, RN, Irene Landry, RN, and Irmgard Von Bockum Dolffs, RN. Landry, later known as Landry Kirby, served as a nurse anesthetist at HSS until the early 1960s—a period of over 30 years.

Wagner left R&C in 1939 and moved to Tupper Lake, New York, and continued to practice anesthesia at hospitals in the surrounding communities. Wagner joined the American Society of Anesthesiologists (ASA) in 1948, and interestingly, he finished his career as the coroner of Tupper Lake in the early 1950s.

During Wagner's tenure, there was a plethora of surgical advances at R&C. In 1931, 1,672 orthopaedic procedures and 1,432 hernia surgeries were performed. Although anesthetics were provided for those cases, the anesthesia service was generally ignored by the hospital. The Annual Report of 1931 listed the departments at R&C and included Orthopaedics, Hernia, Medicine, Urology, X-Ray, Laboratory, and Physiotherapy.

By 1939, however, more attention was afforded to the anesthesia service at the hospital. Statistics were kept on the number and types of anesthetics provided: 1,949 inhalational, 166 spinal, and 498 local. Patient safety played an increasingly important role as well. Explosions caused by the combination of static electrical sparks and flammable anesthetics such as cyclopropane remained a constant hazard. New anesthetic technologies, such as the use of helium to assist in patients with respiratory obstruction, were introduced. Finally, anesthetists at HSS began to publish case reports in journals on observations during orthopaedic anesthesia.[11] A transformation in the role of anesthesia at HSS had begun.

In 1939, Charles L. Burstein, MD, joined the staff at R&C and was immediately appointed to the position of supervisor of anesthesia. Burstein's arrival ushered in a new era in anesthesia care at the Hospital for Special Surgery (newly named in 1940). Born in Paris, France, on April 22, 1906, Burstein came to the United States in 1916 and received his BS degree from New York University in 1928. Following his marriage to Loretta Lipschitz in 1930, the couple returned to France so that Burstein could attend medical school at Université de Paris Faculté de Médecine, where he graduated in

1934. Upon graduation, Burstein sought to enter the up-and-coming specialty of anesthesiology.

During the first two decades of the twentieth century, anesthetists were, for the most part, surgeons, nurses, or other individuals who had some interest and skill in providing anesthesia care. However, in the late 1920s and early 1930s, Ralph Waters, MD, at the University of Wisconsin developed one of the earliest formal training programs and academic models in anesthesiology, organizing 3-year apprenticeships in the practice of anesthesia. This residency training included clinical practice, as well as didactics and medical student instruction.[12] One of Waters's brightest protégés was Emery A. Rovenstine, MD.

Modern Anesthesia Takes Root

Emery Andrew Rovenstine is widely considered one of the founding fathers of modern anesthesia in the United States. After graduating from Indiana University Medical School in 1928, he studied anesthesiology under Waters in Madison. In 1935, Arthur Wright, MD, Chairman of Surgery at Bellevue Hospital, recruited Rovenstine to New York City upon Waters' recommendation.[12] Two years later, Rovenstine was appointed Professor of Anesthesiology at New York University School of Medicine.[13]

Over the next two decades, Rovenstine was instrumental in mentoring many future leaders in anesthesiology. One of his first trainees was Burstein. Some of Burstein's contemporaries at Bellevue included John Adriani, MD, Virginia Apgar, MD, Stuart Cullen, MD, and Lewis Wright, MD. This group, as well as the next several residency classes, became known as "Rovenstine residents."[13]

Rovenstine was also appointed to the staff at HSS in 1945. During those years, Rovenstine had a private clinic, practicing therapeutic and diagnostic regional blocks in New York City. He also taught regional anesthesia courses at Bellevue Hospital.[12] The HSS Department of Anesthesiology's roots in the science and the practice of regional anesthesia can therefore be traced back to Rovenstine and his predecessor, Gaston Labat, MD, at Bellevue.

Following O'Dowd's departure from HSS in 1942, Burstein was, in name, the sole physician anesthesia provider at HSS until 1949—although several nurse anesthetists, including Irene Landry Kirby, maintained their practice at HSS through those years, providing much of the anesthetic care. In actuality, between 1942 and 1944, Burstein was on a leave of absence from HSS to serve in the military during World War II.

More than any other event in history, this war acted as a catalyst for the growth and development of anesthesiology as a medical specialty in the United States.[14] The number of anesthesiology training programs increased from 37 in 1940 to 217 in 1950. The American Board of Anesthesiology, established by the American Medical Association in 1938, gave credit for 1 year of residency training for anesthesia service in the military. The shift from nurse-provided care to physician-provided care was spurred by the fact that most nurses at the time were female, and women's roles in the combat military at the time were limited. Therefore, the armed services organized training programs in anesthesia, which focused on male physician involvement.

Burstein received the Bronze Star for Meritorious Service during the war. This honor, established in 1944, was awarded to an individual who had distinguished himself by heroic or meritorious achievement or service.

Burstein returned to HSS in 1945 and began the transformation and advancement of the anesthesia service. Upon his arrival at HSS in 1939, five articles were published by the anesthesia service at the hospital. By 1945, 35 of the 154 reports that were published by staff at HSS were written by physicians in the Anesthesia Department. Burstein was directly involved in a multitude of clinical and laboratory research projects, often collaborating with Rovenstine and other colleagues at New York University. He published dozens of articles on topics ranging from new general anesthetics to techniques in regional anesthesia and pain management.

Some of his earliest work set the foundation for research at HSS that would be performed 50 years later. His article in the first edition of *Anesthesiology,* on the physiology of total spinal blockade, and his study on postural blood pressure changes during spinal anesthesia, published in *Anesthesia and Analgesia* in 1939, are two such examples.[15,16] Burstein continued to collaborate with Rovenstine, maintaining an academic appointment at the New York University College of Medicine.

In 1949, Burstein published a major textbook entitled *Fundamental Considerations in Anesthesia.* This book was widely considered a comprehensive text on the pharmacology, physiology, and pathophysiology of problems that may be observed during the course of clinical anesthesia. The second edition, published in 1955, included a number of new drug preparations as well as information on the expanded use of electrocardiographs and electroencephalographs in the practice of anesthesia.

1944: The HSS Department of Anesthesia Is Founded

By 1944, it was clear that the practice of anesthesiology at HSS was gaining respect, both within the institution and beyond. During that year, the Medical Board designated the Anesthesia Service as the Department of Anesthesia. In 1946, Burstein was granted a seat on the Medical Board, signifying the importance of anesthesiology to HSS and recognizing his contributions to the institution. Detailed statistics were kept on the types of anesthetics administered. Most anesthetics were inhalational, with a small minority being spinal. Local and intravenous anesthetics accounted for the remainder.

Over the next 20 years, the department continued to expand the role of physician anesthesiologists. John Fox, MD, Robert Byers, MD, Andrew Kerr, MD, Gerald Millstein, MD, and Arthur Lee-Roy, MD, joined the department. In 1955, HSS, in an agreement with New York Hospital–Cornell Medical Center, limited its care to orthopaedic patients. Although Burstein continued to perform and publish clinical and laboratory research in collaboration with Rovenstine and others, clinical practice and care became the primary focus, at the expense of academic achievement.

In 1965, Anita Haack Goulet, MD, was appointed to the staff at HSS (Fig. 2). Like the three other anesthesiologists on staff, she was a diplomate of the American Board of Anesthesiology. She thus became the first woman in the Department of Anesthesia to be a fully trained, board-certified anesthesiologist.

Goulet was born in 1927 and graduated from the New York University College of Medicine in 1952. She completed an internship at Kings College Hospital in Brooklyn and a residency in anesthesiology at New York Hospital in 1955. Goulet practiced anesthesia at New York Hospital and Memorial Hospital until 1965, when she was appointed to the staff at HSS. She published several clinical studies and remained on staff at HSS until 1979. Upon her death in 2007, a scholarship was endowed in her name at New York University for those who "possess a deep and abiding commitment to the role of women in the medical profession."

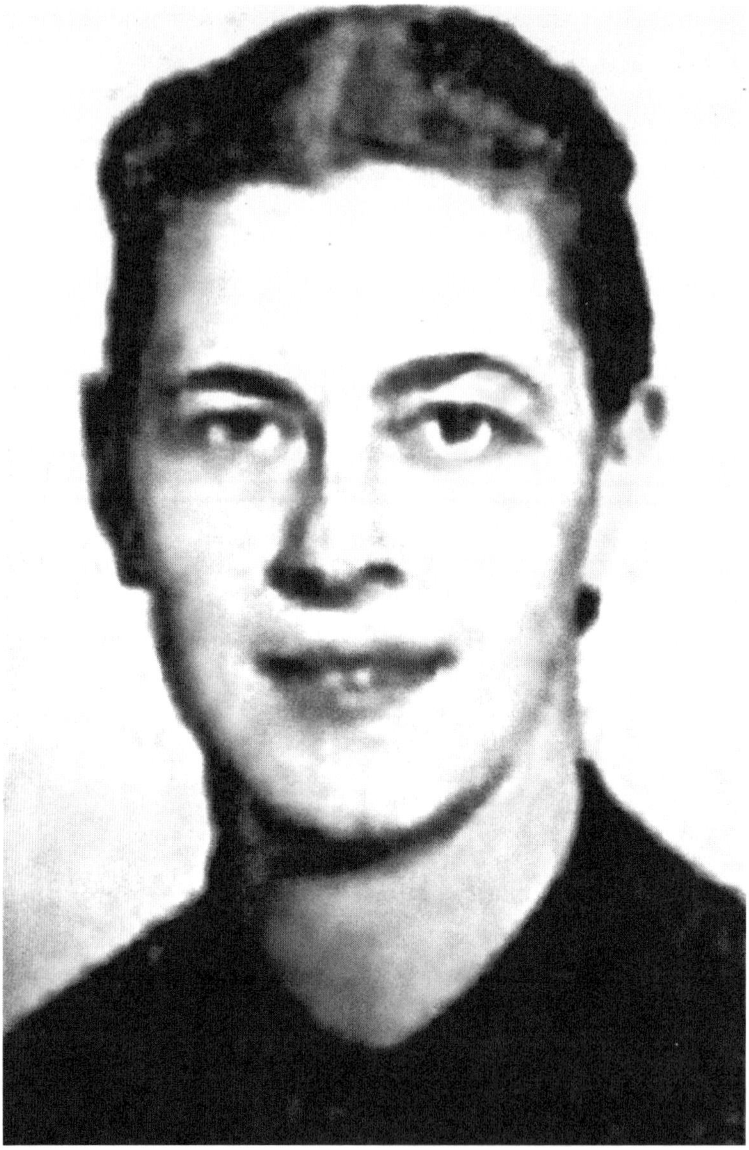

Fig. 2 Anita Goulet, MD, first woman anesthesiologist at R&C (circa 1960). (From *Anesthesia and Analgesia*, vol. 39, Nov–Dec 1960)

The 1960s saw continued advancement in the clinical and academic practice of anesthesia at HSS. Burstein continued to publish clinical and laboratory research. In 1965, 2,196 anesthetics were performed, including 1,776 general anesthetics, 220 regional blocks, and 15 spinals. In 1966, residents from New York Hospital began to rotate through the operating rooms at HSS. This was the beginning of a continuing relationship that would last for the next half century. The following year, medical students from Cornell University Medical

Table 1 Anesthesiologists Recruited to HSS: 1960s–Present

Late 1960s
Yvonne DeSouza, MD
Stephanie Lichtenstein, MD
Sylvia Pescatore, MD
Barnard Robbins, MD
William A. Seibert, MD
Earnest Stern, MD

1970s
Helen Bacanovic, MD
George Balint, MD
Elina Lobrin-Farcon, MD
Thomas Miles, MD
Changkiat Ong, MD
Joseph Shahmoon, MD

1980s
Michael A. Gordon, MD
Douglas S. T. Green, MD
Richard L. Kahn, MD
Richard S. King, MB, ChB
Jeffrey Y. Ngeow, MB, BS
H. Keith Pinchot, MD
Thomas J. Quinn, MD, MBA
James J. Roch, MD
Steven Seidman, MD
Nigel E. Sharrock, MB ChB
Michael K. Urban, MD, PhD
William F. Urmey, MD
Victor M. Zayas, MD

1990s
James D. Beckman, MD
Thomas J. J. Blanck, MD
Marie-Louise Caloustian, MD
Bradford E. Carson, MD
Mary F. Chisholm, MD
Chris R. Edmonds, MD
Stephen N. Harris, MD
Kethy Jules-Elysee, MD
Vincent R. LaSala, MD
Andrew C. Lee, MD
David L. Lee, MD
Gregory A. Liguori, MD

Table 1 (*continued*)

Leonardo Paroli, MD, PhD
Paul Rodericks, MD
Philip J. Wagner, MD
Seth A. Waldman, MD
Jacques T. YaDeau, MD, PhD
2000s
Jonathan C. Beathe, MD
Devan D. Bhagat
Kathryn R. DelPizzo, MD
Christopher A. Dimeo
Naomi Dong, MD
Sean Garvin, MD
Enrique A. Goytizolo, MD
Robert Griffin, MD
Carrie R. Guheen, MD
Semih Gungor, MD
Michael C. Ho, MD
Simon G. Ho, MD
David H. Kim, MD
Vladimir Kramskiy, MD
Yi Lin, MD, PhD
Spencer S. Liu, MD
Daniel Maalouf, MD, MPH
Stavros Memtsoudis, MD, PhD
John G. Muller, MD
Fani Nhuch, MD
Michael Nurok, MB, ChB, PhD
Joseph A. Oxendine, MD
Swetha Pakala, MD
Christine Peterson, MD
Cephas P. Swamidoss, MD, MPH
Lauren H. Turteltaub, MD
David Y. Wang, MD, MS, MPH

College came to HSS, where they were "taught regional nerve blocks and given lectures on circulatory reflexes."[17] The department continued to expand, with the recruitment of physician anesthesiologists (Table 1). Fox was appointed assistant director of the department in 1968.

In 1967, the surgeon-in-chief's annual report noted that the Anesthesia Department was responding to "an increasing demand for diagnostic and therapeutic nerve blocks."[17] This was the informal origin of what would become the Chronic Pain Service at HSS. At about the same time, David

B. Levine, MD, returned to HSS after completing a scoliosis fellowship in California. Working with Burstein, he encouraged the use of electrocardiographic monitoring during all operative cases. He also organized a "step-down" pediatric care unit, which, along with the post-anesthesia care unit, would be the precursor of critical care initiatives that would develop over the next half century at HSS.

One of the accomplishments of the department noted in the 1969 Annual Report was the adoption of a common Anesthetic and Recovery Room Record by all Cornell-associated hospitals. Documentation of medications and vital signs during an anesthetic had been considered vital for many years. As early as the first decade of the twentieth century, anesthesiologists documented what occurred in the operating rooms. At R&C, information about the operative patient was recorded on an "anesthetic card" that was started on the wards and then pinned to the gown of a patient prior to entering the operating suite. The anesthetist would complete the card and paste it into the medical record.[1] The evolution of the anesthetic record would continue for the next century.

On November 1, 1970, at the age of 64 years, Charles Burstein retired as the director of the Anesthesia Department. He had served in that capacity for 31 years. Under his leadership, the department grew from a small group of nurses and surgeons who casually practiced anesthesia, to a fully recognized department of specialty-trained physicians who made anesthesiology their chosen profession. Burstein died in Palm Beach, Florida, on December 27, 1986.

Second Department Director: John Lawrence Fox, MD

In 1970, John Lawrence Fox, the assistant director of the Anesthesia Department, was appointed Acting Director of Anesthesia at HSS. Two years later, he was promoted to director. Fox was born on October 12, 1917, in Brooklyn, New York, and attended Xavier High School in New York City. He went to St. John's University and graduated from New York Medical College in 1943. Following an internship at St. Catherine's Hospital in 1944, Fox served as captain in the 236-305 General Medical Corps of the U.S. Army during World War II, in the European Theatre.

He received his New York medical license in 1945 and, in 1948, spent 6 months as the first resident in anesthesia at HSS. Following another 6 months in anesthesia at the Bronx Veterans Administration Hospital, he was recruited by Burstein to HSS as an assistant attending anesthesiologist in 1949. Fox remained on staff at HSS until 1954, when he received his board certification in anesthesia, and left HSS for an appointment at St. Claire's Hospital. He rose through the ranks from assistant to associate attending and was appointed as an attending anesthesiologist at St. Claire's in 1964. In 1965, he was recruited back to HSS by Burstein and surgeon-in-chief Robert Lee Patterson. In a letter to Fox on October 5, 1964, Burstein wrote, "You are the one I would select and recommend to take over the directorship of the Department when I retire in 1970 or 1971."

During Fox's first year as director, approximately 2,900 operations were performed at HSS. There was a five-bed recovery room staffed by the Anesthesia Department. Fox recruited six anesthesiologists in the 1970s and another two in the 1980s (Table 1). During that time, the practice focused on clinical care. Few, if any, research studies were performed. Residents from Cornell continued to rotate through the operating rooms, and slowly, anesthesiologists began to perform more frequent regional anesthetics.

The utilization of spinal anesthesia for orthopaedic procedures increased from less than 1% in 1965 to 15% in 1981.[18] Other centers around the country, however, had realized the benefits of regional anesthesia for orthopaedics and promoted its use more aggressively. Daniel C. Moore, MD, and John J. Bonica, MD, in Seattle, Alon P. Winnie, MD, in Chicago, and Leroy D. Vandam, MD, and Benjamin G. Covino, MD, in Boston were pioneers in the clinical use of regional anesthesia during that time.[19] Despite the leadership position achieved by HSS in orthopaedics, regional anesthesia remained an afterthought with respect to its potential role in contributing to medical and surgical outcomes at the institution. That vision would change significantly in 1986.

Fox retired from the position of director of anesthesia at HSS on September 1, 1986. In announcing his retirement, surgeon-in-chief Philip D. Wilson, Jr. noted, "Dr. Fox will be remembered for his skillful and attentive care to his patients and for successfully expanding the staff of his Department to match the increasing Hospital's operative case load after he became Chief." Following his retirement, Fox moved to Sag Harbor, Long Island, and later to Charlotte,

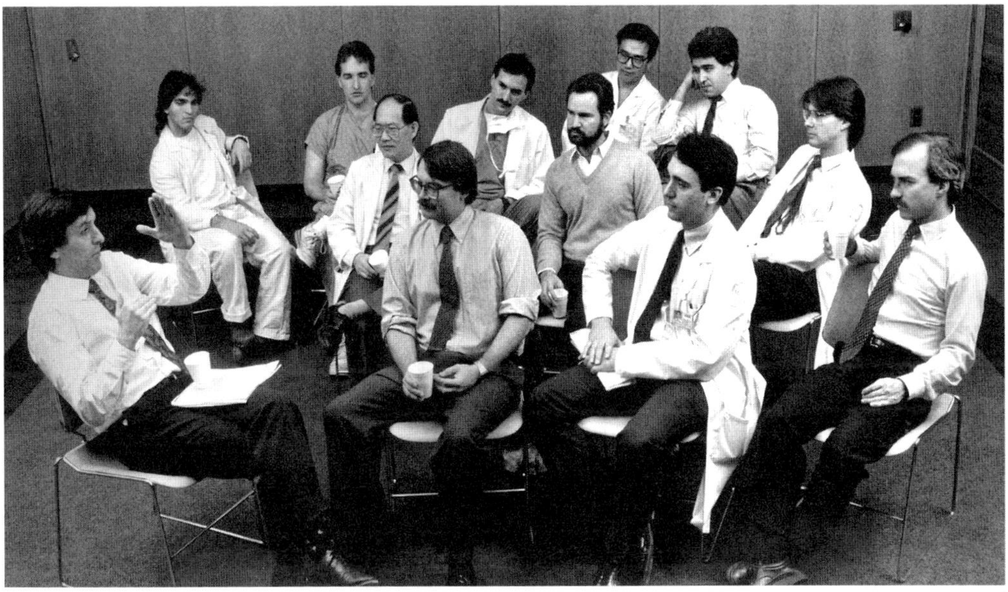

Fig. 3 Nigel Sharrock, MB, ChB, and HSS Anesthesiology Staff (1989). (Courtesy of Brad Hess, professional photographer)

North Carolina. He remained on the honorary staff in Anesthesiology at HSS until his death on January 6, 2001.

Expanding the Use of Regional Anesthesia

In 1986, after Fox's retirement, Nigel Sharrock, MB, ChB, was appointed director and anesthesiologist-in-chief at HSS (Fig. 3). Sharrock was born in Nelson, New Zealand, and received his medical degree from Otago Medical School. Following a rotating internship at Wellington Hospital, he traveled to New York, where he completed his residency in anesthesia at Albert Einstein Medical School. He was then appointed to the attending staff at Peter Bent Brigham Hospital of Harvard Medical School in Boston. Vandam, chairman at Brigham at the time, instilled in Sharrock an appreciation for the applications and benefits of regional anesthesia.

In 1977, Sharrock returned to New York to join the attending staff at Lenox Hill Hospital, where he continued to practice regional anesthesia for a variety of surgical procedures. He began to publish clinical studies and observations involving regional techniques. He became very interested in developing a full academic department and program and realized that Lenox

Hill, as a private community hospital, was not the appropriate environment for that concept.

Sharrock is recognized today as the founder of the modern regional anesthesiology practice at HSS. In 1986, regional anesthesia was used for less than 15% of all surgical procedures at HSS. By 2010, that proportion increased to 85%. Sharrock not only practiced regional anesthesia but also studied its effects on both medical and surgical outcomes. The use of regional anesthesia significantly improved outcomes while markedly decreasing morbidity and mortality, including substantially reduced blood loss and thromboembolic complications.[20]

Under Sharrock's direction, the anesthesiology practice at HSS began to promote the exclusive use of regional anesthesia for orthopaedic surgery and pain management. Sharrock initiated several changes in the management of patients during the perioperative period, including increased use of invasive, hemodynamic monitoring during surgery, extended postoperative scrutiny for several days for patients with severe comorbidities, and the use of postoperative epidural analgesia for pain management.

Converting the mindset of HSS administration, nurses, support staff, and particularly orthopaedic surgeons to the benefits of regional anesthesia in orthopaedics was complicated. Sharrock identified the primary concerns of each group and addressed them individually. His belief was that the most important first step was to recruit the most talented attending staff from prestigious institutions and training programs and teach them effective and efficient regional anesthetic techniques.

Kevin Sanborn, MD, the anesthesiology residency director at Columbia Presbyterian Hospital, joined HSS in 1986 and was appointed assistant director. Sanborn remained on staff at HSS until 1993, when he accepted another position at St. Luke's Roosevelt Hospital. Through Sanborn's contacts, Sharrock was able to recruit talented graduates of the Columbia residency program (Table 1). Other physicians with an interest in regional anesthesia and pain management joined the department over the next few years (Table 1).

Victor Zayas, MD, who had trained in both pediatrics and anesthesia, became the first director of pediatric anesthesia at HSS. Jeffrey Ngeow, MB, BS, with fellowship training in pain medicine, formalized a Chronic Pain Program, which was first conceived in the late 1960s under Burstein. William

Urmey, MD, would later become the first medical director of ambulatory surgery when the center opened with two operating rooms in 1990.

Sharrock set high expectations for the Attending Staff. He expected all to be board-certified and to advance the practice of regional anesthesia, believing it to be the optimal technique for most orthopaedic patients. Under Sharrock's leadership, the use of regional techniques continued to expand. He espoused the use of hypotensive epidural anesthesia for hip replacement surgery to minimize perioperative complications and improve both anesthetic and surgical outcomes. By the early 1990s, the use of regional blocks for shoulder procedures was common practice as well.

In 1987, Richard King, MB, ChB, a graduate of Dundee University Medical School in Scotland and a practicing anesthesiologist in Australia and New Zealand, joined HSS as the first fellow in regional anesthesia. Fellowship training in regional anesthesia, which at the time was quite rare, became more popular over the next few decades. King remained on staff at HSS following his fellowship.

Recognizing the need to better address the acute pain management needs of the postsurgical population, Sharrock implemented the Acute Pain Service (APS) in 1990. On March 4, 1991, the first patients were treated on the service. Rom Stevens, MD, an anesthesiologist who trained in the Navy, joined HSS and was appointed the first director of the APS. Due to family reasons, Stevens left HSS in 1992. Approximately 1,300 patients were treated by the APS in 1991—a number that would grow to nearly 12,000 by 2010.

With the surgical volume slowly increasing, the department also continued to expand in the early 1990s, adding Chris Edmonds, MD, a pediatric specialist; Seth Waldman, MD, a pain specialist, and Kethy Jules-Elysee, MD, a pulmonologist and anesthesiologist. Gregory Liguori, MD, arrived in 1993.

A Commitment to Research

Sharrock's arrival at HSS spurred a resurgence of clinical research as well. Burstein's commitment to clinical and laboratory investigations, as well as his collaborations with Rovenstine at New York University, had been replaced by a focus on clinical anesthetic care for orthopaedics under Fox in the 1970s. Upon his arrival, Sharrock implemented several studies to investigate the physiology of regional anesthesia and its effects on both medical and surgical outcomes. These studies were remarkably similar to original work performed by Burstein 40 years earlier. Most of Sharrock's research was collaborative, working with his surgical and medical colleagues to evaluate thrombogenesis following orthopaedic surgery.

Notably, Sharrock's research has been particularly recognized in the orthopaedic community, as he is the recipient of many prestigious awards, including the Hip Society Award and the Charnley Award.[21] Sharrock remains on staff at HSS today as clinical professor of anesthesiology and senior scientist. While maintaining his very active clinical practice, he continues to perform research and mentor young trainees and faculty in the department.

1995: Thomas J. J. Blanck, MD, PhD, Takes the Helm

In 1993, the Anesthesia Department was restructured. Michael Urban, MD, PhD, was appointed director of clinical operations, and Sharrock assumed the role of director of education and research. Thomas J. J. Blanck, MD, PhD, was appointed director and chair of the department in 1995. Blanck had received his medical degree from the University of Pennsylvania School of Medicine in 1970. He then did his internship at the Children's Hospital of Philadelphia. Blanck completed a clinical fellowship in biochemistry at the National Institute of Mental Health before graduating from Yale University's anesthesia residency program in 1977. Following appointments at Johns Hopkins and Cornell, he assumed the directorship of the department in 1995.

At the same time, HSS was undergoing a major expansion in its physical plant. The "new building" over the FDR drive was in its final stages of completion. That expansion resulted in an increase in the number of operating rooms and the need to recruit additional anesthesiologists (Table 1). Over the next few years, the clinical volume of anesthetics increased significantly, to 15,663 cases in 2001.

Blanck had vast experience in bench science and research. When he came to HSS, he instituted the Excitable Tissues Research Lab, which investigated the manner in which anesthetics perform biochemically and molecularly and how they affect end organs. Investigators in this laboratory sought to describe the mechanism of action of anesthetics. Blanck recruited and collaborated with basic scientists, including Esperanza Recio-Pinto, PhD, Michael Schlame,

MD, and Fang Xu, PhD. Clinical research continued, but a clear shift toward basic science had occurred.

One of Blanck's major accomplishments was the implementation of the department's first regional anesthesia symposium in 1997. This program, which would later be called "Controversies and Fundamentals in Regional Anesthesia," featured didactic sessions and small group workshops. Over the years, this program has become one of the largest educational programs dedicated to regional anesthesia in the country. Over 2,000 individuals have attended the program throughout its existence. Guest faculty have included experts in regional anesthesia from Virginia Mason Medical Center in Seattle, the University of Toronto, Centre Clinical in Soyaux, France, University of California at San Diego, Duke University, Wake Forest-Baptist Medical Center, Mayo Clinic (Minnesota), and Johns Hopkins Medicine.

The final major initiative of Blanck's tenure was the formation of East River Medical Anesthesiologists (ERMA). The early anesthetists at HSS were salaried. Because most of them practiced surgery as a primary profession, the salary was a necessary incentive to encourage their interest in providing anesthesia.[1]

After World War II, the financial arrangement with the hospital was altered. A base salary was provided to anesthetists, and additional incentive income could be earned up to a ceiling. Upon achieving the ceiling, all additional income was given back to the institution. When Sharrock arrived in 1986, the structure changed again to a fee-for-service model, with no guaranteed minimum salary and no ceiling on income. This method incentivized anesthesiologists in a manner similar to that of the surgeons, and resulted in great efficiency and productivity.

By the mid-1990s, the complexities of the healthcare insurance industry and government reimbursement made it clear that a group model was in the physicians' and hospital's best interests. ERMA was incorporated in February 1998. Blanck was its first president, followed for a brief time by Gregory Liguori. In 2002, Victor Zayas was elected ERMA President, and he remains in that position today. Most members of the department joined the corporation, with the final contracts being signed during a department golf outing at the Dyker Beach Golf Course in Brooklyn in 2000.

In August 2001, Blanck left HSS to become director and chair of the Anesthesiology Department at New York University School of Medicine. It was from NYU that Burstein trained more than 60 years earlier. Blanck still holds that position today.

Leadership in the New Millennium: Gregory Liguori, MD

Michael Gordon, MD, who was clinical director in 2002, was appointed acting director of the department after Blanck's departure. An extensive search for a new director and anesthesiologist-in-chief was initiated, and a search committee—which included Russell F. Warren, MD, then surgeon-in-chief, and John Savarese, MD, and Roger Wilson, MD, the chairs of the Anesthesiology Departments at New York–Presbyterian Hospital and Memorial Sloan-Kettering Cancer Center, respectively—was formed. Within a few months, Gregory Liguori was selected as the new director and anesthesiologist-in-chief, formally assuming the directorship in June 2002 (Fig. 4).

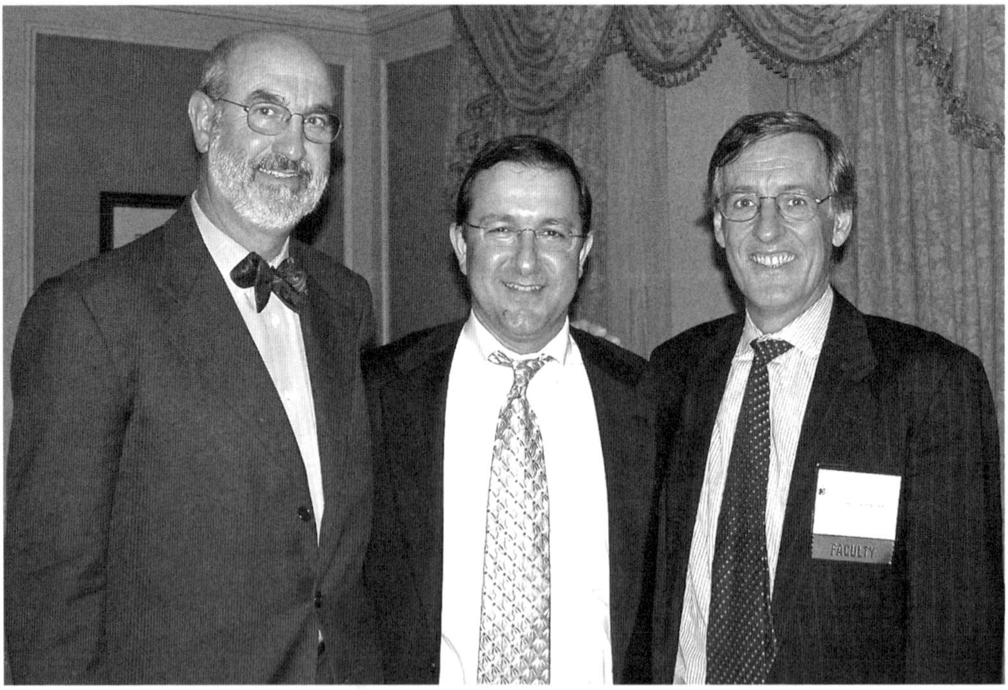

Fig. 4 From left: Thomas J. J. Blanck, MD, PhD, director and anesthesiologist-in-chief, 1995–2001; Gregory A. Liguori, MD, director and anesthesiologist-in-chief, 2002–present; Nigel E. Sharrock, MB, ChB, director and anesthesiologist-in-chief, 1986–1993.

Liguori attended the University of Pennsylvania School of Engineering as an undergraduate and received his medical degree from Cornell University Medical College. Following an internship in medicine at New York Hospital and a residency in anesthesia at Brigham and Women's Hospital, he came to HSS in 1993. Similar to Sharrock, Liguori's interest in regional anesthesia was fostered at Brigham and Women's Hospital by Vandam and Covino. Before his appointment as director and anesthesiologist-in-chief, Liguori held a number of other leadership positions in the department, including medical director of ambulatory surgery and chair of the Quality Assurance Committee, and he was elected as the second president of ERMA in 2001.

By 2002, the orthopaedic, and hence, regional anesthesia practice at HSS was growing exponentially. New operating rooms were being added each year. The diversity of anesthetic procedures increased as well. Over 8,000 neuraxial anesthetics and nearly 6,000 peripheral nerve blocks were performed that year. Cases were becoming more complex, and the range of orthopaedic procedures grew weekly.

Liguori recognized that changes in the clinical practice were necessary, and subspecialization within orthopaedic anesthesia was required. Over the next decade, he recruited specialists to HSS to achieve the high level of care and quality outcomes that were expected by all (Table 1). Kathryn DelPizzo, MD, and Naomi Dong, MD, were recruited to support the growing pediatric patient population. David Wang, MD, Simon Ho, MD, Semih Gungor, MD, and Vladimir Kramskiy, MD, joined the Chronic Pain Program. The increase in complex spine procedures necessitated the recruitment of Joseph A. Oxendine, MD, Michael Ho, MD, Jonathan C. Beathe, MD, and Carrie R. Guheen, MD.

Liguori began a critical care initiative to treat the medically complex patients recovering from surgically complex procedures. Stavros Memtsoudis, MD, PhD, Michael Nurok, MBChB, PhD, Fani Nhuch, MD, and Sean Garvin, MD, specialists in intensive care medicine, were recruited to support this initiative. The APS, initiated under Rom Stevens in 1991, had grown in lock-step with the surgical volume. In 2006, Spencer Liu, MD, was recruited to direct this initiative. Liu had spent the prior decade at Virginia Mason in Seattle and is widely considered one of the foremost authorities in acute pain medicine in the anesthesia community. Under his leadership, the APS would expand to innovative areas, such as recuperative pain medicine.

Finally, the introduction of ultrasound technology expanded the utilization of regional anesthetic applications for orthopaedic surgery. New and previously rare peripheral blocks were now being performed regularly. Liguori continued with extensive recruitment of anesthesiologists to support the growing regional and orthopaedic anesthesia needs of HSS (Table 1).

A Commitment to Education

Another major initiative of Liguori's tenure was the expansion of the graduate medical education program in anesthesiology at HSS. Fellowship training in regional anesthesia at HSS began with King in 1987. At that time, advanced training in regional anesthesia was limited, with a modest amount of interest from quality residency graduates. With the expansion of orthopaedic surgery and the applications for regional blocks, fellowship training exploded. The HSS fellowship developed an international reputation for academic and clinical excellence. Since 2002, over 70 fellows have graduated from the program.

Residency training in regional anesthesia has also expanded. Since 1966, Cornell residents rotated through HSS to learn neuraxial and peripheral nerve blocks. By 2004, the number of residents coming to HSS from Cornell increased to five per month. Around the country, many residencies were having difficulty providing their trainees with adequate numbers of regional anesthetics. One such program was Johns Hopkins. In 2003, the HSS Anesthesia Department entered into an academic affiliation with the Johns Hopkins School of Medicine to provide additional training in regional anesthesia for their senior residents. Over the last decade, the department has also entered into academic affiliations with Harvard Medical School–Massachusetts General Hospital, the University of California, San Francisco, the University of Washington, and Virginia Mason Medical Center.

With Blanck's departure to NYU, Liguori refocused the department's research efforts on clinical initiatives. He appointed Jacques YaDeau, MD, PhD, as Director of Clinical Research, and greatly expanded the infrastructure necessary to perform clinical trials. Collaborations between orthopaedics and medicine that were commonplace under Sharrock led to hundreds of publications on anesthetic and analgesic care for orthopaedic patients.

Today the mission statement of Hospital for Special Surgery's Anesthesiology Department is "to achieve an international leadership role by providing the highest quality anesthetic care and pain management for patients undergoing orthopaedic surgery, to advance the science of regional anesthesia, pain management, and orthopaedic critical care through clinical and translational research, and to promote educational opportunities to all students of regional anesthesiology and pain medicine." It is clear that during the 115 years of anesthesia at HSS, the Department of Anesthesiology has remained focused on these ideals, which embody the great traditions of HSS.

REFERENCES

1. Gibney VP. Anesthetics at the Hospital for Ruptured and Crippled. *Med Rec.* 1908:266.
2. Osborn WH. *Thirty-Seventh Annual Report of the New York Society for the Relief of the Ruptured and Crippled.* New York, NY: New York Society for the Relief of the Ruptured and Crippled; 1900.
3. Sanders J. Bennett's Inhaler. Waring Historical Library Artifact Collection. Available at: http://waring.library.musc.edu.
4. Bastron RD. Albert Heircy Miller: anesthesiology pioneer. *ASA Newslett.* 2005 October;69.
5. Bennett TL. New anesthetic apparatus. *Med J: Weekly J Med Surg.* 1900;57:524–526.
6. Hopkins HR. Practical hygiene. *Buffalo Med J.* 1900;46:87–88.
7. Bull WT, Coley WB. Observations upon the operative treatment of hernia at the hospital for ruptured and crippled. *Ann Surg.* 1898;28:577–604.
8. Bennett TL. The amount of the anesthetic. *JAMA.* 1900;34:708.
9. Vandam L. Early american anesthetists. *Anesthesiology.* 1973;38:264–74.
10. Thomas L. Bennett Memorial Fund. *The New York Medical Week.* 1933:8.
11. *Seventy-Fifth Annual Report of the New York Society for the Relief of the Ruptured and Crippled.* New York, NY: New York Society for the Relief of the Ruptured and Crippled; 1939.
12. Bacon DR, Darwish H. Emery A. Rovenstine and regional anesthesia. *Anesthesiology.* 1997;22:273–275.
13. Hershey SG. The Rovenstine inheritance: a chain of leadership. *Anesthesiology.* 1983;59:455.
14. Waisel DB. The role of World War II and the European theater of operations in the development of anesthesiology as a physician specialty in the USA. *Anesthesiology.* 2001;94:907.
15. CoTui CL, Burstein CL, Ruggiero WF. Total spinal block: a preliminary report. *Anesthesiology.* 1940;1:280–291.
16. Burstein CL. Postural blood pressure changes during spinal anesthesia: a preliminary experimental report. *Anesth Analg.* 1939:18:132–139.

17. Patterson RL. *One Hundred and Fourth Annual Report of the New York Society for the Relief of the Ruptured and Crippled.* New York, NY: New York Society for the Relief of the Ruptured and Crippled; 1967.
18. *Annual Report of the New York Society for the Relief of the Ruptured and Crippled.* New York, NY: New York Society for the Relief of the Ruptured and Crippled; 1981.
19. Mulroy MF. Daniel C. Moore, MD, and the renaissance of regional anesthesia in North America. *Region Anesth Pain Med.* 2011;36:625–629.
20. Sharrock NE, Cazan MG, Hargett MJ, Williams-Russo P, Wilson PD Jr. Changes in mortality after total hip and knee arthroplasty over a ten-year period. *Anesth Analg.* 1995;80:242–248.
21. Sharrock NE, Go G, Harpel PC et al. The John Charnley Award: thrombogenesis during total hip arthroplasty. *Clin Orthop Relat Res.* 1995;(319):16–27.

CHAPTER 16

RADIOLOGY AND IMAGING (1905–2012)

HELENE PAVLOV, MD, FACR

IN 1895, WILHELM ROENTGEN WAS studying the passage of an electric current through a gas at low pressure. That November, he discovered that if he enclosed the discharge tube in a sealed black carton to exclude light and if he placed a paper plate coated with barium platinocyanide in the path of the rays in a dark room, the rays became fluorescent. He immobilized his wife's hand on such a prepared plate and placed it in the path of these rays. Upon developing the photographic plate, he saw an image of her bones and soft tissues and her ring. He called this image a "roentgenogram," and because the nature of this experiment was not known, he called these fluorescent rays "x-rays."

In January 1896, x-rays were described as being able to generate dense bodies impenetrable to light waves and to produce an image. These x-rays were a subject of much excitement, as evident in the following:

X-ACTLY SO!
The Roentgen Rays, the Roentgen Rays,
What is this craze?
The town's ablaze
with the new phase
of x-ray's ways.

I'm full of daze,
Shock and amaze;
For nowadays
I hear they'll gaze

Thro' cloak and gown—and even stays,
These naughty, naughty Roentgen Rays.

—Wilhelma, *Electrical Review*
April 17, 1896

Three years after the discovery of the x-ray, in 1899, the Hospital for the Ruptured and Crippled bought its first x-ray machine. In the *Record and Chronicle*, Virgil P. Gibney stated, "The pathological laboratory and photographic rooms, equipped with an x-ray machine, are presided over by men trained in their respective departments, and it gives me pleasure to report progress."

The first radiologist, Fred R. Albee, MD, was employed from 1905 to 1911, with roentgenologist Byron C. Darling, MD, joining the staff in 1911. In 1915, Darling reported, "In a Hospital where bone and joint diseases are so prevalent, a patient needs at least one diagnostic x-ray examination, [and] in many instances, repeated ones. This department should therefore be one of the strongest and most efficient in the Hospital."

He also reported a connection between the mouth and teeth as an underlying cause of arthritis and saw future research in x-rays of the teeth. In the 53rd Annual Report (1916), Gibney referenced dentistry: "with the aid of the x-ray laboratory, we have been able to discover the cause of infection in many of the obscure diseases involving joints." By 1928, it was recognized that "in dealing with pathologic conditions of bones and joints, the X-Ray Department is of the greatest importance. In many cases of difficult interpretation, the roentgenogram may be the determining factor in establishing the diagnosis. This is especially true in bone sarcoma."

The volume of x-rays in 1917 was 3,820, multiplying nearly sixfold to 22,052 by 1928. In 2011, approximately 265,000 imaging examinations are performed annually at Hospital for Special Surgery (HSS). The HSS Department of Radiology and Imaging continues to provide expert insight into the diagnosis and management of orthopaedic and rheumatologic diseases and conditions. The department has 39 conventional and fluoroscopic x-ray rooms, 2 computed tomography (CT) scanners with 3D capability, 4 ultrasound (US) units, and 10 high field-strength magnetic resonance imaging (MRI) units. There are 14 board-certified radiologists, all with musculoskeletal subspecialty expertise.

Department Leadership

Albee was the radiologist in charge of the x-ray laboratory from 1905 to 1911, followed by Darling in 1911. Percy C. Ashley, a layman and technician, served as spokesperson for the x-ray laboratory from 1917 to 1921, with Darling identified as a "consultant roentgenologist." Captain Louis F. Kuntz provided x-ray services in 1924, the same year radiologist Harvey M. Imboden, MD, joined the staff.

Although there were x-ray machines at the hospital for 27 years, x-ray was considered a laboratory or a technical specialty until 1926, when the Department of Radiology was officially established. Raymond W. Lewis, MD, was appointed the first director and served from 1926 to 1951; however, he did not become a full-time staff member until June 1, 1938, when he transferred his private practice to the hospital.

Upon his retirement, Lewis was replaced by Harold Jacobson, MD. Jacobson's tenure was brief, lasting from 1952 until 1954, when he left HSS to become director of Radiology at Montefiore Hospital in the Bronx. Charles Breimer, MD, was appointed interim Chief, serving from 1954 to 1957, but he also had a private office and was a member of the Special Committee on Radiology of the New York County Medical Society. He therefore spent only a few hours a day in the department.

In the spring of 1955, after completing his tour of duty as the chief and the only radiologist at the Army Hospital in Fort Eustis, Virginia, Robert H. Freiberger, MD, began civilian life as assistant radiologist in the Radiotherapy Department of Columbia Presbyterian Hospital in New York City. Six months later, realizing he preferred diagnostic radiology, Freiberger applied for a position at HSS. He was interviewed at the hospital on 42nd Street by the surgeon-in-chief, Philip D. Wilson Sr., MD, and was offered the position of director of the Department of Radiology.

Freiberger, a modest man, felt he lacked sufficient experience in orthopaedics and rheumatology to assume the position of director and asked that his appointment be postponed until he felt better qualified. Wilson agreed, and Freiberger began his illustrious career on June 15, 1955, working as a radiologist at the new current hospital location. After 2 years, Freiberger was re-offered the position of director of the Department of Radiology, and this time he confidently accepted.

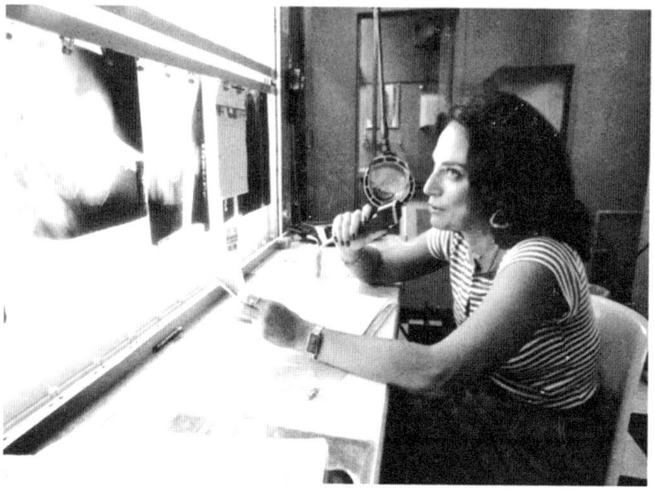

DEPARTMENT OF RADIOLOGY AND IMAGING®

Fig. 1 Helene Pavlov, MD, dictating an x-ray report as a radiology fellow in 1977. She designed a department logo (right) and initiated it in 1997, when she became the first woman at HSS to chair a department. (From Hospital for Special Surgery Archives)

Freiberger led the department from 1957 until he stepped down in 1988 and remained on staff until he retired in 1997. He was consistently referred to as an ultimate professional, leading with patience, wisdom, and humor and eager to share his knowledge.

Jeremy Kaye, MD, an HSS attending radiologist before leaving to go to Vanderbilt University Medical Center in 1976, returned to HSS in 1988 as director of the Department of Radiology. In 1996, Kaye resigned and returned to Vanderbilt University to serve as professor and chairman of the Department of Radiology at that institution.

Russell Warren, MD, surgeon-in-chief, formed a search committee for a new director and interviewed many outstanding candidates from around the nation, along with internal candidate Helene Pavlov, MD. In April 1996, while interviewing for a new assistant, Pavlov described the state of the department as one of being in "flux." On April 1, 1997, Warren called Pavlov and told her she had the job. Pavlov became one of the first, if not the first, female directors of a clinical department at HSS.

Her first order of business was to change the title of director to "radiologist-in-chief," to better reflect the value that radiology provides to the overall success of HSS. Additionally, Pavlov asked for and received the Board of Trustees' approval to rename the Department of Radiology and Nuclear Medicine as the "Department of Radiology and Imaging" to more accurately reflect radiology advances and those anticipated for the 21st century. Believing that branding is essential, Pavlov designed a logo for the department, which was approved by the board and trademarked (Fig. 1).

Physical Plant and Technological Advances

At the end of the jubilee year of HSS (1913), the 50th Annual Report discussed the move to the new quarters, referencing the X-Ray Department as being "well equipped." By the second year in the new facilities, the impact of radiology to clinical care and the cost were summarized as follows: "The slight increase in running cost over the old building is more than compensated by in part due to improvements in the methods of treatment—for example, the x-ray photographs so necessary in [the] treatment of bone disease now involve an annual expense of about $2,000, which a few years ago was not thought of."

In 1921, improved resolution of the "deep parts" of the body, such as the hips and spine, was enabled with a "Bucky diaphragm" installation. Intensifying screens and film replaced plates, which equated to shorter exposure time and more economical production costs, as film costs considerably less than plates. A film filing system was installed in 1924. By 1940, the storage space for films was exhausted, and a copying camera (microfilm) was purchased to make miniature photographic reproductions.

In the 78th Annual Report (1941), Raymond Lewis reported that the "reduction of x-ray film to small rolls of photographic film saves an immense amount of storage space." Over 18,000 x-ray film examinations performed between 1931 and 1934 were photographed in miniature, greatly reducing the required storage space. A terminal digit filing system replaced numerical filing for both x-ray films and reports in 1967, allowing for current studies to be maintained in a smaller storage area while the more remote cases were warehoused for retrieval as needed.

In 1935, the X-Ray Department was remodeled on the West Wing of the lower floor, and the number of examinations increased 15% compared with 1934. William B. Coley, MD, surgeon-in-chief, reported: "Dr. Raymond W. Lewis and members of the working force took much pleasure, and pride in their new X-ray Department with improved facilities after working for so long with the previous antiquated equipment."

Coley, internationally recognized as a pioneer in cancer research and as the "father of cancer immunotherapy," was interested in establishing an X-Ray Therapy Department and wanted to try diagnosing cancer using organic iodine compounds and x-ray visualization, as was being done in Europe. According to Coley, the X-Ray Department was "complete in all respects, except x-ray therapy." With government approval and a $7,000 patient donation, x-ray therapy apparatus was installed in September 1941. It was the last unit available, with none expected to be manufactured until the war was over. The war impacted the department in other ways, too, as materials for making film were used for rocket powder; x-ray film therefore had to be used sparingly.

Facilities to rapidly develop x-rays were installed in 1936 underneath the operating room amphitheater, which allowed for "an immediate check on the position of bones and correction of deformities secured at the time of operation." Laminographic (later known as "tomographic") equipment was installed in 1940 to identify new applications for skeletal imaging, and was quickly recognized as being useful for visualizing lesions that were not evident on routine x-rays.

By 1948, hospital requirements for x-ray examinations again outgrew physical capacities. As there was insufficient space available for growth and expansion, the emphasis was on greater efficiency for output within existing facilities; therefore, hours of operation were extended from 5 to 7 PM. Secretarial staff hours were staggered, and part-time technician services added.

As reported by Wilson Sr., "There was minimal employee turnover or lost man hours due to illness; examinations were carried out usually on the same day as the requisitions or within 24 hours, recognizing the loyalty and devotion of the technical and clerical staff." Limited and nonexpandable facilities continued to be identified in the 1950 and 1954 Annual Reports, increasing the anticipation of the move to the new hospital location.

HSS had moved to its current location just prior to Freiberger's arrival in 1955. At that time, the X-Ray Department consisted of a central work area on the first floor; four x-ray rooms (two equipped for fluoroscopy), a large darkroom, two film processors, a file room, and two small offices. There was a large room next to the radiologists' offices for film interpretation.

In 1958, tomograms (to identify lesions not otherwise seen) and a device to permit weight-bearing foot x-rays were introduced. By 1962–1963, image intensifiers replaced the mandatory requirement for the radiologist to sit in the dark and wear red goggles for a half an hour to enable their eyes to adapt to the dark before performing a fluoroscopic procedure. The image intensifier reportedly "brightens the fluoroscopic image 3,000 times." Cine or motion pictures of normal diseased joints for evaluation of operatively fused joints were also introduced.

Until 1958, x-ray films were hand-processed in liquid chemicals, requiring hours to allow the film to dry—hence the "wet reading" for STAT interpretation, as the film would be dripping wet. Automatic film processing machines produced a dry film in 6.5 minutes and enabled permanent dry films to be interpreted by the radiologist on the wards within hours of ordering the examination. A Polaroid x-ray processing unit was purchased for the operating room, which produced good-quality prints in 10 seconds and was used for procedures requiring x-ray control. By 1967, the film processing machine (X-Omat) produced a dry x-ray in just 90 seconds.

Goran C. H. Bauer, MD, a Swedish orthopaedic surgeon and director of research, invited Lars Andren, MD, a radiologist from University of Lund in Malmo, Sweden, to be a visiting associate professor of radiology for 2 months in 1963. During this visit, Andren demonstrated his technique for knee arthrography to the HSS Radiology staff. Freiberger was intrigued and subsequently went to Sweden as the guest of the chairman of radiology of Malmo University Hospital, becoming an expert in the technique of knee arthrography.

In 1964, a pilot project of 100 knee arthrograms for the diagnosis of torn knee cartilages was undertaken. Between 1966 and 1967, the number of knee arthrograms doubled, and arthrograms of other joints were investigated. Eventually, fluoroscopic-controlled knee arthrography using the image intensifier was performed, and HSS sponsored annual knee arthrography courses that attracted radiologists from around country, with standing-room-only capacity. Freiberger became known as the "father of arthrography," and a textbook, *Arthrography*, by Freiberger et al. was published in 1979.

Freiberger saw multipanel viewing units called "Philips alternators" used in Sweden (Fig. 1), and in 1967 they were used at HSS to facilitate interpretations of x-rays. The department had two such alternators, each holding 300 films, with a third alternator on order. The hanging and removing of films was initially performed by radiology technologists and later became the responsibility of file clerks. The radiologists dictated reports that were transcribed; because the reports were hard copies, a mistake in the report required retranscription.

Through the trip to Sweden, Freiberger was also introduced to a new method of myelography using a water-soluble medium. Freiberger and J. Paul Harvey, MD, an HSS Orthopaedic Resident (class of 1957) and staff orthopaedist, introduced a Swedish method of myelography to HSS. They used a Swedish contrast medium for myelography that required the injection of

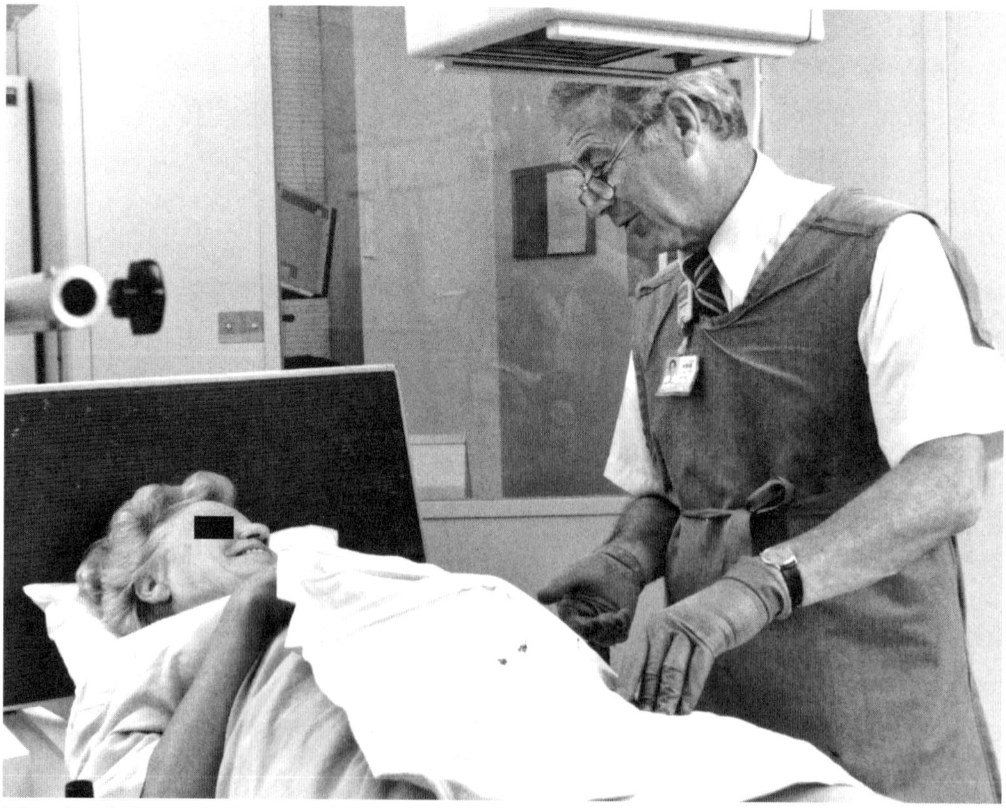

Fig. 2 Robert Freiberger, MD, after completing a hip arthrogram in 1977. (From Hospital for Special Surgery Archives)

spinal anesthesia. The patient had to be inclined, head up during filming, and was paralyzed below the waist. The doctors, along with the Department of Physiology at Cornell University Medical College, performed spinal nerve conduction tests during the myelogram. It was subsequently decided that the disadvantages outweighed the advantages, and this technique was discontinued.

At that time and for years to come, myelography was performed using an oil-based contrast agent, which, despite attempts to remove it at the end of the examination, left a few drops of residue that could be visualized on spinal x-rays for years following the examination. Myelography today uses a water-soluble contrast agent that is significantly less toxic. Although myelography has been replaced by MRI in most facilities today, most spine surgeons at HSS rely on both types of imaging examinations.

The Division of Interventional Radiology (IR) uses image guidance under fluoroscopy, CT, and ultrasound. The chief of the Division of IR and Ultrasound is Gregory Saboeiro, MD; the division includes a nurse practitioner, two physician assistants, and several nurses. It is an extremely busy service, performing myelograms, discograms, facet and other spinal injections, and also aspirations and injections of all joints. Biopsies are also performed in this division using appropriate image guidance at the site of involvement. Technologies have improved considerably over the years, and state-of-the-art radiation dose-reduction techniques are now utilized in all procedures employing ionizing radiation.

Nuclear medicine at HSS using a radioactive fluorine isotope and a rectilinear scanner with opposing crystal detectors was introduced by Bauer during the late 1960s and was housed on the fifth floor of the Caspary Research Building. In 1975, a crystal gamma camera and an online computer were purchased through a generous private gift. Robert Schneider, MD, already a board-certified radiologist, became board-certified in nuclear medicine and was named chief of the Nuclear Medicine Division. Schneider was also appointed radiation safety officer for HSS. The division was closed in 2010, as most of the nuclear medicine examinations performed at HSS had been replaced by either by MRI or CT examinations.

In 1970, the surgical suites and recovery room required heavy-duty electrical lines to permit the use of adequate x-ray equipment, including image intensifiers and disc storage. A program to initiate computerization in the department for patient work data, to be combined with x-ray request and report forms, was introduced in 1971.

In the early 1980s, hospital construction allowed for expansion of the operating rooms and the Radiology Department. Timing, however, was problematic: in an attempt to decrease the cost of medical care, the New York State legislature enacted a law limiting the number of units of expensive medical equipment that hospitals could purchase. This resulted in a delay in the HSS acquisition of a CT scanner until 1982.

The first single-slice CT scanner required two rooms: one for the scanner and a second temperature-controlled room for the computer and data storage equipment. The computer stored the data digitally, and axial images were reformatted into coronal, sagittal, and other display formats. This new expansion divided the department into outpatient services performed on the first floor, and inpatient services and CT examinations performed on the fourth floor.

As time went by, CT scanners became much more powerful and faster, and eventually the second room was no longer required. HSS updated its CT equipment several times over the years. As of 2012, there were two state-of-the-art scanners—64- and 16-slice units—both with low-dose technology, increased signal-to-noise ratio, and 3D capability. In 2012, the 64-slice unit received ACR accreditation, and Eric Bogner, MD, was appointed chief of the Division of CT.

Radiation dose reduction is a primary focus of the department and especially of the CT Division. Software, hardware, and various postprocessing techniques are utilized to achieve the highest quality images with the lowest patient dose possible. Postprocessing techniques can yield 3D color images when such enhancement is requested for improved patient communication and/or presurgical planning.

In 1989–1990, HSS acquired its first MRI unit, culminating a 4-year effort to gain authorization from the New York State Department of Health. The MRI Division is housed in the basement, given the magnetic restrictions of weight and positioning. MRI uses high field-strength magnets instead of ionizing radiation and provides exquisite soft tissue detail. This technology, coupled with the nontraditional vision of Hollis G. Potter, MD, chief of the MRI Division, opened up new vistas for the evaluation of cartilage, tendons, ligaments, muscles, bone marrow, the brain and spinal cord, and peripheral nerve pathology. MRI applications for orthopaedic patients grew exponentially.

The MRI Division was initiated in 1997, and the second MRI unit was added in 1998. The number of high field-strength units with state-of-the-art gradients grew to 3 in 2003, 5 in 2004, 7 in 2007, and 10 in 2012.

In the 1990s, further growth demanded improved patient turnaround. Limited space facilitated the opening of HSS-affiliated private offices, examination areas, and a general x-ray unit in the newly constructed Belaire Building in 1991. Since the Belaire Building was not part of the hospital, the facilities required licensing as a private practice. Belaire Radiology, PC, was established within 2 months; all equipment was licensed and inspected, and Belaire Radiology, PC, opened with Kaye as president, Pavlov as vice president, and Mary Giesa, RT, as practice administrator. Pavlov became president of Belaire Radiology, PC, in 1997.

In 1996–1997, inpatient and CT examinations were consolidated on the fourth floor, and outpatient examinations were performed on the first floor; all imaging services other than MRI were housed on the third floor of the main hospital. When the Belaire Radiology, PC x-ray facility converted to hospital space in 2004, all of those were incorporated into the HSS Department of Radiology and Imaging. Today, Giesa is an assistant director in the department and is in charge of radiology registration for the main campus.

Before and during the acceptance and validation of MRI, single- and double-contrast (contrast agent and air) arthrography of the shoulder was used to diagnose rotator cuff injuries. In 1998, Pavlov recruited Ronald Adler, PhD, MD, to HSS as chief of the Ultrasound Division, bringing the expertise required to establish quality musculoskeletal ultrasound. The Ultrasound Division grew precipitously, once the hospital's referring surgeons and rheumatologists realized the benefit and improved outcomes associated with highly accurate diagnostic capabilities and the use of interventional guided targeted medication injections to treat conditions such as tendonosis, bursitis, and neuromas—without ionizing radiation. Adler resigned in 2011 and Saboeiro was appointed chief of the Division of Ultrasound.

Teleradiology was instituted at HSS when Richard Herzog, MD, joined the staff in 2000 as Chief of the Division of Teleradiology. Using teleradiology, HSS radiologists now apply their musculoskeletal imaging expertise to examinations that were performed elsewhere. Herzog and his team work with multiple out-of-state orthopaedic practices. No HSS images are outsourced for interpretation.

A major change in imaging occurred in the early 2000s with the conversion from analog (film) to digital image capture—i.e., computed radiography and direct radiography. This transition from film to digital was required to enable the subsequent conversion to a Picture Archive Communication System

(PACS) in 2005. A PACS system had to be selected, purchased, and installed. Light boxes throughout the hospital and in the multiple hospital satellites, physician offices, clinics, operating and conference rooms—and anywhere else images were viewed—were replaced with digital monitors, cables lines, and computers. Training on the PACS system was required for the entire hospital staff, including physicians, surgeons, trainees, and nurses. This effort was successful thanks to the extensive collaboration between the Information Technology (IT) and Radiology Departments. The PACS team is headed by Tai DeNunzio, assistant director of the Department of Radiology and Imaging IT Systems.

The transition away from film brought many changes and challenges. Film, dark rooms, and chemical storage facilities were no longer needed. The film file room was once the hub of the Radiology Department, with nonstop delivery and return of film folders (Fig. 3). From the early 1970s through the end of the 20th century, Lincoln Champagne and Jose Martinez, along with a dedicated crew of file clerks, maintained the file room. Today, Teddy Simmons and Terry Williams (the latter honored as the HSS Employee of the Month in 2010) remain part of this team. Due to the change in their responsibilities, file clerks were renamed Image Records Clerks to more accurately describe their duties. At the time of this writing, the Image Records team was managed by Henry Caban.

Conversion from film to digital images and the establishment of PACS required a complete remodeling of the radiology reading room for ergonomically filmless interpretation. Speech or voice dictation was introduced in 2006. PACS enabled images to be instantly available and displayed on monitors to physicians throughout the hospital by 2006–2007 and in the operating room by 2008. All HSS images and reports are currently available for viewing by multiple physicians simultaneously, improving efficient consultations between radiologists and the referring physicians.

As of 2011, the Department of Radiology and Imaging is located in separate sites, including the third floor and basement in the main hospital, the Belaire Building, River Terrace, East River Professional Building, Omni in Queens, and at East 72nd and 75th Streets.

Radiologists, Technologists, and Other Staff

The first radiologists at HSS, as discussed earlier, were Fred Albee, Byron Darling, and Dustin Hobbs, followed by Alberto Inclan, MD, in 1915. In

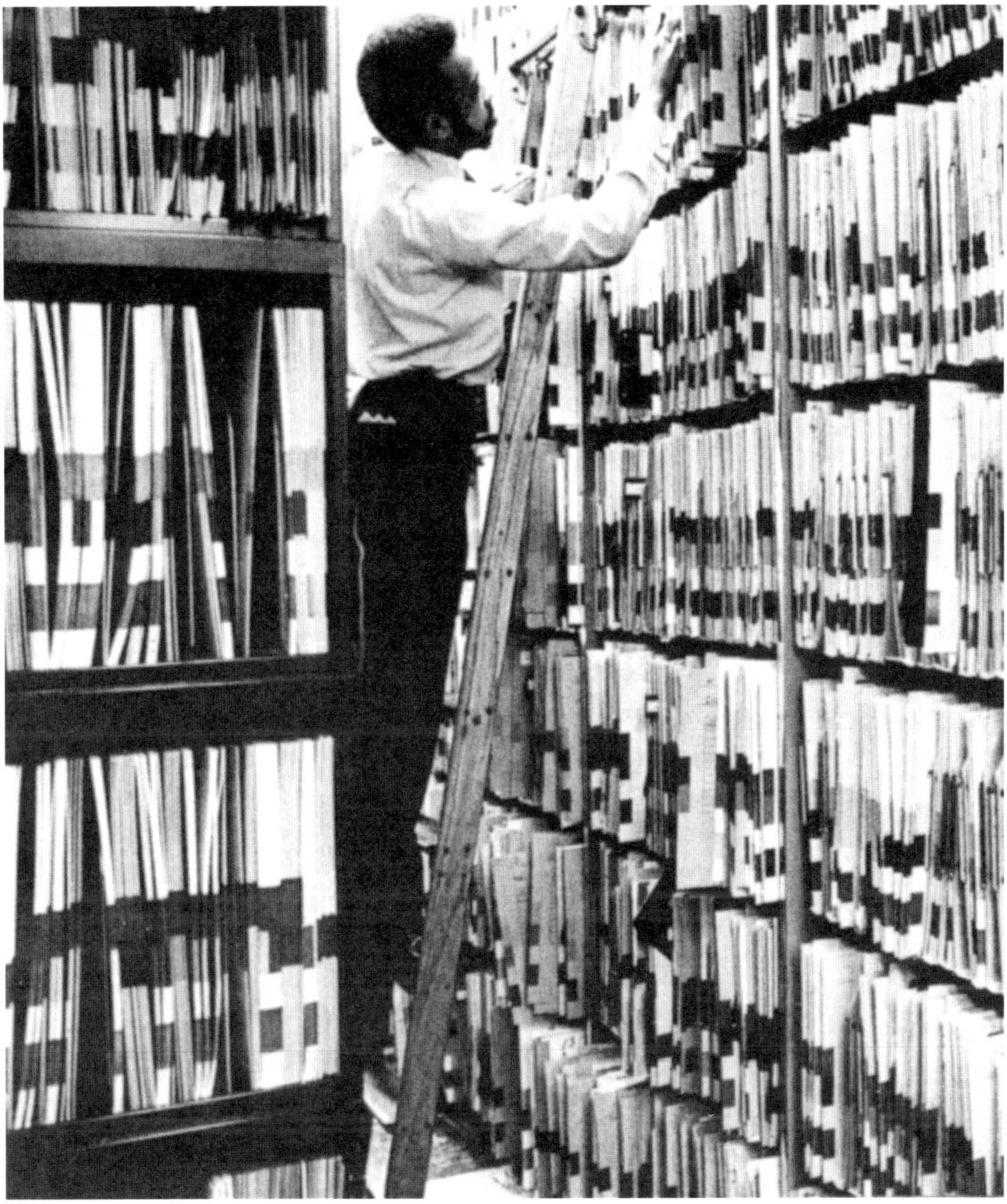

Fig. 3 Terry Williams, Image Record Clerk, in 1970, seeking a patient film jacket in the main file room. (From Hospital for Special Surgery Archives)

1924, Chief Technician Tina Rocke, assistant technician Grace McCullough, Clerk K. M. Grant, and roentgenologist Harry M. Imboden, MD, composed the staff. William Coley cited his indebtedness to Imboden in the 62nd Annual Report in 1925, "because he made regular visits to the Hospital, and has been willing at all times to aid in the diagnosis of x-ray films, and all of his services have been rendered without compensation." Unable to make a full-time commitment, Imboden remained on staff as a consultant when Raymond Lewis became director in 1926.

Ramsey Spillman, MD, joined the department in 1934 as associate roentgenologist. Ruth E Snyder, MD, was listed as associate roentgenologist and radiation therapist in 1945, and Robert Freiberger started working at HSS in 1955.

In 1960, x-ray technologists could not maintain their positions if they were pregnant (due to the potential risks of radiation to the fetus). Therefore, a temporary position became available, and Dola Polland was hired to fill it. She had intended to go to medical school like her older brother, who became a radiologist, but World War II intervened. Instead, Polland trained to become a radiology technologist at Beth Israel Hospital in Newark, New Jersey. Although Polland was initially hired for a temporary position, Freiberger asked her to remain.

Another long-term dedicated employee in the department was Marilyn Bierer, RT, a technologist from 1966 to 1985. She helped train many fellows in fluoroscopic technique and safety. She subsequently left HSS to attend law

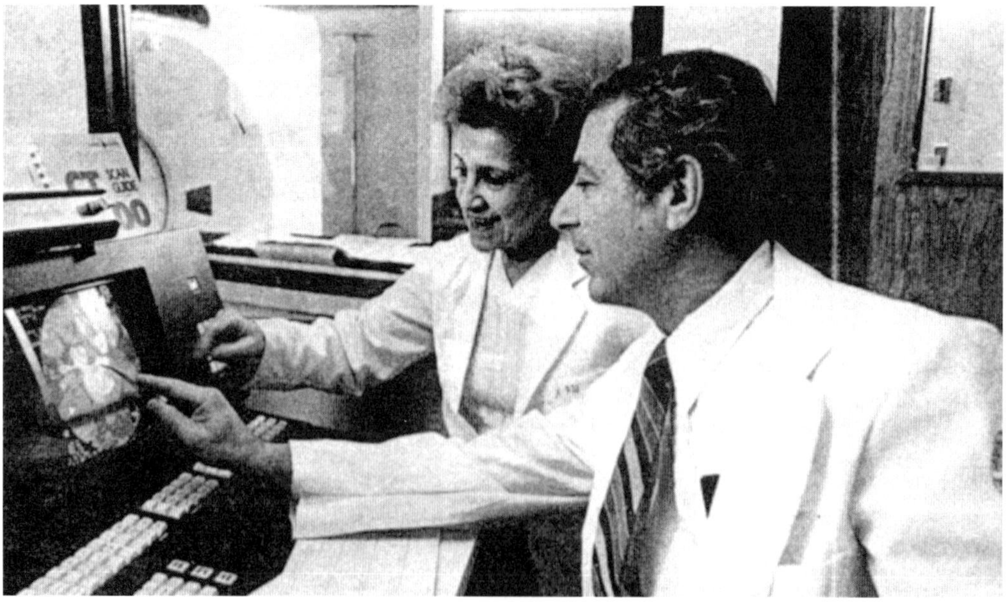

Fig. 4 Robert Freiberger and Dola Polland in 1987, reviewing images on the CT workstation. (From Hospital for Special Surgery Archives)

school in San Diego, where she currently has a successful law practice. Gerald Jaffess, RT, was coordinator and chief of Technical Services in 1967.

Polland advanced to become the senior technologist and controlled both inpatient and outpatient flow through the department (Fig. 4). During the 1970s, x-ray technician students from New York Hospital, Memorial Sloan-Kettering Cancer Center, and Hostos Community College rotated through HSS for training. Polland was instrumental in hiring two New York Hospital radiology technologists she trained—Ralph Bianco, the current HSS vice president of operations, and Ed White, assistant vice president of radiology (Fig. 5).

For Polland, HSS was her first and only job. Although retired in 1987, she maintained her technologist license until 1996 and was periodically drafted back to work as a technologist when the department was shorthanded. Polland works at HSS to this day as a much loved member of the HSS volunteer staff.

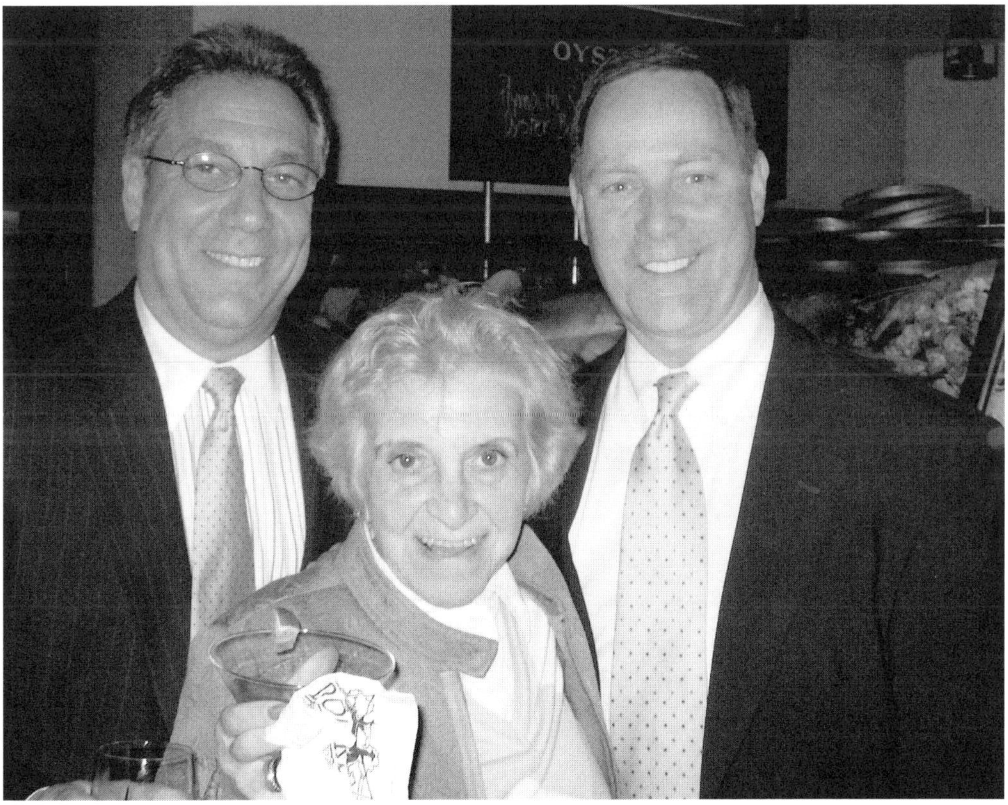

Fig. 5 (From left) Ralph Bianco, Dola Polland, and Ed White at an HSS 15–25 Year Club Annual Dinner. (From Hospital for Special Surgery Archives)

In 1962, Paul Killoran, MD, a graduate of the New York Hospital–Cornell University Medical College residency program, joined Freiberger as a full-time radiologist. An increase in the number of procedures in 1964 necessitated the addition of Thane Asch, MD, and Mordecai Halpern, MD, as attending roentgenologists, and Charles Reid, DVM, as a research consultant.

Freiberger hired Waltrand Gisela Blasberg-Ryan, MD, immediately upon graduation from her HSS fellowship in July 1968, making her the first female attending radiologist at HSS. She left in 1970 to have a family. When Killoran left in 1968 to become chief of radiology at the Rockland Maine Hospital, Margaret Harrison-Stubbs, MD, joined the department.

Bernard Ghelman, MD, started in 1969, and he was joined a year later by Jeremy Kaye, MD. James C. Hirschy, MD, and Nancy S. Hoge, MD, were recruited to be radiologists to Outpatient Department, and both worked part-time. Robert Schneider joined the HSS Faculty in 1973 as chief of nuclear

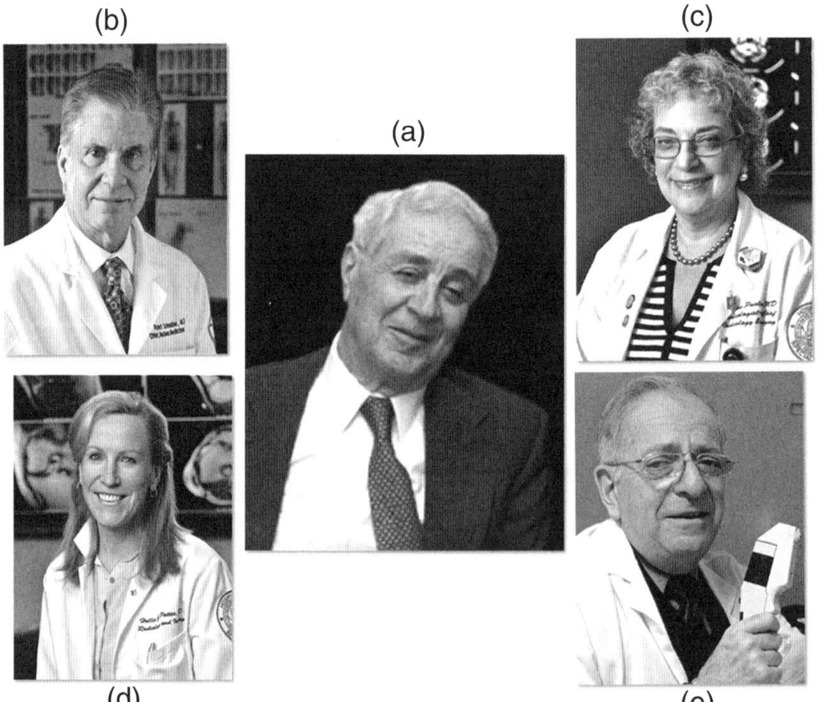

Fig. 6 Robert H. Freiberger, MD (a), surrounded by Robert Schneider, MD (b), Helene Pavlov, MD (c), Hollis G. Potter, MD (d), and Bernard Ghelman, MD (e). (From Hospital for Special Surgery Archives)

medicine and radiation safety officer. Amy B. Goldman, MD, joined 2 years later and was part of the department until 1998. Helene Pavlov joined the staff in July 1977, following completion of her HSS Musculoskeletal Radiology Fellowship. Ghelman, Schneider, and Pavlov all remain in the department today (Fig. 6).

Over the following years, other radiologists were hired—several immediately upon completion of the HSS Musculoskeletal Radiology Fellowship, some returning to HSS years later, and others from various other training programs and universities.

Service Commitment

HSS radiologists and members of the staff have consistently demonstrated service commitment to professional societies and have become officers and committee members in most of the major local, national, and international imaging and orthopaedic societies. In recognition of the significant orthopaedic imaging research and educational contributions of Freiberger, Pavlov, and Potter, each was granted the rare honor of radiologists as Associate Members in the American Academy of Orthopaedic Surgeons. Potter is also a member of the American Association of Sports Medicine (AAOSM), the Hip Society, and the Knee Society.

Freiberger (retired HSS Radiologist Emeritus), Goldman (former HSS radiologist), Miller, and Pavlov each held the elected position of President of the New York Roentgen Society. Pavlov, Carolyn Sofka, MD, and Eric Bogner, MD, have served as counselors and/or alternate counselors to the American College of Radiology for New York City, and delegates and/or alternate delegates representing the New York State Roentgen Society to the ACR.

The International Skeletal Society is a prestigious collaboration of dedicated subspecalized musculoskeletal radiologists, pathologists, and surgeons. Freiberger was a founding member. Theodore Miller was president of the society in 2006, and Schneider, Pavlov, Adler, and Sofka are currently active members.

Maureen R. Firth, regulatory and quality manager for the department, served as president of the Association of Medical Imaging Management (AHRA) in 2005. She was elected chair in 2010 and vice chair in 2011 of the AHRA Education Foundation.

Douglas N. Mintz, MD, a member of the HSS Department of Radiology and Imaging from 1998 (following completion of his HSS Musculoskeletal

Radiology Fellowship) until 2010, when he left to work Miami Baptist Hospital. However, he maintained his ties to HSS, and served as secretary-treasurer of the HSS Alumni Association until 2011. As of November 2012, Mintz returned to HSS and the department of radiology and imaging.

Education

The X-Ray Department was always committed to the HSS academic mission of education and research. X-rays were quickly incorporated into teaching, with "stereopticon lantern" projections of select cases used at monthly meetings. In 1919, the hospital purchased an apparatus for making lantern slides from radiographs, enabling the department to do this work without charge. Raymond Lewis attended all Monday morning conferences of the orthopaedic staff and contributed interesting cases each week.

Freiberger felt strongly that the role of academic radiologists was to educate our colleagues at HSS and around the world in the state-of-the-art diagnostic imaging of musculoskeletal diseases. The main reading room had an entire wall of light boxes used for teaching and clinical review of x-ray films by orthopaedic surgeons and visiting clinicians. A small adjacent area held a box and camera to photograph interesting or rare cases and prepare slides for teaching conferences and publications. Another entire wall of the reading room was dedicated to the teaching file film collection. These x-rays are still valuable and are being considered for inclusion in our digital teaching file collection.

The education of the fellows and residents of multiple disciplines has always been recognized as an important part of the department's responsibility. In the early years, orthopaedic residents and fellows each received 3 months of instruction in x-ray interpretation. In the 1960s and through the early 2000s, HSS radiologists traveled to New York Hospital to be trained in the interpretation of trauma films with the radiology residents. Today, second- and third-year New York–Presbyterian Hospital radiology residents and first-year HSS orthopaedic residents rotate through the department for dedicated musculoskeletal imaging training. Theodore T. Miller, MD, was appointed director of Resident/Medical Student Training in 2008 and oversees the resident curriculum.

The Musculoskeletal Radiology Fellowship at HSS is the oldest of its kind in the country, established in 1967. The first fellow was Blasberg-Ryan. Upon completion of her 1-year fellowship, she was invited to stay on as an assistant attending radiologist. Harrison-Stubbs was offered a staff position by Freiberger in July 1968 but continued to be listed as a fellow until the HSS Medical Board met in August/September 1968, and New York State granted her a license that November. At that time, she became the second female attending and second fellow on the HSS alumni list.

The Musculoskeletal Radiology Fellowship accepted one fellow a year until in 1969, when the department accepted two—Damiano Dumas, MD, and Terry Hudson, MD. When Pavlov began her fellowship in July 1976, she overlapped the last 6 months of the fellowship of Donald Sauser, MD. The fellowship positions have grown over the years, consistent with the increase in staff and examination volume.

In the early years of the Musculoskeletal Radiology Fellowship, the director's assistant was the administrator for the fellows. A stricter oversight of residencies and fellowships was mandated, and an Academic Education Coordinator position was created. In 1998, Pavlov appointed her administrative assistant, Marcia Budd, to that position. She remained in that position until her retirement in 2007, providing guidance and mentoring to the fellows.

In 2001, Sofka (HSS Musculoskeletal Radiology Fellowship graduate in 2000) was appointed director of Education and Fellowship Training for the department to ensure the continued growth and reputation of the fellowship program. Under her guidance, the Musculoskeletal Radiology Fellowship achieved ACGME accreditation in 2009. Today, there are two fellowship offerings: the General Musculoskeletal Fellowship and a Dedicated Orthopaedic MR Fellowship, for which we receive approximately 100 applications annually. The bar for acceptance into the radiology fellowship programs is high, and only about 40 fellow candidates are selected annually to interview for the coveted seven annual positions.

Attesting to the department's commitment to the training of future subspecialized musculoskeletal radiologists since 1967, over 100 general Musculoskeletal Radiology Fellows and approximately 10 dedicated Orthopaedic MR Fellows have graduated from the Department of Radiology and Imaging Fellowship program (Table 1).

In recognition of the impact that Freiberger has had on musculoskeletal radiology at HSS and both nationally and internationally, Pavlov instituted the

Table 1 Fellowship Graduates

1967–1968	Waltrand Gisela Blasberg-Ryan, MD
1968–1969	Margaret Harrison Stubbs, MD
1969–1970	Sigmund (Simon) Mittler, MD
	Damianos Doumas, MD
1971–1972	Robert Dussault, MD
1973–1974	Terry M. Hudson, MD
1975–1976	Donald Sauser, MD
1976–1977	Helene Pavlov, MD
1977–1978	Bilha Chesner-Fish, MD
1978–1979	Gerald Vienne, MD
1979–December 1980	Jamshid Tehranzadeh, MD
1981–1982	Robert C. Hewes, MD
1982–1983	Ann M. Abenavoli, MD
1983–1984	Lynne Steinbach, MD
1984–1985	Tod G. Abrahams, MD
1985–1986	Mark R. Goldberg, MD
1986–1987	David J. Rubenstein, MD
	Bonnie Lemberg, MD
1987–1988	Andrew Collins
	Harris Freed, MD
1988–1989	Susan Schraft, MD
1989–1990	Marcia Blacksin, MD
1990–1991	Hollis G. Potter, MD
1991–1992	Jacqueline C. Hodge, MD
1992–1993	Kathleen Finzel, MD
	Theodore T. Miller, MD
1993–1994	Hilary Ruth Umans, MD
	Kevin R. Math, MD
1994–1995	Jill H. Kingsley, MD
	Doohi Lee, MD
1995–1996	Elizabeth Gaary, MD
	Peter Gusmer, MD
	Julie Schatz, MD*
1996–1997	Pamela Burdett, MD
	Michael S. Thorpe, MD
	James Linklater, MBBS*

Table 1 *(continued)*

1997–1998	Mark Decker, MD
	Douglas N. Mintz, MD
	David Connell, MBBS*
1998–1999	Caroline Rodriguez, MD
	Charles Tsai, MD
	Britton Limes, MD (6 months)
1999–2000	Marc S. Weinstein, MD
	Carolyn M. Sofka, MD
2000–2001	Ketan Davae, MD
	Geoffrey Tashjian, MD
	Simi R. Anidjar, MD
	Timothy Hooper, MBBS* (resigned in April 2001)
	Angela Berning, MBBS
2001–2002	Steve Ling, MD
	Anthony Notino, MD
	Steve Sharon, MD
	Wendy Brown, MBBS*
2002–2003	Ziyad Haddad, MD
	Dennis Lin, MD
	Hiren Patel, MD
	Lauren Ernberg, MD
	Stephanie, Ho, MD**
2003–2004	Olga Bauman-Fishkin, MD
	Liat Kaplan, MD
	Jonathan Luchs, MD
	Tej Dugal, MBBS*
	Ian Tsou, MD** (visiting)
2004–2005	Richard Batz, MD
	Martha Danon, MD
	Gene Han, MD
	Sinchun Hwang, MD
	Gregory Saboeiro, MD
	Li Foong Foo, MD, MRCP, FRCR**
2005–2006	Aditya Daftary, MD
	Gregory Timm, MD
	Amir Mehdizade, MD

Table 1 *(continued)*

	Sebastian Fung, MBBS*
	Gina Ciavarra, MD
	Li Foong Foo, MD, MRCP, FRCR**
2006–2007	Mike Abiog, MD
	Qi Chen, MD
	Dan Feinberg, MD
	Alex Maderazo, MD
	Madhavi Kaza, MD (Battineni)*
	Li Foong Foo, MD, MRCP, FRCR**
2007–2008	Jarett Burak, MD
	Anthony Chang, MD
	Le Roy Chong, MBBS
	Jean Jose, MD
	Patrick Lee, MD
	Scott Lehto, MD
	Brandon Black, MD*
2008–2009	Timothy W. Deyer, MD
	Cono W. Gallo, MD
	Kevin Johnson, MD
	Valeriy Kheyfits, MD
	Michael H. Ngo, MD
	Anuraag Sahai, MD*
2009–2010	Graham Campbell, MD
	Yoshimi Endo, MD
	Akira M. Murakami, MD
	Harlan Stock, MD
	Hsiu Su, MD
	Gregory Wilde, MD
	Tom Hash, MD*
2010–2011	Timothy Chen, MD
	Christina Geatrakas, MD
	Sapna Jain, MD
	Ralph Pinchinat, DO
	Yvonne Moreno, MD
	Brendan Skonieczki, MD
	Catherine Hayter, MBBS*

Table 1 *(continued)*

2011–2012	Alissa J. Burge, MD
	Mauricio de la Lama, MD
	Eric Feldmann, MD
	Talia Friedman, MD
	Andrew Gargiulo, MD
	Himanshu Patel, MD
	Andrew Plodkowski, MD
	Razia Rehmani, MBBS
	Catherine Hayter, MBBS* (6 months)
2012–2013	Jan Fritz, MD
	Shari T. Jawetz, MD
	Judith L. Kaplan, MD
	Michael L. Loftus, MD
	Anukul Panu, MD
	Aubrey J. Slaughter, MD
	Brett Lurie, MBBS**

Annual Robert H. Freiberger lecture series in 1997. Over the years, outstanding lecturers have offered presentations to the HSS community (Table 2). Pavlov also established the Robert H. Freiberger Academic Center and Library in 2002 (internally referred to as "The Freiberger") as a quiet area and a musculoskeletal imaging resource center, with journals, textbooks, online reference material, videos, and so forth for our fellows, physician colleagues, and patients.

A Web site is maintained through the center and its staff. Two monthly features are extremely popular on the HSS Web site: Imaging Case of the Month, edited by Bogner, and Ultrasound Case of the Month, edited by Saboeiro. Other patient education materials and information about the department, imaging procedures, examinations, staff, and imaging aspects of various orthopaedic diseases, and conditions can be found on the Web site and are updated regularly.

Research

An academic department must both initiate and collaborate on quality research for advances to be made that improve patient care. Freiberger has been an avid clinical researcher and was the first to identify the association of stomach ulcers

Table 2 Honorary Speakers: Annual Robert H. Freiberger Lecture Series

Richard Herzog, MD, FACR	May 28, 1999
Bruno D. Fornage, MD	April 28, 2000
Robert G. Dussault, MD	May 18, 2001
Lawrence M. White, MD, FRCPC	May 10, 2002
John Mathis, MD, MSc	May 30, 2003
Thomas P. Sculco, MD	May 14, 2004
Diego Jaramillo, MD, MPH	April 22, 2005
Kenneth Buckwalter, MD	April 21, 2006
Daniel I. Rosenthal, MD	April 27, 2007
Christopher J. Palestro, MD	May 16, 2008
Sharmila Majumdar, PhD	May 15, 2009
Carlo Martinoli, MD	May 14, 2010
Douglas Beall, MD	May 13, 2011
Christine B. Chung, MD	May 18, 2012

and avascular necrosis with steroid use. Hollis Potter (HSS graduate in 1991) was appointed director of research in the department in 2000 to address the increased mandated documentation and heightened rules of engagement regarding Institutional Review Board (IRB) and HIPAA compliance. Potter Chairs the Department Clinical Research Panel (CRP) and provides insight and guidance for research projects in which imaging has a major role in outcome determinants. This panel includes Richard Herzog, Theodore Miller, the department's Clinical Research Manager, and Barbara Bosco (representing the Clinical Research Department). Herzog represents Radiology on the HSS IRB review panel.

There are many ongoing research projects in the department. Under Potter, direction utilization of MRI in orthopaedics has flourished. The MRI Division has numerous active research projects funded by Cornell University in Ithaca, General Electric Healthcare, the National Institutes of Health, and private donors. The MRI research team, including Mathew F. Koff, PhD, assistant scientist, has pursued many clinical and basic science investigations, including the detection of preclinical changes in cartilage and the identification of MRI criteria to predict arthoplasty loosening. In 2012, Potter was honored with the Stephanie and Chase Coleman chair, MR Research.

Research in ultrasound has included the evaluation of the efficacy of ultrasound contrast agents to detect the development of microvascular blood vessels and flow patterns, and the relationship between vascularity and the healing process and tendon regeneration following surgery and trauma. In addition, ultrasound researchers are exploring the images and quantitative differences in the shear elastic modulus of soft tissues following compressive forces.

Other investigators have explored orthopaedic applications for multiplanar (CT-like) images obtained while the patient is weight-bearing, with specific focus on identifying previously undetected sources of foot and ankle pain. These and other research projects are performed under a Strategic Research agreement between HSS and Philips Medical Systems.

Awards and Recognition

Over the years, the HSS radiologists have received numerous honors and awards related to research and education (Table 3). The faculty serves as principal investigators or co-investigators on many federal, corporate, and society grant-supported research studies. They are also the recipients of individual endowed research funding.

In 2011, there were more than 300 peer-reviewed publications, presentations of original research, book chapters, invited articles, posters, and electronic exhibits produced by members of the Department of Radiology and Imaging. HSS radiologists serve as reviewers of scientific exhibits and on the Scientific Program Committees of most of the major peer-reviewed scientific assemblies, and as reviewers for various prestigious peer-reviewed radiology, orthopaedic, and subspecialty journals. Several of our radiologists are editors or assistant editors and serve on the advisory editorial boards of elite peer-reviewed journals, including the *Musculoskeletal Journal of HSS*, *American Journal of Orthopaedics*, *Journal of AAOS*, *Spine*, and *Sports Health*.

In Summary

In the 1943 *Record and Chronicle*, Raymond Lewis wrote, "Either on account of the war (or name your own scapegoat), the volume of work in the sinecure X-ray Department continues its practically uninterrupted, and apparently limitless, growth. Whether the thing should be turned to the endocrinologists for study of the pituitary; whether we should radiate the epiphyses or do

Table 3 Highlighted Research and Educational Honors/Awards

Ronald Adler, PhD MD	
General Electric Foundation Award	1976
NIH National Research Service Award; James A. Shannon Award	1979, 1995
SRU Annual Laurence A. Mack Research Award	2001
American Shoulder and Elbow Society—Neer Award	2006
New York Magazine—"Best Doctors," Castle Connolly "America's Top Doctors"	2009, 2010
Castle Connolly's "Top Doctors New York Metro 13th Edition"	2008–2011
Castle Connolly's "America's Top Doctors"	2008–2011
Eric Bogner, MD	
HSS Teacher/Mentor of the Year	2009
HSS Honorable Mention Teacher/Mentor of the Year	2010
EFORT Jacques Duparc Award (co-author)	2010
Li Foong Foo, MD, MRCP, FRCR	
"HAP" Paul Award (co-author)	2008
Charles L. Christian Fellow Award for Musculoskeletal Research (co-author)	2005
Richard J. Herzog, MD, FACR	
Alpha Omega Alpha Medical Honor Society	1971
International Society Study for the Lumbar Spine Lumbar Spine Research Award	2009
North American Spine Society—Top Research Paper	2009
Selected one of Philadelphia's "Top Docs" by *Philadelphia Magazine*	1996, 1999
Best Doctors in America	2004–2011
Theodore Miller, MD, FACR	
The Roentgen Award, Vanderbilt University School of Medicine	1987
The Corinne Farrell Prize, "Best Paper" International Skeletal Society	1991
Radiology Editor's Recognition Award for Reviewing with Distinction	1999–2003
Radiologic Society of North America (RSNA)—Certificate of Excellence in Design, Certificate of Merit	2005, 2006

Table 3 *(continued)*

International Skeletal Society, Presidents Medal	2006
Castle Connolly's "Top Doctors New York Metro, 11th–14th Editions"	2008–2011
Helene Pavlov, MD, FACR	
American Roentgen Ray Society (ARRS)—Certificate of Merit	1981
Radiologic Society of North America (RSNA)—Honorable Mention, 1980, 1983	1980, 1983
9th Annual Eastern Orthopaedic Association Award for Spinal Research	1987
69th Annual Meeting of the HSS Alumni Association, Philip D. Wilson Award	1987
70th Annual Meeting of the HSS Alumni Association, Lewis Clark Wagner Award	1988
Association of Bone and Joint Surgeons—Nicholas Andry Award "For Outstanding Achievement in the Field of Orthopaedic Surgery"	1994
North American Spine Society Award for Outstanding Research Paper in Orthopaedics	1997
Orthopaedic Research Society/AAOS Elizabeth Winston Lanier Kappa Delta Award	2004
New York Magazine—"Best Doctors in New York" Diagnostic Radiology	2000, 2001, 2011
Consumers' Research Council of America: Guide to America's Top Radiologists	2002, 2003, 2006, 2007
Castle Connolly's "Top Doctors: New York Metro Area"	2000–2011
Castle Connolly "America's Top Doctors"	2010
Hollis G. Potter, MD	
Alpha Omega Alpha Medical Honor Society	1985
The American Orthopaedic Association, Gary G. Winzelberg Memorial Research Award	1994
77th, 79th, and 82nd Annual Meetings of the HSS Alumni Association	1995, 1997, 2000
Philip D. Wilson Award	1995, 1997, 2000
American Orthopaedic Society of Sports Medicine AOSSM—Cabaud Award for Excellence in Basic Science	2005

Table 3 (*continued*)

Charles L. Christian Fellow Award for Musculoskeletal Research	2005, 2006, 2011
Radiologic Society of North America (RSNA)—Certificate of Merit	2006
Association of Bone and Joint Surgery Nicholas Andry Award "For Outstanding Achievement in the Field of Orthopaedic Surgery"	2007
EFORT Jacques Duparc Award (co-author)	2010
New York Magazine—"Best Doctors"	2008–2010
Castle Connolly's "America's Top Doctors'	2010
Castle Connolly's "Top Doctors New York Metro, 11th–14th Editions"	2008–2011
Gregory Saboeiro, MD	
Alpha Omega Alpha Medical Honor Society	1988
HSS Department of Radiology Teacher/Mentor Fellow Award	2010
Castle Connolly's "Top Doctors, New York Metro Area"	2008–2011
New York Magazine—"Best Doctors"	2008–2011
Robert Schneider, MD	
Robin Watson Award for Teaching of NYPH Radiology Residents	2002
HSS Department of Radiology Fellows Teaching Award	2008, 2010
Carolyn Sofka, MD	
Guide to America's Top Physicians	
Consumer Research Council of America	2005
Guide to America's Top Radiologists	
Consumer Research Council of America	2002, 2003, 2006

epiphysiodesis; whether to call in a vitamin expert; or whether to just cut down the food intake, we're at a complete loss to know. The cowbird fledgling has darn near pushed us all out the nest."

Clearly, while written tongue in cheek, the growth of the X-Ray Department has continued as predicted. Lewis' choice of the adjective "sinecure" (definition: a job or position that provides a regular income but requires little or no work) to describe the X-Ray Department, however, is far from accurate. The sustained growth in the department has throughout the years kept pace with hospital growth because of the dedicated hardworking and patient-focused radiologists and staff. The mission of the Department of Radiology and Imaging continues to be the provision of top-quality clinical imaging expertise, the conduct of cutting-edge research in all imaging modalities, and the education of future radiologists and colleagues regarding the benefits that quality image acquisition and interpretation provide to patient care.

Our radiologists continue to be consultants to HSS orthopaedic surgeons and rheumatologists and contribute to the reputation, the bottom line, and the overall success of the institution. If history repeats itself, it is safe to anticipate that the department will continue to grow beyond its facilities. Given the increased sensitivity and specificity of MRI, ultrasound, CT, and x-rays—combined with unlimited access to digital images, radiologists' expertise, and intense collaboration with physicians fostered by the HSS environment—the future clinical, teaching, and research opportunities and accomplishments of the Department of Radiology and Imaging remain infinite.

ACKNOWLEDGMENTS

For extensive review of historical data, interviewing former and special department personnel, writing the original draft, rereading, and editing multiple versions, and providing commentary and suggestions, a special thank you to the invaluable assistance provided by Marcia Budd.

For typing and retyping multiple manuscript versions, creating charts and tables, and always with a "no-problem" smile, a heartfelt thank you to my assistant, Tawana Hayes.

For putting up with endless hours researching data, writing, editing, and allowing for my distractions, a special acknowledgement and thank you to my husband, Harvey Zeichner, Esq, PsyD, and daughter Dalas Zeichner, for their understanding and support.

REFERENCES

1. Adler RS, Sofka CM, Positano RG. *Atlas of Foot and Ankle Sonography*. Philadelphia, PA: Lippincott Williams & Wilkins; 2004.
2. Freiberger RH, Kaye JJ, Spiller J. *Arthrography*. Upper Saddle River, NJ: Prentice Hall; 1979.

3. Goldman AB, Dines DM, Warren RF, Ghelman B. *Shoulder Arthrography: Technique, Diagnosis, and Clinical Correlation.* Boston, MA: Little, Brown and Company; 1982.
4. Halpern B, Herring SA, Altchek D, Herzog R. *Imaging in Musculoskeletal and Sports Medicine.* Malden, MA: Blackwell Science; 1997.
5. Lewis RW. *The Joints of the Extremities: A Radiolographic Study.* Notes on Non-Routine Methods, Non-Routine Ideas, and Less Common Pathology. Springfield, L: Charles C. Thomas Publisher; 1955.
6. Manaster BJ, et al. *Diagnostic and Surgical Imaging Anatomy: Musculoskeletal.* Philadelphia, PA: Lippincott Williams & Wilkins; 2006.
7. Miller TT, Schweitzer ME. *Diagnostic Musculoskeletal Imaging.* New York, NY: McGraw-Hill Medical Pub. Division; 2005.
8. Pavlov H, Burke M, Giesa M, Seager KR, White ET. *Orthopaedist's Guide to Plain Film Imaging.* New York, NY: Thieme Medical Publishers, Inc.; 1999.
9. Pavlov H, Ghelman B, Vigorita VJ. *Atlas of Knee Menisci: An Arthographic-Pathologic Correlation.* Upper Saddle River, NJ: Prentice Hall; 1983.
10. Pavlov H, Torg JS. *The Running Athlete: Roentgenograms and Remedies.* Chicago, IL: Year Book Medical Publishers; 1987.
11. Sofka CM. *Musculoskeletal Radiology: Past, Present, and Future.* Philadelphia, PA: Saunders; 2009.

CHAPTER 17

RESEARCH (1955–2011) SIX DEGREES OF SEPARATION

ADELE L. BOSKEY, PHD

"SIX DEGREES OF SEPARATION" IS the belief that everyone in the world is separated from everyone else by six links. Reviewing the history of the Research Division at the Hospital for Special Surgery (HSS), this chapter will repeatedly illustrate the existence of close links between the Research Division and the clinical staff that have created the unique character of HSS. Research themes introduced during the early history of the Research Division are tied (in some cases, by fewer than six degrees) to active areas of investigation today.

The Beginnings of the Research Division

The orthopaedic surgeons who directed HSS from its infancy always recognized the importance of research. In the HSS original headquarters, research laboratories were part of the main hospital. In 1955, when the HSS moved to its present site on the East River between 70th and 71st Streets, Philip D. Wilson Sr., MD, retired as surgeon-in-chief and assumed the position as the first director of research. Wilson was convinced of the importance of basic science research to enhance patient care at the hospital. He established the Philip D. Wilson Research Foundation to support the development of a new research building and its activities.

In 1956, the construction of the Alfred H. Caspary Research Building marked the beginning of a new era in orthopaedics, in which the specialty of orthopaedics would benefit from ever-deeper grounding in basic research. This center, along with a university affiliation, positioned HSS to become a world leader in the fields of musculoskeletal research, biomechanics, and rheumatic diseases.

The Caspary Research Division at HSS was opened in 1958 by Eugene Lance, MD, PhD, who recognized the need for an academic orthopaedic hospital to play a significant role in orthopaedic and musculoskeletal research. The official opening on November 17, 1960, attracted dignitaries from the City of New York. Wilson was joined by Sanford Atwood, PhD, provost of Cornell University, and George B. Kistiakowsky, PhD, special assistant to the president (Dwight D. Eisenhower) of the United States for Science and Technology, in giving talks at the event. Trained as a chemist, Kistiakowsky is best known for his research with the Manhattan Project, as well as his studies in thermodynamics, spectroscopy, photochemistry, and chemical kinetics. In 1972, he received the Priestley Medal, the highest award presented by the American Chemical Society.[1]

The Caspary Research Building became the hub of HSS laboratory investigation and, with renovation and expansion over the years, remains so today.

A History of Research Leadership

As the first director of research, Wilson was responsible for recruiting a larger research staff than had existed when research was first done in the main hospital building. He set the paradigm for the functions of the research director: supervision of all research activities, recruitment and retention of faculty, fundraising, teaching, and mentoring. As the Research Division grew, those functions did not change, but the responsibilities became shared by more individuals.

Since 1955, there have been seven directors of research and two chief scientific officers (CSOs) (Fig. 1). In 1999, the Board of Trustees created the CSO position, which features similar responsibilities to those of the previous director of research position but with direct reporting authority to the board. (Directors of research had reported to the surgeon-in-chief.) Directors of research either migrated from successful orthopaedic leadership positions in the hospital or rose through the ranks from positions within the Research Division. CSOs, to date, have been recruited from other institutions.

The second director of research was Goran C. H. Bauer, MD, a Swedish orthopaedic surgeon who served from 1962 to 1967, leaving in 1969 to become chairman of orthopaedics at the University of Lund in Sweden. Bauer was

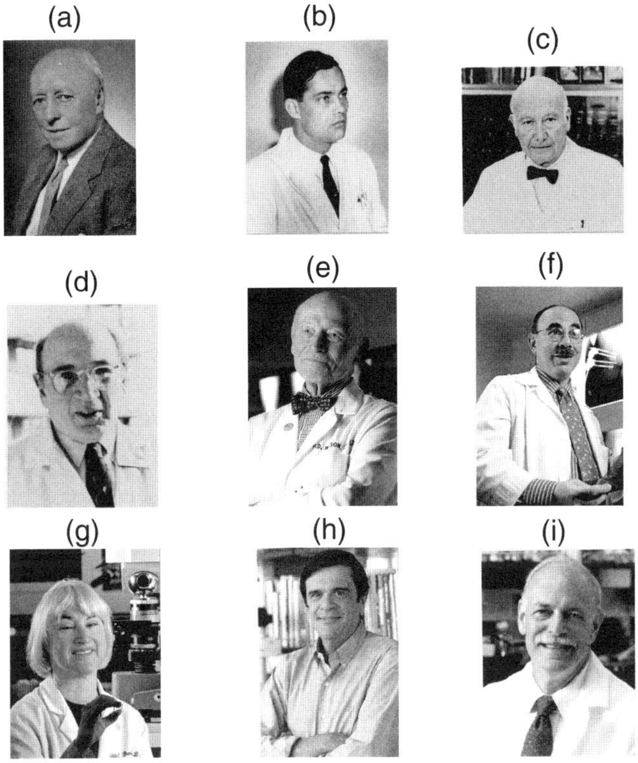

Fig. 1 Directors of research: Philip D. Wilson Sr., MD, 1955–1962 (a); Goren C. H. Bauer, MD, 1962–1969 (b); Robert C. Mellors, MD, PhD, 1969–1985 (c); Aaron S. Posner, PhD, 1985–1987 (d); Philip D. Wilson Jr., MD, 1987–1990 (e); Joseph M. Lane, MD, 1990–1993 (f); Adele L. Boskey, PhD, 1993–2002 (g). Chief scientific officers: Francesco Ramirez, MD, 2002–2006 (h), and Steven R. Goldring, MD, 2006–present (i). (From Hospital for Special Surgery Archives)

interested in physiology, pharmacology, and bone pathology. He was known for introducing bone-seeking isotopes into diagnostic medicine[2] and also for establishing the first national quality registry in the world when he returned to Sweden. The registry tradition started by Bauer in Europe now exists at HSS, with a number of large and small registries accessible by computer available to the research and clinical communities. The first registry at HSS was for the study of lupus and included serum samples for analyses. Thus, an idea pioneered by a former research director when he returned to Sweden came home to roost at HSS.

Robert C. Mellors, MD, PhD, who had been associate director of research and head of the Pathology Laboratories, became the director of research in

July 1969 and remained in that role for 16 years. Mellors had obtained his BA, MS, and PhD degrees from Case Western Reserve University in Ohio. Parenthetically, the six degrees of separation relate to the current chair of mechanical engineering at Case Western Reserve University, Claire M. Rimnac, PhD, who did her postdoctoral fellowship with Timothy Wright, PhD, at HSS and was part of the HSS research faculty almost 25 years ago. In 1989, she and Wright won a Kappa Delta Award for their work on polyethylene joint components. She thus shared with Mellors the affiliation with Case Western as well as the honor of this prestigious prize: Mellors had received a Kappa

Table 1 Major Orthopaedic Research Awards Received by HSS Research Staff

Shands Award—presented by the AAOS and ORS for contributions to orthopaedics and the devotion of a significant portion of a professional lifetime to furthering knowledge in the field of musculoskeletal disease

Albert Burstein, PhD (1989)

Adele L. Boskey, PhD (2010)

Donald Bartel, PhD (2011)

Kappa Delta Awards—presented by the Kappa Delta Society at the AAOS/ORS meeting

Robert C. Mellors, MD, PhD (1962): Rheumatoid Arthritis and the Cellular Origin of Rheumatoid Factors

Aaron S. Posner, PhD (1977): The Relation of Synthetic Amorphous Calcium Phosphate to Bone Mineral Structure

Adele L. Boskey, PhD (1979): Calcium Acidic Phospholipid Phosphate Complexes in Tissue Mineralization

Andrew J. Weiland, MD (1986): Fate of Vascularized Bone Grafts

Steven P. Arnoczky, PhD (1987): The Meniscus: Its Repair and Replacement

Timothy M. Wright, PhD, Donald L. Bartel, PhD, and Clare M. Rimnac, PhD (1989): Surface Damage in Polyethylene Total Joint Components

Joseph S. Torg, MD, Helene Pavlov, MD, and Albert Burstein, PhD (2004): The Pathomechanics, Pathophysiology and Prevention of Reversible and Irreversible Cervical Spinal Cord Injury: Results of a Thirty-Year Clinical Experience

ORS Women's Leadership Award—presented by the Women's Leadership Forum of the ORS for significant contributions to orthopaedic research and leadership within the ORS.

Adele L. Boskey, PhD (2008)

Jo A. Hannafin, MD, PhD (2009)

Delta Award in 1962 for his discovery of the cellular origin of rheumatoid factors (Table 1).

Mellors received his MD from Johns Hopkins University in 1944. He was trained in immunopathology and initially held a position at Memorial Sloan-Kettering Cancer Center, and then at HSS, where among his numerous achievements was the use of immune microscopy to demonstrate the pathogenesis of immune complex vasculitis and systemic lupus erythematosus. This marked the start of lupus research at HSS, which would become an area of international recognition for the Research Division.

Aaron S. Posner, PhD, succeeded Mellors as director of research in 1985. Posner's expertise was in crystal structure determination; after he received his PhD from the Polytechnic Institute of Brooklyn, he served in the U.S. Air Force. He then completed a fellowship at the National Institutes of Health (NIH), where he was involved in determining the crystal structure of hydroxyapatite, the geologic analogue of bone mineral.[3] He joined the HSS Research Division in 1963.

Among Posner's notable contributions was the description of the first mineral deposits in bone as noncrystalline or amorphous (amorphous calcium phosphate, ACP).[4] Although there is still some debate as to whether ACP is present in adult bone, recent studies by researchers at the Weizmann Institute (Israel) have demonstrated that there is some ACP in embryonic bones.[5] Independent of this debate, ACP is the starting material for most of the coatings now used on orthopaedic implants. Posner was the first principal investigator on an NIH training grant used to provide research experience to HSS residents. He was succeeded as PI on that grant by Joseph M. Lane, MD, and then by Wright.

Adele L. Boskey, PhD (who would become director of research in 1993), joined the Research Division 15 years before Posner became director of research to work as his postdoctoral fellow. She had met Posner when he presented a seminar at Harvard, while Boskey was a graduate student in physical chemistry/crystallography at Boston University. Posner had been invited to give the seminar by Melvin J. Glimcher, MD, an orthopaedic surgeon holding the Peabody Chair at Children's Hospital, Boston, who would eventually join the HSS Board of Trustees. Glimcher's research focused on the physical chemistry of bone, and Boskey's recruitment to Posner's laboratory and entry into the mineralized tissue field heralded the start of her long collaboration with Glimcher, his students, and his daughter, Laurie, who in 2011 was appointed dean of Weill Cornell Medical College.

There would be many other links to Glimcher. He became a member of the HSS Board of Trustees in 2001, joining 1981 Nobel Prize in Physiology and Medicine Laureate Torsten Wiesel, MD, who had joined the board in 2000. Later, Richard Brand, MD, and Carl F. Nathan, MD, became members of the HSS Board of Trustees in 2002 and 2004, respectively. These links to the Glimcher family are yet another illustration of six degrees of separation.

Posner retired as director of research in 1987. During his tenure, however, he established faculty meetings with the directors of the different basic science laboratories who assisted in management of the Research Division. He also hired a full-time research manager to monitor research financials and grants, as well as government-mandated approvals and records. The responsibilities of one person in 1987 are now performed by a staff of at least six individuals.

Posner was succeeded by Philip D. Wilson Jr., MD, who stepped down from the position of surgeon-in-chief in 1989 (the same position held by his father 35 years earlier) to become director of research. As surgeon-in-chief, Wilson Jr. had expanded the Biomechanics Department, which then became a center for computer-assisted design (CAD/CAM). He recruited an expert bone electron microscopist, Stephen B. Doty, PhD, as a member of the Research Division. Doty supervised the hospital's electron microscopes, which were then located in the Pathology Laboratories under Peter Bullough, MD, and was actively involved in the analysis of the effects of space flight on bone properties. Wilson Jr. maintained the Faculty Council structure, with a representative from each of the research disciplines within the building.

When Wilson Jr. retired as director of research, he became more active in fundraising for the Research Division and he is still active in that arena. His successor as director of research was Lane, an orthopaedic surgeon with research training experience from the NIH and the University of Pennsylvania. Lane's main area of interest has been metabolic bone disease and fracture healing. He served as director of research for only 2 years, leaving HSS to take a position as Chairman of Orthopaedics at the University of California at Los Angeles. He returned to HSS 2 years later to take on a more active role in his own research and in clinical medicine.

The First Woman to Take the Helm

When Lane left, Adele Boskey was a member of the Research Faculty Council and was appointed director of research, a position she held from 1993 to 2002 and the first (and to date, only) woman to do so. Her own research interests had started out under Posner's tutelage, investigating the stabilizers of ACP. She then expanded her focus to study the mechanism of biologic calcification and the formation of mineralized tissues (a grant she maintained for 37 years), eventually moving from the study of lipids in calcification to the roles of other macromolecules. This grant led to "spin-offs" in the cell culture field—such as studies of the importance of cells for the regulation of bone formation—and the study of osteoporosis.

Boskey's late husband played bridge with a spectroscopist. While playing cards, Richard Mendelsohn, PhD (of Rutgers University), would suggest collaborating with Boskey. "Isn't there some pathology problem that we could address using spectroscopy?" he would ask her. After many years, they sought to determine the compositional properties of bone (bone quality) that contributed to fracture risk. Those investigations led them to introduce the technique of infrared imaging to the musculoskeletal field and to define risk factors for bone fragility that could be derived from those data.[6] Today they are continuously revamping these techniques but are still using them to determine the relative effects of different osteoporotic therapies.

As director of research, Boskey maintained the Faculty Council, and with their help, she rewrote the Research Division By-Laws and added a clinician scientist to the Faculty Council—the start of the enhancement of clinical research at HSS. She also recruited a director of research administration, who is now a vice president for research. She wrote and received a grant to modernize the second floor of the research building and brought to the attention of the Board of Trustees the need for facilities improvement and research staff expansion.

In 2001, with the help of the newly elected Faculty Council, new laboratories were created, Core Facilities were expanded, and a new lupus research center was established (Fig. 2). Ongoing construction of the sixth, seventh, and ground floors prepared the way for a scaling up of research activities. The

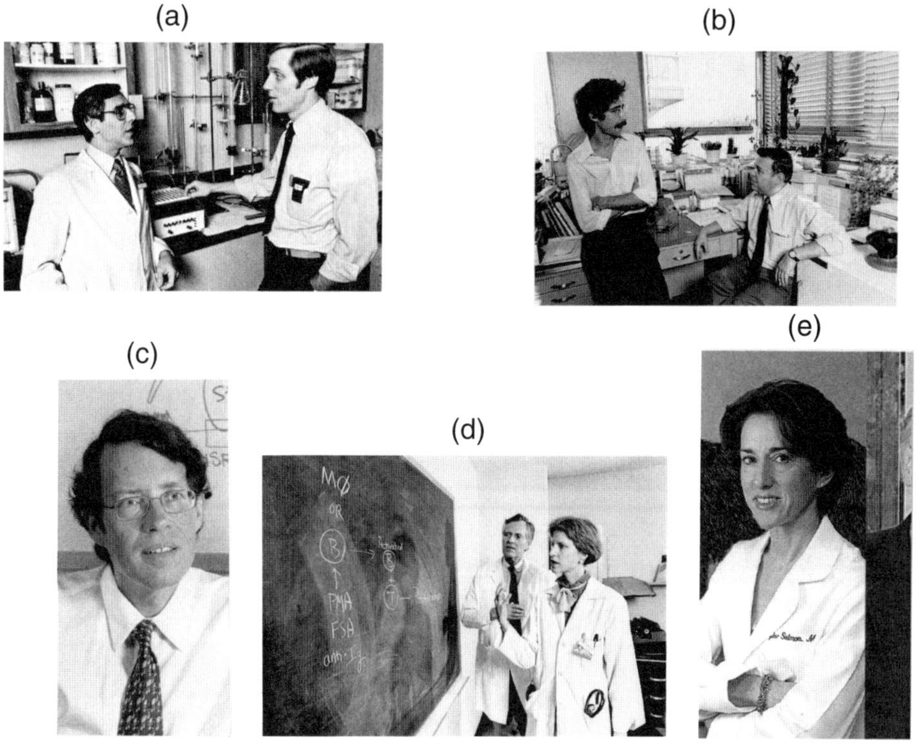

Fig. 2 Key contributors to HSS research: Immunology (1985). Michael Lockshin, MD, and Robert Kimberly, MD (a, from left to right); Keith Elkon, MD, and Larry Kagan, MD (b, from left to right); Lionel Ivashkiv, MD (c); Charles Christian, MD, and Mary K. Crow (Peggy), MD (d); Jane Salmon, MD (e). (From Hospital for Special Surgery Archives)

Faculty Council in 2001 consisted of Mary Crow, MD; Doty and Wright, representing basic science; and Jo Hannafin, MD, Lane, and Hollis Potter, MD, as clinician investigators. As director of research, Dr. Boskey chaired the Faculty Council.

In 1993, HSS became the first NIH-sponsored Specialized Center of Research in Lupus. In 2001, with support from Katherine and Arnold Snider of Rheuminations, Inc., HSS inaugurated the Mary Kirkland Center for Lupus Research—one of the most significant events that occurred during Boskey's leadership. The Kirkland Center provides support for intramural basic and clinical research at HSS and pilot research grants focused on lupus.[7]

The Advent of the Chief Scientific Officer

In June 1998, the Board of Directors of the Hospital held a research retreat, and in 1999, they approved a strategic plan for research and established a 5-year fundraising campaign to support it. They declared that the Research Division should be reorganized into individual laboratories, collectively headed by a CSO instead of a director of research.

It took almost 4 years to recruit the first CSO: Francesco (Checco) Ramirez, PhD, from Mount Sinai Hospital, who received a mandate to enhance research quality and improve the financial platform. His research interests were related to the molecular basis of connective tissue diseases—in particular, Marfan syndrome and osteogenesis imperfecta. He was recognized worldwide as a leader in the molecular genetics of human connective tissue disorders and identified the genetic cause of Marfan syndrome.[8,9] Ramirez held the St. Giles Chair in genetics while at HSS.

Upon his arrival, he created a series of task forces to carry out that reorganization. He established Programs in Autoimmunity and Inflammation, Musculoskeletal Integrity, Genetics and Tissue Regeneration, and Applied Orthopaedic Sciences. Each program consisted of one or more laboratories, and each had a group of target diseases that linked them to the HSS patient population.

For example, the Autoimmunity and Inflammation Program covered systemic lupus, rheumatoid arthritis, and osteoarthritis. The Musculoskeletal Integrity Program targeted the more common conditions of osteoporosis and osteoarthritis, to the rarer skeletal dysplasias and osteogenesis imperfecta. It was the umbrella organization for Hard and Soft Tissue Development and Degeneration and Repair and consisted of the Mineralized Tissues Laboratory, the Soft Tissues Laboratory, and the Biomedical Mechanics and Biomaterials basic science program. It also was the home for the Orthopaedic Scientist Incubator, where research was allowed to develop with future research grants. The incubator established such clinician researchers as Mathias P. Bostrom, MD, Scott A. Rodeo, MD, Chisa Hidaka, MD, and Aaron Daluiski, MD. The Musculoskeletal Integrity Program was also home to the Research Cores, which provided education and facilities to hospital- and university-based investigators.

The Applied Orthopaedic Program had more general clinical goals: restoring normal joint function, improving implant performance, and establishing the integrity of musculoskeletal structures. The Genetics Program did not exist at the time, and a search for a director of that program commenced in 2002.

During his tenure as CSO, Ramirez introduced a Clinician Scientist Program. He recruited three new investigators to the HSS research staff:

1. Carl Blobel, PhD, who studies a family of membrane-anchored metalloproteases called ADAMs (a disintegrin and a metalloprotease) and their roles in tissue degeneration and regeneration, rheumatoid arthritis, and angiogenesis.[10]
2. Inez Rogatsky, PhD, who is a member of Blobel's Program in Arthritis and Tissue Degeneration, explores the importance of glucocorticoids in inflammation and the molecular mechanisms, cofactors, and targets of their actions.[11]
3. Theresa Lu, MD, PhD, is an immunologist who examines blood vessels of the lymphoid tissues and their contributions to the delivery of oxygen and micronutrients to cells and to immune function.[12]

Ramirez left HSS in 2005 to become the Head of the Child Health Institute of New Jersey at the Robert Wood Johnson University Hospital.[13] He was succeeded in 2006 by Steven Goldring, MD, a rheumatologist and professor of medicine at Harvard Medical School and chief of rheumatology at Beth Israel Deaconess Medical Center. Goldring had received his medical degree from Washington University School of Medicine and has had a longstanding interest in the role of the osteoclast in bone and cartilage destruction. He too established a Faculty Council that included representatives of all hospital services, and he soon initiated meetings with the Program Heads to outline new directions and recruitment plans. He inspired closer collaborations between clinicians and basic science researchers, helping to enhance the Clinician Scientist track in the Research Division. In December 2011, Goldring was named the first Richard L. Menschel Research Chair.

In 2009, Goldring asked Lionel Ivashkiv, MD, who had been the director of basic science research under Ramirez, to assume the position of associate CSO. At about the same time, Robert N. Hotchkiss, MD, was appointed the director of clinical research.

Pioneering Achievements

A number of patented orthopaedic devices came out of research conducted at HSS in the Bioengineering Laboratory, which was first established in 1965 when Bauer provided laboratory space and funds to purchase the first testing equipment. Harlan Amstutz, MD, was the first to work in the laboratory, when he was an NIH fellow.[14] Amstutz collaborated with researchers from Polytechnic Institute of Brooklyn, the Department of Tribology at Columbia University, the NASA-Lewis Tribological Laboratory in Cleveland, and mechanical engineers at New York University. The results of HSS's first study in biomechanics were published in 1968.[15] Amstutz recruited Peter S. Walker, PhD, from England as a project engineer. Soon after Walker took over, a prototype of a knee replacement was developed, leading to the evolution of the HSS total condylar knee replacement—the first knee replacement designed at the hospital. The major designers were (alphabetically) Allan E. Inglis Sr., MD, John N. Insall, MD, Chitranjan S. Ranawat, MD, and Peter S. Walker, PhD. The design was completed in 1974 and patented in 1980. Implants for the elbow and wrist developed at HSS soon followed.[16]

Not long after the release of the total condylar knee replacement, surgeons and patients were seeking an implant with a greater range of motion than the 90 degrees provided by the total condylar knee. In 1978, Insall and Albert Burstein, PhD, developed the Insall-Burstein posterior stabilized knee. This knee was patented in 1981, and like the total condylar knee, it rapidly achieved worldwide use. Today, HSS holds 72 patents resulting from HSS research efforts in bioengineering and other areas.

As noted earlier, the Research Division would also make HSS a world leader in the study of systemic lupus erythematosus. The application of registries to predict patient outcomes was first introduced at HSS by Jane Salmon, MD, and Robert Kimberly, MD, circa 1985, when they established the Lupus Registry and Repository. Use of this registry over the past 30 years has resulted in more than 33 publications by HSS and outside investigators. Salmon and Kimberly used DNA from the Lupus Registry and Repository to identify one of first genes associated with the increased risk and severity of lupus.[17] Samples from the collection have been shared with HSS and outside investigators studying biomarkers of lupus, and with international consortia to define the genetics of the disease.

This registry system served as the paradigm upon which other rheumatologic and orthopaedic registries at HSS were developed. More than 40 years later (in 2011), a Center for Musculoskeletal Outcomes and Patient-Oriented Research was established at HSS. The mission of this center is to incorporate rigorous research investigation into the delivery of orthopaedic and rheumatology patient care and the outcomes of that care. The center has been headed most recently by Wright and Art Sedrakyan, MD, PhD, formerly with the U.S. Food and Drug Administration.

Laboratory Expansion

As the hospital's research efforts expanded over the decades, so did the number of laboratories. In 1960, there were three divisions of research:

1. The Division of Rheumatic Diseases, headed by Richard Freyberg, MD, had four research laboratories: Clinical Studies, the Laboratory for the Study of Collagen, the Laboratory for the Study of Fibroblasts, and the Rheumatic Diseases Laboratory.
2. The Orthopaedic Division, headed by Wilson Sr. included the Laboratory for Clinical Studies, Laboratory for Study of Disorders of Bone Metabolism (headed by Paul Saville, MD, 1926–2010), Laboratory for Mineral Metabolism (headed by Felix Bronner, PhD), and Laboratory for Analytical Biochemistry.
3. The Immuno-Pathology and Microbiology Division, directed by Mellors, housed laboratories on immunopathology (also directed by Mellors), immunochemistry (led by Leonhard Korngold, PhD), and ultrastructure, virology, and hematology (headed by Klauss Mayer, PhD, 1925–2011).[18]

As many readers know, Saville was known for his development of animal models of osteoporosis, even before the need for such models was recognized. Furthermore, he carried out investigations of the effects of modulators of bone formation, such as fluoride, on the mechanical strength of bone before the Research Division included a Biomechanics Department. Today such mechanical studies are actively pursued in the Research Division, recognizing that osteoporosis is a major economic burden in the United States and that animal models are efficient ways to evaluate new therapeutics.

Bronner was widely recognized for his studies of calcium metabolism. He served on the faculty at HSS and Cornell University Medical College from 1956 to 1963, when he joined the University of Connecticut, where he remained until he retired in 1984. During his academic career, he published more than 120 articles on nutrition and calcium metabolism and stimulated recent studies of "calcium mimetics" for the treatment of metabolic bone disease. He still attends meetings and reminds presenters about the importance of calcium in all stages of life.[19]

Korngold was trained as a bacteriologist, but having worked on immunology at Memorial Sloan-Kettering Cancer Center before joining HSS, he concentrated on the immunology of proteins involved in multiple myeloma and identified numerous diagnostic methods. In fact, a strand of the immunoglobulin molecule is named after him.[20]

Mayer spent the majority of his career at HSS and the neighboring institution of Memorial Sloan-Kettering, where he served as director of hematology while maintaining his affiliation with HSS.

By 1980, there were eight different laboratories in the Research Division (Table 2). The research interests of each of these eight laboratories can easily be tied to most of the three that existed 20 years prior, with the exception of the Biomechanics and Comparative Orthopaedics Laboratory.

By 2001, the research enterprise had expanded to 11 laboratories (Table 3). Ten years later, there were 5 research programs and 20 laboratories, not including the laboratories of clinician investigators who belong to these programs (Fig. 3 and Table 4).

These laboratories continue to focus on elucidating the mechanisms of the diseases that affect HSS patients, including, but not limited to, autoimmune diseases, lupus, osteoarthritis, osteoporosis, and conditions of impaired healing—many of the same conditions that were the focus of the early HSS

Table 2 1980 Research Division Laboratories

Department of Biomechanics
Laboratory of Comparative Orthopaedics
Laboratory of Ultrastructural Biochemistry
Laboratory of Connective Tissue Research
Laboratory of Orthopaedic Pathology
Department of Medicine Laboratory
Laboratory of Experimental Pathology
Immunochemistry Laboratory

Table 3 2001 Research Division Laboratories and Their Leaders

Ultrasound Research: Ronald S. Adler, MD, PhD
Mineralized Tissues Laboratory: Boskey
Immunoregulation Laboratory: Crow
Cytokine Signaling and Inflammation: Ivashkiv
T-Cell Signal Transduction Laboratory: Philip King, PhD
Clinical Outcomes Research: Robert Marx, MD
Arthroplasty Research Laboratory: Bryan J. Nestor, MD
Immunoreceptor Biology: Luminita Pricop, MD
Inflammatory Effector Mechanisms Laboratory: Salmon
Soft Tissue Research: Torzilli
Biomedical Mechanics and Molecular Design: Wright

Table 4 2011 Research Programs and Laboratories and Their Leaders

Arthritis and Tissue Degeneration Program (Blobel)
Laboratory of Cell-Cell Signaling in Disease and Tissue Regeneration (Blobel)
Laboratory of Cellular Signaling and Immune Regulation (Xiaoyu Hu, MD, PhD)
Laboratory of Cytokine Signaling and Inflammation (Ivashkiv)
Laboratory of Osteolysis Research (Paul Edward Purdue, PhD)
Laboratory of Steroid Hormone Receptors and Inflammation (Inez Rogatsky, PhD)
Autoimmunity and Inflammation Program (Crow)
Autoimmunity-Immunoregulation Laboratory (Crow)
Immunotherapy Laboratory
Inflammatory Effector Mechanisms Laboratory (Salmon)
Molecular Mechanisms of T-Cell Dysfunction in Autoimmunity (Alessandra Pernis, MD)
Lymphoid Tissue Organization and Function Laboratory (Lu)
Flow Cytometry Laboratory (Sergei Rudchenko, PhD)
Musculoskeletal Integrity Program (Boskey)
Mineralized Tissues Laboratory (Boskey)
Laboratory for Musculoskeletal Imaging and Spectroscopy (Philipp Mayer-Kuckuk, PhD)
Bone Adaptation (Bostrom)
Analytical Microscopy (Doty)
Infrared Imaging (Boskey)
Cell Signaling (Wei Zhu, PhD)
Tissue Engineering, Regeneration, and Repair Program (Torzilli)
Laboratory of Cartilage Biology (Mary Goldring, PhD)
Laboratory of Functional Tissue Engineering (Suzanne Maher, PhD)
Soft Tissue Research Laboratory (Torzilli)
Department of Biomechanics (Wright)

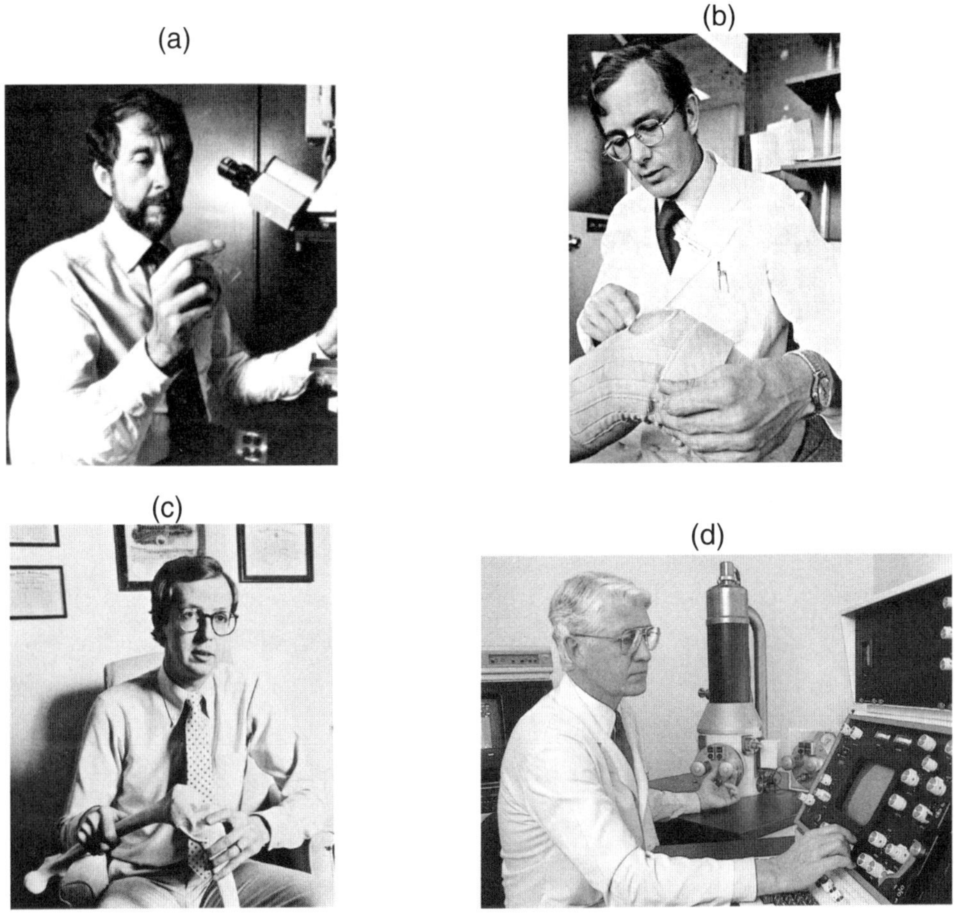

Fig. 3 Key contributors to research at HSS: comparative orthopaedics, pathology, and analytical microscopy. Peter Bullough, MD, 1985 (a); John Marshall, MD, 1970s (b); Steve Arnoczky, DVM, 1985 (c); Steven Doty, PhD, 1989 (d). (From Hospital for Special Surgery Archives)

Research Division laboratories. What has changed, most notably, are the techniques by which these studies are pursued, the closer link between the bench and the bedside, and the introduction of advanced biostatistical tools into these studies. In 2007, Stephen Lyman, PhD, established the Epidemiology and Biostatistics Core to assist with epidemiologic studies and study design in both the hospital and the Research Division.[21]

The Research Division Today

The Research Division remains on its original site, but the interior of the building was renovated into modern laboratory spaces in the 1990s to allow for expansion of the research faculty while providing new recruits with state-of-the art equipment for basic science, orthopaedic, and rheumatologic investigations. Thanks to an NIH reconstruction grant, the second floor was remodeled in 1999 into facilities equipped for molecular biology, cell culture, and flow cytometry. The modernizing of the 40-year-old research facility was then expanded to all seven floors of the building.

Additionally, the receipt of an NIH Core Center grant in 1999, under the Direction of Wright, led to the creation of new facilities for analytical microscopy, biomechanics, and imaging, including micro-CT and in vivo molecular imaging. This Core grant was used to support the research of orthopaedic clinicians and basic scientists, with 70% of the pilot grants being converted to NIH investigator-initiated awards to three clinicians and four basic scientists.

A unique feature of the Research Division has been its close ties with the Cornell University Campus in Ithaca, and in particular, the Sibley School of Mechanical and Aerospace Engineering. While recruiting for a director to replace Walker, the engineering school was consulted, and they suggested Donald L. Bartel, PhD, and Burstein as members of a search committee (Fig. 4). After the committee convened, Burstein indicated he was interested in the position. He was officially appointed in 1972, and he and Bartel established a linkage program that, almost 20 years later, became the paradigm for other programs between the Medical College and the Ithaca campus.

Bartel served as an adjunct member of the Biomechanics Department at HSS until his retirement in 2009, working closely with Burstein and his successor, Wright, on device design, student and resident teaching, and grant proposals. Bartel's role as the Sibley School of Engineering representative on the HSS faculty was assumed by Marjolein van der Meulen, PhD, who had been active in HSS research since she joined the Ithaca faculty.

This collaboration is but one example of "off-campus" HSS research. HSS investigators have always maintained close ties with collaborators at other institutions. Moreover, space limitations have led to biomechanics and other laboratories being moved "off-site" to the Dana Center on East 73rd Street, two blocks from the Caspary Research Building. These moves have occurred twice in the history of the Research Division, and while initially somewhat

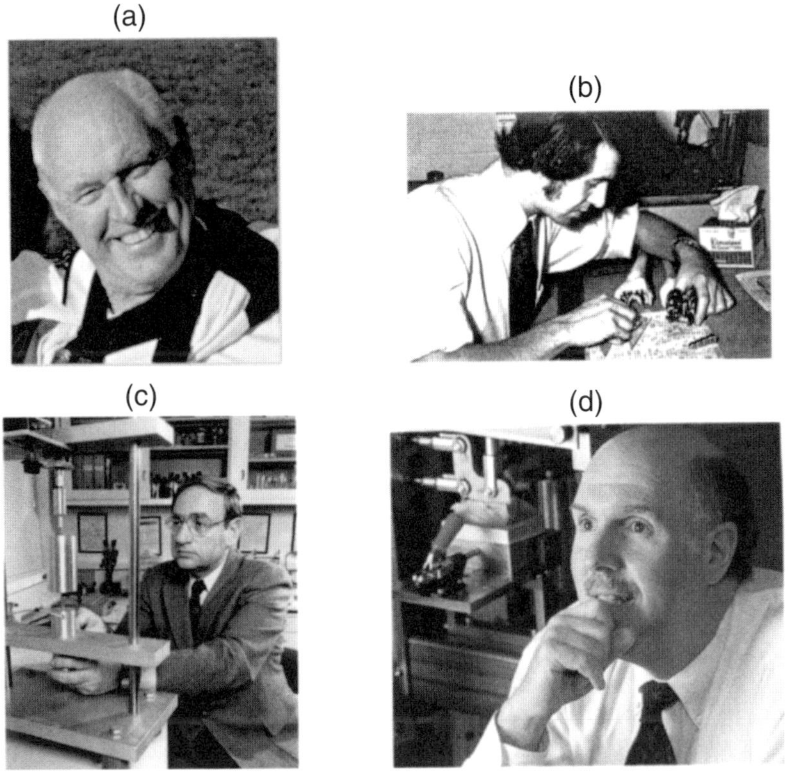

Fig. 4 Key contributors to HSS research: biomechanics. Harlan Amstutz, MD (a), was appointed the first director of biomechanics (1966–1970). Other directors were (b) Peter Walker, PhD (1970–1975), (c) Albert Burstein, PhD (1976–1991), and (d) Timothy Wright, PhD (1991–present). (From Hospital for Special Surgery Archives)

disruptive, the laboratories that moved have understood the space constraints and accepted the separation.

The expansion of research staff, programs, and laboratories in the Research Division was also accompanied by an almost exponential rise in grant funding. In 1960, when the Caspary Research Building opened, grants from all research resources (NIH, other agencies and foundations, and estates and trusts) totaled $202,420 (Fig. 5). By 1972, grants from NIH and endowments amounted to just over $1 million. By 1981, the Research Division received $1.5 million from the NIH alone. In 2000, HSS received $4.75 million in total NIH funds, and in 2010, even with reduced federal spending, HSS was awarded $17.5 million in federal support.[22]

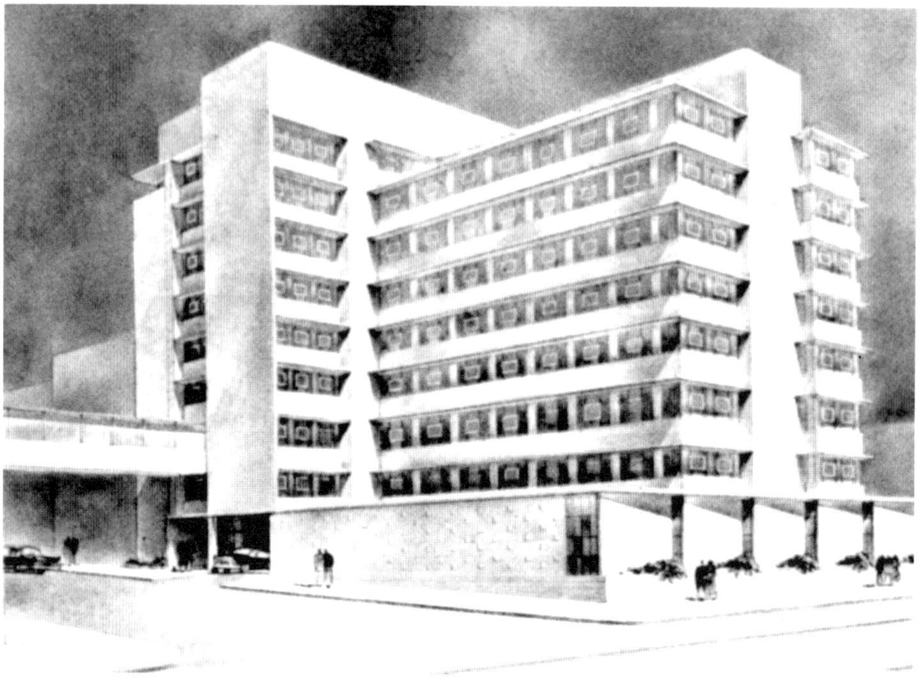

Fig. 5 The Caspary Research Building design includes seven floors, but only five were initially constructed. Two additional floors were added in 2002. The bridge crossing 71st Street joins the Research Building to the main hospital. (From Hospital for Special Surgery Archives)

REFERENCES

1. *History of the Priestley Medal 1972: George B. Kistiakowsky (1900–1982).* Chem Eng News. 2008;86:14.
2. Bauer GCH, Urist MR. *The use of radionuclides in orthopaedics: radionuclide scintimetry of the skeleton.* Clin Orthop Relat Res. 1993;287:3–12.
3. Kay MI, Young RA, Posner AS. *Crystal structure of hydroxyapatite.* Nature. 1964;204:1050–1052.
4. Boskey AL. *Amorphous calcium phosphate: the contention of bone.* J Dent Res. 1997;76:1433–1436.
5. Mahamid J, Sharir A, Gur D, Zelzer E, Addadi L, Weiner S. *Bone mineralization proceeds through intracellular calcium phosphate loaded vesicles: a cryo-electron microscopy study.* J Struct Biol. 2011;174:527–535.
6. Boskey AL, Mendelsohn R. *Infrared spectroscopic characterization of mineralized tissues.* Vib Spectrosc. 2005;38:107–114.
7. Wilson PD Jr., Levine DB. *Hospital for Special Surgery. A brief review of its development and current position.* Clin Orthop. 2000;374:90–105.

8. Ramirez F, Pereira L, Zhang H, Lee B. *The fibrillin–Marfan syndrome connection.* Bioessays. 1993;15:589–94.
9. *Ramirez named chief scientific officer at Hospital for Special Surgery*. Available at: www.hss.edu/newsroom_11317.asp.
10. *Profile for Carl Blobel, MD, PhD*. Available at: http://www.hss.edu/research-staff_blobel-carl.asp.
11. *Profile for Inez Rogatsky*. Available at: http://www.hss.edu/research-staff_rogatsky-inez.asp.
12. *Profile for Theresa Lu*. Available at: http://www.hss.edu/research-staff_lu-theresa.asp.
13. *Robert Wood Johnson Medicine*. 2006;Summer:37.
14. Amstutz HC, Sissons HA. *The structure of the vertebral spongiosa*. J Bone Joint Surg Br. 1969;51:540–50.
15. Amstutz HC. *Polymers as bearing materials for total hip replacement.* A friction and wear analysis. J Biomed Mat Res. 1968;3:547–568.
16. *Mary Kirkland Center for Lupus Research*. Available at: www.hss.edu/mary-kirkland.asp.
17. Salmon JE, Millard S, Schachter LA, Arnett FC, Ginzler EM, Gourley MF, Ramsey-Goldman R, Peterson MG, Kimberly RP. *Fc gamma RIIA alleles are heritable risk factors for lupus nephritis in African Americans*. J Clin Invest. 1996: 97:1348–1354.
18. *Ninety-Eighth Annual Report of the New York Society for the Relief of the Ruptured and Crippled.* New York, NY: New York Society for the Relief of the Ruptured and Crippled; 1961.
19. *Felix Bronner obituary*. Available at: http://www.the-aps.org/livinghistory/cvs/bronner.pdf.
20. *Leonhard Korngold obituary*. Available at: http://www.legacy.com/obituaries/wickedlocal-brewster/obituary.aspx?n=leonhard-korngold&pid=146392337.
21. *Discovery to recovery: clinical and research highlights at HSS; 2010 Fall.* Available at: http://www.hss.edu/files/D2Rfall2010.pdf
22. Available at: http://projectreporter.NIH.gov/reporter.cfm.

CHAPTER 18

RHEUMATOLOGY AT HSS: THE BEGINNING (EMPHASIS ON 1924–1995)

CHARLES L. CHRISTIAN, MD

Rheumatology Becomes a Subspecialty

"RHEUMATISM," A TERM FOR A category of illness, had its origin in antiquity, when disease was thought to result from the abnormal flux and flow of body humors, but the term "rheumatologist"—a physician with a special interest in the care of patients with musculoskeletal disease—did not arise until rather recently.

When the author of this chapter came to Hospital of Special Surgery in 1970, his titles were physician-in-chief, chairman of medicine, and director of rheumatic diseases. His predecessor, Richard H. Freyberg, MD, was also called director of rheumatic diseases (and neither would have introduced himself as a "rheumatologist" then), while before Freyberg, R. Garfield Snyder, MD, was director of the Arthritis Clinic.

Rheumatology would earn formal recognition as a clinical subspecialty in the United States following two key events: the approval by the American Board of Internal Medicine of subspecialty certification in Rheumatology in 1971 and the change in name of the American Rheumatism Association (ARA) to the American College of Rheumatology (ACR) in 1988.

The Early Years of Rheumatology at the Hospital for the Ruptured and Crippled

The two dominant figures in the early history of Hospital for the Ruptured and Crippled (R&C)—James Knight and Virgil P. Gibney—would qualify as rheumatologists according to the definition above. Many of Knight's patients in the earliest days of R&C likely had bone and joint tuberculosis, whereas others had a variety of congenital and acquired musculoskeletal problems.

Gibney and 10 other prominent physicians organized the New York Polyclinic Medical School in 1882, and the same year, he and a group of physicians and surgeons founded the Practitioner's Society of New York. Members of the Practitioner's Society met in their homes several times a year (in rotation) for a scientific program followed by dinner. Proceedings were published in *The Medical Record.*

Gibney enjoyed both the professional and the social aspects of membership, and from 1882 to 1888, he made 11 presentations on such topics as joint diseases and constitution treatment, Pott's disease, fibrous ankylosis of the shoulder and syphilitic joint disease. At the first meeting of the society in May 1882, Gibney's paper was entitled "The Sequelae of Measles, with Special Reference to the Development of a Strumous Diastheses." In his view, measles was associated with a variety of illnesses, including many now recognized as tuberculosis or other inflammatory conditions; no one present at the meeting was aware of Koch's identification of the tubercle bacillus, reported two months earlier. (For that matter, many physicians in America did not accept the infectious nature of tuberculosis for several years.) The skin lesions now associated with rheumatic syndromes and the cutaneous eruptions characteristic of systemic childhood arthritis, lupus erythemas, postrubella arthropathy, and so forth might have been the basis for Gibney's mistaken belief in the relationship between measles and "strumous diastheses."[a]

Gibney began practicing at R&C without any postdoctoral training. Subsequent interests and experience led him to the emerging field of orthopaedic surgery, and after 6 years of service, his title was changed from "assistant" to "house surgeon." Knight did not share Gibney's opinion that surgical treatment of some patients with arthritis was indicated and fired him in 1884 when Gibney published his text on hip disease.[1] (The early days of Knight and Gibney are chronicled in chapter 2.)

Rheumatology Enters the 20th Century

The first effort to organize an international campaign against rheumatism failed because of the exigencies associated with World War I. In 1913, at the

First International Congress on Physical Therapy, the Dutch physician Jan van Breemen advocated a worldwide effort to study and control rheumatic diseases. In Europe, the early leaders in rheumatology were physiatrists or hydrologists, many associated with spas, while virtually all leaders in America were internists. Van Breemen proposed the formation of an international institute and the preparation of a report to be considered in 1917 when the Congress was scheduled to meet in St. Petersburg.

The plan laid dormant until 1925, when van Breeman's proposal was re-examined. Two years later, at the meeting of the International Society of Medical Hydrology, an International Committee Against Rheumatism was established. In 1928, after several European countries had formed national committees, "Le Ligue International contre Rhumatisme" (The International League Against Rheumatism) was organized.

Physicians in North America began to meet in 1928, establishing the American Committee for Control of Rheumatism. At its first national meeting in New Orleans in 1932, its name was changed to the American Association for the Study and Control of Rheumatism. The name changed again (1936–1937) to the American Rheumatism Association (ARA). Of the 150 members in 1937, some 45 attended the meeting in Atlantic City that year (Fig. 1). All were men, and almost all were internists living along the eastern seaboard of the United States. (In contrast, attendance at ACR meetings since 2008 has exceeded 10,000, with more than half coming from overseas, and women are very well represented in the membership.)

R. Garfield Snyder: 1924 to 1944

The son of a Methodist clergyman, Snyder was born in Thamesville, Ontario, Canada in 1881. He graduated from the University of Toronto Medical School in 1904, came to New York in 1908, and served as assistant pathologist at the Russell Sage Institute of Pathology for 3 years. He was then appointed attending physician to the City Hospital of New York and professor of medicine at the New York Polyclinic Medical School. In 1924, his final year, Gibney—then surgeon-in-chief at R&C—recruited Snyder to be the director of the new Arthritis Clinic. The two men likely became acquainted via their New York Polyclinic Medical School appointments. Snyder thus became the first director of the first arthritis clinic in New York (Fig. 2).

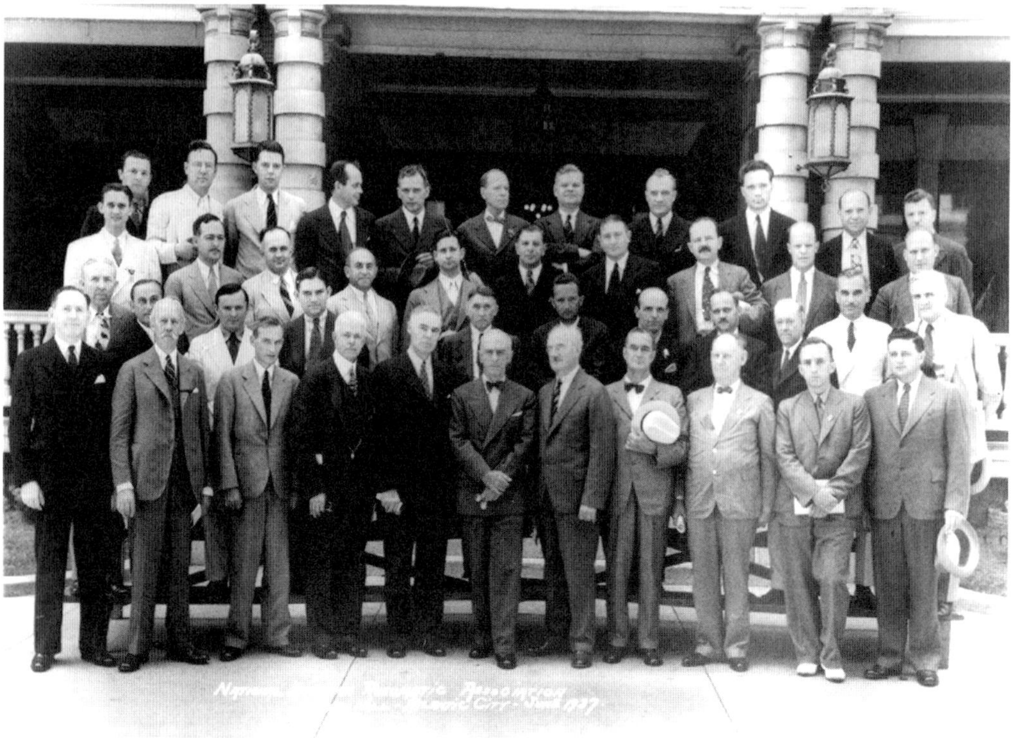

Fig. 1 Attendees at the meeting of the ARA in Atlantic City, June 1937 (mislabeled "National American Rheumatic Association" by the photographer). Early founders of the ARA are in the bottom row, beginning fourth from the left: Ernest Irons, Loring Swain, Russell Cecil, Homer Swift, Ralph Pemberton, and (far right) W. Paul Holbrook. All listed in the front row (except Homer Swift) were early presidents. Others who served as presidents include Otto Steinbocker (row two, second from the left); L. Maxwell Lockie (row three, fifth from left); Charles Short (row three, second from right); Philip Hench (back row, third from left), Walter Bauer (back row, fourth from left); M. Henry Dawson (back row, fifth from right), and Ralph Boots (back row, fourth from right). Robert Osgood, an orthopaedist from Boston and a founding member of the association, is in the middle of the back row. Connie Traeger (voluntary attending at HSS) is in the back row (far right). Second from right in the front row is Lemoyne Kelly, New York Hospital rheumatologist, who was a frequent collaborator with R. Garfield Snyder (first chief of the HSS Arthritis Clinic).

In the mid-1920s, there was scant scientific inquiry regarding rheumatology. The dominant hypothesis was that foci of bacterial infection (in diverse sites) caused chronic arthritis. In fact, a common synonym for rheumatoid arthritis was "chronic infectious arthritis." Foci of infection were sought in the sinuses, teeth and tonsils, and in the respiratory, gastrointestinal, and genitourinary tracts. Surgical drainage or removal of infected sites was recommended.

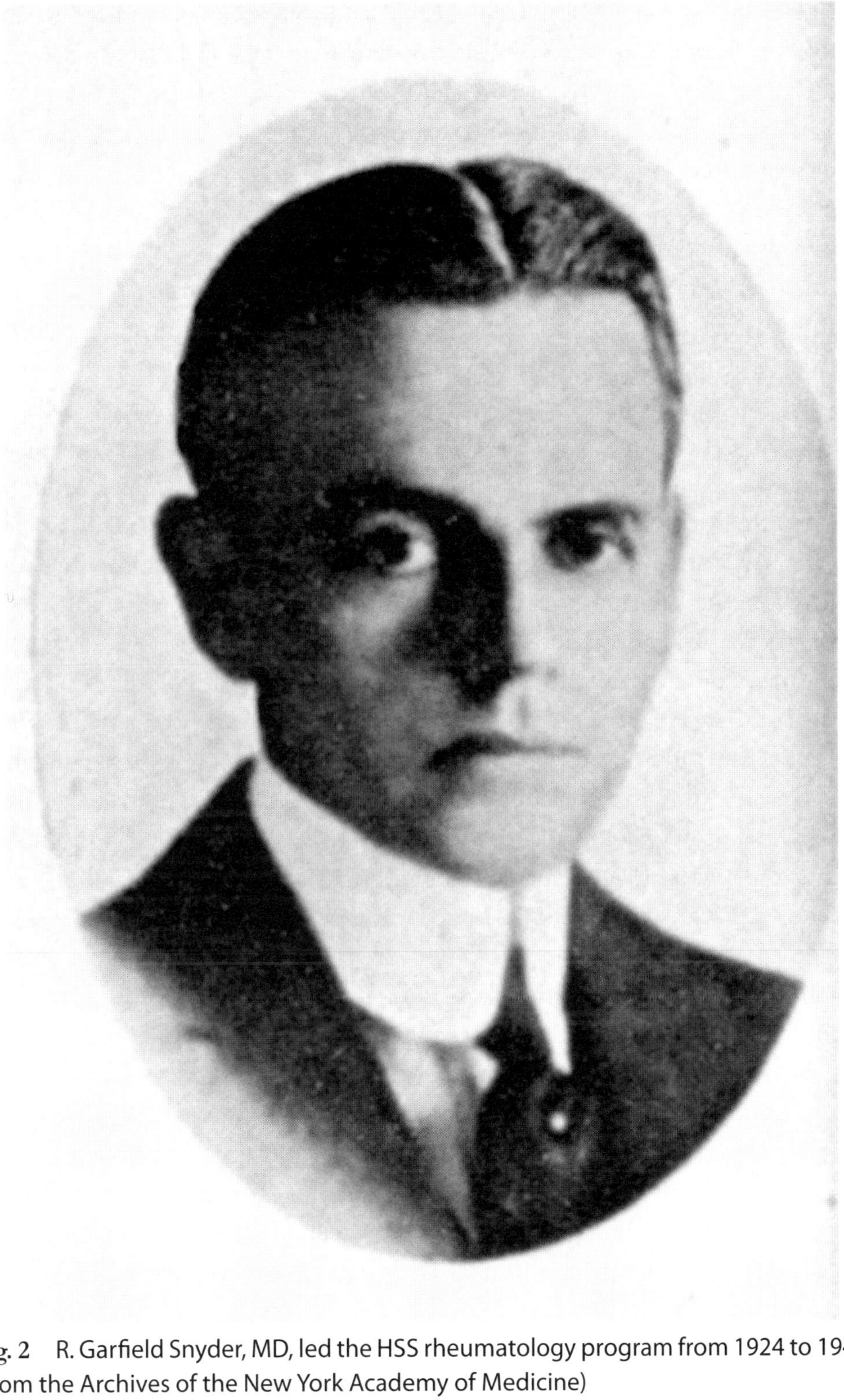

Fig. 2 R. Garfield Snyder, MD, led the HSS rheumatology program from 1924 to 1944. (From the Archives of the New York Academy of Medicine)

The 1925 roster of Arthritis Clinic staff included Mrs. Cora Gunther, "Research Worker in Bacteriology of Teeth and Mouth." In the 1927 Annual Report of R&C, it was noted that, having detected focal infection, "it has not been possible to eliminate them in each case for two reasons: (1) patients naturally fear that a fatal result will result from surgical interference, and (2) others claim that they cannot afford the extra expense of a few days in the Hospital." Vaccination with killed bacteria was a common treatment for rheumatoid arthritis, with some physicians favoring autogenous vaccines (bacteria cultured from individual patients).[b]

In his early years, Snyder published therapeutic studies (including those on vitamin D, cinchophen, and gold compounds) and reviews on sinusitis and colon stasis in association with arthritis and the efficacy of colonic irrigation.[c]

Snyder's office was at R&C on East 42nd Street. At the outset of his service, another physician, Augusta Rucker, MD, was listed as assistant attending physician in the Arthritis Clinic. By 1929, she and two other physicians (Connie H. Traeger, MD, and M. C. Shearer, MD) were all associate attending physicians.

In 1932, the list of associate attendings included Rucker, Traeger, and two others (N. W. Osher, MD, and C. A. Zoll, MD). Traeger and Zoll were coauthors with Snyder on publications. The record is not clear regarding the relationship of the associate attendings to the program, but they were almost certainly volunteers in the Arthritis Clinic who maintained outside offices as private practitioners. (In the early 1950s, Traeger was still an active volunteer physician at HSS.)

Scattered throughout annual reports from the 1930s are references to the impact of the "severe financial depression in the city" on the hospital. The 1937 report noted that a "special Arthritis Fund is urgently desired in order to help pay the cost of treatment and to finance research." In the 1930 report, it was reported that the entrance fee for the Arthritis Clinic had been increased to $3.00, with subsequent visits costing $1.00; total daily income to the clinic ranged from $25 to $30.

Snyder was also responsible for the recruitment and representation of physicians from other clinical specialties, such as urology, gynecology, otorhinolaryngology, dental surgery, neurology, and dermatology/syphilology. Some clinics met twice weekly, dermatology/syphilology once weekly, and others "by appointment." Orthopaedic and arthritis clinics could refer patients to an obesity clinic that met three times weekly, with visits totaling 4,085 in 1937. (No data are available, however, regarding the success of weight loss regimens.)

During the years of American involvement in World War II, a publication entitled "Record and Chronicle. Maintained by HSS for Dispensing the Family

Gossip to our Members with the Armed Services" was circulated monthly to HSS personnel overseas. The editors were Drs. Snyder, Wagner, Hansson and Carr, who called themselves the "Four Horsemen."

In one issue (volume II, number 17, October 1, 1943) contributed by "Pop" Snyder, it was announced that Carr (whose duties included financial management) had joined the Navy; the editorial group then numbered three. There were joking references to the belief that the homeland staff were working much harder than those in the military. There was an admission that the editors did some of their "hard work" in vacation spots (such as Rockland, Maine)—a mild complaint. Wagner (who made hotel arrangements for them) always signed in as "Lewis Clark Wagner and Party," and there was speculation (2 years before the defeat of Japan) when the war might end.

Snyder described his fellow editors as follows: Carr as "good-looking, dashing (rather stout), reddish moustache and never-ending infectious smile"; Wagner as a "quiet, good looking (but slightly corpulent) Southerner with that naughty twinkle in his eye"; and Hansson as a "tall, thin doctor with the erect figure, cold blue eyes, youthful complexion, crew-cut gray hair, [a] good looking Swede." As for himself, he wrote, "Pop Snyder doesn't look so bad himself. He dresses as smartly as ever and has the ever present bachelor's button or carnation in his buttonhole." He signed off, "Well so long boys. As the New York Times says, this is all the news that's fit to print."

Sadly, less than 6 months following that communication, Snyder had a more final "sign off"; he died unexpectedly on February 25, 1944, at age 63 years while visiting Palm Beach, Florida. His obituary in the *Annals of Internal Medicine* indicated gastric ulcer as the cause of death.

R. Garfield Snyder: In Summary

The 20 years that R. Garfield Snyder served at HSS were not tranquil times, characterized by extended financial depression, World War II, and the absence of any extramural support of patient care, medical research, and training. Conditions were not permissive of innovation in any of these spheres. Snyder was a well-trained internist, essentially working solo, who was challenged to learn more about rheumatic disease at a time when the tools required for scientific inquiry were still yet to come.

Richard H. Freyberg: 1944 to 1970

While Gibney essentially hand-picked R. Garfield Snyder, MD in 1924 as the first director of the HSS rheumatic disease program, evidence suggests that Philip D. Wilson Sr., MD, chose Snyder's successor: Richard H. Freyberg, MD in 1944.

Richard Freyberg was valedictorian of his high school class in Goshen, Indiana. He was a star basketball player, attended the University of Michigan, served as captain of the track team, and was one of the leading middle distance runners nationally during the 1920s. After medical and postgraduate training in Ann Arbor, he joined the faculty there, and in 1937, was appointed as the first director of the Rackham Arthritis Research Unit.

His research efforts focused on calcium and phosphorus metabolism and the pharmacokinetics of gold compounds. During the 1930s, several laboratories had reported perturbations of sulfur metabolism in patients with rheumatoid arthritis and suggested that administration of sulfur, in various forms, was therapeutic. Freyberg and his colleagues laid these claims to rest in careful and thorough studies, concluding that "no evidence of sulfur deficiency or abnormality in sulfur metabolism was found to exist in patients with rheumatoid arthritis" and that there was "no biochemical or metabolic indication of need for, or benefit from, sulfur medication in the treatment of rheumatoid arthritis."[2]

How and why did Freyberg, age 40 years in 1944, come to HSS? In a profile published in *HSS Horizon* (volume 1, number 3), he indicated that he desired to "broaden the scope of his work." He knew HSS was seeking someone to lead the rheumatic disease program. A surgical colleague at Michigan who had been a Harvard roommate of Wilson probably played a role in Freyberg's recruitment. There is no record of discussion nor communication between Freyberg and Wilson, but before the end of the year, Freyberg had accepted an invitation to come to New York as HSS director of rheumatic diseases.

In addition to space for arthritis clinics and Freyberg's office, rooms in the hospital on East 42nd Street were remodeled and converted to laboratory space suitable for research. Records indicate, however, that his main goal at the outset (and for some time) was the establishment of a state-of-the-art clinical service and a training program for rheumatology fellows.

Bernard Rogoff, MD, returning from military duty in New Guinea, shared an office and practice with Freyberg. Rheumatic disease research was about to experience a sea change, and Freyberg, with his expertise in metabolic studies, was well positioned to be a major player.

Freyberg served as president of the ARA (1948–1949) and as chairman of the Seventh International Congress on Rheumatic Diseases when it met in New York in 1949. At this meeting, the first report of the dramatic effects of cortisone treatment in rheumatoid arthritis patients was presented.[3] Freyberg was one of five clinical investigators outside of the Mayo Clinic chosen to extend and confirm the efficacy of cortisone, thus launching the first clinical trial of cortisone therapy in New York at HSS.

During his tenure at HSS, Freyberg was a leading participant in several prominent activities (Fig. 3):

- He served on a committee of the National Research Council that recommended the formation of a national voluntary agency to support arthritis education and research.
- He recruited one of his patients (Floyd B. Odlum, a leader in the financial community and CEO of Atlas Corporation) to be the founding chairman of the Arthritis and Rheumatism Foundation.
- He was a consultant and advisor pertinent to Congressional passage of the Omnibus Medical Research Act in 1950, which authorized formation of the National Institute of Arthritis and Metabolic Disease (NIAMD) and the NIH Clinical Center in Bethesda, and greatly expanded extramural NIH Training and Research Programs. Freyberg was a member of the first Advisory Council of NIAMD and served again from 1955 to 1957.
- He was elected president of the Pan American League Against Rheumatism (1953–1957).
- He played a major role in the establishment of the journal *Arthritis and Rheumatism* and in the selection of its first editor, William S. Clark, MD.

Richard Freyberg's role at HSS changed when the hospital moved to East 70th Street in 1955 and began its affiliation with New York Hospital (NYH) and Cornell University Medical College. During the first decade of his service (on East 42nd

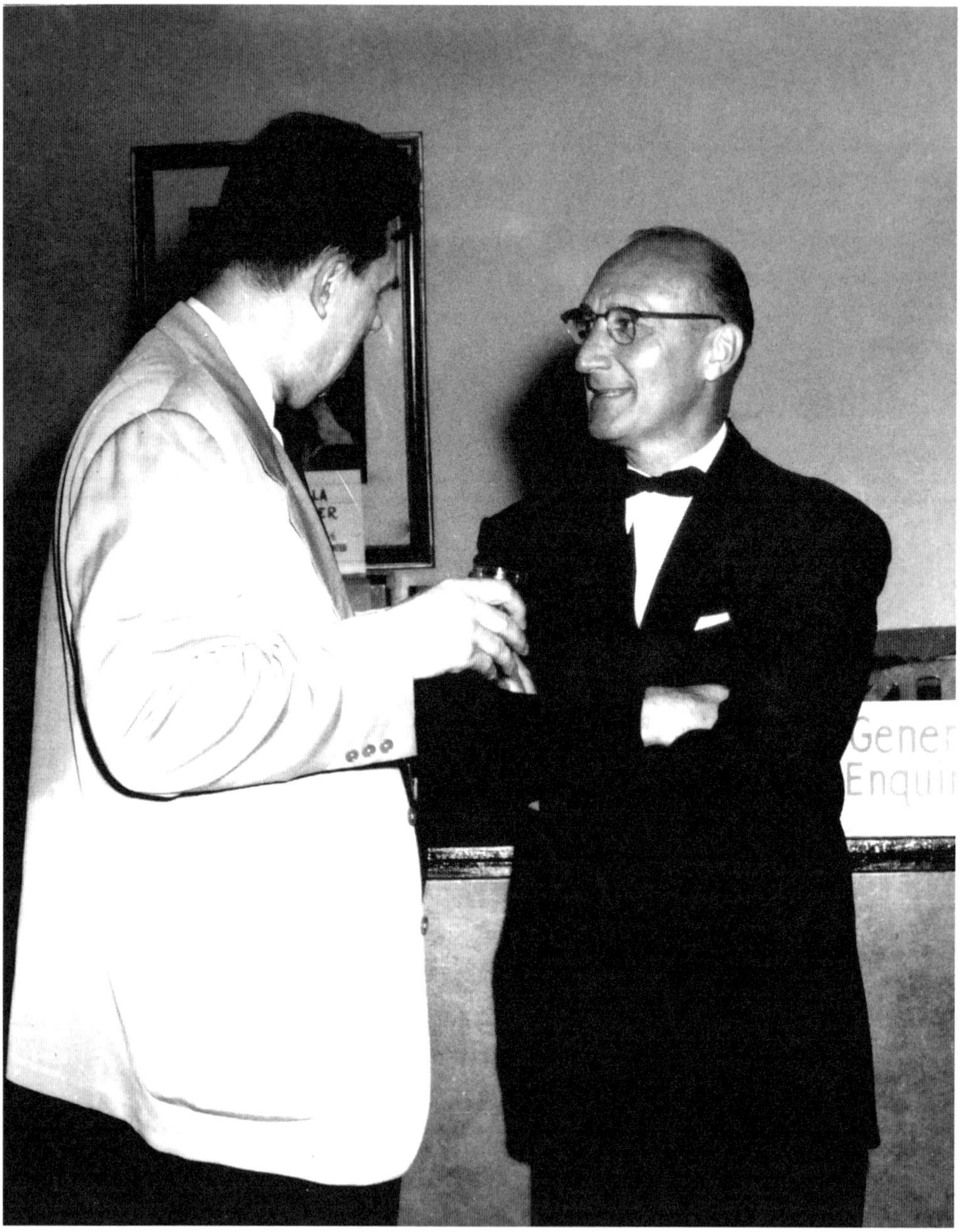

Fig. 3 Toronto, 1958: Richard H. Freyberg, MD (right), speaking with Philip S. Hench, MD, ScD (1950 Nobel Laureate). Freyberg led the HSS rheumatology program from 1944 to 1970.

Street), there was a degree of isolation from the scientific resources of a university medical center. In time, the association with Cornell would foster a wider range of opportunities. Simultaneously, there would be an explosion of new concepts and techniques pertinent to the study of rheumatic disease (Table 1).

In the new setting, the many attending physicians at NYH were available as consultants to HSS, and NYH medical residents were assigned to serve rotations on the HSS inpatient rheumatology service. In the mid-1960s, when

Table 1 Discoveries Relevant to Rheumatology Research

1940s	**1950s**
Immunofluorescent microscopy	Immune tolerance
DNA transformation	Clonal selection theory
Coombs technique	Radioimmune assay
Experimental allergic encephalopathy	Ion-exchange chromatography
Rheumatoid factor (rediscovery)	Murine lupus (NZB)
LE cell described	Thyroid autoimmunity
Cortisone therapy for rheumatoid arthritis	IgG structure
	Immune complex disease
	Autoimmunity, new concepts
	Structure of DNA

1960s	**1970s**
Genetic code	Monoclonal antibodies
Role of thymus in immune regulation	Recombinant technology
B/T-lymphocyte concept	T-cell subsets (monoclonal antibodies)
T-cell rosette technique	MHC spondyloarthropathy, rheumatoid arthritis, and lupus
MHC-linked immune response genes	FcR functions
Restricted endonucleases	Interferon α/lupus
Gel filtration chromatography	Hepatitis B-associated vasculitis
Crystal-induced arthropathy	

1980s	**1990s**
PCR technique	HIV biology
Anti-phospholipid syndrome	Apoptosis
Gene knockout technique	FAS defect/autoimmunity
Neonatal lupus	Microarray technique
Methotrexate for rheumatoid arthritis	C1q deficiency/lupus
	Anti-TNF therapy for rheumatoid arthritis

there was concern about the support and supervision of NYH residents during their HSS rotations, Martin Gardy, MD, a general internist from NYH, was hired to address that need.

The rheumatology attending staffs of HSS and NYH were fused, complementing the HSS professional staff (Fig. 4). The NYH staff included William Kammerer, MD, Robert Lintz, MD, Marion Tyndall, MD, Emmanuel Rudd, MD, Sidney Rothbard, MD, Abraham Jacobson, MD, and William Robbins, MD. Robbins had postdoctoral research training at the Rockefeller University, and had participated in some of the earliest studies of autoimmunity in patients with systemic lupus. Rothbard was involved in immunologic studies of collagen in experimental models of disease. Establishment of an NIH Rheumatic Disease Training Program allowed for expansion of clinical and research fellowships.

The opening of the Caspary Research Building at HSS in 1960 provided an opportunity to develop laboratory-based research, which had enjoyed only modest success in the rheumatology field. The recruitment of George Heller, MD, an immunologist at the Bronx VA Center, was planned, but he died before his expected arrival at HSS. For a year or two, Ralph Heimer, PhD, a Columbia University-trained proteoglycan chemist, established a laboratory to study rheumatoid arthritis serological phenomena and then accepted a position at Jefferson Medical College. Jose Granda, MD, PhD, was accepted as a fellow in 1966; he was involved in studies of proteolytic enzymes in inflammatory joint fluid, and later served as chief of rheumatology in a VA Medical Center in Michigan.

A unique activity at HSS was initiated in the mid-1960s: the Comprehensive Arthritis Program (CAP), a venture led by Freyberg and Straub. CAP was built around a weekly consultative clinic that brought together faculty representing rheumatology, orthopaedics, nursing, allied health professionals, house staff, fellows, and students. It also featured an inpatient service for patients selected for surgical rehabilitation—usually prosthetic arthroplasty. CAP became the prototype program for multispecialty collaboration in education, research, and patient care relative to chronic arthritis. After five decades, it is still in play at HSS and is now called the Surgical Arthritis Program.

Richard H. Freyberg: In Summary

During his quarter decade of service to HSS, Freyberg was a preeminent clinician/teacher, a very skilled and conscientious physician, and a much-admired

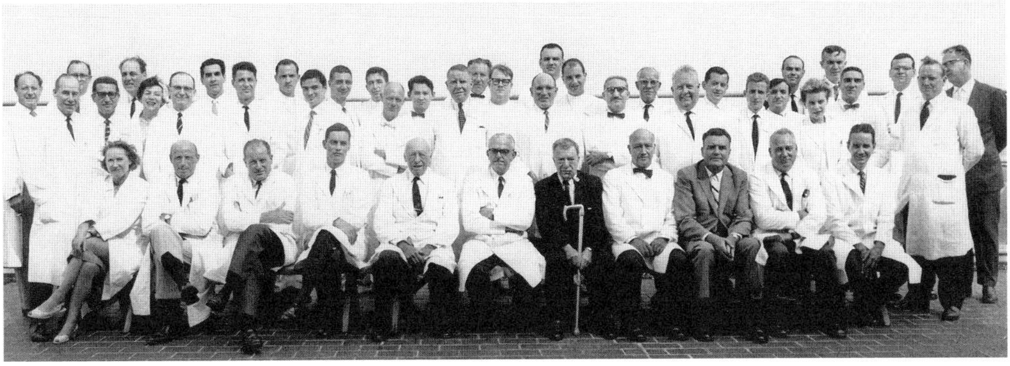

Fig. 4 1962: HSS professional staff on the rooftop of HSS. (From Hospital for Special Surgery Archives)

academic leader, both nationally and internationally. He made important observations as a clinical investigator early in his career, but laboratory research was not his forte. Freyberg would establish an NIH-funded postdoctoral training program, but he passed on opportunities to promote laboratory-based rheumatic disease research.

For 3 years after Freyberg retired, he maintained a small practice in New York. He left for Palm Desert, California, where he helped establish the Arthritis & Rheumatism Wing of the Eisenhower Medical Center. He retired to Venice, Florida, in 1976, and died in 1999 at age 94 years.

Charles L. Christian: 1970 to 1995

Charles L. Christian, MD (the author of this chapter), was born in Wichita, Kansas, on July 10, 1926. After being educated in local public schools, he served in the navy from 1944 to 1946, where he had his first experience as a medical professional (as an operating room technician). Following his military service, he attended and graduated from Wichita State University and Case Western Reserve School of Medicine, completing postdoctoral training at Columbia-Presbyterian Medical Center.

Christian joined the faculty of Columbia College of Physicians & Surgeons, succeeded his mentor (Charles A. Ragan Jr., MD) as director of the Edward Daniels Faulkner Arthritis Clinic, and attained tenure rank in 1969. In 1970, he accepted the positions of physician-in-chief at HSS and professor of medicine at Cornell University Medical College.

Summarizing his decision to move from Columbia to Cornell, he noted that

- Although both institutions were highly regarded, the climate for developing multidisciplinary programs was (at that time) more favorable at Cornell.
- A special opportunity existed at HSS for establishing a unique partnership between rheumatology and orthopaedics in patient care, education, and research.
- There was agreement from HSS management to fund additional faculty positions.
- Henry G. Kunkel, MD, a much admired scientist at Rockefeller University, volunteered his support for collaborative research and research training.

Christian started at HSS on January 1, 1970. Four younger colleagues from Columbia arrived the following July 1: Lawrence J. Kagen, MD, Robert W. Lightfoot Jr., MD, Michael D. Lockshin, MD, and Paul E. Phillips, MD (Fig. 5). They had all served as rheumatic disease fellows at Columbia. Two fellows were appointed at HSS: Graham R. V. Hughes, MD (from England), and Stefano Bombardieri, MD (from Pisa, Italy).

HSS leadership made a very large commitment by taking on five new academic full-time faculty who would be spending a significant part of their time doing research. There was no prior institutional experience with such an arrangement. The HSS Board was a little nervous regarding the financial commitment. Strong support came from the surgeon-in-chief, Robert Lee Patterson Jr., and two board members—Philip Bastedo (President) and Marshall Rawle. In addition to the new recruits, members of the HSS/Cornell faculty who continued to serve included William Kammerer, Bernard Rogoff, Martin Gardy, Emmanuel Rudd, William Robbins, Robert Lintz, Sidney Rothbard, Abraham Jacobson, Jose Granda, and Edgar Desser—all as voluntary staff.

Productivity during Christian's tenure as director of the Rheumatic Disease Program can be measured by assessing progress in four overlapping and interdependent areas: training of fellows, research, the development of a

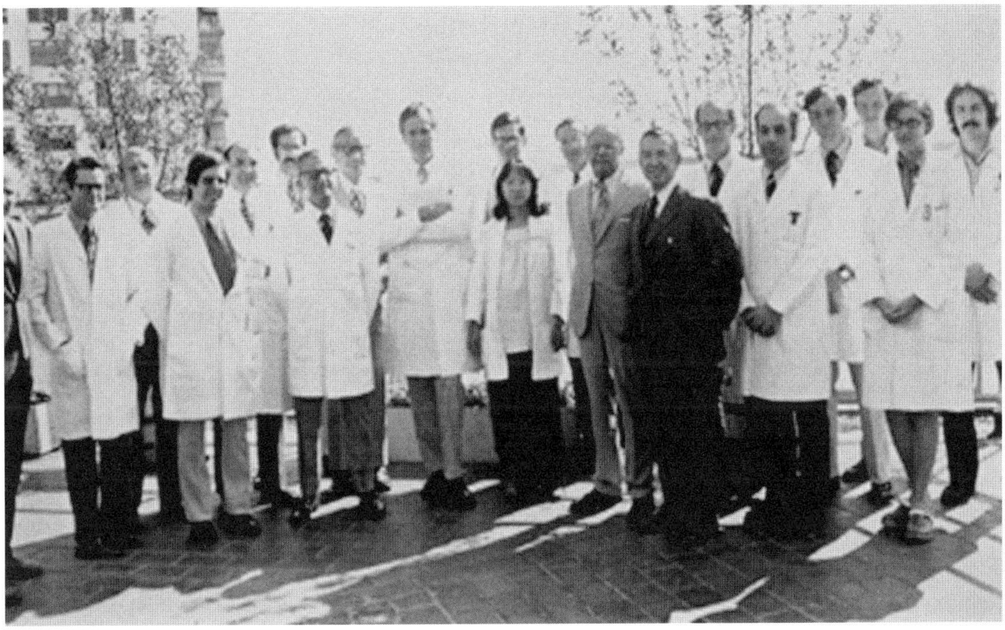

Fig. 5 Rheumatology staff and fellows on the HSS roof in 1972. From left: Jose Granda, Marcos Rivelis, Michael Lockshin, Martin Gardy, Sidney Block, Bernard Rogoff, Herbert Koteen, Charles Christian, William Gough, Teresita Go, Paul Phillips, William Kammerer, Carl Bernsten, Robert Lightfoot, Ron Saykaly, John Sergent, Andrew Eisenhauer, Patricia Redecha, and Michael Knapp. (From Hospital for Special Surgery Archives)

multipurpose arthritis center, and experience with a practice plan for hospital-based academic physicians.

Training

Talented trainees—whether headed for roles in clinical medicine, research, teaching, or some combination thereof—are critically important for academic programs to achieve high quality. Trainees "pick up" new leads and tips, challenge their mentors and keep them honest, carry heavy responsibilities for guiding younger colleagues (students, house officers, and junior fellows), and constitute the most important pool of candidates for faculty recruitment. A list of trainees who were in fellowship status in 1995 or before appears in Table 2.

Fourteen former trainees (as of 1995) were HSS faculty; nine had directed major rheumatology programs in the United States or abroad; three were destined to serve as ACR Presidents (John Sergent, MD, Allan Gibofsky, MD, and

Table 2 Rheumatology Fellows: 1970 to 1995

Anderson-Imbert, Anabel	1971–1973	Magid, Steven K.	1979–1981
Ashany, Dalit	1988–1991	Magsaam, Juergen	1986–1988
Beary, John F. III	1978–1980	Mancuso, Carol	1989–1991
Bhardwaj, Nina	1984–1987	Marcus, Ralph J.	1974–1976
Bini, Paolo	1988–1989	Markenson, Joseph	1975–1977
Block, Sidney	1973–1975	McDougal, J. Steven	1973–1974
Bombardieri, Stephano	1970–1971	McDougal, J. Steven	1977–1978
Bonfa, Eloisa	1984–1987	McNally, Jeremy	1994–1997
Bucala, Richard	1988–1991	Mevorach, Dror	1995–1998
Chang, David	1991–1994	Mysler, Eduardo	1992–1995
Chartash, Elliot	1985–1988	Onel, Karen	1992–1995
Chatpar, Prem	1983–1985	Paget, Stephen A.	1975–1977
Clarkson, Sarah B.	1983–1985	Parris, Ted M.	1979–1981
Crow, Mary K. (Peggy)	1981–1983	Philip, George	1988–1990
DelGiudice-Asch, Gina	1990–1993	Polk, J. Robert	1979–1981
Drappa, Jorn	1995–1998	Porges, Andrew	1989–1992
Edberg, Jeffrey	1990–1992	Russell, Linda	1992–1995
Elkon, Keith	1981–1982	Russo, Pamela W.	1987–1989
Fafalak, Robert	1990–1992	Salmon, Jane E.	1981–1983
Furie, Richard	1983–1985	Saykaly, Ronald J.	1972–1974
Georgescu, Liviu	1994–1996	Scarpa, Nicholas	1983–1985
Go, Terisita	1973–1975	Schnapp, Jerome J.	1971–1972
Golombek, Steven	1984–1986	Schned, Eric	1979–1981
Gottlieb, Alice	1982–1984	Schwartzman, Sergio	1985–1988
Gough, William W.	1972–1974	Sergent, John S.	1972–1974
Gratwick. Geoffrey	1975–1977	Spiera, Robert F.	1992–1995
Greisman, Stewart	1984–1986	Stern, Richard	1975–1976
Harisdangkul, Valee	1971–1973	Stevenson, Jon T.	1980–1982
Hasler, Paul	1989–1991	Teitel, Ariel	1989–1992
Hughes, Graham RV	1970–1971	Vaishnow, Akshay	1995–1998
Inman, Robert D.	1977–1979	Wainstein, Eduardo	1993–1996
Jover, Juan	1985–1988	Walsh, Mary Beth	1977–1979
Kaell, Alan T.	1981–1983	Waxman, Jack	1971–1993
Kassan, Stuart S.	1976–1978	Weiss, Allen	1975–1977
Kimberly, Robert P.	1977–1979	Whitman, H. Hal	1978–1980
Kirou, Kyriakos	1995–1998	Yee, Arthur M. F.	1993–1996
Lans, David	1987–1989	Young, James W.	1982–1984
Lawson, John	1987–1989	Zagon, Gary	1990–1993
Levy, Roger	1987–1989	Gibofsky, Allan	1977–1979

Mary K. (Peggy) Crow, MD); and two would become HSS physician-in-chief (Stephen Paget, MD, and Crow).[d] Other fellows would, via various pathways, achieve distinguished careers (Fig. 6).

Thomas J. A. Lehman, MD, was recruited in 1987 to establish the HSS Division of Pediatric Rheumatology. He also served as Chief of Pediatric Rheumatology at New York Hospital. Providing the services of a state-of-the-art clinical center, he has trained more than 20 pediatric rheumatologists, several of whom are directing programs in the United States and abroad. In 2007, Lehman received the American Academy of Pediatrics' James T. Cassidy Award for excellence in teaching and patient care and the training of the next generation of pediatric rheumatologists.

Research

In the 1950s and 1960s, coincident with expanded federal support of research and research training, new concepts, and insights greatly expanded opportunities

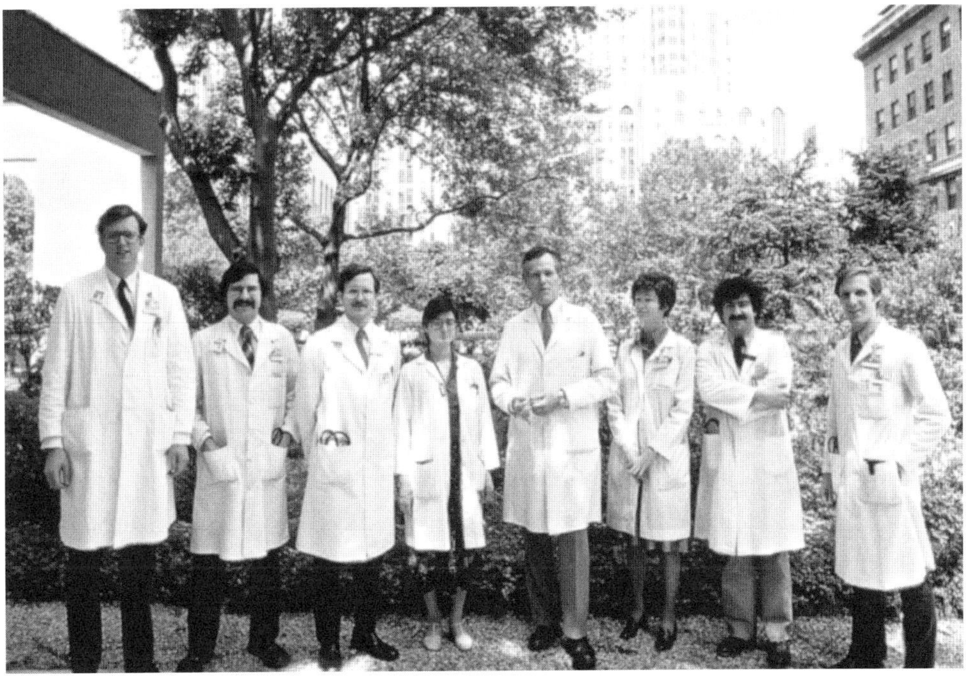

Fig. 6 HSS rheumatology fellows with Charles Christian on the Rockefeller University campus in 1979. From left: Hal Whitman, Robert Inman, John Beary, Stephanie Korn, Charles Christian, Mary Beth Walsh, Allan Gibofsky, and Robert Kimberly. (From Hospital for Special Surgery Archives)

for the study of rheumatic diseases. In particular, there was new evidence supporting the immunologic mediation of tissue inflammation and injury and features associated with rheumatoid arthritis, systemic lupus erythematosus (SLE), Sjögren syndrome, vasculitis, and other autoimmune diseases (Table 1).

In the search for potential stimuli of the immune system, investigators' attention focused on microbial factors. With some illnesses, there were explicit links—such as hemolytic streptococci and acute rheumatic fever, *Borrelia* species in Lyme disease, hepatitis B infection and systemic vasculitis, chlamydia, and gram-negative bacterial infection in seronegative arthritis, and a variety of autoimmune manifestations of hepatitis C infection. In other situations, the connection between infection and the pathogenesis of rheumatic disease remained hypothetical.[4]

Christian's research, which began at Columbia, centered on a variety of areas and generated new data on the link between immunity and rheumatic disease:

- He demonstrated that rheumatoid factor reactivity with gamma globulin preparations was dependent on the presence of aggregates in the latter; that aggregates of gamma globulin could be increased by chemical and heat treatment; and that such aggregates simulate properties of immune complexes, activate complement, and induce inflammatory lesions *in vivo*.

- He showed that hyperimmunization of rabbits with bacteria induced antibodies reacting with gamma globulin and DNA.

- He reported that the response of rabbits to daily intravenous administration of heterologous serum albumin was variable. One group was immunologically tolerant, another group made large amounts of precipitating antibody, and a third group produced large amounts of nonprecipitating antibody. Only the latter group manifested features of chronic serum sickness.

Of the other new faculty arriving in 1970, Paul Phillips had previous experience in virologic research. He initiated a program seeking evidence to link viral infection to SLE.[5] He also developed a tissue culture model for in vitro studies of rheumatoid synovial explants.[6] Christian, Lockshin, and Sergent extended studies of the association of hepatitis B virus with systemic vasculitis.[7] Later, Robert Inman, MD (who came to HSS as a fellow in 1977), demonstrated that both hepatitis B antigens and corresponding antibodies were present in circulating immune complexes in such patients[8] (Fig. 5).

The biological properties of immune complexes in rheumatic disease patients and in experimental models of disease were determined in studies involving Christian, Inman, Robert P. Kimberly, MD, and J. Stephen McDougal, MD (a fellow beginning in1973).[9,10] Lockshin and Sidney Block, MD (a fellow beginning in 1973), with collaborators in Cornell and Rockefeller laboratories, conducted a classic study of SLE in twin pairs (both homozygous and dizygous).[11,12] The study clearly documented the power of genes, with concordance in two thirds of monozygous twins, and also the power of environmental factors, since some identical twin pairs were discordant for disease.

Lockshin, in collaboration with scientists at the University of Oklahoma, later demonstrated that the "well" subjects in discordant pairs tended to have the same profile of autoantibodies manifesting in their "sick" twin siblings, albeit at lower levels.[13] His laboratory was also involved in early studies documenting impaired cellular immunity in people with rheumatic disease.[14]

Kagen's interests focused on muscle disease, particularly inflammatory myopathy. His documentation of myoglobulinemia in such subjects was the stimulus for his 1973 monograph entitled "Myoglobin. Biochemical, Physiological and Clinical Aspects."[15] (see Fig. 2, chapter 17, photo of Kagen). Inman and Eric S. Schned, MD (a fellow from 1979 to 1981), characterized the immune reactants in infectious endocarditis—a model of immune complex disease of known etiology.[16, e]

As rheumatology-related research interests at HSS to explore the immunopathogenesis of rheumatic disease continued circa 1970, dramatic new insights and concepts were unfolding that would bolster the field, including new knowledge regarding the

- biology of cytokine networks
- definition of receptor/ligand relationships
- knowledge of immune response genes
- associations of major histocompatibility complex (MHC) antigens with rheumatic diseases

- relationship of apoptosis (programmed cell death) to health and disease
- new dimensions of cellular immunity (T/B lymphocyte compartments, T-cell subsets, dendritic cells, and so forth)
- new insights regarding autoimmunity (with an expanded list of autoantibodies, some which are distinctly pathogenic, and differentiation of "benign" and "pathologic" patterns of autoimmunity)
- better definition of hypercoagulant pathology
- recognition of the power of genes as risk factors for the development of disease.

In short, medical research became molecular.

In the early 1980s, several clinical scientists (younger than the 1970 group) were recruited to the rheumatology program: Drs. Crow and Kimberly, Keith B. Elkon, MD, Steven M. Friedman, MD, and Jane E. Salmon, MD. All but Friedman had served as HSS fellows. Friedman graduated from Cornell University Medical College and served his medical residency at New York Hospital, and his research training was completed at Harvard and Columbia.[f]

All five members of this group were gaining expertise in the techniques of molecular biology. They formed collaborative relationships with each other, as well with other scientists, clinicians, and fellows. There were particularly close investigative ties between Crow and Friedman and between Kimberly and Salmon.

Elkon, a native of South Africa, arrived at HSS in 1982 after several years at London's Hammersmith Hospital, where Christian first met him. Early in his U.S. experience, Elkon was an apprentice to senior scientists at the Roche Institute in order to learn, at the bench, the techniques of molecular biology. He defined the molecular character of cellular targets of some autoantibodies[17,18] and was a major contributor to knowledge about apoptosis and its role in normal homeostasis and the development of autoimmunity.[19] In 1993, Elkon received an NIH Specialized Center of Research (SCOR) grant for the study of SLE (see Fig. 2, from chapter 17, photo of Elkon). He was successful in recruiting one of his former U.K. colleagues, E. A. Gharavi, to provide technical support and to continue Gharavi's studies of the antiphospholipid syndrome (APLS).[g]

Before joining forces, both Crow and Friedman had pursued studies of the cellular elements of immune regulation. As a laboratory technician before entering medical school, Crow had discovered and studied the autologous mixed lymphocyte reaction, and then other aspects of immune regulation.[20,21] Friedman's research interest focused on allospecific human helper T-cell lines that amplify B- and T-cell responses.[22] Crow and Friedman maintained individual research interests and were also natural and productive collaborators (Fig. 7).

As a research trainee at the NIH before his arrival at HSS as a fellow in 1977, Kimberly had participated in studies demonstrating a striking impairment of splenic phagocyte function in patients with SLE. That discovery set the stage for a systematic and sustained effort to determine the basis for this phenomenon.[23] Salmon (who came to HSS as a fellow in 1981) joined forces with Kimberly. She had some research training as a predoctoral student at Columbia College of Physicians and Surgeons. Their partnership generated an amazing trove of information regarding the structure, genetic control, heterogeneity, and function of Fc (gamma) receptors[24] (Fig. 8).[h]

Lionel B. Ivashkiv, MD, came to HSS later than the clinical scientists described above, joining the HSS and Cornell faculties in 1992 after rheumatology and

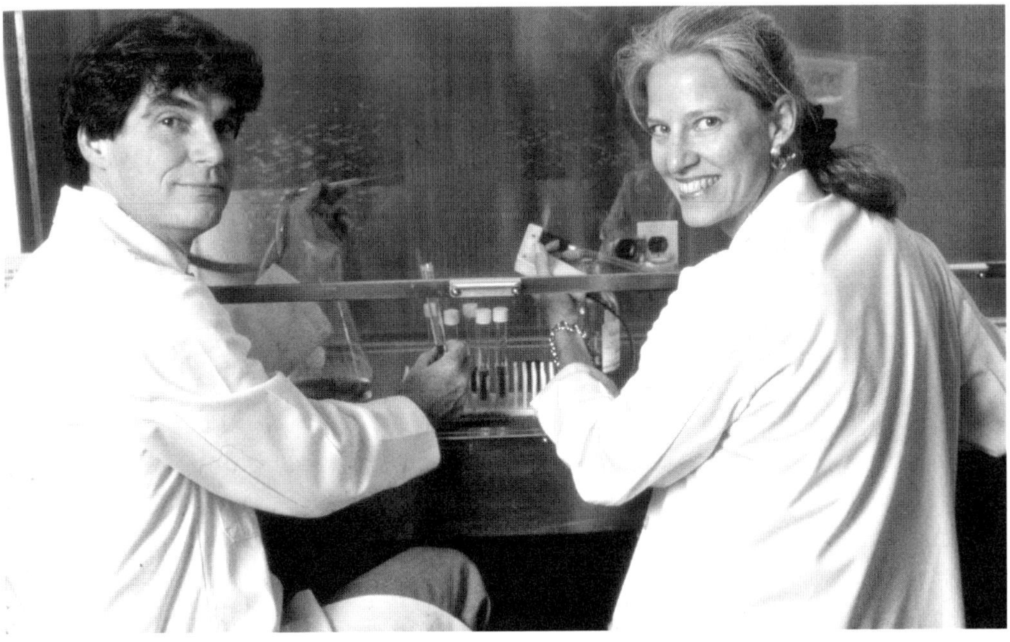

Fig. 7 1988: Mary K. (Peggy) Crow, MD, and Steven M. Friedman, MD, were research collaborators at HSS. (From Hospital for Special Surgery Archives)

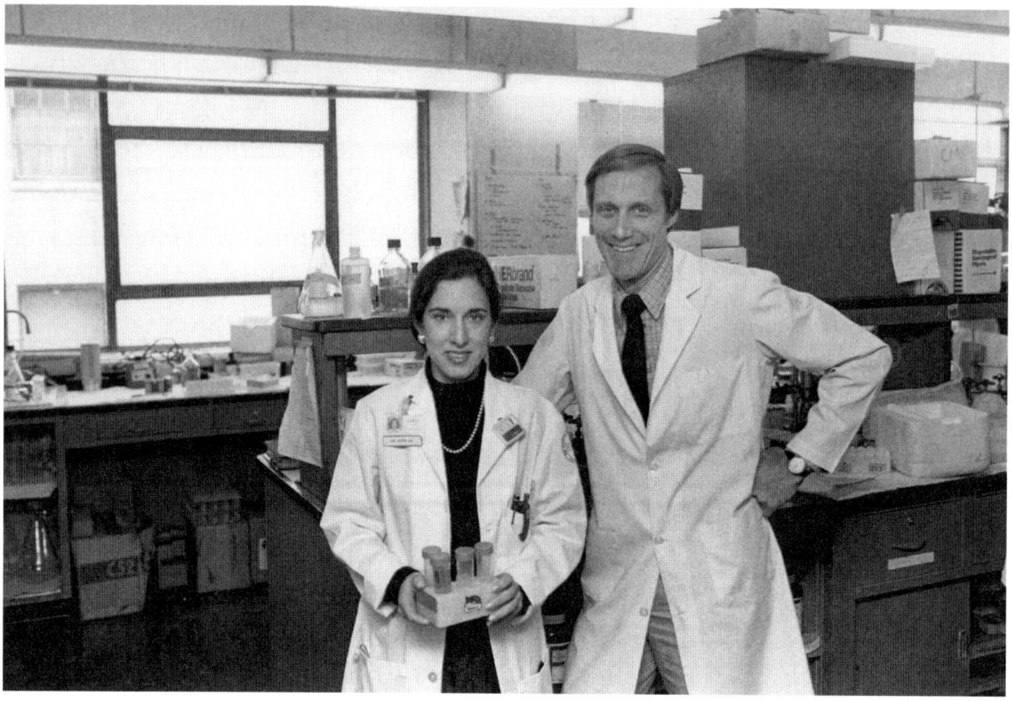

Fig. 8 1988: Robert P. Kimberly, MD, and Jane E. Salmon, MD, were an integral part of the rheumatology research effort at HSS. (From Hospital for Special Surgery Archives)

research fellowships at Brigham and Women's Hospital and Harvard Medical School (Fig. 9). His research mentor at Harvard was Laurie H. Glimcher, MD.[i] Ivashkiv's research experience in Boston focused on the regulation of class II MHC genes. In the HSS/Cornell environment, he shifted to studies pertinent to inflammation, tissue destruction, and repair and to cytokine/chemokine regulation of such processes. He has an enviable record in establishing collaborations with Rockefeller and Cornell scientists, in gaining extramural support of his research, and in achieving success in attracting talented trainees.[j]

In addition to their research, the clinical scientists in the rheumatology program at HSS have had important collateral functions: they maintain some contact with bedside and clinical conference activities; they serve as role models for students, house officers, and fellows; and they educate (and are educated by) more clinically oriented faculty and trainees. Their bibliographies contain dozens of names of coauthors who were fellows, younger faculty, and clinical colleagues.

The study of APLS is an example of the productive interplay between bedside observations and scientific inquiry. HSS faculty (past and present) played key roles in the development of the concept.[k]

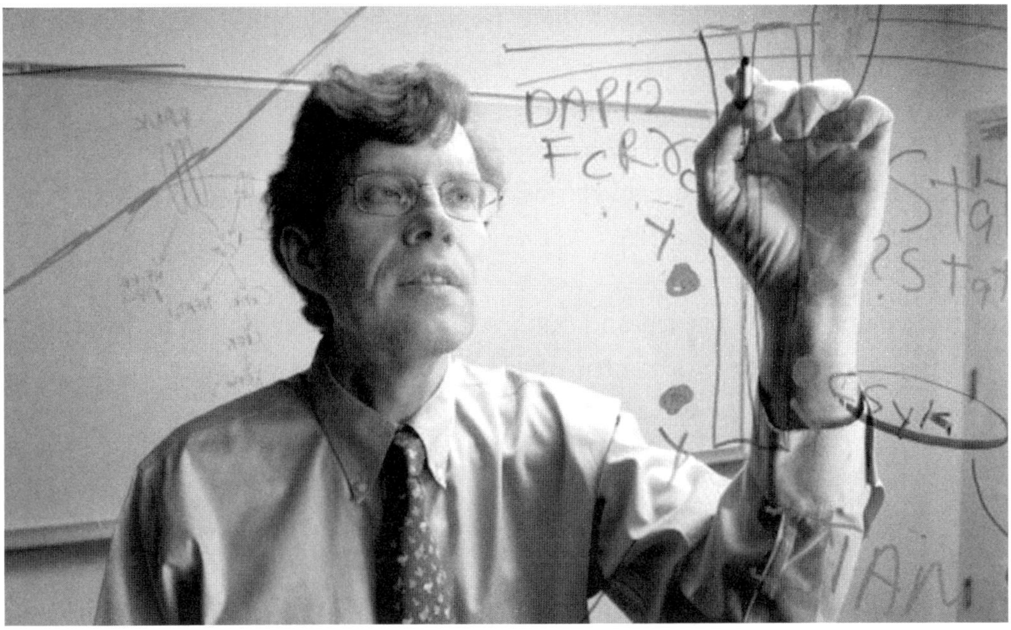

Fig. 9 2009: Lionel B. Ivashkiv, MD, came to HSS in 1992 to study inflammation, tissue destruction, and repair and their roles in rheumatic diseases. (From Hospital for Special Surgery Archives)

The list of HSS faculty members supporting the laboratory research mission has continued to grow and includes (in addition to those mentioned above) Lisa Sammaritano, MD, Kyriakos Kirou, MD, and Allan Gibofsky, MD, JD. There is an even larger list of talented academic physicians involved in patient care and bedside research.

Establishment of the Multipurpose Arthritis Center

Congressional passage of the Arthritis Act in 1975 resulted in a number of advances in arthritis research, including the founding of the National Arthritis Advisory Board (with Christian as the first Chairman of the Board), initiation of NIH Multipurpose Arthritis Centers (MAC), funding of research epidemiology programs, support of data systems, and promotion of new therapies, including prosthetic arthroplasties.

HSS received funding to become one of 13 MACs (and the only one in the mid-Atlantic area) through three cycles: 1978–1983, 1986–1991, and then 1991–1996 (Fig. 10). Rheumatology, orthopaedic, and biomechanical research programs were augmented by the establishment of core facilities (including

Cell Culture, Cytofluorograph, Patient Registry, Serum, and DNA Repository and Research Methodology).

MAC provided funding of multiple new ventures, such as

- establishment of an intramural biostatistics program (led by Margaret Peterson, PhD)
- development of patient and public education programs, led by John P. Allegrante, PhD (Director of Health Education at Columbia)[1]

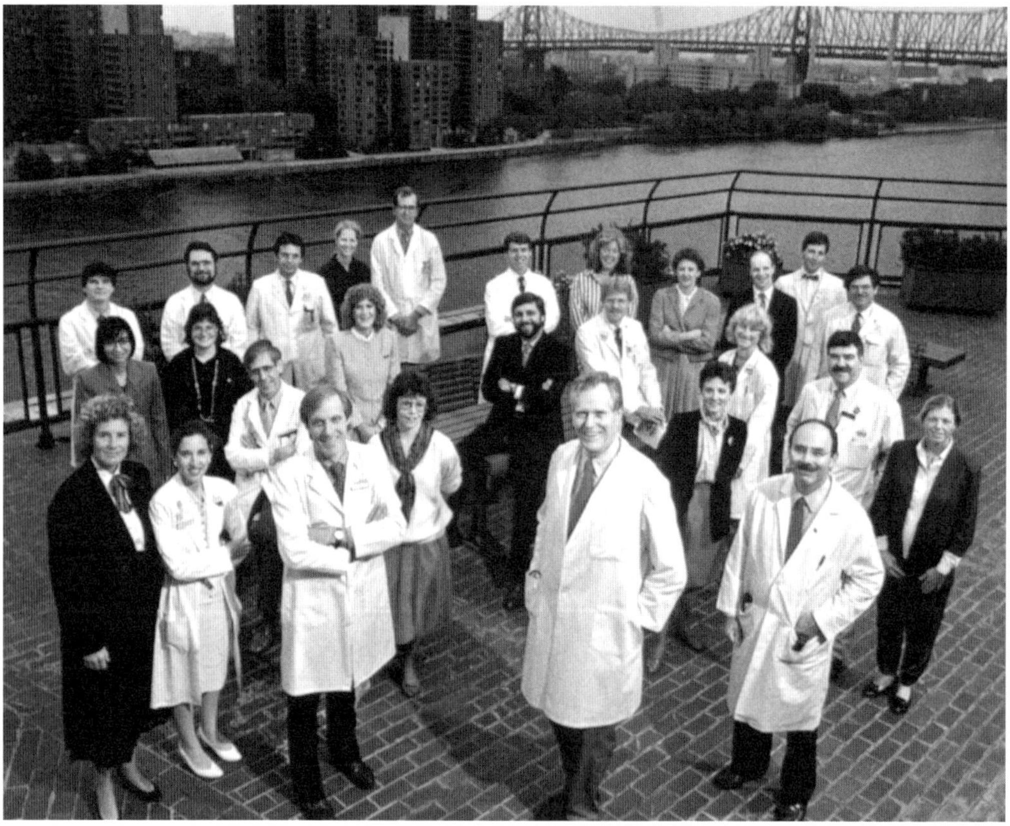

Fig. 10 Multipurpose Arthritis Center Staff on the HSS roof in 1988. Outer ring, clockwise, beginning front row, far left: Marita Murrman, Nina Bhardwaj, Steven Friedman, Thomas Lehman, C. Ronald MacKenzie, Peggy Crow, Steven Arnoczky, Norman Johanson, (person not identified), Pamela Quigley, Elliot Chartash, John Healy, Stephen Paget, Allan Gibofsky, Karen Gordon, Joseph Lane, Charles Christian, Robert Kimberly, and Jane Salmon. Inner core, beginning far left: Deborah Majerovitz, Michael Lockshin, Tracey Revenson, Kathleen Schiaffino, John Allegrante, Peter Torzilli, Suzanne Oullette Kobasa, and Adele Boskey. (From Hospital for Special Surgery Archives)

- establishment of programs for the study and management of psychosocial problems associated with rheumatic disease (directed by Suzanne Oullette Kobasa, PhD, Graduate School, City University of New York)
- fortification of the capacity of HSS faculty to participate in epidemiological and health-related research (through a program led by Mary E. Charlson, MD, Director of Cornell Clinical Care Research, and Stephen Paget).

NIH funding of MACs tapered and then ceased entirely by the end of the 1990s. But the decade of support allowed HSS to confirm and expand its commitment to excellence in research, education, and patient care and to incorporate some of the lessons learned into the institution's mission. Essentially all of the innovations developed with MAC support have been maintained—a credit to the leadership of the hospital and its success in generating private funding of programs and endowed chairs.

Organization of the Hospital-Based Physician's Academic Practice Plan

In 1977, with the support of surgeon-in-chief Philip D. Wilson Jr., HSS president Donald S. Broas, and the board, the Hospital-Based Physicians (HBP) Group was organized. It was designed to manage the financial aspects of the medical practice of full-time academic faculty, particularly for those spending a substantial part of their time and effort in patient care.

All practice-related expenses were covered by the hospital, and income was shared according to a formula that compensates the hospital for its costs, the individual physicians, and a research and education fund available to the leadership of the department. The latter fund never had an official name (it could be called "physician-in-chief's account"), and the formula for sharing income over the years has changed. But during Christian's tenure, it played a vital role in funding start-up costs of new research and education ventures, recruitment, and short-term rescue of critically threatened functions, and minimizing the discrepancy of incomes for clinicians versus research-based scientists.

The practice plan enhanced the recruitment of a cadre of premier academic physicians who generated income for the hospital and activated private philanthropic support by providing exemplary patient care. At the outset, there were five physicians in the program; in 1995, there were 22.

Charles L. Christian: In Summary

Christian believes his legacy is the cadre of people (of all stripes) who passed through HSS Rheumatology during his tenure, including those who now have their own legacies—the "multiplier phenomenon." He is enormously in debt to an army of colleagues and to the institution itself for making it possible.

REFERENCES

1. Beekman F. In: *Gibney of the Ruptured and Crippled*, edited by AR Shands Jr. New York, NY: Appleton-Century-Crofts; 1969.
2. Freyberg RH, Block WD, Fromer MF. *Sulfur metabolism and the effect of sulfur administration in rheumatoid arthritis.* JAMA. 1939;113:1160–1166.
3. Hench PS, Kendall EC, Slocumb CH, et al. *The effect of a hormone of the adrenal cortex (17 hydroxy-11 dehydrocorticosterone:compound E) and pituitary adrenocorticorticotropic hormone on rheumatoid arthritis (preliminary report).* Proc Staff Meetings Mayo Clinic. 1949;24:181–297.
4. Hitchon CA, El-Gabalawy HS. *Infection and rheumatoid arthritis: still an open question.* curr opin Rhematol. 2011;23:352–357.
5. Phillips PE, Christian CL. *Myxovirus antibody increases in human connective tissue disease.* Science. 1970;168:982–984.
6. Paget SA, Anderson K, Phillips PE. *Immunopathologic studies of rheumatoid arthritis I. Absence of complement-dependent cytotoxicity of rheumatoid sera for rheumatoid synovial cell cultures.* Arthritis Rheum. 1978;21:249–255.
7. Sergent JS, Lockshin M, Gocke D, Christian CL. *Vasculitis with Hepatitis B antigenemia: long-term observations in nine patients.* Medicine. 1976;55:1–18.
8. Inman RD, McDougal JS, Redecha PB, Lockshin MD, Stevens CE, Christian CL. *Isolation and characterization of circulating immune complexes in patients with hepatitis B systemic vasculitis.* Clin Immunol Immunopathol. 1981;21:264–374.
9. McDougal JS, Redecha PB, Inman RD, Christian CL. *Binding of immunoglobulin G aggregates and immune complexes in human sera to Staphlococci containing protein A.* J Clin Invest. 1979;63:627–636.

10. Kimberly RP, Parris TM, Inman RD, McDougal JS. *Dynamics of mononuclear phagocyte system Fc receptor function in systemic lupus erythematosus. Relation to disease activity and circulating immune complexes.* Clin Exp Immunol. 1983;51:261–268.
11. Block SR, Winfield JB, Lockshin MD, D'Angelo WA, Christian CL. *Studies in twins with systemic lupus erythematosus. I. A review of the literature and presentation of 12 additional sets.* Amer J Med. 1975;59:533–552.
12. Block SE, Lockshin MD, Winfield JB, Weksler ME, Imamura M, Winchester RJ, Mellors RC, Christian CL. *Immunological observations on 9 sets of twins either concordant or discordant for systemic lupus erythematosus.* Arthritis Rheum. 1976;19:545–554.
13. Reichlin M, Harley JB, Lockshin, MD. *Serological studies on twins with lupus erythematosus.* Arthritis Rheum. 1992;35;457–464.
14. Lockshin M, Eisenhauer A, Kohn R, Weksler M, Block S, Mushlin S. *Cell-mediated immunity in rheumatic diseases. II. Mitogen responses in RA, SLE, and other illnesses. Correlation with T and B lymphocyte populations.* Arthritis Rheum. 1975;18:245–250.
15. Kagen LJ. *Myoglobin: Biochemical, Physiological and Clinical Aspects.* New York and London: Columbia Press; 1973.
16. Schned ES, Inman RD, Parris TM, Kimberly RP, Redecha PB, Christian CL. *Serial circulating immune complexes and monocyte phagocyte system function in infective endocarditis.* J Lab Clin Med. 1983;102:947–959.
17. Elkon KB, Culhane L. *Partial immunochemical characterization of the Ro and La proteins using antibodies from patients with the sicca syndrome and lupus erythematosus.* J Immunol. 1984;132:2350–2356.
18. Elkon, KB, Parnassa AP, Foster CL. *Lupus autoantibodies target the ribosomal P proteins.* J Exp Med. 1985;162:459–471.
19. Ashany D, Savir A, Bhardwaj N, Elkon KB. *Dendritic cells are resistant to apoptosis through the Fas (CD95/Apo-1) pathway.* J Immunol. 1999;103:5303–5311.
20. Kuntz MM, Innes JB, Weksler ME. *Lymphocyte transformation induced by autologous cells. IV. Human T lymphocyte transformation induced by autologous or allogeneic non-T lymphocytes.* J Exp Med. 1976;143:1042–1054.
21. Crow MK, Jover JA, Friedman SM. *Direct T helper-B cell interactions induce an early B cell activation antigen.* J Exp Med. 1986;164:1760–1772.
22. Friedman SM, Thompson GS. *Functionally restricted, allospecific human helper T cell lines which amplify either B or cytolytic T cell responses.* J Exp Med. 1983;157:1675–1680.
23. Kimberly RP, Ahlstrom JW, Click ME, Edberg JC. *The glycosyl phosphatidylinositol-linked Fc gamma RIII mediates transmembrane signaling events distinct from Fc gamma RII.* J Exp Med. 1990;171:1239–1255.
24. Salmon JE, Edberg JC, Kimberly RP. *Fc gamma RIII (CD 16) on human neutrophils: alleic variants have functionally distinct capacities.* J Clin Invest. 1990;85:1287–1295.
25. Simantov R, LaSala J, Lo S, Gharavi AE, Sammaritano JE, Silverstein RL. *Activation of cultured vascular endothelium by antiphospholipid antibodies*v. J Clin Invest. 1995;96:2211–2219.

26. Girardi G, Salmon JE. *The role of complement in pregnancy and fetal loss*. Autoimmunity. 2003;36:19–27.

NOTES

a. A dramatic meeting of the Practitioner's Society was the 255th gathering, held in May 1913 at the home of Bacon. The paper of the evening was entitled "General Sepsis of Oral Origin," read by Kinnicutt. The secretary noted, "Discussion was opened by Drs. Dana, Huddleston, Gibney and James. At that point, attention was attracted to Dr. Kinnicutt because of his stertorous breathing. He was unconscious, his face ashen gray and his body still upright but relaxed. After Dr. Kinnicutt had been laid on the couch, Dr. James listened for heart sounds with a stethoscope, then stood erect and said, 'He is dead gentlemen, like a soldier in battle.' Dr. Gibney, sitting quietly to one side, remarked immediately, 'Field of battle, nothing. You talked him to death, James.'"

b. In the 1928 Annual Report, it was noted that various types of vaccines had been studied as treatments for chronic arthritis: "ordinary hemolytic streptococci obtained from the Board of Health, Burbank's vaccine (hemolytic streptococcal obtained from patients with arthritis) and Coley's serum (streptococci combined with bacillus prodigiosus)." Streptococcal vaccine obtained from Parke Davis & Co., and staphylococcal preparations from the Board of Health were also evaluated. It was reported that "Coley's serum when properly administrated gives the best results" (see chapter 6). Eight decades later, there is renewed interest in the possible relationship of periodontal infection (now *Porphyromonas gingivalis*, rather than streptococcal species) in the pathogenesis of rheumatoid arthritis[4].

c. With respect to the association between the digestive system and arthritis, as well as focal infection, there were concerns regarding overeating (particularly carbohydrates), poor elimination, and "inability and unwillingness to undertake a thorough course of colonic irrigation." At R&C, practitioners believed that the latter procedure was effective for treating patients with arthritis, but "the financial outlay of the hospital would be out of all proportions to the benefit derived" (1927 Annual Report).

d. Paget is truly gifted as an academic physician and teacher; he also recognized quality in research and how to support it, and during his 15 years of leadership, private philanthropy to rheumatology increased to unprecedented levels. Crow, at the publication date of this history, had been physician-in-chief for approximately 3 years. It is too early to summarize her role in that capacity, but her service to HSS and the Cornell community began more than 35 years ago. Her scholarship shines in every category of academic life, and the success of her leadership is predictable.

e. Robert D. Inman, MD was a member the HSS faculty for 4 years after completing his fellowship. In 1983, he returned to his native Canada, where he presently serves as professor of medicine at the University of Toronto. He is a pre-eminent authority on the spondyloarthropathies.

f. In 1998, Steve Friedman joined DuPont Pharmaceuticals as executive director of Immunological and Inflammatory Diseases Research. He died on December 26, 2010. At the time of his death, he was senior vice president of Discovery Biology at Incyte Corporation.

g. Since 2001, Keith Elkon has served as head of the Division of Rheumatology at the University of Washington.

h. In 1996, Robert Kimberly moved to the University of Alabama at Birmingham, where he is now professor of medicine and senior associate dean for research. He continues to study the genetic and molecular biology of rheumatic disease. During the proceedings of the 2010 HSS Alumni Meeting, he served as physician-in-chief, pro tempore.

i. Laurie Glimcher became dean of Weill Cornell Medical College in 2012.

j. Lionel Ivashkiv is now professor of medicine and professor of immunology at Weill Cornell Medical College, and the David H. Koch Chair in Arthritis and Tissue Degeneration and associate chief scientific officer at HSS.

k. Graham Hughes returned to the United Kingdom and began to observe and collect patients with two paradoxical manifestations: procoagulant complications (thrombi and emboli) and the presence of a circulating anticoagulant. Some of the patients had SLE, and many also had a false-positive test for syphilis; the reagent common to such tests is cardiolipin, a phospholipid derived from beef heart.

People at the Hammersmith Hospital interacting with Hughes included Gharavi, E. Nigel Harris (a fellow from Jamaica), and Elkon. Observing that an increasing number of autoantibodies were associated with SLE, cardiolipin is a mammalian substance, and some phospholipids have roles in blood coagulation, Hughes and colleagues speculated that APLS might be an autoimmune disease. In the 1983 volume of the *British Medical Journal*, there are multiple reports from these investigators reporting that APLS sera contain antibodies reacting with cardiolipin. The suggested name for the illness was "anti-cardiolipin syndrome," which was later changed to anti-phospholipid syndrome; there has since been advocacy for renaming it "Hughes syndrome."

On the American side of the Atlantic, Lockshin and colleagues were involved in studies of obstetric problems associated with lupus and APLS; their work was energized by Elkon's recruitment of Gharavi. Salmon and colleagues in 1995 reported that anti-phospholipid antibodies activated vascular endothelial cells in culture, and in 2003, she and Guillermina Girardi, PhD (a postdoctoral colleague), demonstrated that vascular injury in an experimental model of APLS was mediated by complement.[25,26]

l. Laura Robbins, currently HSS Senior Vice President, Education & Academic Affairs, began her career at HSS as a colleague of John Allegrante, overseeing patient and community education programs of the Arthritis Center.

CHAPTER 19

RHEUMATOLOGY AND MEDICINE (1995–2010) THE TRANSITION FROM CHARLES L. CHRISTIAN, MD, TO STEPHEN A. PAGET, MD, AS PHYSICIAN-IN-CHIEF AND CHAIRMAN OF THE DIVISION OF RHEUMATOLOGY

STEPHEN A. PAGET, MD

THE YEAR 1995 REPRESENTED a significant shift for Charles Christian, from an internationally recognized basic science and translational physician-scientist and academic "triple threat" to a highly respected clinician, clinician-scientist, and educator. Aside from superb clinical and educational programs in rheumatology and perioperative care, Christian established a Division of Rheumatology that focused on autoimmunity, particularly the nexus between autoimmunity and infectious diseases. He and his scientific faculty, including Peggy Crow, Keith Elkon, Robert Kimberly, Lionel Ivashkiv, and Jane Salmon, continued Christian's career-long interest in furthering our knowledge about autoimmunity, and particularly the immunopathogenesis of systemic lupus erythematosus (SLE). The legacy of the highest quality clinical care and medical education and the focus on basic, translational, and clinical research that Christian left were embraced by Stephen A. Paget, MD, who assumed the helm as chairman of rheumatology in 1995.

Stephen A. Paget, 1995–2010

Stephen Paget was born in Brooklyn, New York, was educated in the local public schools, and received his bachelor of arts degree in biology at Brooklyn College and his medical degree from Downstate Medical Center. He did his residency in internal medicine at the Johns Hopkins Hospital and was a clinical associate in the Arthritis Rheumatism Branch at the National Institute of Arthritis, Musculoskeletal and Skin Diseases (NIAMS), and subsequently completed his rheumatology fellowship at Hospital for Special Surgery (HSS). He joined the faculty in the Division of Rheumatology at HSS in 1978.

While at the National Institutes of Health (NIH), Paget defined T-cell predominance in rheumatoid arthritis (RA) synovial membranes using tissue obtained from surgeries in the HSS comprehensive arthritis program. This singular finding foreshadowed the future development of biological agents for the treatment of RA. He continued his research on the pathogenesis of RA in the laboratory of Paul E. Phillips, MD.

Paget's research interests shifted from the laboratory to the clinical sphere, and he became an associate director of the NIH-funded Cornell Multipurpose Arthritis Center. He focused his research on steroid-induced osteoporosis, systemic vasculitides, RA, joint replacement surgery, premature atherosclerosis in RA and SLE, and hip fractures. In the midst of these activities, Paget became the rheumatology training program director, a forerunner of his interest in advancing medical education and developing an Academy of Medical Educators in the division some years later. Paget was an early member of the Board of the hospital's Medical Indemnity Assurance Company and contributed to its financial stability, expansion, and participation in maintaining quality care programs at HSS.

Rheumatology and Department of Medicine Leadership

Paget worked closely with Peggy Crow, the director of rheumatology research, and C. Ronald MacKenzie, MD, the director of perioperative medicine, to conceptualize and develop many new programs to assure that HSS remained both contemporary and innovative in its approach to patient care, medical education, and research and a world leader. By all metrics, this Division of Rheumatology remained one of the most respected programs in the world. The

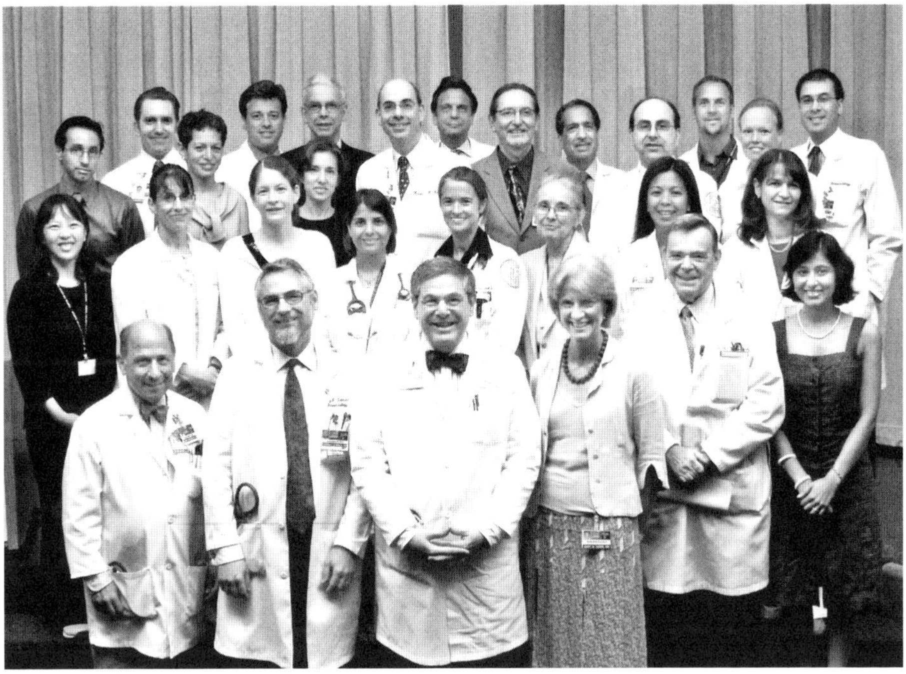

Fig. 1 The HSS Division of Rheumatology is the largest and most respected in the country in the areas of clinical care, education, and research. This photograph shows members of the Division of Rheumatology in the middle of Stephen Paget's tenure as Chairman. In the middle of the first row is the rheumatology leadership, including Thomas Lehman, MD, and Peggy Crow, MD, with the chairman of adult rheumatology, Stephen Paget, MD, in the middle. (From Hospital for Special Surgery Archives)

Perioperative Program enabled the hospital to perform surgeries on even the most complicated cases, under optimal medical conditions, allowing for the best of outcomes and leading to worldwide recognition (Fig. 1).

A Rapidly Changing World Inside and Outside of Medicine

It is important to appreciate the activities, programs, and progress of the Division of Rheumatology in the context of what was happening in the world during these 15 years. There was a profound upheaval in the country's economy; increasing competition for NIH funding; basic and profound changes in the healthcare system, including passing of the Affordable Care Act, an act that gave greater focus to chronic diseases and disease prevention; a spotlight from governmental and private healthcare payers on better-defined health outcomes, the importance of evidence-based medical decision-making, the use of electronic medical records, the development and utilization of medical guidelines, comparative effectiveness research aimed at defining the best possible treatment options, and better value for the dollar; a more knowledgeable and involved patient, due to the impact of the Internet, a 24/7 news cycle, and their increased power in the medical marketplace via satisfaction ratings; personalized medicine and patient access to their files and laboratory tests; physician and hospital profiles displayed on the Internet; technologic advances in the development of biological drugs and small molecules; and a revolution in the power and application of computers, information technology, and science (see Table 1). Paget and his team chose to address each of these head-on as opportunities, and the progress that is described below demonstrates the effectiveness in doing so.

Table 1 Discoveries and Technologies Relevant to Rheumatology: Late 1990s–2010

Immunology and autoimmunity

- Innate immunity, Toll-like receptors, the inflammasome, the role of IL-1 in autoinflammatory disorders*
- TH17 cells, TH17; IL-12/23; IL-18—roles in autoimmune disorders*
- Dendritic cells and their role in autoimmunity and cancer*
- The role of B lymphocytes in SLE, RA, and ANCA-related vasculitides*
- Interferon alpha and its importance in SLE*
- The role of complement in triggering clot formation in APS*
- Monoclonal antibodies
- Improved transplant outcomes
- Biomarkers*
- Small molecules
- Cell cloning

Bone and cartilage biology

- The biology of the osteoclast, osteoblast, osteocyte, and chondrocyte*
- Osteoporosis: its pathophysiology, assessment, and treatment options*

Endothelial cell, vascular biology, and coagulation

- Premature atherosclerosis in RA and SLE due to both the inflammatory milieu and traditional Framingham risk factors*
- Angiogenesis*
- Endothelin receptor biology
- Placental physiology*
- The antiphospholipid syndrome, catastrophic APS*

Table 1 (*continued*)

- Anticoagulants inhibiting thrombin and factor Xa*
- Connection between APS and preeclampsia*

Modern therapeutic options

- Blockade of
  - B lymphocytes: rituximab and belimumab*
  - Transcription factors and tyrosine kinases
  - T lymphocytes and co-stimulation with abatacept*
  - Tumor necrosis factor α, new options*
  - Endothelin receptors in pulmonary hypertension
  - Dendritic cells
  - IL-6 with tocilizumab*
  - IL-12/23
  - IL-17
- Newer treatment agents
  - Rituximab for RA, SLE, and ANCA-related vasculitides*
  - Belimumab for SLE
  - Tocilizumab for RA
  - Alefacept, T-cell blocker in psoriasis and psoriatic arthritis
  - Ustekinumab, IL-12/23 blockade for psoriatic arthritis
  - Small molecules in RA

Disease activity, outcome assessment tools, health information*

- Health assessment/function questionnaires
- Disease activity scores
- Patient-derived disease activity and outcome tools
- Damage scores
- OMERACT: an international initiative to improve outcome measurement in rheumatology
- Health Information Technology (HIT) that fosters the integration of research and clinical data
- Artificial intelligence

New concepts in the study of neurologic disorders

- Imaging technology: MRI, MRA, functional MRI
- Study of neurocognitive dysfunction in SLE*
  - Blood-brain barrier biology*
  - Biology of pain and new treatment options for pain control

(*continued*)

Table 1 *(continued)*

Broader understanding of infectious agents in autoimmune disorders and arthritis
➢ Microbiome
➢ Reactive arthritis and new diagnostic and treatment options
➢ HIV
Genetics, the genome, and modern technology
➢ Human genome project
➢ Haptotype map
➢ Large-scale mapping and sequencing of genomes
➢ Molecular genetics: merging of cell biology and genetics*
➢ Personal genome project
➢ Molecular fingerprinting
➢ Epigenetics*
➢ High-throughput sequencing
➢ Bioinformatics*
➢ Proteomics
➢ Metabolomics
➢ Nanotechnology
Personalized medicine
➢ Creation of an individual's genome map: personal genomics
➢ Correlation of specific genes and proteins with specific diseases
➢ Very simple and inexpensive computing devices with integrated wireless telephone and Internet capabilities
➢ The Semantic Web
Imaging technology
➢ Magnetic resonance imaging*
➢ Ultrasonography*
➢ Magnetic resonance angiography
➢ Positron emission imaging
➢ Bone density measurements*
Anatomical constructs
➢ Understanding the enthesis in the spondyloarthropathies
➢ Appreciation of organ dysfunction as a pathophysiologic model for osteoarthritis*

*Reflects the areas in which HSS rheumatology physician-scientists were involved.

New Initiatives

Paget's tenure as physician-in-chief and chairman of the Division of Rheumatology built on what Christian had so ably started. He developed the following overarching divisional and departmental concepts, goals, and programs:

1. Expansion of the breadth, type, and focus of clinical care in both rheumatology and perioperative care, as demanded by changes in the practice of medicine and rheumatology and a significant expansion of the volume of operative cases and their complexity.
2. A shift to a "Center of Excellence" research model to build powerful research structures in inflammatory arthritis, SLE, vasculitis, and scleroderma, each of which was supported by registries to support the continuum of research, translational research programs, drug trials, and focused teams of rheumatologists with expertise in those specific clinical areas.
3. Broaden the education arm of the division, with the support of clinician-scholar-educators who have expertise in education and research and the development of an Academy of Medical Educators to support their growth and improve the educational prowess of every member of the division teaching medical students, residents, and fellows.

The Clinical Sphere

To assure the highest quality of rheumatology and perioperative care and address the rapidly increasing volume of rheumatology patients and surgeries, the faculty expanded from 30 to 46 members. As always, the partnership with rheumatology and IV infusion unit nurses enabled faculty to deliver the best and most sensitive care to an increasing number of patients, with disease severities ranging from mild to life- and organ-threatening. Marjorie Pangas, RN, Julie Pollino-Tanner, RN, and Linda Leff, RN, represent the best in nursing care, and they and their exceptional staff deserve equal credit for our well-earned reputation and patient outcomes.

Rheumatology had become a largely outpatient subspecialty due to advances in the care of patients with rheumatologic disorders, including the focus on early diagnosis and onset of therapy, treatment aimed at a specific clinical target by employing disease activity measures, and an aggressive treatment paradigm using powerful and immunologically focused immunosuppressive drugs and biological disease modifiers (such as tumor necrosis factor α inhibitors and monoclonal antibodies to T and B lymphocytes). Gone were the days of wheelchairs and, in a profound way, the need for orthopaedic surgery in the care of patients with RA.

Our development of Centers of Excellence in various clinical entities, such as inflammatory arthritis and SLE, led to specialized rheumatologists in those areas who could deliver multidisciplinary, world-class care in the setting of a center to address the complex issues of patients with autoimmune disorders. Whereas in the decades before 1995, many patients with rheumatologic disorders were admitted to HSS or New York–Presbyterian Hospital for the care of severe or unresponsive disease or medication side effects, the shift to outpatient rheumatologic care stimulated the need for an infusion unit to treat patients with newer biological drugs that were given intravenously. The unit was built in the midst of our busy rheumatologic practice and became a vitally important part of our care and a safe environment for ambulatory care of all kinds, allowing patients to be admitted for hours rather than days. As of 2012, there were eight chairs in the infusion unit and 4,000 treatments delivered annually.

In view of the increasing complexity of patients admitted to the hospital, we needed to expand certain services to address specific clinical issues that arose more commonly. Since the age of our patients undergoing joint and back surgeries was increasing, a broadened in-house cardiology presence was necessary. Lawrence Levin, MD, succeeded Irwin Nydick, MD, as director of cardiology.

Psychiatric care had been coordinated by J. Warren Brown, MD, but after his passing, we transitioned to an HSS academic Division of Psychiatry under the leadership of John Barnhill, MD. Barnhill was chief of the Psychiatric Consultation-Liaison Service at New York–Presbyterian Hospital/Weill Cornell Medical Center and is chief of the Division of Psychiatry at the HSS. In these roles, he supervises a team of students and residents who perform psychiatric consultations in both institutions.

As surgical volume increases, the possibility of infection rises, and thus there was a need to expand the Division of Infectious Disease with the hiring of Andrew Miller, MD. Barry Brause, MD, continued to direct this division in a most able and scientific manner, coordinating the HSS program with that of New York–Presbyterian Hospital. His national reputation in the field of musculoskeletal and surgical infections is second to none, and the institutional psyche regarding avoidance and early treatment of infection that he engendered was vital to achieving the best possible patient and surgical outcomes. Every few years, operative volumes leaped by the thousands, and this demanded an expansion and modernization of perioperative care at HSS. This growth coincided with the explosion of the hospitalist model of care in the 1990s, in which a generalist physician cares for and coordinates the care of hospitalized patients, returning the patients to their primary physicians at the time of hospital discharge. Before 2002, perioperative care of the 10,000 to 20,000 orthopaedic surgeries each year at HSS was performed mostly by members of the HSS rheumatology faculty. After that, internists were added specifically to deliver perioperative care, and in 2006, a Hospitalist Program was instituted to assure world-class, 24/7 in-hospital and perioperative care. This program grew significantly over the subsequent years. Perioperative Grand Rounds met monthly to focus on medical and surgical specific topics that enhanced the perioperative physician's grasp of a broad range of issues with an impact upon the medical outcomes of orthopaedic surgery.

One of the most important clinical care innovations developed during this time involved the formation of daily postoperative multidisciplinary rounds coordinated by Edward Parrish, MD, and modeled after the Johns Hopkins Hospital Firm System. This program assured that each postoperative patient receives in-depth attention by a multispecialty team that includes internists, nurses, physician assistants, social workers, and dietitians. This model allowed for improved outcomes, satisfaction, and continuity of care as well as decreased length of inpatient stay.

A renewed focus on ethical issues in the field of rheumatology occurred under the leadership of C. Ronald MacKenzie, whose interest in bioethics grew out of a melding of his former role as chairman of the HSS Institutional Review Board and his affinity for the humanistic aspects of medical practice. He was selected as a faculty scholar in the Ethics Division of Weill Cornell as part of the bioethics training program of Joseph J. Fins, MD. An endowment has been developed to support the C. Ronald MacKenzie, MD, Chair in Ethics and Medicine. In July 2010, the Ethics Forum first appeared in the professional publication, *The Rheumatologist*, a symbol of the ever-increasing importance of the many ethical issues that exist in medicine in general and rheumatology in particular (Fig. 2).

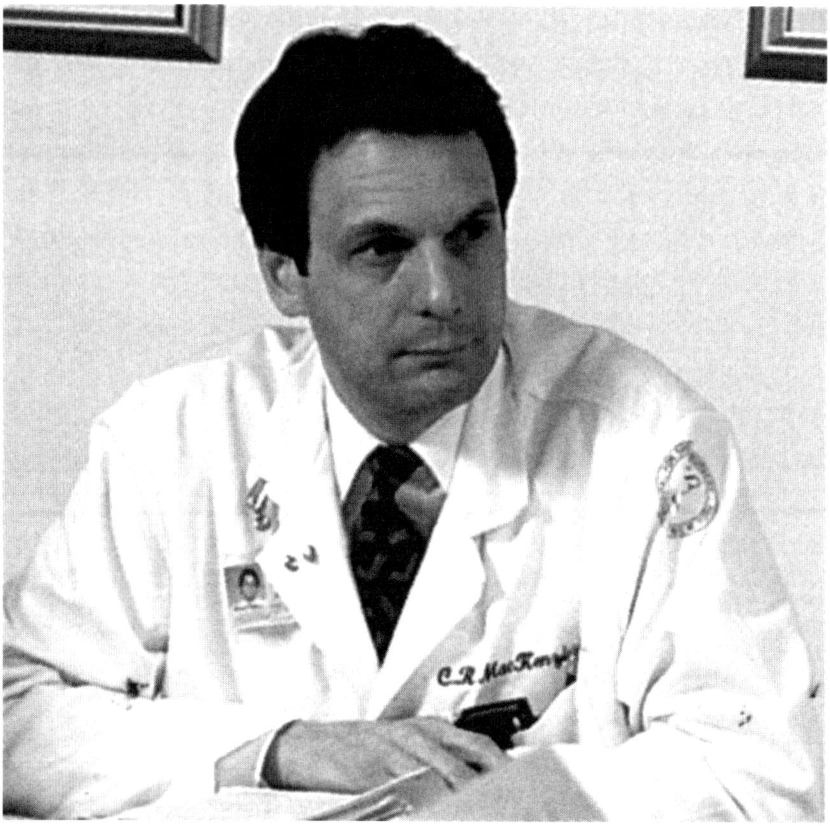

Fig. 2 C. Ronald MacKenzie, MD, is an associate attending physician at Hospital for Special Surgery, the director of medical services for the Spine Care Institute, co-chairman of the HSS Ethics Committee and chair of the American College of Rheumatology Ethics and Conflicts of Interest Committee. Formerly the director of perioperative services at HSS, MacKenzie also was a faculty scholar in the Division of Medical Ethics, Weill Cornell Medical College. (From Hospital for Special Surgery Archives)

Information technology has exploded in its importance in the delivery of care over the past decade. The use of information technology to assure the best outcomes in patient care has been led by Steven K. Magid, MD, a member of the division. He has played a leadership role during the hospital's development and implementation of a new quality review infrastructure, which set in place mechanisms to allow better alignment of strategic goals, sharing of information, and the setting of benchmarks and metrics.

Web development under the leadership of Theodore R. Fields, MD, played an increasingly important role in the dissemination of information both inside and outside of HSS. He served as co-chairman of the hospital's Web Committee and director of the HSS rheumatology Web pages, which feature over 800 articles and a large number of videos, audio material, podcasts, and online CME programs. The rheumatology Web pages attract 280,000 unique users a month.

Collaboration with Roberta Horton, LCSW, ACSW, of the HSS Department of Social Work Programs, led to the development of innovative patient support initiatives, including free programs that reflected our comprehensive approach to care for people with SLE. This included LANtern® (Lupus Asian Network),

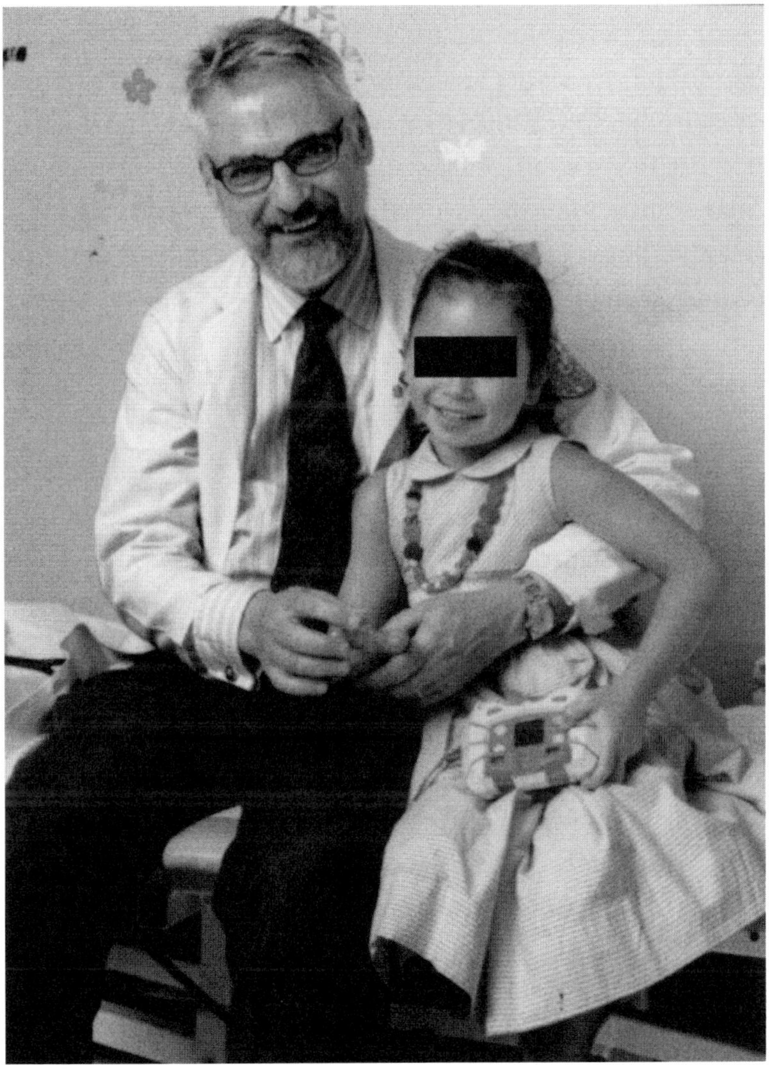

Fig. 3 Thomas Lehman, MD, chairman of Division of Pediatric Rheumatology from 1995 through 2012. During this time, the division grew in size and scope, and the pediatric and adult rheumatology fellowship programs were closely integrated. (From Hospital for Special Surgery Archives)

a free national support and education program for Asian Americans with lupus and their families; monthly in-person chat groups for teens with lupus and their parents; SLE Workshop, a monthly education and support group for people with lupus, along with their family and friends; LupusLine®, a free national telephone peer counseling service focusing on one-to-one support for people with lupus and their families; and Charla de Lupus (Lupus Chat)®, a free national peer health education and support program for Spanish-speaking communities with lupus. Similar support groups have been developed for patients with myositis, scleroderma, and osteoporosis.

There was an important expansion of pediatric rheumatology with the hiring of physician-scientist Theresa Lu, MD, PhD, two new pediatric rheumatologists, and the integration of pediatric rheumatology into the structure of adult rheumatology. Under the leadership of Thomas Lehman, MD, chair of pediatric rheumatology, this division expanded its academic productivity and strengthened its training program (Fig. 3).

Education

A high priority for the division was enhancement of medical education across the continuum through the support of junior faculty clinician-scholar-educators, hiring of new faculty with education prowess, and the ultimate development of an Academy of Medical Educators. Our academy was fashioned after that at the University of California, San Francisco, and was developed to create a stimulating academic environment for educators that enhances the quality of teaching; defines a clear and effective structure for the development and management of education programs at HSS; promotes teaching excellence at all levels for every type of teacher and training situation; elevates the status of medical educators in the HSS Division of Rheumatology; supports faculty career development; encourages ongoing, critical review of all divisional education programs; and creates an innovative medical education grant-funding mechanism.

An example of such a program that arose from one of our clinician-scholar-educators, Jessica Berman, MD, was her development and coordination of a city-wide yearly ROSCE (Rheumatology Objective Structured Clinical Examination), an assessment tool for evaluating rheumatology fellows in areas such as professionalism and patient care skills. Importantly, Michael D.

Lockshin, MD, MACR, has developed a course for Weill Cornell Medical College students on caring for patients with chronic illness, an underappreciated patient population that is rising exponentially as the population ages.

The Rheumatology Fellowship Program

Our main educational goal is to prepare outstanding physicians for leadership positions in academic rheumatology and careers as independent basic and clinical investigators who will make important contributions to advancing the understanding and treatment of rheumatic diseases. This goal demanded renewals of the NIH T32 institutional training grants. Keith Elkon administered the program from 1996 to 2001 and Peggy Crow since 2001.

> Our rheumatology fellowship is dedicated to training the academic rheumatology leaders of tomorrow. With in-depth interdisciplinary training in the management of both common and rare autoimmune, inflammatory, and musculoskeletal disorders, combined with a requirement for completion of a basic or clinical research project, our rheumatology fellows are competitive for faculty positions at leading academic centers. In 2009, we successfully competed for renewal of our NIH-funded T32 Rheumatology Research Training Grant, supporting trainees headed for a career in rheumatic disease research. Nine adult rheumatology fellows—three per year of the 3-year program—and one or two pediatric rheumatology fellows are accepted as trainees and gain experience in the outpatient clinics at HSS and through rotations as rheumatology consultants at New York–Presbyterian Hospital and Memorial Sloan-Kettering Cancer Center. Under the direction of Anne R. Bass, MD, and Alexa B. Adams, MD, who lead the adult and pediatric programs, respectively, the fellowships focus on clinical training in the first year and investigative opportunities in the second and third years. Mentorship committees comprised of faculty members meet with fellows in their first year. Over the next 2 years, the committee assists the primary mentors and fellows with the design and conduct of research and with career planning.

Between 1995 and 2010, we typically received 120 applications each year out of approximately 260 residents applying nationally and chose three of the best, with a total of 45 fellows during this period. As opposed to most 2-year rheumatology programs, designed to conform to the ACGME requirement for two clinical years of training, the HSS fellowship has, since its inception in the 1970s, has been a 2-year program—a reflection of its emphasis on research training. Consistent with our goal of developing national academic leaders, approximately 80% of these fellows remained in academic medicine. Of particular note were eleven whose research was supported by our NIH T32 research training grant, and who went on to productive careers at programs around the country (including ours).

Research

Fundraising to assure the ongoing support of all clinical, educational, and research activities in rheumatology has always been vitally important. In 1998, the Board of Trustees made a significant contribution to the institution's research program by raising $100 million to support the renovation of all seven floors of the research building, as well as the recruitment of new basic science investigators. This led to a $35 million renovation of the Caspary Research Building, providing state-of-the art research laboratory space for all HSS basic science investigators. Other significant fundraising for the Kirkland Center, the Leonard Wagner Charitable Trust's Molecular Core Center and the Barbara Volcker Center for Women and Rheumatic Diseases and from The Kohlberg Foundation, The Rudolph Rupert Foundation, and the Robinson Foundation had a profound impact on the ability of the Division of Rheumatology to recruit new scientists, move basic science, translational and clinical research forward, and assure optimal education in the areas of study. Between 2004 and 2010, $78 million was raised—$44 million from federal grants, $6 million from industry, and $28 million from individual donors, including the Snider family and foundations.

The most important structural change was the development of Centers of Excellence in research that would be self-sustaining; enhance clinical care, education, and research in their domains; foster translational research; and develop registries to support all activities and the naming or recruitment of faculty to direct them. Centers of Excellence include

- The Mary Kirkland Center for Lupus Research and Care: The inauguration of the Mary Kirkland Center for Lupus Research in 2001 through the support of the Katherine and Arnold Snider family provided support for intramural basic and clinical research at HSS and pilot research grants focused on lupus. The Kirkland Center also administered the Kirkland scholars program to honor outstanding lupus investigators who have achieved an international reputation for their scientific accomplishments and collaborative approach to research. By drawing on the extensive patient resources, biomedical expertise, and technology of HSS and its affiliated institutions, investigators at the Kirkland Center had unique opportunities to collaborate with specialists in hematology, cardiology, neurology, and obstetrics, along with outstanding basic scientists, to support a multidisciplinary approach to SLE. HSS has developed the largest registries of adult and pediatric lupus patients in the United States, with more than 1,000 patients enrolled—a unique platform to support basic, translational, and clinical research. This spawned the formation of the Mary Kirkland Center for Lupus Care in 2009. These centers work synergistically and symbiotically to provide excellent patient care for people with lupus and to conduct research that will improve patient care and outcomes in the future. The Mary Kirkland Center for Lupus Care provides comprehensive medical care to people with lupus and antiphospholipid syndrome. Through the Kirkland Center, HSS rheumatologists Doruk Erkan, MD, and Kyriakos Kirou, MD, the center's clinical co-directors, and six additional faculty-level rheumatologists work closely with HSS fellows, nurses, social workers, and physical therapists to provide innovative, comprehensive care to patients with lupus, including 600 adult and child clinic visits per year to people who might not otherwise have access to world-class rheumatologic care. Their success can be best highlighted by the fact that the nearly $15 million donated by the Katherine and Arnold Snider family and Rheuminations, Inc., yielded grant support totaling $67 million and 213 publications between 2003 and 2011.

- The Mary Kirkland Center for Lupus Research Conferences: Three multidisciplinary clinical and research conferences arose from the Kirkland Center, including one in 2003 that focused on a broad range of clinical, research, and therapeutic lupus issues, one in 2006 concentrating on aspects of biological sex and human disease, and a third in 2008 to address the issue of cognitive dysfunction in patients with SLE. In 2011, all of the Kirkland Scholars and their mentees gathered for a 3-day symposium to highlight the outcomes of their research and the research of the young investigators they mentored. Each of these symposia brought together a broad range of clinicians and investigators to tackle current and complicated topics that demand a collaborative approach. These conferences became catalysts for scientists and clinicians to work together to study specific problems and collaborate on grants.

- The Kirkland Scholar Program chose three world-class lupus investigators and mentors per year to be supported with a 3-year stipend to support their work and their mentoring of young investigators. From this venture arose an extraordinarily close collaboration between HSS and scientists across the country and Canada.

- The Lupus Clinical Trials Consortium (LCTC): With financial support and direction by the Katherine and Arnold Snider family, Lockshin and Paget were instrumental in the conceptualization and formation of the LCTC in 2002. Since its inception, HSS has been a member of this collaborative group of 20 academic lupus centers in North America, sharing a specific focus on assuring that new lupus drugs in development come to the bedside and the development of a registry of 2,000 lupus patients that can stimulate and support both clinical and translational research efforts throughout the country.

- The Cardiovascular Disease Prevention Counseling Program for patients with lupus and/or antiphospholipid antibodies (aPL) addresses this population's higher risk for cardiovascular disease compared with the general public. The comprehensive program evaluates traditional cardiac risk factors, such as blood pressure, blood glucose, cholesterol levels, body mass index, diet and exercise habits, smoking status, aPL profile, and medication usage, as well as nontraditional and lupus-specific risk factors. In addition to a cardiovascular risk assessment, the program provides general education and tailored lifestyle recommendations and referrals of patients to nutritionists, physical therapists, and smoking cessation specialists. Currently, nearly 90 patients are enrolled in the program.

- Centers of Excellence in scleroderma, the vasculitides, and inflammatory joint diseases: Scleroderma has become a major focus of investigations at HSS, facilitated by a $1 million research award from the Rudolph Rupert Foundation and the establishment of the Rudolph Rupert Scleroderma Research Center in 2007. Under the direction of Robert

Spiera, MD, and Peggy Crow, these resources have supported an infrastructure for clinical, translational, and basic science research in scleroderma and as well as for community outreach and patient and physician education. Jessica Gordon, MD, a junior faculty member, was hired to expand the activities of this Center. A Vasculitis Center, directed by Spiera, has been focused on groundbreaking studies assessing the role of biological agents in the treatment of antineutrophil cytoplasmic antibody (ANCA)-associated vasculitides. One recent seminal study has demonstrated the equal effectiveness of rituximab and cyclophosphamide in the treatment of the ANCA-related vasculitides and granulomatosis with polyangiitis. The Center for Inflammatory Arthritis and Innovative Biologic Therapies was established in 2009 under the direction of Sergio Schwartzman, MD, and Allan Gibofsky, MD, and is focused on patient care, education, translational research, and pharmaceutical trials. This center evolved from the Gosden-Robinson Early Arthritis Center (created in 2002), one of the few such early arthritis centers in the United States. The Division's Early Arthritis Initiative, a collaborative effort of Rheumatology, Social Work, and Nursing and the only such program in the New York metropolitan area, is committed to the education of the community, local physicians, and individual patients. Over 60 patients are treated at this weekly clinic, where they benefit from the highest quality care provided by a multidisciplinary team that includes clinicians, social workers, a radiologist, and scientists. Lionel Ivashkiv, associate chief scientific officer, and Steven Goldring, MD, chief scientific officer, worked actively as the scientific arm of this center. Collaborative studies with Rockefeller University investigators including one of our previous rheumatology fellows, Dana Orange, MD, include cloning of B-cell receptors and evaluation of T-cell responses in *anti-citrullinated protein antibody* (ACPA)-positive RA.

There was considerable growth in clinical research expertise and training and orthopaedic collaboration with the addition of Lisa Mandl, MD, MPH, and Carol Mancuso, MD. As a member of a national multicenter trial with seven major musculoskeletal centers in the country, Mandl has led a group of HSS researchers investigating the most appropriate treatment for patients who have knee osteoarthritis and a meniscal tear. Since 2007, she has spearheaded the establishment of a hospital-wide total joint replacement registry. The registry is funded through a major Center for Education and Research on Therapeutics grant from the Agency for Healthcare Research and Quality. To date, data on over 22,000 joints have been registered. This collaborative effort between HSS and Weill Cornell Medical College is one of the most comprehensive registries in the United States focusing exclusively on total joint replacement. The data will be used to identify predictors of satisfactory long-term outcomes and will help to determine which surgical practices and implant models are most effective.

Mancuso is a clinical epidemiologist with specific interests in patient-centered clinical research and medical education. As a clinical researcher, she focuses on treatment expectations and outcomes in patients with musculoskeletal conditions, and self-management and quality of life in patients with asthma. Mancuso is actively involved in training physicians to be clinical researchers through her roles as an NIH-sponsored clinical mentor and co-director of the Masters Degree Program in Clinical Epidemiology and Health Services Research at the Weill Cornell Graduate School of Medical Sciences. In collaboration with orthopaedic surgeons at the HSS, she conducted a series of studies to ascertain patients' expectations of orthopaedic surgery. This work led to the development of validated surveys to measure patients' expectations of hip, knee, and shoulder surgery, which have become the gold standards used in national and international outcomes studies.

Research Focus between 1995 and 2010

Under the leadership of Peggy Crow, the HSS Autoimmunity and Inflammation Program has focused on cells and mediators of the immune system that function together in a highly complex network to maintain the integrity of the body in the face of potentially damaging microbes in our environment (Fig. 4). The goals of the Autoimmunity and Inflammation Program at HSS are to characterize the underlying mechanisms that account for autoimmune and inflammatory diseases; determine the immune and inflammatory contributions to musculoskeletal disorders; and identify new targets for therapeutic intervention in autoimmune, inflammatory, and musculoskeletal diseases. When control of the immune system is impaired, autoimmunity, and tissue damage due to inflammation can result. Investigators in the Autoimmunity and Inflammation Research Program have studied the basic mechanisms of immune system function and the role of altered immune system activation, regulation, and effector function in the pathogenesis of systemic autoimmune and inflammatory diseases.

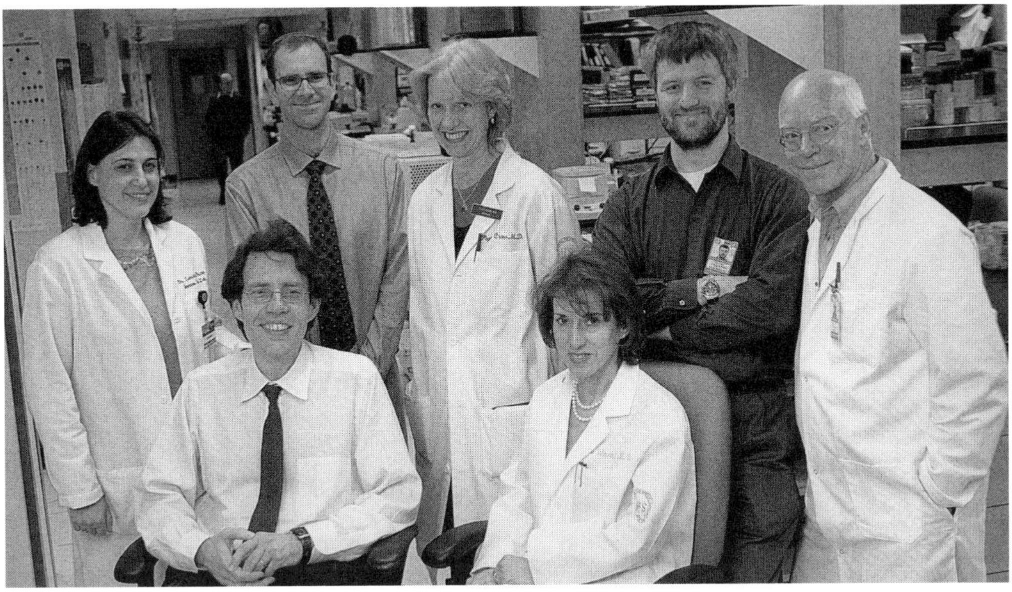

Fig. 4 Rheumatology research leadership, including Peggy Crow (center), Lionel Ivashkiv, and Jane Salmon (first row). These investigators made seminal discoveries related to autoimmune disorders. (From Hospital for Special Surgery Archives)

The prototype diseases studied include SLE, antiphospholipid syndrome, RA, scleroderma, and vasculitis. In addition, inflammatory contributions to musculoskeletal disorders, such as osteoarthritis, have been investigated. Observations from basic research studies have been applied to the care of patients with autoimmune and inflammatory diseases in translational research that aims to identify new therapeutic targets and to develop improved treatments.

An explosion of knowledge and technological advances in the area of autoimmune disorders, immunology, bone and cartilage biology, genetics, and molecular medicine was employed by scientists in rheumatology to better understand disease pathogenesis and to develop new, more focused, and better tolerated therapeutic options. Table 1 lists the scientific trends between 1995 and 2010 and the contribution of HSS rheumatology scientists to these efforts. Table 2 focuses on our research endeavors, including the investigators and their high-impact publications.[1–40]

Paradigm-changing research included the demonstration by Jane Salmon and Guillermina Girardi, PhD, of the role of complement in the antiphospholipid syndrome and clot formation; the important role of interferon alpha in the pathogenesis of systemic lupus defined by Crow and Kyriakos Kirou, MD; the role of inflammation in the causation of premature atherosclerosis in

Table 2 Highlights of Rheumatology Research (1995–2010)

Systemic lupus erythematosus

- Characterization of the central pathophysiologic significance of type I interferon production and interferon-induced gene expression in SLE: Peggy Crow, Timothy Niewold, and Kyriakos Kirou
- Characterization of mechanisms and outcomes of cognitive disorders in patients with SLE and the antiphospholipid syndrome: Michael Lockshin and Elizabeth Kozora
- The prevalence and correlates of accelerated atherosclerosis in SLE and RA: Jane Salmon, Mary Roman, Peggy Crow, Stephen Paget, Michael Lockshin, and Lisa Sammaritano
- Assessment of quality of life in children with SLE: Lakshmi Moorthy and Thomas Lehman
- The effectiveness of the combined use of rituximab and cyclophosphamide in childhood lupus nephritis: Thomas Lehman and Barbara Edelheit

The antiphospholipid syndrome

- Discovery of the fundamental role of complement activation in fetal loss induced by anti-phospholipid antibodies: Jane Salmon and Guillermina Girardi
- Investigation of complement regulatory proteins and regulators of angiogenesis in preclampsia: Jane Salmon
- Predictors of pregnancy outcomes in SLE and the antiphospholipid syndrome: Jane Salmon, Michael Lockshin, Peggy Crow, and Doruk Erkan
- Development of a registry for the catastrophic antiphospholipid syndrome: Doruk Erkan and Michael Lockshin
- Definition of and treatment options for the antiphospholipid syndrome: Michael Lockshin and Doruk Erkan

Rheumatoid arthritis

- Characterization of the complex pathways among distinct signaling pathways, including Toll-like receptors (TLR) and cytokine pathways in the regulation of the inflammatory responses: Lionel Ivashkiv
- Tumor necrosis factor can also suppress aspects of inflammation: Lionel Ivashkiv
- A signal switch hypothesis for cross-regulation of cytokine and TLR signaling pathways: Lionel Ivashkiv

Table 2 *(continued)*

➢ The generation of the B-lymphocyte repertoire in patients with lupus, rheumatoid arthritis, and scleroderma: Eric Meffre
Osteoarthritis
➢ Definition of the role of inflammation in osteoarthritis: Peggy Crow and Carla Scanzello
Vascular biology
➢ Cell-cell interactions which contribute to development of the vascular support system that supports lymph node enlargement and effective immune responses: Theresa Lu
Scleroderma
➢ Molecular pathways and biomarkers in scleroderma: Peggy Crow, Kyriakos Kirou, Robert Spiera, and Jessica Gordon
➢ The use of imatinib mesylate for the treatment of scleroderma: Robert Spiera and Jessica Gordon
Vasculitides
➢ Biological agents in the treatment of ANCA-related vasculitides: Robert Spiera

SLE and RA by Mary Roman, MD, Salmon, Crow, Lockshin, and Paget; the effectiveness of rituximab in the treatment of granulomatosis with polyangiitis (Wegener granulomatosis) and microscopic polyangiitis as defined by Spiera; characterization of the complex pathways among distinct signaling pathways, including Toll-like receptors and cytokine pathways in the regulation of the inflammatory responses, as described by Ivashkiv; the effectiveness of imatinib in the treatment of scleroderma; and Theresa Lu's research demonstrating the role of soluble mediators controlling the development of lymphoid structures (a finding that may generate new ideas for the development of agents that could modulate excessive immune activity).

Collaboration and Collegiality Remain the HSS Watchwords

Throughout its history, HSS has achieved excellence in clinical care, research, and medical education in the fields of orthopaedics and rheumatology by fostering and modeling a collaborative spirit. Stephen Paget's close collaboration with Thomas P. Sculco, MD, who was named surgeon-in-chief in 2003, Steven Goldring, and Thomas Lehman exemplify how a common goal of excellence can generate exceptional outcomes in all components of the academic paradigm.

HSS also operates within the rich academic and research environment of the York Avenue tri-institutional complex, which includes Weill Cornell Medical College (WCMC), Memorial Sloan-Kettering Cancer Center, and the Rockefeller University. A close research, education, and clinical care alliance has enabled the Division of Rheumatology to expand its academic reach in important ways. During this period, we have successfully and increasingly built research collaborations and attained leadership positions in the research training programs of the tri-institutional medical complex, of which HSS has become a recognized essential component. Rich collaborations with faculty at WCMC and members of the Divisions of Cardiology, Hematology, and Pulmonary and Critical Care Medicine, and the Departments of Immunology, Microbiology and Pathology have been vitally important to our work. Ties with WCMC have been especially strengthened by the federal funding of the WCMC's NIH Clinical and Translational Science Center. Peggy Crow served as one of two Coordinating Program Directors for the Center, which is funded by a $49 million NIH grant.

Continued international collaborations with leaders in rheumatology who were previously fellows in rheumatology from Argentina, Spain, Greece, and Brazil have enriched and broadened the character of our research and stimulated new fellows from those countries to join our program. Country-wide collaborations arose in the setting of the Kirkland Center for Lupus Research and multicenter grants such as the PROMISSE study.

Major Transitions

Keith Elkon and Robert Kimberly, two world-class physician scientists, took positions as the chairmen of rheumatology at the University of Washington and the University of Alabama, respectively, in the late 1990s. These two investigators focused their academic careers on the study of autoimmunity and SLE and were founding members of the Kirkland Center for Lupus Research.

In April 1997, the return of Michael Lockshin from his Directorship at the National Institutes of Arthritis, Musculoskeletal and Skin Disease brought a renewed sense of focus on and expertise in SLE and the antiphospholipid

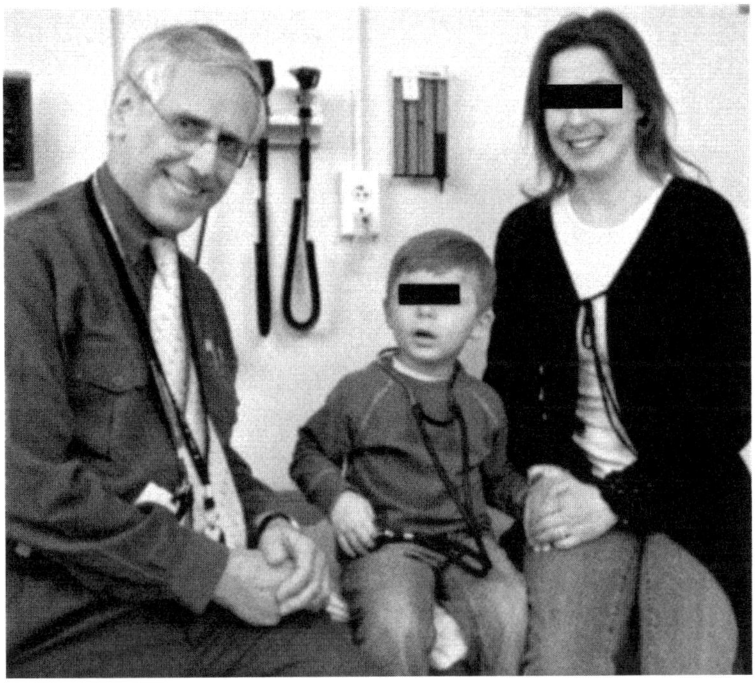

Fig. 5 Michael Lockshin, MD, professor of medicine, with a patient and her child. Lockshin was the director of the Barbara Volcker Center for Women and Rheumatic Diseases and the Kirkland Center for Lupus Research. He was the editor of rheumatology's flagship journal, *Arthritis and Rheumatism*, and a world authority on pregnancy in systemic lupus erythematosus and the antiphospholipid syndrome. (From Hospital for Special Surgery Archives)

syndrome. The creation of the Barbara Volcker Center for Women and Rheumatic Diseases that Lockshin directed, and the ultimate addition of Doruk Erkan, MD, to its staff in 2002, enhanced the division's capacity to carry out world-class investigations into these two disorders and to interact with other more basic and translational HSS scientists, such as Salmon and Crow (Fig. 5).

Lionel Ivashkiv, senior scientist and director of basic research, became the associate chief scientific officer of the HSS Research Division in 2008. His research focuses on the role of cytokines in the pathogenesis of autoimmune disorders, particularly RA and SLE, and he played important roles in both the Kirkland Center for Lupus Research and the Inflammatory Arthritis Center. In his newly created position, Ivashkiv, the David H. Koch Chair in Arthritis and Tissue Degeneration, is charged with developing a long-term strategic plan for basic science research programs; fostering collaborative research among the basic science programs; and enhancing translational research. Ivashkiv has an outstanding record of NIH funding and has made major contributions to the understanding of inflammatory mechanisms in autoimmune and musculoskeletal disorders.

Eric Meffre, PhD, has conducted groundbreaking research investigating the generation of the B lymphocyte repertoire in patients with lupus, RA, and scleroderma. Using sophisticated single-cell polymerase chain reaction technology, Meffre is identifying the points in the B-cell maturation pathway at which B cells from autoimmune disease patients fail to be appropriately deleted. Alterations in the mechanisms of B-cell maturation can result in the persistence of cells that ultimately produce pathogenic autoantibodies.

Theresa Lu studies the mechanisms that account for expansion of the lymphoid system in the setting of immune responses—conditions that can be exaggerated and altered in lupus. Understanding the soluble mediators that control development of these lymphoid structures may yield new ideas for the development of agents that could modulate excessive immune activity. Once the cells and structures of the lupus immune system are in place, development of autoimmunity will depend on activation of those cells by self antigens. Lu's success is best exemplified by her receipt of the American College of Rheumatology's prestigious 2011 Henry Kunkel Young Investigator Award.

Alessandra Pernis, MD, is an outstanding immunologist whose research into lymphocyte signaling pathways has identified candidate therapeutic targets relevant to SLE and inflammatory arthritis. One of the strengths of HSS that attracted Pernis was its well-developed patient resources, which she can access to extend her studies from murine models to patients.

Lawrence Kagen, MD, was an attending rheumatologist and professor of medicine at HSS since the early 1970s, with world-renowned expertise in inflammatory muscle diseases. He retired in 2010. He was the model of the academic triple-threat who was beloved and respected by staff, patients, fellows, and trainees. He brought a unique and scholarly approach to science, medical care, and education and represented the best in medicine and rheumatology. The national reputation of the division throughout his more than 30 years at HSS was a reflection of gifted and caring physicians like Kagen.

National Leadership

As a reflection of the recognition of the Division of Rheumatology and its national impact, members of the division have held key positions in national and international professional organizations, including Crow's presidency of the American College of Rheumatology from 2005 to 2006. Jane Salmon was Chair of the NIAMS Special Grants Review Committee and Chair of the Committee on Research, as well as a member of the Board of Directors of the American College of Rheumatology. She held leadership positions in two important organizations whose missions are to encourage and promote the sharing of education and research—the Federation of Clinical Immunology Societies (FOCIS) and the European League Against Rheumatism (EULAR). She served as secretary-treasurer on the Executive Committee of FOCIS—a federation of some 43 member societies representing 60,000 clinician-scientists throughout the world.

Michael Lockshin was editor of *Arthritis and Rheumatism*, the flagship journal of the American College of Rheumatology, a position of profound significance because of its impact on the world of rheumatology investigation. Stephen Paget was an associate editor of that publication and was the chair of the American College of Rheumatology's Research and Education Foundation's Development Advisory Committee. He was also a member of the Board of Directors of the American Board of Internal Medicine and Chair of its Rheumatology Subspecialty Board. In 2011, he received the American College of Rheumatology's prestigious Distinguished Clinician Scholar Award.

On a national level, Anne R. Bass, MD, program director of the division's Fellowship Training Program, served as chairman of the American College of Rheumatology Training Resources Subcommittee of the Committee on Workforce and Training. Her responsibilities included chairing the panel that rewrites the rheumatology in-training exam and manages the Rheumatology Fellowship Match Program. C. Ronald MacKenzie was appointed to the Ethics and Conflict of Interest Committee of the American College of Rheumatology in 2005, and was named the committee's chairman in 2010. In this capacity, he supports the efforts of and provides guidance to the ACR Board across the range of ethical issues arising in the organization and among its membership.

Faculty Recruitment

From 1995 until 2010, 15 new rheumatology faculty members were hired—specialists in osteoporosis, scleroderma, vasculitis, myositis, pediatric rheumatology, clinical epidemiology, acupuncture and pain medicine, biomarkers, and SLE/antiphospholipid syndrome—with a focus on strengthening research, education, and patient care in specific adult and pediatric rheumatology areas. Clinician-scholar-educators were also brought on board to coordinate rheumatology and resident training programs. During the same time, eight internists and hospitalists joined the staff to broaden the expertise in perioperative medicine and expand the hours of coverage and clinical safety net in the hospital 24/7. The expansion of the division assured HSS of its place as a world leader in patient care, research, and educational efforts related to rheumatology.

REFERENCES

1. Ahmed ST, Ivashkiv LB. Inhibition of IL-6 and IL-10 signaling and STAT activation by inflammatory and stress pathways. *J Immunol.* 2000;165:5227–5237.
2. Chyou S, Ekland EH, Carpenter AC, et al. Fibroblast-type reticular stromal cells regulate the lymph node vasculature. *J Immunol.* 2008;181:3887–3896.
3. Crow MK. Type I interferon in systemic lupus erythematosus. *Curr Top Microbiol Immunol.* 2007;316:359–386.
4. Crow MK. Collaboration, genetic associations, and lupus erythematosus. *N Engl J Med.* 2008;358:956–961.
5. Crow MK. Type I interferon in organ-targeted autoimmune and inflammatory diseases. *Arthritis Res Ther.* 2010;12(Suppl 1):S5.
6. Crow MK. Interferon-alpha: a therapeutic target in systemic lupus erythematosus. *Rheum Dis Clin North Am.* 2010;36:173–186.
7. Crow MK, Kirou KA. Interferon-alpha in systemic lupus erythematosus. *Curr Opin Rheumatol.* 2004;16:541–547.
8. Crow MK, Kirou KA, Wohlgemuth J. Microarray analysis of interferon-regulated genes in SLE. *Autoimmunity.* 2003;36:481–490.
9. Erkan D, Asherson RA, Espinosa G, et al. Long term outcome of catastrophic antiphospholipid syndrome survivors. *Ann Rheum Dis.* 2003;62:530–533.
10. Erkan D, Barbhaiya M, George D, Sammaritano L, Lockshin M. Moderate versus high-titer persistently anticardiolipin antibody positive patients: are they clinically different and does high-titer anti-beta 2-glycoprotein-I antibody positivity offer additional predictive information? *Lupus.* 2010;19:613–619.
11. Erkan D, Harrison MJ, Levy R, et al. Aspirin for primary thrombosis prevention in the antiphospholipid syndrome: a randomized, double-blind, placebo-controlled trial in asymptomatic antiphospholipid antibody-positive individuals. *Arthritis Rheum.* 2007;56:2382–2391.
12. Girardi G, Redecha P, Salmon JE. Heparin prevents antiphospholipid antibody-induced fetal loss by inhibiting complement activation. *Nat Med.* 2004;10:1222–1226.
13. Ivashkiv LB. Type I interferon modulation of cellular responses to cytokines and infectious pathogens: potential role in SLE pathogenesis. *Autoimmunity.* 2003;36:473–479.

14. Ivashkiv LB. A signal-switch hypothesis for cross-regulation of cytokine and TLR signalling pathways. *Nat Rev Immunol.* 2008;8:816–822.
15. Ivashkiv LB. Cross-regulation of signaling by ITAM-associated receptors. *Nat Immunol.* 2009;10:340–347.
16. Ivashkiv LB, Hu X. Signaling by STATs. *Arthritis Res Ther.* 2004;6:159–168.
17. Kirou KA, Lee C, George S, et al. Coordinate overexpression of interferon-alpha-induced genes in systemic lupus erythematosus. *Arthritis Rheum.* 2004;50:3958–3967.
18. Kirou KA, Lee C, George S, Louca K, Peterson MG, Crow MK. Activation of the interferon-alpha pathway identifies a subgroup of systemic lupus erythematosus patients with distinct serologic features and active disease. *Arthritis Rheum.* 2005;52:1491–1503.
19. Kozora E, Hanly JG, Lapteva L, Filley CM. Cognitive dysfunction in systemic lupus erythematosus: past, present, and future. *Arthritis Rheum.* 2008;58:3286–3298.
20. Lockshin MD. Pathogenesis of the antiphospholipid antibody syndrome. *Lupus.* 1996;5:404–408.
21. Lockshin MD. Biology of the sex and age distribution of systemic lupus erythematosus. *Arthritis Rheum.* 2007;57:608–611.
22. Meffre E, Salmon JE. Autoantibody selection and production in early human life. *J Clin Invest.* 2007;117:598–601.
23. Meffre E, Wardemann H. B-cell tolerance checkpoints in health and autoimmunity. *Curr Opin Immunol.* 2008;20:632–638.
24. Niewold TB, Hua J, Lehman TJ, Harley JB, Crow MK. High serum IFN-alpha activity is a heritable risk factor for systemic lupus erythematosus. *Genes Immun.* 2007;8:492–502.
25. Roman MJ, Devereux RB, Schwartz JE, et al. Arterial stiffness in chronic inflammatory diseases. *Hypertension.* 2005;46:194–199.
26. Roman MJ, Moeller E, Davis A, et al. Preclinical carotid atherosclerosis in patients with rheumatoid arthritis. *Ann Intern Med.* 2006;144:249–256.
27. Roman MJ, Salmon JE. Cardiovascular manifestations of rheumatologic diseases. *Circulation.* 2007;116:2346–2355.
28. Roman MJ, Shanker BA, Davis A, et al. Prevalence and correlates of accelerated atherosclerosis in systemic lupus erythematosus. *N Engl J Med.* 2003;349:2399–2406.
29. Salmon JE, de Groot PG. Pathogenic role of antiphospholipid antibodies. *Lupus.* 2008;17:405–411.
30. Salmon JE, Girardi G. Antiphospholipid antibodies and pregnancy loss: a disorder of inflammation. *J Reprod Immunol.* 2008;77:51–56.
31. Salmon JE, Girardi G, Holers VM. Activation of complement mediates antiphospholipid antibody-induced pregnancy loss. *Lupus.* 2003;12:535–538.
32. Salmon JE, Roman MJ. Accelerated atherosclerosis in systemic lupus erythematosus: implications for patient management. *Curr Opin Rheumatol.* 2001;13:341–344.
33. Salmon JE, Roman MJ. Subclinical atherosclerosis in rheumatoid arthritis and systemic lupus erythematosus. *Am J Med.* 2008;121(Suppl 1):S3–S8.

34. Spiera RF, Gordon JK, Mersten JN, et al. Imatinib mesylate (Gleevec) in the treatment of diffuse cutaneous systemic sclerosis: results of a 1-year, phase IIa, single-arm, open-label clinical trial. *Ann Rheum Dis.* 2011;70:1003–1009.
35. Spiera RF, Mitnick HJ, Kupersmith M, et al. A prospective, double-blind, randomized, placebo controlled trial of methotrexate in the treatment of giant cell arteritis (GCA). *Clin Exp Rheumatol.* 2001;19:495–501.
36. Stone JH, Merkel PA, Spiera R, et al. Rituximab versus cyclophosphamide for ANCA-associated vasculitis. *N Engl J Med.* 2010;363:221–232.
37. Tzeng TC, Chyou S, Tian S, et al. CD11c(hi) dendritic cells regulate the re-establishment of vascular quiescence and stabilization after immune stimulation of lymph nodes. J Immunol. 2010;184:4247–4257.
38. Webster B, Ekland EH, Agle LM, Chyou S, Ruggieri R, Lu TT. Regulation of lymph node vascular growth by dendritic cells. *J Exp Med.* 2006;203:1903–1913.
39. Yee AM, Hotchkiss RN, Paget SA. Adventitial stripping: a digit saving procedure in refractory Raynaud's phenomenon. *J Rheumatol.* 1998;25:269–276.
40. Yuan W, DiMartino SJ, Redecha PB, Ivashkiv LB, Salmon JE. Systemic lupus erythematosus monocytes are less responsive to interleukin-10 in the presence of immune complexes. *Arthritis Rheum.* 2011;63:212–218.

PART III

CHALLENGES

Study the past if you
would define the future.

—Confucius
(551–579 BCE)

CHAPTER 20

HSS VALUE PROPOSITION

LOUIS A. SHAPIRO, PRESIDENT AND CHIEF EXECUTIVE OFFICER, HOSPITAL FOR SPECIAL SURGERY

THE HOSPITAL FOR SPECIAL SURGERY'S (HSS) vision to lead the world as the most innovative source of medical care, a premier research institution, and a most trusted educator is becoming a reality, as we now celebrate the extraordinary milestone of 150 years of enhancing the mobility of countless lives. What is the key to HSS's longevity, and how can its success and stellar reputation be sustained for another century and a half?

One answer can be found in the HSS value-based model. This model has allowed the institution to build on its strengths and continuously improve results for its patients.

It is composed of five interlocking elements. At the center is our unique culture, surrounded by specialization, best practices, volume, and academics. I will review each in this chapter, demonstrating why HSS will survive and thrive into the next century.

1. Culture

> The way a team plays as a whole determines its success. You may have the greatest bundle of individual stars in the world, but if they don't play together, the club won't be worth a dime.
>
> —Babe Ruth

According to Webster, culture is defined as "the set of shared attitudes, values, goals, and practices that characterizes an institution or organization." Culture is at the core of what makes HSS special.

For any organizational model to succeed, it must be built on a strong culture with defined values. Internal culture, perhaps more than any other factor, drives performance, as evidenced in a study in the *Annals of Internal Medicine*.[1] For a hospital to perform well, all employees must be focused and aligned in their goals. Everyone at HSS, no matter what their job, comes together as a team every day to accomplish what is needed. We all work toward the same endpoint: improving the mobility and quality of life of all our patients.

Service Excellence

Providing patients with an unsurpassed hospital experience is at the heart of HSS's culture and mission. Employees are trained in service excellence, and hired because service is part of their personal value systems.

We continue to elevate the quality of service, and at every level of the organization, we consistently deliver a patient experience that is unparalleled. Our patients expect this, and we expect this of ourselves. Based on patient feedback, for 17 consecutive quarters at the time of this writing. HSS inpatient satisfaction scores on "likelihood to recommend" to others have been in the 99th percentile, compared with other Magnet Hospitals in the Press Ganey patient satisfaction database. This is one indicator of the high level of patient satisfaction with service delivery. These exceptional scores speak volumes about our employees' commitment to excellence and their tireless efforts to deliver the highest level of service to our patients each day.

A successful medical outcome is our top priority, and to achieve this, the entire organization needs to be dedicated to meeting not only the clinical, but also the emotional needs of our patients and their families. The best evidence of this can be seen in the letters we receive from patients. Here are excerpts from some of these letters:

> Today is four weeks from the date of my surgery, and I wanted to tell you how pleased I was with the care I received at HSS. As a special note to my surgeon

> and anesthesiologists, I have only raves with the way they interacted with my family and treated me. From the intake through the surgical procedure to the nurse who took care of me in the PACU and the nursing staff on the floor, they all responded to my requests and needs in a friendly, professional, and timely manner. The gentlemen who cleaned the room were also friendly and respectful. When my roommate was discharged, I was very impressed with the way his bed was cleaned. It appeared that every nut and bolt was washed.
>
> Not only is my doctor great, but he has a warm and caring personality that makes you feel very comfortable and secure. He and his staff are the kindest, most sympathetic, and caring professionals.
>
> The nursing and other personnel were so calming, efficient, and happy that they eased any fears I may have had.
>
> In the five days I was at HSS, I interacted with 50 to 60 doctors, nurses, and support staff. Everyone was very responsive and competent. The HSS culture is far and away the best I have experienced.

Achieving this level of service excellence is a result of the committed focus by all members of the HSS family. Patient satisfaction survey scores, comments, and individual letters from patients are taken very seriously as measures of service excellence by the HSS leadership team.

To ensure continuous improvement, the Service Excellence Council at HSS meets monthly to discuss the latest patient satisfaction survey results and to highlight department initiatives and best practices. This is also an opportunity for staff recognition, as those who have made improvements in their scores are publicly recognized.

Many departments have internal committees that analyze patient satisfaction scores and comments, suggesting and implementing improvements based on results. For example, the Nursing Department implemented, among other things, hourly rounding; reorganized floors into smaller units so that all patient rooms are closer to nursing stations; instituted a self-governance structure based on nursing councils; and created a career ladder that gives all nurses the opportunity, based on experience and commitment to professional activities and education, to apply for advancement. In 2011, HSS became the first hospital in New York State to achieve its third consecutive designation as a Magnet Hospital by the American Nurses Credentialing Center, the gold standard for nursing excellence.

Providing quality patient care in our areas of specialization leads to a high degree of patient satisfaction. HSS continually improves its best practices to enhance the patient experience. We have clearly shown our ability to maintain and improve patient satisfaction scores. Although we are pleased with our accomplishments, we remain relentless in our focus to improve upon our foundation of excellence.

Employee Engagement

A commitment to achieving excellence requires that everyone in the organization is motivated and inspired to work toward that goal. All individuals must trust that the organization cares about them. Building that trust requires a great deal of time, energy, and commitment, from the CEO and the entire leadership team, and it pays off.

Employee engagement drives culture and is a foundation of the HSS model. Our people are critical to our success, and their engagement in everything we work toward is fundamental to retaining and growing a workforce that is committed to our mission and vision. Employee engagement initiatives at HSS are developed and implemented through thoughtful planning and analysis by a hospital-wide committee, composed mostly of frontline staff. Many initiatives are developed around the core goals of communication and employee support, enrichment, and recognition.

HSS uses the Gallup survey to assess employees' level of engagement. In 2011, scores were the highest in the hospital's history. Engaging everyone at HSS has created a shared outlook in which all employees work toward the highest level of service attainable. This is critical to maintaining our position of strength in the marketplace because only engaged employees will strive toward continuous improvement. In 2012, our hospital was a recipient of the prestigious Gallup Great Workplace Award, which recognizes the most engaged workplaces in the world.

Employee engagement scores have continued to improve. The overall composite score increased from 3.74 in 2007 to 4.14 in 2012, placing HSS in the 73rd percentile among hospitals participating in the Gallup survey. HSS survey response rates have also increased, from 69% in 2007 to 81% in 2012. Importantly, the ratio of engaged staff to actively disengaged staff has now reached 6.88:1, with Gallup noting that a ratio of 4:1 marks the tipping point at which organizations begin to see positive gains in productivity, profitability, and satisfaction outcomes.

Hands-on leadership is essential to engagement. Walking around the hospital, visiting patients, recognizing employees—in short, modeling the behavior of respect and communicating and inspiring everyone to share the mission of excellence are key ingredients to our success. Employees should come to work everyday with a personal commitment to an organization's mission. At HSS, each employee receives a copy of the Strategic Plan summary and understands his or her role in that plan. They recognize the critical connection between individual goals and the success of the organization.

2. Specialization

> Each man is capable of doing one thing well. If he attempts several, he will fail to achieve distinction in any.
>
> —Plato

Specialization is a key factor in the hospital's past and future success. Our capabilities and accomplishments in the specialized areas of orthopaedics, rheumatology, and their related specialties set us apart from all other hospitals.

The 1974 article "Focused Factories," published in *Harvard Business Review*, first shed academic light on the specialty concept from a manufacturing perspective: Some organizations that are able to specialize and focus can produce better outcomes and create higher value than those that do not.[7] This approach has been credited with helping to revive U.S. manufacturing in the 1970s and has more recently been adopted by the service sector. Its premise is that attempting to do many tasks may compromise all of them, while focusing and specializing provides an opportunity to concentrate resources and strategies toward producing a better product that meets market needs. In other words, do one thing, and do it exceptionally well. As a specialty institution, we are able to focus all of our attention on musculoskeletal medicine, and our physicians and scientists are leaders in their fields.

Research in our specialty areas is integral to the hospital's vision as our scientists engage in collaborative investigations that translate to real improvements in patient care. HSS invests in both basic and clinical research programs. HSS scientists publish annually in scholarly journals, advancing the science of musculoskeletal medicine.

The HSS Research Division is committed to the concept of "bench-to-bedside," in which clinical and laboratory research often create a cycle of discovery. Scientists discover a new disease mechanism in the laboratory that ultimately results in the development of new therapeutic interventions, which are finally studied in clinical trials and translated to patient care. HSS surgeons collaborate with biomechanical engineers to pioneer new treatments and evaluate current practices for improving patients' mobility and quality of life. Our laboratory scientists have discovered molecules that serve as new therapeutic targets for rheumatoid arthritis, lupus, and other autoimmune diseases.

Investment in patient registries and in comparative effectiveness research is also a high priority. Our 43 active patient registries have enrolled 84,000 people to date. Patient-reported outcomes data from these registries will allow our scientists and physicians to better understand musculoskeletal diseases and conditions and ultimately improve upon the standard of care.

HSS is at the forefront of the national movement focused on elevating awareness of osteoarthritis, as well as the research, patient care, and innovation necessary to improve outcomes in patients experience this disease. Osteoarthritis affects more than 27 million Americans and is expected to increase in prevalence as the 78.2 million baby boomers age and life expectancies increase. Total joint replacement is still the only cure for end-stage arthritis.

Previous chapters have discussed the amazing story of how a group of HSS physicians pioneered the modern-day knee replacement in the 1960s and 1970s. Today, our scientists and engineers continue to develop new and improved implants for the knee, hip, elbow, shoulder, wrist, and spine. Simultaneously, HSS scientists are researching the disease mechanisms behind osteoarthritis so they can develop new treatment options, potentially reducing the need for joint replacements in the future. In 2011, HSS hosted an international summit on osteoarthritis led by co-directors Steven Goldring, MD, and Timothy Wright, PhD, which was attended by a multidisciplinary group of scientific leaders from around the world who shared current research, opportunities for future investigation, the newest diagnostic tools and treatment, public health strategies, and information on prevention of this disease.

For 150 years, our physicians and scientists have innovated medical techniques that have improved the way people move. The hospital's Research Division is internationally recognized as a leader in both patient-centered outcomes research and laboratory research of autoimmune and musculoskeletal diseases.

3. Best Practice

> Don't be afraid to give up the good to go for the great.
> —John D. Rockefeller

HSS has the privilege of specializing and thus has the obligation to be extraordinary. Anything less is not an option. It is critical that leadership has a laser-like focus on excellence. The goal is to lock in the current level of achievement, and then refocus on moving up to the next level.

Our focus enables us to fine-tune our processes, which contribute to our quality. Multidisciplinary teams regularly work to improve safety in the operating rooms and have developed protocols to further reduce the hospital's already very low infection and complication rates. Surgical teams have developed and implemented four surgical safety checklists designed especially for orthopaedic surgery. Because all operating rooms are used for orthopaedics and because our perioperative protocols are targeted to orthopaedic surgery, we are able to implement and standardize safety protocols across the board.

At HSS, getting it right the first time is best for the patient, and also reduces costs by avoiding infections and other expensive complications and readmissions. Our 30-day readmission rates are significantly lower than the New York City average for spinal surgery and hip and knee replacement.

While HSS's clinicians achieve excellent outcomes and low complication rates, they never stop evaluating and analyzing their practices and instituting improvements. The hospital has instituted a full range of mechanisms to improve quality and safety on an ongoing basis and to encourage staff to immediately identify and improve systemic problems. We have established a quality coordinating committee, co-chaired by an orthopaedic surgeon and a rheumatologist, which is charged with developing patient safety and performance improvement projects across the hospital. The hospital's peer-review process includes members from every specialty who review safety issues or administrative policies and procedures that may not be physician-specific or even specialty-specific but impact orthopaedic care provided by the whole team. This collaborative, multidisciplinary approach is extremely successful, as all members of this HSS team are trained in some aspect of musculoskeletal medicine, with the expertise and common focus to improve the quality of care provided.

In 2011, HSS launched a new area on the hospital's Web site for Quality and Safety, providing consumers with specific benchmarking data they need to know to make the most informed healthcare decisions. We are proud of our results, and making this information easily accessible to the public provides us with an opportunity to share the outcomes we are tracking and our commitment to the highest levels of quality. Consumers can find our outstanding results, for example, in reducing pain and increasing mobility following hip and knee arthroplasty, as well as our low rates of infection.

Our best practices have attracted numerous patients from all walks of life, including those whose livelihoods and reputations depend upon their physical performance. An elite group of professional sports teams utilize HSS and its physicians, including the World Champion New York Giants football team, New York Mets baseball team, New York Knicks, and Brooklyn Nets basketball teams, New York Liberty women's basketball team, and New York Red Bulls soccer team. Elite athletes also come to HSS from other professional teams in a variety of sports from across the country and around the globe.

HSS sports medicine specialists provide medical coverage for U.S. Rowing and USA Swimming and serve on the U.S. Olympic Committee medical staff team. HSS is the official hospital of the Professional Golfers' Association (PGA) of America, partnering on a health and wellness platform at the Ryder Cup, PGA Championship, and Senior PGA Championship. The hospital is an orthopaedic consultant to the New York Road Runners Club and the ING New York City Marathon. Our physicians also care for a number of collegiate teams as well as New York City high school teams, participating in the Public School Athletic League, covering their games, and holding clinics for players.

4. Volume

> The only source of knowledge is experience.
> —Albert Einstein

In healthcare, volume is related to quality in two ways: (1) frequently performing a procedure with successful results builds expertise and (2) a reputation for this expertise creates a growing demand for our services. The hospital has earned its world-class reputation by maintaining best practices and service excellence.

More patients come to us from across the country and around the world each year. Our patient volume has grown more than 36% in the past four years, and in 2011, our surgeons performed nearly 26,000 orthopaedic surgeries with over 300,000 outpatient visits. Nearly 6,000 patients traveled from beyond the tri-state area to HSS, including 630 international patients from nearly 80 countries—an increase of almost 12% over 2010.

Medical research has demonstrated that the more you do something, the better you do it. For example, studies have specifically shown a strong link between higher hip and knee surgical volumes performed by physicians and hospitals and better outcomes. High volume is an important indicator of quality, one of the measures we make available to the public on our Web site. Medicare data show that HSS surgeons perform more than twice as many hip and knee replacements than the second highest volume hospital in the country. In New York State, HSS performed more than 3,500 total hip replacements, whereas the hospital with the next highest volume performed just over 1,000. These numbers mean that procedures that are rarely performed elsewhere are relatively common for HSS surgeons.

Our extraordinary results have been well recognized: *U.S. News & World Report* named HSS the number one hospital in the country for orthopaedics and number two for rheumatology in its 2011 "America's Best Hospitals" issue.

5. Academics

> Education's purpose is to replace an empty mind with an open one.
> —Malcolm Forbes

HSS's commitment to excellence in education extends deep into our history, exemplified by the establishment of the first orthopaedic residency training program in the country. We welcome superior faculty members to the staff every year.

Our orthopaedic residency and fellowship programs continue to be two of the most highly competitive training programs, attracting the best and brightest physicians from across the country and around the world. In 2012, HSS received more than 600 residency applications, the most in the hospital's history. From this highly competitive group, just 8 residents were chosen. We have 18 fellowship programs educating 81 fellows, 42 of whom are in the orthopaedic specialties and 14 in rheumatology.

Other chapters have discussed our educational programs at length, demonstrating the deep commitment to advancing the field through discovery and teaching. As a world leader, our influence extends beyond the United States. We have several international clinical fellows coming to HSS from countries such as Greece, Germany, and China. Nearly 400 visiting physicians rotate through HSS, learning from our experts. We have embarked on several international partnerships with organizations in Brazil and China, providing educational expertise to help strengthen their orthopaedic programs.

From our historical roots to the present day, HSS has trained some of the finest physicians in the country and abroad. Our commitment to excellence in education is ingrained in our mission and vision and contributes to our leadership in helping to shape the future of musculoskeletal medicine around the world.

The Future

As we continue to fulfill our vision as the leader in patient care, research, and education related to orthopaedics and rheumatology, we anticipate continued demand for our services, with increasing numbers of people traveling to HSS for care from beyond our regional area—independent of changes in the external healthcare environment. In keeping with the HSS value-based model, here is a look into what we are doing over the next several years.

The development of the 2015 Strategic Plan focuses on five major topics:

- Support and align a world class medical staff
- Operational excellence: Invest in quality and efficiency
- Advance through research and innovation
- Serve as the most trusted educator
- Enable growth and extend the HSS brand.

Two foundational strategies include investing in information technology systems and elevating employee engagement.

At the time this chapter is being written, details of healthcare reform are still unknown. Preparation for the likelihood that changes will take place has HSS focusing on several significant areas, including (1) the impact on physicians in terms of revenue and costs, which are key to our strategic topic of maintaining alignment and supporting a world-class staff; (2) revenue impact on the hospital and implications for patient care, teaching, and research; (3) systems capabilities for the hospital to ensure that we have the specific information technology systems and skills needed to meet meaningful use and handle bundled payments; (4) cost implications for the hospital, including rising costs of implants, medications, and labor; (5) demonstrating value and differentiating what the hospital offers to consumers and payors, so we capture market share and command a premium in the market; (6) as an employer, controlling costs and recruiting and retaining top talent; and (7) implications for the HSS mission, value proposition, and growth strategy.

HSS, which protects and builds upon its legacy while adapting to change, will remain successful far into the future.

Conclusion

The HSS's model—built on its unique culture, specialization, best practices, volume, and its position as an independent academic medical center—has allowed us to achieve consistently remarkable results and high patient satisfaction. The hospital's unique culture and talented people will continue to drive improvements in our specialty area based on this model, always creating new standards of excellence and taking what is great to extraordinary.

REFERENCES

1. Curry LA, Spatz E, Cherlin E, et al. What distinguishes top-performing hospitals in acute myocardial infarction mortality rates? A qualitative study. *Ann Intern Med.* 2011;154:384–390.
2. Skinner W. The focused factory. *Harvard Bus Rev.* 1974;52:113–121.11.

CHAPTER 21

THE CHANGING ROLE OF THE SURGEON-IN-CHIEF AT HOSPITAL FOR SPECIAL SURGERY

THOMAS P. SCULCO, MD

THE HOSPITAL FOR RUPTURED AND CRIPPLED, now known as Hospital for Special Surgery (HSS), celebrates its 150th anniversary on May 1, 2013. The incredible history of this unique institution spans three different centuries. James Knight was the founder, first chief, and the moving force behind its inception in 1863. He housed the first patients, primarily disabled children, in his home in the Lower East Side of New York City.

The original name for the hospital was the New York Society for the Relief of the Ruptured and Crippled. Renamed Hospital for Special Surgery, HSS has since grown to become the largest musculoskeletal institution in the world. Our scope now includes patients of all ages with all types of bone and joint diseases. We provide conservative and surgical management of individuals afflicted with arthritis (inflammatory and degenerative), traumatic and sports injuries, congenital and developmental diseases, and all varieties of spinal disease. Throughout our history, the hospital's chief goal has been to relieve pain and restore function and mobility to all who come seeking care.

This continues to be the mission of HSS. Today hundreds of thousands of patients are treated each year, and over 26,000 operative procedures are performed. Ours is a special hospital, just as our name implies, devoted solely to improving the quality of life of our patients.

The role of the surgeon-in-chief has changed significantly throughout the history of HSS. In fact, James Knight was not a surgeon at all and was vigorously opposed to surgical therapy for the crippling diseases he treated. Some would say he had good reason: surgery at that time was associated with significant risk. There were no antibiotics, so when infection occurred, it was often catastrophic. Many patients who contracted infection ultimately died or required disabling amputations. They often lived a miserable life of chronic pain, with draining sinuses and severe bone destruction from infection.

During the Civil War, amputation was commonly performed on the battlefield for gunshot wounds involving the limbs to eradicate a potentially infected focus, which was usually fatal. In additional, the era of anesthesia was relatively new, and many surgical procedures were extremely painful and were reserved only for life-threatening conditions.

Knight was a skilled craftsman, with much of his knowledge passed down from his father, who worked in the fabrication of munitions. In his book *Orthopaedia*, one of the first orthopaedic textbooks, Knight does not mention surgical treatment at all and solely describes various braces and traction devices used to correct spinal and limb deformities. Knight described his treatments as "surgico-mechanics" and believed it to be the best and safest way to treat skeletal deformities. He also believed that the mission of the new hospital should be to make its benefits "available to the poorest in the community."[1] Knight had an extraordinary knowledge and understanding of soft tissue and muscle forces as causes for deformity, and he was a great teacher of conservative measures to deal with these crippling conditions.

As the first leader of Hospital for the Ruptured and Crippled (R&C), Dr. Knight had a small number of medical assistants and worked closely with the Board of Managers, directing all aspects of day-to-day medical activities. Since the initial hospital was domiciled in his brownstone, he took personal responsibility for everything, including the hygiene, nutrition, therapy, and medical treatments for patients. This extensive role continued when the hospital expanded and moved to East 42nd Street in 1870. He wore the hats of both administrator and medical director.

In 1871, when Virgil Gibney joined R&C as Knight's assistant, he originated the role of surgeon-in-chief and introduced surgical treatment for bone and joint diseases. Born in Kentucky, Gibney became the second leader of R&C and was to firmly establish it as an orthopaedic institution. He believed that there was a role for surgery in the treatment of musculoskeletal disease and spent time at Bellevue observing Lewis Sayre. There he learned surgical techniques for various types of hip disease, particularly tuberculosis and pyogenic infection.

Gibney was impressed with the results of surgery, and in 1884, he published the textbook *Diseases of the Hip* while still working with Knight. In the very last chapter, entitled "Operative Treatment in Chronic Articular Osteitis of Hip," he briefly mentions the role of surgery as a treatment for hip infection. This infuriated Knight, who summarily dismissed Gibney from the staff of the hospital. In 1887, after James Knight's death, the Board of Managers asked Virgil Gibney to return as chief of R&C, a position that he held until 1924.

Gibney transformed the hospital in many ways and defined the role of surgeon-in-chief. The hospital was exclusively directed by him. He supervised the building of the new hospital in 1912 and increased the size of the medical staff. He created two surgical services—one for orthopaedic surgery and a second for the repair of hernias, under the direction of William T. Bull, a well-known general surgeon. Gibney expanded the role of the surgeon-in-chief and emphasized the academic and clinical importance of the position. He was a strong leader and implemented his vision for education, research, and clinical care at the new hospital. He created the first orthopaedic residency program in the United States in 1888.

As surgeon-in-chief, Gibney helped set the direction for orthopaedic surgery, and his influence extended well beyond the walls of R&C. He was a powerful force in establishing orthopaedic surgery as a true surgical discipline and was one of the founding members of the American Orthopaedic Association. He served as its first president, and he was the only surgeon to serve in this role twice. His goals as surgeon-in-chief were achieved by his strength of character and his innovative skill and vision. Like all great leaders, he wanted to have talented faculty around him. This was particularly true of Royal Whitman, who joined the staff in 1899. A giant among orthopaedic surgeons, Whitman's textbook on orthopaedic surgery was the definitive guide for decades, and his teaching ability, knowledge of orthopaedic surgery and pursuit of excellence were legendary.

Virgil Gibney evolved the role of surgeon-in-chief, and as its leader, he directed the medical and administrative operations of the hospital. There was no administrative leadership at R&C except for Gibney, and as the scope of the hospital expanded, he realized he needed assistance in running it. In 1916, the first administrative superintendent (Joseph D. Flick) joined the hospital to help with day-to-day management.

Gibney's tenure as Chief carried the institution through World War I. In 1922, an article in the *New York Times* commemorated his 50-year affiliation with R&C by stating that over 500,000 patients had been treated while he was at the hospital. It also noted that 165 orthopaedic surgeons were trained under his direction and that 35 of them had teaching appointments at medical schools.

Gibney pioneered surgery as a treatment for bone and joint diseases. He established R&C as an important orthopaedic center for patient care and learning. In 1924, after serving as surgeon-in-chief for 37 years, and in ill health, Gibney retired. William Coley, a general surgeon on the R&C staff who was famed for his development of a "vaccine" made from bacteria and injected into sarcomas (with dramatic improvement in some patients), succeeded Gibney. Coley will always be remembered for his incredible work on immunotherapy and the "Coley's Toxins" he developed to treat malignant lesions. Despite his brilliance, however, the orthopaedic divisions did not thrive under Coley's direction, and the Great Depression also severely impacted the hospital.

Coley was followed by another general surgeon, Eugene H. Pool, in 1933. He was an interim appointment to help recruit an orthopaedic surgeon as the new surgeon-in-chief. The appointment of Philip D. Wilson Sr., a Harvard professor of orthopaedic surgery, as surgeon-in-chief marked the next major evolution of the hospital and redefined the role of its leadership.

Philip D. Wilson continued to develop and evolve the role of surgeon-in-chief. He stressed the importance of a medical school affiliation and strengthened the relationship with Columbia University's College of Physicians and Surgeons. He was appointed clinical professor of orthopaedic surgery and sought academic appointments for all members of his staff. He reorganized orthopaedics into adult and pediatric services. He expanded the staff and encouraged subspecialization.

John Cobb was recruited as chief of the Scoliosis Service. He emphasized the need for attending coverage in the clinics, and the importance of teaching of residents in the operating room and clinics by the attending staff. Wilson initially believed that the hospital could serve as a center for complex surgery in many different areas, and the name was changed to the Hospital for Special

Surgery in 1940 to reflect this idea. Although the reputation of the hospital as an orthopaedic center continued to grow under his leadership, however, other surgeries were not performed.

A strong leader, Wilson increased the academic and research strength of HSS. He served as a key member of the Medical Corps during World War II and was a dominant force in hip surgery. He also became the third president of the American Academy of Orthopaedic Surgeons in 1934. Wilson recognized that the hospital should cover all aspects of bone and joint disease, and he recruited Richard Freyberg to develop a rheumatology service in 1944. He recognized the importance of research, and after retiring as surgeon-in-chief, he became chief of research and strengthened all aspects of the research effort.

Wilson had negotiated the new academic relationship with Cornell University Medical College and supervised the move to East 70th Street. He was a visionary who catapulted HSS into a leadership role in clinical care, graduate education, and research related to orthopaedic surgery. He broadened the scope of the hospital and led its expansion to its present location in 1955.

Those who followed as surgeons-in-chief, T. Campbell Thompson and Robert Lee Patterson, continued to expand the size and excellence of the staff at HSS. It was the advent of the era of joint replacement, which allowed HSS to achieve international recognition as a major center of orthopaedic care. Philip D. Wilson Jr., who became surgeon-in-chief in 1972, was a renowned hip surgeon on the staff and president of the AAOS. He attracted surgeons and engineers with an innovative spirit and outstanding clinical skill. John Insall, Chitranjan Ranawat, Allan Inglis, and Eduardo Salvati, along with Wilson Jr. were the driving forces working with exceptional engineers Peter Walker, Albert Burstein, and Timothy Wright to develop a new and improved series of implants. Wilson Jr. brought this multinational group together, and under his leadership, joint replacement services at HSS grew and excelled to become arguably the best in the world. This growth marked an important role of the surgeon-in-chief: to build a center of orthopaedic excellence that was strong both nationally and internationally.

Andrew Weiland succeeded Wilson Jr. in 1990 and reached outside the institution to further enhance the quality of the staff. He recruited David Helfet in trauma from Johns Hopkins and Robert Hotchkiss in hand surgery from San Antonio. Weiland's most important contribution was bringing stellar orthopaedic surgeons from other institutions to HSS.

Russell Warren, MD, became surgeon-in-chief in 1993 and led a needed expansion of the hospital. He built the best sports medicine program in the world. Creative and armed with boundless intellectual curiosity, Warren clarified the need for basic and clinical research as key components of HSS. He set a high standard and defined the surgeon-in-chief as being a committed educator, inquisitive researcher, and outstanding clinician.

When I was appointed surgeon-in-chief in May 2003, significant changes in the health care environment made the role of surgeon-in-chief even more complex. The current position of surgeon-in-chief at HSS represents an amalgam of those who have served previously. The role has evolved, just as medicine has changed so dramatically in the past 150 years. Certainly the most important role of the surgeon-in-chief, which has not changed, is the key responsibility to ensure that all patients who come to HSS receive the best quality care. As patient volume has increased, and with it the complexity of cases, this has become a complicated task. We have also had many external influences, managed care being one, which have driven down the length of stay. Just 20 years ago, a joint replacement would require a stay in the hospital of two weeks, and the patient would remain in bed for three to four days. Today, patients are often up on the operative day and leave the hospital in 2 to 3 days. Nearly half of all surgeries are performed as ambulatory procedures, leading to an increase in operating rooms from four in the 1970s to 35 by 2012.

In the aftermath of the Libby Zion case, restriction in resident work hours led to the recruitment of physician assistants (more than 100 at HSS today) and hospitalists to provide patient care. We have created an entire division of perioperative medicine to oversee and monitor the medical management of our patients. Complications will always occur, but today they are evaluated far more rigorously, and procedures and processes have been developed to reduce their occurrence.

As in the past, the paramount role of the surgeon-in-chief, serving also as medical director, is the unending pursuit of excellence in patient outcomes. The days of the surgeon-in-chief directing the day-to-day operations of the hospital are over, and an expanded administrative staff, headed by a CEO, works closely with the surgeon-in-chief to constantly improve the quality of care HSS provides, with strong financial underpinnings and always an emphasis on patient safety. This has been a needed and successful evolution that has greatly improved the quality of what we do and has led to a steadily rising level of patient satisfaction.

Another challenge that has become increasingly complex for the surgeon-in-chief is the leadership of a diverse department of almost 100 orthopaedic surgeons—all outstanding in what they do, all with strong ideas, and personalities and lead them toward common goals. This is not an easy task in the current era of reduction in physician reimbursement and the different needs of orthopaedic subspecialties. The collegiality and daily interaction with a small staff in the past has been replaced by a department comprised of 10 divisions organized by subspecialty, and many of these divisions are larger than entire orthopaedic departments in other centers. As a new surgeon-in-chief, I felt it necessary to implement a new infrastructure to manage the ever-increasing size and complexity of the Orthopaedic Surgery Department. No longer can the surgeon-in-chief direct all activities—clinical care, research, and education—without the help of colleagues who assume important leadership roles and run these important divisions.

As surgeon-in-chief, I have always believed that each one of our subspecialty divisions should be the best in the world, and it is this constant striving for excellence that has made our staff so great. Further delegation of responsibility and leadership to the clinical chiefs of the 10 clinical subdivisions is also key to the success of the surgeon-in-chief's leadership today. The Service Chiefs are responsible for all issues on their services: clinical care, education, and curriculum for fellows and residents, and clinical and basic research. Reporting occurs through the Service Chief Council, chaired by the surgeon-in-chief, and regular meetings to review activities on the service with the surgeon-in-chief. As of 2012, the entire clinical operation was directed by Charles Cornell, who has led an effort that is so pivotal to the care of patients who come to HSS for a special experience.

It has been my goal as surgeon-in-chief to encourage leadership and creativity among the talented faculty at HSS. An executive committee was therefore formed, with directors of the clinical divisions, academic training, orthopaedic research, and faculty development. These directors are responsible for all aspects of their departments.

The academic mission of the Orthopaedic Surgery Department has grown significantly and is currently chaired by Mathias Bostrom, MD. The residency consists of 40 residents, and the orthopaedic fellowship program is currently at 42, with fellows assigned to all of the clinical services. There are an additional 43 fellows in nonorthopaedic specialties at HSS. Bostrom is aided by Edward Craig, director of the orthopaedic residency. With over 600 applicants each year, the orthopaedic residency selection process is an overwhelming task, ably led by Riley Williams III. An academic infrastructure to allow cross-fertilization from the various clinical services has improved the curriculum for both residents and fellows.

To be the best musculoskeletal hospital in the world, it is necessary to commit significant resources and place emphasis on both clinical and basic research. It is vital to the success of the institution for the surgeon-in-chief to be fully committed to the excellence of clinical investigation. Steven Goldring as chief scientific officer and Jo Hannafin as director of orthopaedic research have developed a nationally recognized basic and clinical research effort.

Philanthropy also plays a crucial role in funding these research programs, and one of the roles of the surgeon-in-chief is to be active in this area. One of my main interests has been the development of a program to support our young clinician scientists and basic scientists. Recent philanthropic funding of an innovative Kellen Clinician Scientist Program evolved from the development of an outstanding plan to fund our clinician scientists in all disciplines at HSS. It has also been my goal to increase the number of academic chairs at HSS, which increased to 21 endowed chairs by 2012, with 7 being added in orthopaedic surgery in the last 8 years.

The surgeon-in-chief of the largest and most focused musculoskeletal center in the world should be a leader in global care. The volumes and quality of operative and nonoperative treatments performed at HSS allow benchmarks and clinical pathways to be developed, which can improve international orthopaedic and musculoskeletal care. One of my goals has been to increase the role of HSS globally. The creation of the *HSS Journal* and *Grand Rounds from HSS—Management of Complex Cases* has promoted the sharing of our clinical, educational, and research accomplishments with the international orthopaedic community.

Seeing a need for international collaboration and encouraged by a former fellow at HSS, I founded the International Society of Orthopaedic Centers here at HSS, which comprises 16 largest academic orthopaedic departments in the world. The surgeon-in-chief has the responsibility to ensure that these collaborations and sharing of knowledge occur. It is part of the mission of HSS to lead the world in clinical care, research, and education in musculoskeletal disease.

The role of the surgeon-in-chief has indeed evolved over the last 150 years. Each prior chief has provided important contributions to what HSS is today. There is certainly more complexity and more patients needing care at HSS, but the primary goal of the surgeon-in-chief, as it has always been, is to lead the medical staff to a higher level of excellence. Delegation and decentralization of leadership are now necessary to empower outstanding staff to lead important components of the institution. We live in a global society, one without borders, and it is important for HSS to reach out and share our achievements and discoveries with the world. To lead such a talented staff, the surgeon-in-chief must be a communicator and must lead by example. He must always "do the right thing," regardless of the fact that not all constituents will be pleased. He must articulate the message that what is good for HSS is good for the staff, and what is good for the staff should be good for HSS.

Only by working together with common goals of excellence can the unique and preeminent position of HSS be ensured. We have been blessed with extraordinary leadership in our history, and the future surgeons-in-chief carry the responsibility to maintain the legacy of excellence that is HSS.

REFERENCE

1. Wilson PD Jr., Levine, DB. Hospital for Special Surgery. A brief review of its development and current position. *Clin Orthop.* 2000;374:90–105.

ACKNOWLEDGMENTS

THIS BOOK HAS COME TO publication because of the support and confidence of Laura Robbins, Thomas Sculco, and Louis Shapiro; additional funding from the HSS Autumn Benefit Committee, chaired by Cynthia Sculco; as well as the support those who follow.

In compiling the 150-year history of Hospital for Special Surgery, originally named the Hospital for the Ruptured and Crippled, I am grateful to acknowledge those behind the scenes, the dedicated individuals not necessarily recognized who have helped make this story a personal and informative account of the anatomy of a hospital.

As assistant vice president of Education & Academic Affairs, Martha O'Brasky has made her entire staff available to help when needed. Among them were Colleen O'Shea, Jennifer Lyden, Christopher James, and Christopher Famularo.

Marcia Ennis, director of Education Publications and Communications, has been key in guiding me through the logistics of seeking out a publisher and learning the steps necessary to arrive at the day when the completed draft was submitted for layout. She carefully reviewed the entire manuscript, making important suggestions for the final copy. Her staff, including Alane Clemens, Christina Fisher, Paggie (Shin-Ping) Yu, and Elza Tamazashvili, were always ready to assist. Natanya Gayle, managing editor for the *HSS Journal* was also always available to offer her assistance.

A history book depends heavily on facts and verifying those facts from the past. When that past extends as far back as the era of the Civil War, retrieval of full articles is often challenging. I have been fortunate to be assisted with referencing and technical help by Tim Roberts, our then medical librarian, and his able and cooperative staff: Indira Garcia, Karla Felix, archivist Pamela Kerns, and volunteer Lynne Calman. I am also very grateful to Arlene Shaner, acting curator and reference librarian for historical collections at the New York Academy of Medicine, for her availability, willingness, and expertise in tracking down remote publications. She has made the Malloch Rare Book Room very accessible to my staff and myself.

Maureen Bogle, director of HSS medical staff, allowed me to review old hospital and staff files and shared facts from the past that often went undocumented. When confronted by an unusual situation, I could always call on Nancy Bischoff, with whom I worked in the 1990s when she directed medical education at the hospital, and with whom I have continued to have a very special relationship. Since 2006, I have made a new friend in Bradley L. Coley Jr., who has related many stories about his grandfather, William Bradley Coley, the third surgeon-in-chief at R&C; about his father, Bradley L. Coley, attending surgeon at R&C; and about his aunt, Helen Coley Nauts, who founded the only foundation supporting cancer immunology research.

There were a number of sections in the book for which I could not have written in-depth accounts without special input from both professional and administrative hospital staff. The origin and workings of the Biomechanics Department were detailed so vividly with invaluable information and photos by Philip D. Wilson Jr., MD, Harlan Amstutz, MD, Peter Walker, PhD, and Timothy Wright, PhD. This element of the hospital embodied the principle of scientists and surgeons working closely together at a grass roots level to further research in the musculoskeletal field—the principle that Philip D. Wilson Sr., MD, felt so strongly about and proposed when the Caspary Research Building opened in 1960. Stephen Goldring, MD, ably assisted by Rise Schwab, PhD, executive director of the Research Department, described the many changes in the HSS Research Division since Goldring became chief scientific officer. Nursing has always been critical in patient care, dating back to the days of James Knight, MD, when his wife and daughter first assisted him. It was before the time of formal nursing schools. Mary McDermott, assistant vice president of nursing, and Stephanie Goldberg, senior vice president for patient care services, were most helpful in detailing current nursing structure at HSS. Pamela Katkin, director of the Physician Assistants (PA) Department, supplied me with a list of over 100 PAs and described their current function in the hospital.

I am also most grateful to Susan Flics, assistant vice president, Executive Offices, for her description of the changes and current structure of the Case Management and Social Work Programs. Eden Kalman, food services director, was very enthusiastic in describing how the delivery of food to patients and staff has evolved over the years. I particularly want to thank Wendy Yondorf, director of volunteers, who has been so spirited and informative in researching the history of volunteers at R&C and HSS.

Violet Yuen, administrative practice manager, and JeMe Cioppa, vice president of rehabilitation, supplied valuable information about their department. My special gratitude goes to my longtime and very close friend, Leon Root, MD, head of the Department of Rehabilitation, who helped me recall the early developing years of the Rehabilitation Department and who shared an office with me on the third floor of HSS for many years, when I was actively practicing orthopaedic surgery before 1995.

The cooperation of the department and service heads—including Barry Brause, MD, Infectious Diseases; Michael J. Klein, MD, Pathology and Laboratory Medicine; S. Robert Rozbruch, MD, Limb Lengthening; and Joseph H. Feinberg, MD, Physiatry—has been critical in documenting changes in their respective fields. Each has enthusiastically assembled information that I would never have been able to uncover alone.

Crucial in the development and refinement of cardiopulmonary medicine at HSS have been three colleagues who have worked closely with me since 1967, managing difficult medical conditions of children and adults with spinal deformities. They were James P. Smith, MD, a superb pulmonary clinician; Irwin Nydick, MD, one of the best cardiologists I know; and Thomas King, MB, BCh, MD, another world-renowned expert in pulmonary medicine. Peggy Crow, MD, has brought changes in the Department of Medicine since she took over as physician-in-chief in April 2010.

I am particularly grateful to Marion Hare, Catherine Krna, Martha O'Brasky, and Laura Robbins for reviewing the three chapters covering the years 1990 to 2013 for potential errors and omissions. Beth Demel, assistant director of communications, critically reviewed all 21 chapters in the last stages of editing. Her comments added a special element in correct word usage, for which I am most appreciative. Rosie Foster, my copy editor, has not only been able to find all my spelling and grammatical errors, but she was able to streamline my drafts into a flowing style, consistent with my skills as a historian and a surgeon. She went above the call of duty. It was obvious to me that Rosie was as enthusiastic as I was to make this book factual, interesting, and appealing to hospital staff, alumni, patients, and friends of Hospital for Special Surgery as well as our colleagues worldwide.

With more than 150 images documenting the history of HSS, a great number of photos were taken originally by Brad Hess, professional photographer, who has lived with the hospital for more than 30 years—as it emerged from a small orthopaedic hospital to the number one orthopaedic hospital in the United States. I am so grateful to Brad for capturing the heart of HSS.

My special thanks to my eight contributors of the last seven chapters who were so willing to donate their time and energy, researching the history in their fields and expressing to me their unexpected satisfaction from all their endeavors.

In my mind, these chapters are what put the icing on the cake. I especially wish to thank Richard Rothschild, president of Print Matters, Inc., and his editorial and production team for their guidance in making the process of publication run smoothly. They worked with our staff at HSS with grace, skill, and efficiency, for which I shall always be indebted.

For over 50 years, my wife, Janet, has been at my side—sometimes as a critic, sometimes as an editor—but always in support of my personal and professional goals. For being at my side, I shall always cherish her presence.

Lastly, I am most indebted to Richard Menschel, my longtime supporter and friend, and Philip Wilson Jr., my mentor, colleague, and friend for over five decades, for agreeing to write the forewords.

David B. Levine, MD

APPENDIX
NAMES FROM THE PAST

NAME	BRIEF BIOGRAPHY	CHAPTER(S)
LeRoy C. Abbott, MD (1890–1965)	First chairman of the new Department of Orthopaedics at University of California, San Francisco (1949).	11
Fred H. Albee, MD (1876–1945)	Pioneer in bone grafting circa 1906. Chief of surgery, New York Postgraduate Medical School. First radiologist at R&C (1905–1911).	10
William Arnold, MD (1925–1984)	Chief of New York Hospital Combined Fracture Service (1973–1984).	11
Percy C. Ashley (N/A)	A laymen and technician, Ashley served as a spokesperson for the X–Ray Laboratory from 1917 to 1921, with Byron Darling, MD, identified as a "consultant roentgenologist."	16
Kim Barrett (1911–1976)	Head medical librarian from 1941 to 1976, when she died from pancreatic cancer. When the library was struck by fire on Saturday, August 3, 1974, Barrett—assisted by Alexander Hersh, MD—relentlessly worked to save the collections of books, which she called "her children."	14
Philip Bastedo (1908–1987)	New York City attorney. R&C Board President (1958–1972).	9

NAME	BRIEF BIOGRAPHY	CHAPTER(S)
Goren Bauer, MD (1924–1994)	Second director of research (1962) and chief of Knee Service at HSS. He was trained in Malmo, Sweden, and did his thesis on kinematics. At HSS, he initiated the practice of nuclear medicine. In 1969, he left HSS to return to Sweden to be professor of orthopaedics and chairman of the Department of Orthopaedics at Lund University, a post he held for 20 years until he retired in 1989.	10, 16, 17
Wooster Beach, MD (1832–1916)	Promoted a type of medical practice based on herbs. He called it "eclectic medicine."	4
Fenwick Beekman, MD (1882–1962)	A member of the famous New York Beekman family, he was an R&C attending surgeon and first chairman of the Medical Library Committee in 1935. He also served as president of the New York Historical Society.	7
George Bennett, MD (1885–1962)	Professor of orthopaedic surgery, Johns Hopkins Medical School, he trained as a house surgeon at R&C in 1909.	7, 8, 10
Thomas Linwood Bennett, MD (1869–1932)	First anesthetist and instructor at R&C in 1897. Introduced the Bennett respirator in R&C in 1899.	15
Joseph Colt Bloodgood, MD (1867–1935)	Johns Hopkins surgeon who concentrated on cancer, warning the public to become aware of melanoma and other cancers.	6
Carlisle S. Boyd, MD (1881–1971)	Medical attending physician on R&C Staff (1912–1929).	8
Charles W. Breimer, MD (1911–1960)	Director of roentgenology, HSS (1954–1957).	10, 16
Donald S. Broas (1940–2000)	President of HSS from 1977 to 1991, during which time he led a modernization project, including creation of the Belaire Building.	9
Buckminster Brown, MD (1819–1891)	With his father, John Ball Brown, MD, in 1861, he opened a small private hospital: The House of the Good Samaritan in Boston. First physician in the United States to limit his practice to orthopaedics.	2

NAME	BRIEF BIOGRAPHY	CHAPTER(S)
William Tillinghouse Bull, MD (1849–1909)	First in the country to specialize entirely in surgery. Joined New York Hospital staff 1884. Chief of Hernia Department at R&C. One of the foremost surgeons in the United States.	3, 6, 7, 9
Sterling Bunnell, MD (1882–1957)	In 1946, Bunnell was founder and first president of the American Society for Surgery of the Hand, established as a result of World War II hand injuries.	10
Carl G. Burdick, MD (1880–1946)	Appointed chief of general surgery at HSS in 1935.	7
Charles Burstein, MD (1906–1986)	Joined R&C Staff 1939. First director of anesthesiology at R&C (1943). Retired in 1970.	8, 15
Rolla Campbell, MD (1920–2008)	Orthopaedic attending at HSS and Roosevelt Hospital for many years. He tempered his serious professional career with fun, laughter and jokes. Just before he died, he published a book of his life in the same light vein, called *High Jinks of a Feckless Youth.*	10
Andrew Carnegie (1835–1919)	Founded Carnegie Steel Company. Second richest man in America after John D. Rockefeller. Philanthropist.	2
John M. Carnochan, MD (1817–1887)	Professor, New York Medical College. Founding R&C staff.	1, 5
Alfred Caspary (1877–1955)	Philanthropist. One of the most noted philatelists in the world and collector of ceramics. Owned A. H. Caspary & Co., a member of the New York Stock Exchange. He donated to HSS more than $25 million (in 2010 dollars), including $1.5 million to build the Caspary Research Building in 1960, and willed his Catskill fishing estate as well. With his previously deceased wife, Margaret Caspary, they made major contributions to The Rockefeller University (the blue-domed Caspary Auditorium is named in their honor) and they contributed the funds to build the Animal Medical Center in New York City. Both Caspary and his wife were patients of Philip D. Wilson Sr., MD, and Lee Ramsay Straub, MD.	10

NAME	BRIEF BIOGRAPHY	CHAPTER(S)
John Charnley, MD (1911–1982)	Professor of orthopaedic surgery at Manchester Royal Infirmary in England (1972). At the Centre for Hip Surgery in Wrightington, England, he introduced the principles of low friction arthroplasty of the hip. He received many awards and honors, including being knighted in 1977 and became a legendary orthopaedic surgeon in the world as the developer of total hip replacement surgery.	11
David Clayson, PhD (1934–2001)	Head of psychology at New York Hospital–Cornell Medical Center (1968–1993). Appointed attending psychologist at HSS in 1967.	11
John R. Cobb, MD (1903–1967)	Appointed a fellow at R&C in the mid-1930s by Philip D. Wilson Sr., MD. The Scoliosis Service was instituted in 1947, with Cobb as chief. He introduced a measurement for scoliosis (the "Cobb angle") and became world-renowned.	7, 10
William A. Cochrane, FRCS (1893–1944)	Staff member at the Royal Infirmary in Edinburgh, Scotland. Authored text of *Orthopaedic Surgery* in 1926, and, jointly with Philip D. Wilson Sr., MD, *Fractures and Dislocations* in 1925.	7
Ernest Amory Codman, MD (1869–1940)	Boston surgeon and cancer expert who founded the Bone Sarcoma Registry in 1920, a step toward patient outcomes management. At Massachusetts General Hospital, he instituted the first morbidity and mortality conferences, which led to his loss of staff privileges at the hospital.	6
Wallace Cole, MD (1888–1973)	Replaced Philip D. Wilson Sr., MD, as director of American Hospital in Britain in 1941. Professor of orthopaedic surgery at University of Minnesota.	8
Bradley L. Coley, MD (1892–1961)	Second chief of the Bone Service at Memorial Hospital (1933). Attending Surgeon at R&C (1949). Professor of surgery, Cornell University Medical College. Published textbook called *Neoplasms of Bone.*	6, 7

NAME	BRIEF BIOGRAPHY	CHAPTER(S)
William B. Coley, MD (1862–1936)	Third surgeon-in-chief at R&C (1925–1933). Trained at New York Hospital under William Bull, with whom he advanced the surgical treatment of hernias at R&C. First chief of the Memorial Hospital Bone Service and founder of the field of cancer immunotherapy.	3, 6, 7, 9, 16
Calvin Coolidge (1872–1933)	30th U.S. president (1923–1929). Republican lawyer from Vermont.	6, 7
William Cooper, MD (1909–1970)	Clinical professor of orthopaedic surgery, Cornell University Medical College. Attending orthopaedic surgeon for 30 years. Susan Greenwall director of rehabilitation medicine and chief of the Cerebral Palsy Clinic at HSS. Medical director, Cerebral Palsy Center of Nassau County.	10, 12
Harvey Cushing, MD (1869–1939)	World-famous neurosurgeon who became professor of surgery at Harvard Medical School in 1912. Cushing disease was named after him.	7
Byron C. Darling, MD (1875–1926)	Roentgenologist at R&C (1911–1916).	5,16
Elizabeth (Bessie) Dashiell (1873–1891)	William Coley diagnosed and treated a sarcoma of Bessie Dashiell, close friend of John D. Rockefeller Jr. Her death 6 months later led to a friendship and common goal between Coley and Rockefeller to cure cancer.	3, 6
Carleton I. Dederer, MD (1880–1975)	Cornell University undergraduate degree (1904). MD degree from Columbia University College of Physicians and Surgeons (P&S, 1907). At R&C from 1910 to 1913. Records show that his name when graduating from P&S was Isaac Carleton Dederer.	15
Dominic A. Desanto, MD (1904–2000)	Appointed assistant pathologist in 1934, he became director of laboratories in 1937, following John P. McWhorter.	8

NAME	BRIEF BIOGRAPHY	CHAPTER(S)
John Doherty, MD (1926–1999)	Attending orthopaedic surgeon and chief of the Scoliosis Service at HSS. Chief of Fracture Service at New York Hospital.	10
James Douglas, PhD (1837–1918)	Canadian mining engineer and philanthropist, giving some $600,000 to Memorial Hospital. Introduced radium to Memorial Hospital. Supporter of James Ewing. President of Phelps-Dodge Company.	6
Samuel S. Duryea (1893–1979)	President of Board of Managers at HSS (1948–1958) who successfully led negotiations between HSS and New York Hospital–Cornell University Medical College.	9
Dwight D. Eisenhower (1890–1969)	34th U.S. president (1953–1961). He had previously been a five-star general in the U.S. Army during World War II, and served as supreme commander of the Allied forces in Europe.	17
Charles Elliot (1834–1926)	21st president of Harvard University (1869).	4
Hazel Evans, RN (1901–1995)	Served as HSS operating room supervisor from 1941 to 1967, the longest in this position in the history of the hospital.	10
James Ewing, MD (1866–1943)	First professor of clinical pathology at Cornell University Medical College (1899). Elected medical director of Memorial Hospital (1931). At first a friend of Coley's, but then opposed his treatment of advanced cancers with Coley's Toxins.	6
Laura B. Flawn, MD (1953–2001)	Trained as an orthopaedic resident (1982) and scoliosis fellow (1983) at HSS. Named chief of orthopaedics at Breckenridge Hospital in Austin, Texas, in 1993, she died in an automobile accident in 2001.	10
Abraham Flexner, PhD (1866–1959)	Brother of Simon Flexner. Published famous report in 1910 on quality of medical schools in the United States.	4

NAME	BRIEF BIOGRAPHY	CHAPTER(S)
Simon Flexner, MD (1863–1946)	Pathologist who chaired the Rockefeller Institute Board in 1903.	4
Joseph D. Flick (1872–1937)	Appointed R&C superintendent (1916–1937) at age 44 years.	5, 6, 8
John Fox, MD (1917–2001)	Second director of Department of Anesthesia at HSS (1970–1987).	11, 15
Henry Frauenthal, MD (1862–1927)	Founded the Hospital for Deformities and Joint Diseases with brother Herman in 1906.	1, 2
Herman C. Frauenthal, MD (1866–1942)	Founded the Hospital for Deformities and Joint Diseases with brother Henry in 1906; first surgeon-in-chief.	1
Richard H. Freyberg, MD (1904–1999)	Appointed chief of internal medicine and pediatrics (1944). Director of rheumatology and rheumatology research in the 1960s. He was a founder of the Arthritis Foundation.	8, 17
Steven M. Friedman, MD (1946–2010)	In the 1984, Friedman joined the HSS rheumatology staff and collaborated with Peggy Crow in the research laboratory. He graduated from Cornell University Medical College in 1972 and completed his medical residency at New York Hospital.	18
Edward Gallie, MD (1882–1959)	Professor of surgery and dean of the medical school at Toronto University 1936. Trained as a house surgeon at R&C in 1906.	8
Sidney S. Gaynor, MD (1905–1987)	New York Yankees team physician (1948–1976). Chief orthopaedic surgeon, Lenox Hill Hospital (1956).	11
Robert A. Gibney, MD (1816–1874)	Father of Virgil Gibney.	3
Virgil P. Gibney, MD (1847–1927)	Second surgeon-in-chief of R&C (1887–1924). Orthopaedic surgeon who trained under Lewis Sayre, MD. Established the first operating room in R&C in 1889. Founding member and first president of the American Orthopaedic Association (AOA) (1887).	2, 3, 4, 5, 6, 9

NAME	BRIEF BIOGRAPHY	CHAPTER(S)
Frank Glenn, MD (1902–1982)	Chief of surgery at New York Hospital (1947–1967).	9
Joel E. Goldthwait, MD (1866–1961)	First chief (1899) and founder of the Massachusetts General Hospital Outpatient Clinic. Chief of Orthopaedic Section (1917), American Expeditionary Force in Britain. Major general in the U.S. Army.	7
Anita Haack Goulet, MD (1927–2007)	First woman in the HSS Department of Anesthesiology to be a fully trained anesthesiologist.	15
Oliver R. Grace (1912–1992)	Financier who collaborated with Helen Coley Nauts to found the Cancer Research Institute in 1953.	6
John Cleve Green (1800–1875)	First president of the R&C Board of Managers (1864–1874).	1, 2
Robert B. Greenough, MD (1871–1937)	Assistant professor at Harvard Medical School. Volunteer for the American Ambulance in Neuilly, France. Surgeon-in-chief at Collis P. Huntington Memorial Hospital.	7
Samuel Hahnemann (1755–1843)	German physician who founded homeopathy.	4
William Stewart Halstead, MD (1852–1922)	Surgeon in the "Big Four" and a founder of Johns Hopkins University School of Medicine.	4
Kristian G. Hansson, MD (1890–1962)	Led the first Department of Physiotherapy, which was established in 1924. A 1923 graduate of Cornell University Medical College, Hansson had the special honor of giving the first Coulter Memorial Lecture at the 29th Annual Session of the American Congress of Rehabilitation Medicine on September 5, 1951.	6, 18
Warren Harding (1865–1923)	29th U.S. president (1921–1923). Conservative newspaper publisher.	6
Robert Hartley (1796–1881)	Secretary of the Association for Improving the Condition of the Poor.	1, 2

NAME	BRIEF BIOGRAPHY	CHAPTER(S)
J. Paul Harvey, MD (1922–2010)	HSS resident and HSS staff member. Introduced a Swedish method of myelography to HSS. First full-time chair of orthopaedic surgery at University of Southern California School of Medicine (1964), stepping down in 1974 to continue as professor in the department until he retired in 1992.	16
Milton Helpern, MD (1902–1977)	Appointed R&C pathologist and director of laboratories (1946). Served as chief medical examiner of the City of New York (1954–1973). Professor and chairman, Department of Forensic Medicine, New York University School of Medicine (1954–1974). Considered the world's greatest medical detective and authority in forensic medicine.	8
Alexander Hersh, MD (1909–2005)	Began his orthopaedic residency at R&C in 1943. Chief of the Clubfoot Clinic for over 30 years. Retired from the HSS active staff in 2003.	9, 12
Mildred Hilson (1898–1994)	Fundraiser, grand patron, and perennial chairwoman of HSS's annual benefits. The Belaire plaza was dedicated to her 1989.	10
Dustin Hobbs, MD (1882–1918)	Radiologist in 1911.	16
Thomas I. Hoen, MD (1903–1978)	HSS neurosurgical attending. Received his MD degree from Johns Hopkins and trained at Peter Bent Brigham Hospital in Boston and the Neurological Institute of Montreal.	9
Joseph Peter Hoguet, MD (1882–1946)	Educated at Harvard Medical School, he interned at St. Luke's Hospital. Chief surgeon at French Hospital (1917) and attending surgeon at R&C. Professor of clinical surgery at Cornell University Medical College. He suffered an amputation of his lower left arm in a car accident. Medical director of the 1939 World's Fair.	6

NAME	BRIEF BIOGRAPHY	CHAPTER(S)
L. Emmett Holt, MD (1855–1924)	Chief of pediatrics at Presbyterian Hospital (1888). Professor of diseases of children, Columbia University College of Physicians and Surgeons (1901–1922). Wrote the textbook *Diseases of Infancy and Childhood.*	4
Herbert Hoover (1874–1964)	31st U.S. president (1929–1933). Mining engineer who was ineffective 8 months after the Wall Street crash of 1929.	6
Johns Hopkins (1795–1873)	Railroad owner, Baltimore and Ohio. Philanthropist who funded Johns Hopkins University.	4
David Horwich, MD (1901–1975)	Chief of the Club Foot Service circa 1947.	11
John F. Hylan (1868–1836)	New York City mayor (1918–1926). Tammany Hall candidate, supported by William Randolph Hearst.	5
Gavril Ilizarov, MD (1921–1992)	Russian orthopaedic surgeon who introduced the circular external fixation device in the 1950s.	8, 17
Harry Imboden, MD (1879–1951)	R&C volunteer consultant radiologist (1924).	16
Alberto Inclan, MD (1888–1965)	Radiologist in 1915.	16
Verne T. Inman, MD, PhD (1905–1980)	Second chair, Department of Orthopaedics, University of California San Francisco (1957–1970). Started a biomechanics laboratory and studied locomotion.	11
John Insall, MD (1930–2000)	Chief of HSS Knee Service. World-renowned knee surgeon.	10
Gen. Stonewall Jackson (1824–1863)	Met with General Robert E. Lee on May 1, 1863, to plan the Battle of Chancellorsville. Accidently shot by his own military on May 2 and died after eight days.	1

NAME	BRIEF BIOGRAPHY	CHAPTER(S)
Bernard Jacobs, MD (1924–1992)	Chief of HSS Spine Service and Bronx Veterans Hospital Orthopaedic Department. Married in later life to Ingrid Andersson, director of the HSS operating room.	11
Harold Jacobson, MD (1912–2001)	Director of radiology at R&C (1952–1954).	16
Edward G. Janeway, MD, LLD (1841–1911)	Professor of pathology and practical anatomy at Bellevue Hospital Medical College (1869). New York City health commissioner (1875–1888).	4
F.M. Jeffries, MD (1865–1943)	Part-time R&C staff member (1914–1929). Pathologist and head of the laboratories. Professor of pathology and bacteriology at New York Polyclinic Medical School and Hospital.	5
Edward Jenner (1749–1823)	An English physician credited as the pioneer of the smallpox vaccine, who thus introduced vaccination into the medical world.	6
Sir Robert Jones (1857–1933)	Born in Wales and nephew of Hugh Owen Thomas, Jones was the most famous orthopaedic surgeon in Britain, using x-ray in the treatment of fractures.	3
Frida Kahlo (1907–1954)	Famous Mexican painter, best known for her self-portraits. At age six, she developed polio. Patient at HSS for spine surgery for injuries sustained during a serious bus accident. Volatile marriage with the famous Mexican artist Diego Rivera.	9
F. Wilson Keller (1897–1954)	Administrator of R&C (1941–1954). Inaugurated the HSS newsletter *Record and Chronicle* in 1942.	8
Howard Kelly, MD (1859–1943)	Gynecologist in the "Big Four" and a founder of Johns Hopkins University School of Medicine.	4
John F. Kennedy (1917–1963)	35th U.S. president (1961–1963). Overwhelmed with chronic back pain, he underwent a number of operations. Philip D. Wilson performed an L5–S1 posterior fusion and left sacroiliac fusion on October 21, 1954 at the HSS on 42nd Street.	9

NAME	BRIEF BIOGRAPHY	CHAPTER(S)
Francis Scott Key (1779–1843)	Wrote lyrics for *The Star-Spangled Banner* based on an 1814 poem.	1
Norman T. Kirk, MD (1888–1960)	Major general. Served as U.S. army surgeon general (1943–1947). First military doctor to be certified by the American Board of Orthopaedic Surgery and to become a member of the American Academy of Orthopaedic Surgeons.	8
George Kistiakowsky, PhD (1900–1982)	Invited speaker at the opening of the HSS Caspary Research Building in 1960. Received his PhD in physical chemistry from the University of Berlin in 1925 before emigrating to the U.S. to teach first at Princeton University and then at Harvard University, where he remained for the rest of his career.	10, 17
Samuel Kleinberg, MD (1885–1957)	Studied scoliosis under Royal Whitman, MD. Later on staff at Hospital for Joint Diseases. Moved from R&C and became chief of service at the Hospital for Deformities and Joint Diseases (1927).	3, 4
James Knight, MD (1810–1887)	First surgeon-in-chief and founder of R&C (1863–1887). He was a general practitioner.	1, 2, 3, 4, 5
Leonhard Korngold, PhD (1921–2010)	Bacteriologist who worked on the structure of immunoglobulins while in the HSS Research Division.	17
Henry G. Kunkel, MD (1916–1983)	Joining the Rockefeller Institute in 1945, Kunkel became professor in 1975. In the late 1950s, he introduced the concept of autoimmunity in the demonstrable context of disease with his studies of rheumatoid arthritis. He was the first to characterize the rheumatoid factor as an antibody.	14
Gerhard Küntscher, MD (1900–1972)	German surgeon who perfected intramedullary nailing for femoral fractures during World War II.	8
Capt. Louis F. Kuntz MD (N/A)	Radiologist at HSS in 1921.	16

NAME	BRIEF BIOGRAPHY	CHAPTER(S)
Fiorello H. LaGuardia (1882–1947)	Three-term liberal Republican mayor of New York City (1934–1945).	7
Eugene M. Lance, MD (1933–1993)	Founder of the HSS Research Division. Orthopaedic resident, class of 1964. Trained with Nobel Laureate Peter Medawar in London, and then returned to the attending staff of HSS before leaving to take a position at Shriners Hospital in Honolulu in 1974.	17
Richard S. Laskin, MD (1940–2008)	On HSS staff from 1991 to 2008, he became the first editor of the *HSS Journal* in 2005.	12
Gen. Robert E. Lee (1807–1870)	Commander of the Confederate army at the Battle of Chancellorsville, the day R&C opened its doors to its first patient.	1
Raymond Lewis, MD (1889–1976)	First full-time roentgenologist and director of Department of Radiology at R&C (1926–1951).	7, 16
Frederick Liebolt, MD (1905–1996)	Chief of Orthopaedic Service at New York Hospital when HSS became affiliated. Established a chair of premedical sciences at the University of Arkansas, where he received his BA degree in 1925.	9
Wan Ngo Lim, MD (1920–2004)	Chief of pediatrics at HSS (1965–1984). Worked closely with Leon Root and David B. Levine.	10
Sir Joseph Lister (1827–1912)	English surgeon who discovered carbolic acid's antiseptic properties, publishing his work in 1867.	1, 6
Eva Locke, MD (1874–1954)	A surgeon in the R&C Hernia Service who became the first female anesthetist at R&C (1918–1919).	15
Cleanthe E. Logotheton (1891–1986)	Directress of nursing at HSS (1942–1954). In her retired life, she patented a bobby pin.	11

NAME	BRIEF BIOGRAPHY	CHAPTER(S)
John Edward (Jack) Lovelock, MD (1910–1949)	Assistant director of physiotherapy under Hansson. Born in New Zealand, Lovelock was awarded a Rhodes Scholarship to Oxford University and later obtained a medical degree from St. Mary's Medical School in London. In the 1936 Berlin Olympic Games, he set a world record in the 1500 meters, and became New Zealand's first Olympic gold medalist in athletics. In 1949, suffering from the flu, he became dizzy and fell in front of a subway car at the Church Street Station in Brooklyn, and was killed instantly.	12
John Marshall, DVM, MD (1936–1980)	Founded the first sports medicine clinic in the country at HSS in 1971. World-renowned sports medicine surgeon by age 44 years. He was killed in a private plane crash in 1980 on the way to the Winter Olympics near Lake Placid, New York.	10, 11
Klaus Mayer, MD (1925–2011)	Director of hematology at Memorial Sloan Kettering Cancer Center. He ran the HSS Blood Bank and Hematology Research Laboratory in the HSS Research Division.	17
Charles Mayo, MD (1865–1939)	With his older brother William James Mayo, MD, one of the founders of the Mayo Clinic in 1919.	6
Charles McBurney, MD (1845–1913)	Surgeon-in-chief, Roosevelt Hospital. Published classic paper on approach to appendicitis in 1889.	4
Lawrence McK Miller (1890–1970)	Secretary of R&C Board of Managers. Announced name of Hospital for the Ruptured and Crippled to be changed in 1940 to the HSS. Longest-serving board member. Remembered for his warmth and delightful sense of humor.	8
John P. McWhorter, MD (1867–1936)	Appointed first full-time chief pathologist and director of laboratories at R&C (1929). Assistant professor of surgery at Columbia University Medical School.	6

NAME	BRIEF BIOGRAPHY	CHAPTER(S)
Robert Mellors, MD, PhD (1916–2007)	Appointed director of clinical laboratories in 1958 and chief pathologist and director of research at HSS in 1969. He retired in 1984.	10, 17
John P. Mitchel (1879–1924)	At age 34 years, became the youngest New York City mayor ever (1914–1918).	5
Joseph Moldaver, MD (1899–1982)	HSS director of neurology from 1954 until 1971, when he was replaced by Peter Tsairis, MD, as full-time director of neurology until 1995. In 1969, Moldaver, clinical professor of neurology at the Columbia University College of Physicians and Surgeons, went into mandatory retirement from Columbia in 1969.	14
J. Pierpont Morgan (1837–1913)	Financier, banker, and philanthropist.	2
Robert Moses (1888–1981)	Master builder of 20th century. Built tunnels, highways, bridges, and the 1939 and 1964 World's Fairs. Promoted United Nations headquarters in Manhattan.	7
Valentine Mott, MD (1785–1865)	Professor of surgery, Columbia University (1809). Founding faculty, University Medical College (New York University School of Medicine) in 1841. Founding R&C staff.	1
Ella Murdock (1855–1915)	First chief nursing officer (matron) at R&C (1896–1911). Graduate of Bellevue Hospital School of Nursing.	5
Helen Coley Nauts (1907–2000)	Championed the goal of her father, William Bradley Coley, MD, in developing a vaccine to treat cancer. Founded the Cancer Research Institute in 1953. Wrote an unpublished history of her father (manuscript is over 350 typed pages, with an introduction by her nephew, Bradley "Pete" Coley Jr.).	6

NAME	BRIEF BIOGRAPHY	CHAPTER(S)
Charles S. Neer II, MD (1917–2011)	Having completed his orthopaedic residency in 1949 at Presbyterian Hospital and College of Physicians and Surgeons of Columbia University, founded the Shoulder Service in 1970 and served until his retirement in 1990 as emeritus professor of orthopaedic surgery. He was founding president of the American Shoulder & Elbow Surgeons and founding chairman of the board of trustees of the *Journal of Shoulder and Elbow Surgery*.	13
James Nicholas, MD (1921–2006)	HSS orthopaedic resident (class of 1952). Part of the team of surgeons who operated on Senator John F. Kennedy's spine in 1954. Started the HSS Metabolic Bone Clinic. Founder of Sports Medicine Center in 1973 at Lenox Hill Hospital, where he served as chief of orthopaedic surgery.	9, 11
Florence Nightingale (1820–1910)	Established first school of nursing in 1860 at St. Thomas Hospital in London, England.	5
John O'Dowd, MD (1891–1953)	R&C anesthetist (1920–1942).	15
Sten-Erik Olsson, DVM (1921–2000)	Swedish veterinarian who was director of the HSS Animal Laboratory in the 1960s. In 1968, he resigned and returned to Sweden.	11
William Church Osborn (1892–1951)	President of R&C Board of Managers (1910–1925 and 1928–1937).	4, 5, 8
William H. Osborn (1821–1894)	Fifth president of R&C Board of Managers (1888–1890). Railroad tycoon.	2, 3, 4
Robert B. Osgood, MD (1873–1956)	President of AOA (1920). Chief of Children's Hospital/Massachusetts General Hospital program circa 1922.	7
William Osler, MD (1849–1919)	Physician-in-chief in the "Big Four" and a founder of Johns Hopkins University School of Medicine.	4

NAME	BRIEF BIOGRAPHY	CHAPTER(S)
Willard Parker, MD (1800–1884)	Professor of surgery, Cincinnati and Columbia University College of Physicians and Surgeons. Bellevue Hospital staff. Founding R&C staff.	1
Louis Pasteur (1822–1895)	French chemist who supported germ theory of disease.	1, 6
Russell H. Patterson, MD, Sr. (1890–1993)	Brother of Robert Patterson Jr. and senior surgeon at New York Hospital.	10
Robert Lee Patterson, Jr., MD (1907–1994)	Seventh surgeon-in-chief at HSS.	3, 8
General John J. Pershing (1860–1948)	Appointed general of the armies in 1919, the highest rank in the U. S. Army. The only other individual with this rank was George Washington; commemorated in 1976 at the bicentennial celebration.	7
Sir Harry Platt (1886–1986)	Professor of orthopaedics at the Royal Infirmary of Manchester in England. Helped Philip D. Wilson Sr., MD, set up the American Hospital in England during World War II.	8
Eugene H. Pool, MD (1874–1949)	Fourth surgeon-in-chief at R&C. Professor of clinical surgery at Columbia University College of Physicians and Surgeons (1915–1938) and Cornell University Medical College (1932–1947).	6, 9
J. Lawrence Pool, MD (1906–2004)	Son of Eugene Pool. Professor and chair of neurosurgery department at Columbia University (1949).	7
Edward Tuckerman Potter (1831–1901)	Famous ecclesiastic architect. Designed second R&C building at 42nd Street and Lexington Avenue, which opened in 1870.	1, 2
Joseph Pulitzer (1847–1911)	Hungarian-American publisher of the *New York World*. Crusaded against big business and corruption. Pulitzer Prize named after him.	4
Charles Reed, DVM (1933–2009)	Radiology research consultant at HSS.	16

NAME	BRIEF BIOGRAPHY	CHAPTER(S)
Cornelius "Dusty" Rhoads, MD (1898–1959)	Headed Medical Division of Chemical Warfare during World War II. Medical director, Memorial Hospital. Promoted chemotherapy. Opponent of Coley's Toxins.	6
John Ridlon, MD (1852–1936)	Longest tenured officer of the AOA. Moved from New York to Chicago in 1889. President of AOA (1899).	3
Jacob Riis (1849–1914)	Police reporter for the *New York Tribune*. Brought about changes for people in New York City living in extreme poverty.	3
Diego Rivera (1886–1957)	Prominent Mexican artist and active communist. His frescos established the Mexican Mural Renaissance. From 1913 to 1917, he embraced cubist art after Picasso and Braque. Volatile marriage to artist (and HSS patient) Frida Kahlo.	9
Peter Cyrus Rizzo II, MD (1903–2001)	HSS attending orthopaedic surgeon. His twin sons both trained in orthopaedics at HSS: Peter Cyrus Rizzo III, MD, and Thomas Rizzo, MD.	9
Peter Cyrus Rizzo III, MD (1931–1987)	Twin brother of Thomas Rizzo, MD, he was an HSS orthopaedic resident (class of 1961). He was killed by a disgruntled New York City fireman in a New York City courthouse.	11
Thomas Rizzo, MD (1931–2010)	Son of Peter Cyrus Rizzo II, MD, and father of Peter F. Rizzo, MD, who also trained as an orthopaedic resident at HSS. Thomas was an HSS orthopaedic resident (1959) and orthopaedic fellow (1962).	11
Percy W. Roberts, MD (1867–1937)	Orthopaedic surgeon at R&C; treated tuberculosis.	6
John D. Rockefeller (1839–1937)	Founded Standard Oil Company in 1870. World's richest man. Spent 40 years in retirement creating targeted philanthropy.	2, 3, 4, 6

NAME	BRIEF BIOGRAPHY	CHAPTER(S)
John D. Rockefeller, Jr. (1874–1960)	The only son of John D. Rockefeller. Developed Rockefeller Center on Fifth Avenue in New York City.	3, 6
Wilhelm Conrad Roentgen (1845–1923)	German physicist who discovered x-rays in 1895.	4, 16
Franklin D. Roosevelt (1882–1945)	32nd U.S. president (1933–1945). Established the New Deal in the Depression years. Led the country during World War II.	7
Theodore Roosevelt (1858–1919)	26th U.S. president (1901–1909).	5
Theodore Roosevelt Sr. (1831–1878)	The father of U.S. President Theodore Roosevelt and paternal grandfather of America's First Lady, Eleanor Roosevelt.	1
Preston Pope Satterwhite, MD (1867–1948)	Appointed anesthetist and assistant surgeon in the Hernia Service at R&C in 1901. Graduate of Bellevue Medical College in 1898.	4, 15
Paul D. Saville, MD (1926–2010)	Directed the Metabolic Bone Disease Laboratory in the 1960s. Best known for his evaluation of osteoporosis using animal models.	17
Philip Sawyer (1868–1949)	York & Sawyer architectural firm. Designed R&C building on 42nd Street between First and Second Avenues.	5
Lewis Sayre, MD (1820–1900)	First professor of orthopaedics in the United States, Bellevue Medical College.	1, 2, 3
Horatio Seymour (1810–1886)	18th New York governor. Urged supporters of the New York City draft riots of 1863.	1
Newton Melman Shaffer, MD (1846–1928)	Trained by Knight. Chief of first orthopaedic department in a general hospital in United States (1872) at St. Luke's Hospital. Succeeded Charles Taylor, MD, at New York Orthopaedic Hospital (1876). First professor of orthopaedic surgery at Cornell University Medical College (1900).	1, 3

NAME	BRIEF BIOGRAPHY	CHAPTER(S)
Alfred R. Shands, MD (1876–1941)	Trained at R&C. Graduated 1894. Father of Alfred R. Shands Jr.	3, 4, 5
Alfred R. Shands, Jr., MD (1899–1981)	Medical director of Alfred I. Dupont Institute for Crippled Children in Wilmington, Delaware.	3
Marius Smith-Peterson, MD (1886–1953)	Chief of orthopaedic surgery at Massachusetts General Hospital (1929).	7
William Lent Sneed, MD (1881–1941)	Vanderbilt University School of Medicine (1910). R&C anesthetist (1912–1915). On R&C staff as a surgeon until 1931.	15
R. Garfield Snyder, MD (1881–1944)	Appointed chief of R&C Arthritis Clinic, which was established for the first time, in 1924.	8
Ramsey Spillman, MD (1891–1968)	Radiologist at HSS (1934–1943).	16
Richard M. Stark (1932–2007)	HSS resident (class of 1963). Director of orthopaedic surgery at North Shore University Hospital.	10
Aaron Steele, MD (1835–1917)	Orthopaedic surgeon in St. Louis; was the prime mover organizing the AOA.	3
Richmond Stephens, MD (1890–1958)	Interned at New York Hospital. Served in World War I at Base Hospital #9 (1917–1919).	7
Lee Ramsay Straub, MD (1913–1994)	Executive assistant to surgeon-in-chief Philip D. Wilson Sr., MD. First chief of Hand Service. Co-founder and co-chief with Richard Freyberg, MD, of the Comprehensive Arthritis Program (CAP).	9, 10, 12
Jonathan Sturges (1802–1874)	First R&C board member, followed by eight of his descendants (Osborn family).	1, 4
Charles Fayette Taylor, MD (1827–1899)	Orthopaedic surgeon who founded New York Orthopedic Dispensary and Hospital (1866) with Theodore Roosevelt, Sr.	1, 2
Henry Ling Taylor, MD (1857–1923)	Chief of the Second Division of Orthopaedics at R&C (1921).	5, 12

NAME	BRIEF BIOGRAPHY	CHAPTER(S)
Hugh Owen Thomas (1834–1891)	Welsh surgeon; considered the father of orthopaedic surgery in Britain.	3
T. Campbell Thompson, MD (1902–1986)	Sixth surgeon-in-chief at HSS (1955–1963). Resigned during a period when relations between HSS and New York Hospital were threatened.	3, 7, 8, 9, 10
Wisner Townsend, MD (1857–1916)	R&C staff member. Published article on flat feet in 1903.	3
Walter Truslow, MD (1871–1958)	First to treat scoliosis at R&C in 1899, when he held classes for scoliosis patients in a gymnasium.	3, 12
William H. Van Buren, MD (1819–1883)	Founding R&C staff member. Surgeon to New York Hospital, Bellevue Hospital, R&C and St. Vincent's Hospital. Professor of anatomy at New York University. Married daughter of Valentine Mott.	1
Cornelius Vanderbilt (1794–1877)	Owned shipping companies and railroad companies. Built Grand Central Terminal.	3, 4
Cornelius Vanderbilt II (1843–1899)	Favorite grandson of Cornelius Vanderbilt. In 1885, he succeeded his grandfather and his father, William H. Vanderbilt, as head of the New York Central Railroad. He was a member of the R&C Board of Managers.	3, 4
Konstantin Veliskakis, MD (1923–2005)	Gibney Scoliosis Fellow with John Cobb, MD, in 1957; continued working with him for seven years until Cobb retired. Veliskakis was an attending orthopaedic surgeon at HSS until his death. A skilled, innovative surgeon with superior wit and a deep interest and knowledge in the field of scoliosis, he authored many peer-reviewed articles and exhibits at the American Academy of Orthopaedic Surgeons annual meetings.	14
Rudolph Virchow, MD (1821–1902)	German pathologist. Father of modern pathology. Over 15 medical terms are named for him.	1

NAME	BRIEF BIOGRAPHY	CHAPTER(S)
Preston Wade, MD (1901–1982)	Co-chief of combined New York Hospital–HSS Fracture Service (1955–1968). Received Cornell University Medical College's Alumni Award of Distinction in 1956 (the highest award of his Alma Mater). President of the American College of Surgeons (1969–1970). New York Hospital acting chief of surgery (1970). With Robert Lee Patterson Jr., MD, Wade preserved the affiliation between HSS and New York Hospital–Cornell University Medical College, which had been threatened.	10
Earl Calvin Wagner, MD (1886–1955)	First supervisor of anesthetics and first chief of service at R&C (1934).	15
Lewis Clark Wagner, MD (1897–1974)	Partner of Virgil Gibney. Award at HSS is in his name. Instituted annual Golf-Tennis Day at HSS.	4, 5, 6
Robert F. Wagner Jr. (1910–1991)	New York City mayor (1954–1965) whose administration saw the creation of the City University of New York system, the development of Lincoln Center, and Shakespeare in Central Park.	9
James J. "Jimmy" Walker (1881–1946)	New York City mayor (1926–1932). Facing prosecution for extortion, he resigned from office and fled to Europe.	5, 6
Charlton Wallace, MD (1872–1947)	Clinical professor of orthopaedic surgery, Cornell University Medical College. Established East Side Free School for Crippled Children (1905–1913). Assistant Surgeon at R&C.	6
Robert F. Weir, MD (1838–1927)	Attending surgeon at Roosevelt Hospital (1873–1883, reappointed in 1898). Surgeon to New York Hospital (1876–1898).	3
William Henry Welch, MD (1850–1934)	Pathologist in the "Big Four" and a founder of Johns Hopkins University School of Medicine.	4
Stanford White (1853–1906)	One of the most famous architects at the turn of the 20th century.	4

NAME	BRIEF BIOGRAPHY	CHAPTER(S)
Royal Whitman, MD (1857–1946)	Orthopaedic surgeon who wrote the most comprehensive textbook on orthopaedics, first published in 1901. Chief of First Division, Orthopaedic Department at HSS (1921).	3, 4, 5, 6, 7, 12
Sylvia Green Wilks (1870–1951)	Married Mathew Astor Wilks in 1909. Her mother, Hetty Green, was considered to be the richest woman in the world.	9
May Wilson, MD (1891–1971)	New York Hospital pediatric cardiologist. Mentor to Wan Ngo Lim, MD (not related to Philip D. Wilson).	10
Philip D. Wilson Sr., MD (1886–1969)	Fifth surgeon-in-chief at R&C. Changed the name of the hospital in 1940 to the HSS. He was the founder and first director of the HSS Research Division. He performed a spine fusion in John F. Kennedy when he was a U.S. Senator.	3, 6, 7, 8, 9, 10, 17
Woodrow Wilson (1856–1924)	28th U.S. president (1913–1921). Won the 1912 presidential election over Theodore Roosevelt. President of Princeton (1902–1910). Governor of New Jersey (1911–1913). A Democrat, he was the only president to hold a PhD degree.	5, 6
Fernando Wood (1812–1881)	Mayor of New York City (1854 and 1860). Supported Confederacy and advised New York City to secede from the Union and declare itself a free city.	1
Edward York (1863–1928)	York & Sawyer architectural firm. Designed R&C building on 42nd Street between First and Second Avenues.	5
T. Gordon Young (1916–2005)	HSS executive administrator (1954–1977). Very popular with the hospital staff.	9

CONTRIBUTORS

Adele L. Boskey, PhD
Starr Chair in Mineralized Tissue Research
Director
Musculoskeletal Integrity Program
Research Division
Hospital for Special Surgery
New York, New York
Professor
Department of Biochemistry
Weill Cornell Medical College
New York, New York
Professor
Department of Physiology, Biophysics, and Systems Biology
Weill Cornell Medical College
New York, New York
Professor
Sibley School of Mechanical and Aerospace Engineering
Cornell University
Ithaca, New York
Professor
Mechanical Engineering
City College of New York
New York, New York

Charles L. Christian, MD
Physician-in-Chief Emeritus
Hospital for Special Surgery
New York, New York
Adjunct Professor
Department of Medicine
Division of Rheumatic Disease
Weill Cornell Medical College
New York, New York

Mary J. Hargett, BSci
Administrative Director of Education
Department of Anesthesiology
Hospital for Special Surgery
New York, New York

Gregory A. Liguori, MD
Anesthesiologist-in-Chief
Director, Department of Anesthesiology
Hospital for Special Surgery
New York, New York
Clinical Associate Professor
Department of Anesthesiology
Weill Cornell Medical College
New York, New York

Stephen A. Paget, MD
Physician-in-Chief Emeritus
Director
Rheumatology Academy of Medical Educators
Hospital for Special Surgery
New York, New York
Professor
Department of Medicine
Division of Rheumatic Disease
Weill Cornell Medical College
New York, New York

Helene Pavlov, MD, FACR
Radiologist-in-Chief
Department of Radiology and Imaging
Hospital for Special Surgery
New York, New York
Professor of Radiology
Department of Radiology
Professor of Radiology in Orthopaedic Surgery
Weill Cornell Medical College
New York, New York

Thomas P. Sculco, MD
Surgeon-in-Chief and Medical Director
Hospital for Special Surgery
New York, New York
Professor
Department of Orthopaedic Surgery
Weill Cornell Medical College
New York, New York

Louis A. Shapiro
President and Chief Executive Officer
Hospital for Special Surgery
New York, New York

INDEX